Geriatric
CLINICAL
ADVISOR

Geriatric CLINICAL ADVISOR

Instant Diagnosis and Treatment

TOM J. WACHTEL, M.D., F.A.C.P.

Division of Geriatrics
Rhode Island Hospital
Professor of Community Health and Medicine
Brown Medical School
Providence, Rhode Island

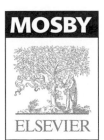

MOSBY

ELSEVIER

MOSBY
ELSEVIER

1600 John F. Kennedy Blvd.
Ste 1800
Philadelphia, PA 19103-2899

GERIATRIC CLINICAL ADVISOR: INSTANT DIAGNOSIS AND TREATMENT   ISBN-13: 978-0-323-04195-9
ISBN-10: 0-323-04195-7

Notice

Knowledge and best practice in this field are constantly changing. As new research and experience broaden our knowledge, changes in practice, treatment, and drug therapy may become necessary or appropriate. Readers are advised to check the most current information provided (i) on procedures featured or (ii) by the manufacturer of each product to be administered, to verify the recommended dose or formula, the method and duration of administration, and contraindications. It is the responsibility of the practitioner, relying on his or her own experience and knowledge of the patient, to make diagnoses, to determine dosages and the best treatment for each individual patient, and to take all appropriate safety precautions. To the fullest extent of the law, neither the Publisher nor the Editor assumes any liability for any injury and/or damage to persons or property arising out of or related to any use of the material contained in this book.

The Publisher

Library of Congress Cataloging-in-Publication Data

Wachtel, Tom J.
    Geriatric clinical advisor : instant diagnosis and treatment / Tom J. Wachtel.
        p. ; cm.
    Includes bibliographical references and index.
    ISBN 0-323-04195-7
    1. Geriatrics—Handbooks, manuals, etc. I. Title.
    [DNLM: 1. Geriatrics—Handbooks. WT 39 W114g 2007]
    RC952.55.W33 2007
    618.97—dc22   2006045520

Acquisitions Editor: Rolla Couchman
Developmental Editor: Mary Beth Murphy

Printed in the United States of America
Last digit is the print number: 9 8 7 6 5 4 3 2 1

Associate Editors

FRED F. FERRI, M.D., F.A.C.P.
Clinical Professor
Department of Community Health
Brown Medical School
Providence, Rhode Island
SECTION I: DISEASES AND DISORDERS,
SECTION II: DIFFERENTIAL DIAGNOSIS,
SECTION III: CLINICAL ALGORITHMS,
SECTION IV: LABORATORY TESTS AND INTERPRETATION
OF RESULTS

CYNTHIA HOLZER, M.D, C.M.D.
Director, Geriatric Education
Roger Williams Medical Center
Providence, Rhode Island
Assistant Professor of Medicine
Boston University School of Medicine
Boston, Massachusetts
SECTION V: CLINICAL PREVENTIVE SERVICES

LYNN MCNICOLL, M.D.
Division of Geriatrics
Rhode Island Hospital
Providence, Rhode Island
SECTION I: DISEASES AND DISORDERS

JOHN B. MURPHY, M.D.
Division of Geriatrics
Rhode Island Hospital
Providence, Rhode Island
APPENDIX 1: SYSTEMS OF GERIATRIC CARE

AMAN NANDA, M.D., C.M.D.
Assistant Professor in Medicine
Brown Medical School
Providence, Rhode Island
APPENDIX 2: TOOLS OF GERIATRIC ASSESSMENT

TOM J. WACHTEL, M.D., F.A.C.P.
Division of Geriatrics
Rhode Island Hospital
Professor of Community Health and Medicine
Brown Medical School
Providence, Rhode Island
SECTION I: DISEASES AND DISORDERS,
SECTION II: DIFFERENTIAL DIAGNOSIS,
SECTION III: CLINICAL ALGORITHMS,
SECTION IV: LABORATORY TESTS AND INTERPRETATION
OF RESULTS,
APPENDIX 1: SYSTEMS OF GERIATRIC CARE

Contributors

PHILIP J. ALIOTTA, M.D., M.S.H.A., F.A.C.S.
Clinical Instructor
Department of Urology
School of Medicine and Biomedical Sciences
State University of New York at Buffalo
Buffalo, New York
Medical Director
Center for Urologic Research of Western New York
Williamsville, New York

GEORGE O. ALONSO, M.D.
Director
Department of Infection Control
Elmhurst Hospital Center
Elmhurst, New York
Instructor in Medicine
Mount Sinai School of Medicine
New York, New York

MEL L. ANDERSON, M.D., F.A.C.P.
Clinical Assistant Professor of Medicine
Brown Medical School
Providence, Rhode Island

PATRICIA AREAN, PH.D.
Associate Professor
Department of Psychiatry
University of California, San Francisco
San Francisco, California

MICHAEL G. BENATAR, M.B.CH.B., D.PHIL.
Assistant Professor of Neurology
Department of Neurology
Emory University
Atlanta, Georgia

SUSAN BERNER, M.D.
Geriatrics Fellow, Department of Family Medicine
University of Cincinnati College of Medicine
Cincinnati, Ohio

LYNN BOWLBY, M.D.
Attending Physician
Division of General Internal Medicine
Rhode Island Hospital
Clinical Instructor of Medicine
Brown Medical School
Providence, Rhode Island

MARIA A. CORIGLIANO, M.D., F.A.C.O.G.
Clinical Assistant Professor
Department of Obstetrics and Gynecology
State University of New York at Buffalo
Buffalo, New York

STEPHEN CORREIA, PH.D.
Dementia Research Fellow
Department of Psychiatry and Human Behavior
Brown Medical School
Providence, Rhode Island

JOHN E. CROOM, M.D., PH.D.
Clinical Fellow in Neurology
Harvard Medical School
Beth Israel Deaconess Medical Center
Boston, Massachusetts

CLAUDIA L. DADE, M.D.
Attending Physician
Division of Infectious Diseases
Elmhurst Hospital Center
Elmhurst, New York
Instructor in Medicine
Mount Sinai School of Medicine
New York, New York

GEORGE T. DANAKAS, M.D., F.A.C.O.G.
Clinical Assistant Professor
Department of Obstetrics and Gynecology
State University of New York at Buffalo
Buffalo, New York

AMAR DESAI, M.D., M.P.H.
Resident Physician
Department of Internal Medicine
University of California, San Francisco
San Francisco, California

JEFFREY S. DURMER, M.D., PH.D.
Assistant Professor, Department of Neurology
Director, Emory Sleep Laboratory
Director, Egleston Children's Hospital Sleep Clinic
Emory University School of Medicine
Atlanta, Georgia

GARY EPSTEIN-LUBOW, M.D.
Postdoctoral Research Fellow
Department of Psychiatry and Human Behavior
Brown Medical School
Staff Psychiatrist
Butler Hospital
Providence, Rhode Island

MARK J. FAGAN, M.D.
Director
Medical Primary Care Unit
Rhode Island Hospital
Associate Professor of Medicine
Brown Medical School
Providence, Rhode Island

GIL M. FARKASH, M.D.
Assistant Clinical Professor
State University of New York at Buffalo
School of Medicine
Buffalo, New York

MITCHELL D. FELDMAN, M.D., M.PHIL.
Associate Professor of Clinical Medicine
University of California, San Francisco
Division of General Internal Medicine
San Francisco, California

FRED F. FERRI, M.D., F.A.C.P.
Clinical Professor
Department of Community Health
Brown Medical School
Providence, Rhode Island

GLENN G. FORT, M.D., M.P.H.
Clinical Associate Professor of Medicine
Brown Medical School
Chief
Infectious Diseases
Our Lady of Fatima Hospital
North Providence, Rhode Island

MICHAEL P. GERARDO, D.O., M.P.H.
Post-Doctoral Research Fellow
Brown Medical School, Center for Gerontology and Health
Care Research
Brown University Geriatric Medicine Fellow
Rhode Island and Miriam Hospitals
Providence, Rhode Island

SUSAN E. HARDY, M.D., PH.D.
Assistant Professor
Geriatric Medicine
University of Pittsburgh School of Medicine
Pittsburgh, Pennsylvania

MIKE HARPER, M.D.
Associate Professor of Medicine
Division of Geriatrics
Department of Medicine
San Francisco Veterans Affairs Medical Center
University of California, San Diego
San Diego, California

TAYLOR HARRISON, M.D.
Neuromuscular Fellow
Department of Neurology
Emory University
Atlanta, Georgia

SHARON S. HARTMAN, M.D., PH.D.
Clinical Associate
Department of Neurology
Emory University
Atlanta, Georgia

HOLLY M. HOLMES, M.D.
Instructor
University of Chicago
Chicago, Illinois

CYNTHIA HOLZER, M.D., C.M.D.
Director, Geriatric Education
Roger Williams Medical Center
Providence, Rhode Island
Assistant Professor of Medicine
Boston University School of Medicine
Boston, Massachusetts

JASON IANNUCCILLI, M.D.
Department of Medicine
Brown Medical School
Providence, Rhode Island

RICHARD S. ISAACSON, M.D.
Director, Research Unit in Medical Education
Associate Medical Director
Wien Center for Memory Disorders and Alzheimer's Disease
Assistant Professor of Medicine
University of Miami—Leonard M. Miller School of Medicine
Departments of Medical Education, Internal Medicine, and
    Neurology
Mount Sinai Medical Center
Miami Beach, Florida

BREE JOHNSTON, M.D., M.P.H.
Associate Professor of Medicine
Division of Geriatrics
Department of Medicine
Veterans Affairs Medical Center
University of California, San Diego
San Diego, California

MELVYN KOBY, M.D.
Associate Clinical Professor of Medicine
Department of Ophthalmology
University of Louisville School of Medicine
Louisville, Kentucky

E. GORDON MARGOLIN, M.D.
Professor, Internal Medicine and Geriatrician
University of Cincinnati College of Medicine
Cincinnati, Ohio

DANIEL T. MATTSON, M.D., M.S.C.(MED.)
Clinical Fellow in Neurology
Beth Israel Deaconess Medical Center
Harvard Medical School
Boston, Massachusetts

LYNN MCNICOLL, M.D.
Division of Geriatrics
Rhode Island Hospital
Providence, Rhode Island

LONNIE R. MERCIER, M.D.
Clinical Instructor
Department of Orthopedic Surgery
Creighton University School of Medicine
Omaha, Nebraska

DENNIS J. MIKOLICH, M.D., F.A.C.P., F.C.C.P.
Chief
Division of Infectious Diseases
VA Medical Center
Clinical Associate Professor of Medicine
Brown Medical School
Providence, Rhode Island

RAM R. MILLER, M.D.C.M., M.S., F.R.C.P.C.
Assistant Professor
University of Maryland School of Medicine
Division of Gerontology
Department of Epidemiology and Preventive Medicine
Baltimore, Maryland

ARVIND MODAWAL, M.D., M.P.H., M.R.C.G.P.
Associate Professor
Department of Family Medicine, Section of Geriatrics
University of Cincinnati College of Medicine
Cincinnati, Ohio

JOHN B. MURPHY, M.D.
Division of Geriatrics
Rhode Island Hospital
Providence, Rhode Island

AMAN NANDA, M.D., C.M.D.
Assistant Professor in Medicine
Brown Medical School
Providence, Rhode Island

TAKUMA NEMOTO, M.D.
Research Associate Professor of Surgery
State University of New York at Buffalo
Buffalo, New York

PRANAV M. PATEL, M.D.
Clinical Associate Instructor, Division of Cardiology
Department of Medicine
Brown Medical School
Providence, Rhode Island

PETER PETROPOULOS, M.D.
Department of Veterans Affairs
Providence, Rhode Island

ARUNDATHI G. PRASAD, M.D.
Clinical Instructor
Department of Obstetrics and Gynecology/Resident Education
State University of New York at Buffalo
Women's and Children's Hospital
Buffalo, New York

HARLAN G. RICH, M.D.
Director of Endoscopy
Rhode Island Hospital
Associate Professor of Medicine
Brown Medical School
Providence, Rhode Island

SEAN I. SAVITZ, M.D.
Clinical Fellow in Neurology
Harvard Medical School
Chief Resident in Neurology
Beth Israel Deaconess Medical Center
Boston, Massachusetts

JOSEPH W. SHEGA, M.D.
Assistant Professor, Division of Hematology/Oncology
Northwestern University
The Feinberg School of Medicine
Chicago, Illinois

CLIFFORD MILO SINGER, M.D.
Associate Professor of Psychiatry
Director, Insomnia and Chronobiology Clinic
Vermont Regional Sleep Center
University of Vermont College of Medicine
Burlington, Vermont

U. SHIVRAJ SOHUR, M.D., PH.D.
Clinical Fellow in Neurology
Harvard Medical School
Chief Resident in Neurology
Beth Israel Deaconess Medical Center
Boston, Massachusetts

JOHN A. STOUKIDES, M.D., R.PH.
Director of Geriatrics
Roger Williams Medical Center
Providence, Rhode Island
Clinical Assistant Professor of Medicine
Boston University School of Medicine
Boston, Massachusetts
Adjunct Associate Professor of Pharmacy and Nursing
University of Rhode Island
Kingston, Rhode Island

JULIE ANNE SZUMIGALA, M.D.
Clinical Instructor
Department of Obstetrics and Gynecology
State University of New York at Buffalo
Buffalo, New York

LAURA TRICE, M.D.
Medical Director
Trihealth SeniorLink
California, Kentucky

EROBOGHENE E. UBOGU, M.D.
Assistant Professor of Neurology
Case Western Reserve University School of Medicine
Staff Neurologist
Louis Stokes Cleveland Veterans Affairs Medical Center
Cleveland, Ohio

TOM J. WACHTEL, M.D., F.A.C.P.
Division of Geriatrics
Rhode Island Hospital
Professor of Community Health and Medicine
Brown Medical School
Providence, Rhode Island

WEN-CHIH WU, M.D.
Assistant Professor of Medicine
Brown Medical School
Cardiologist
Providence VA Medical Center
Providence, Rhode Island

BETH J. WUTZ, M.D.
Clinical Assistant Professor of Medicine
Division of Internal Medicine/Pediatrics
Kajeida Health–Buffalo General Hospital
State University of New York at Buffalo
Buffalo, New York

MADHAVI YERNENI, M.D.
Staff Physician, Academic Medical Center
Miriam Hospital
Pawtucket, Rhode Island

CINDY ZADIKOFF, M.D.
Fellow, Movement Disorders
Morton and Gloria Shulman Movement Disorders Center
Toronto Western Hospital
Toronto, Ontario

The editors would like to dedicate this book to their families and friends.

Contents

Detailed Contents

SECTION I   Diseases and Disorders

SECTION II **Differential Diagnosis**

SECTION III   Clinical Algorithms

SECTION IV   Laboratory Tests and Interpretation of Results

SECTION V Clinical Preventive Services

APPENDIX 1 Systems of Geriatric Care

APPENDIX 2 Tools of Geriatric Assessment

Diseases and Disorders

BASIC INFORMATION

DEFINITION

Elder abuse is the willful infliction of physical pain or injury; emotional pain, injury, humiliation, or intimidation; exploitation or misappropriation of money or property; or neglect by the designated caregiver. In general, three basic categories of elder abuse exist: domestic elder abuse (or abuse in the home); institutional elder abuse (abuse that occurs in nursing homes, foster homes, group homes, board and care facilities); and self-neglect.

Seven types of abuse are described:
- Physical abuse: inflicting of physical pain or injury, including hitting, slapping, or restraining
- Sexual abuse: inflicting of nonconsensual sexual activity of any kind
- Psychologic abuse: inflicting mental anguish, including intimidation, humiliation, ridicule, or threats through verbal or nonverbal means
- Financial abuse: improper use of the resources of any older person without the elder's consent for another's benefit
- Abandonment: desertion of an elderly person by the responsible caregiver
- Neglect: failure to fulfill a caretaking obligation, including provision of food, a safe living environment, health care, hygiene, or basic custodial care
- Self-neglect: behavior of an elderly person that threatens the elder's health or safety

There is considerable variation between states regarding the definitions of abuse and reporting requirements for specific subtypes of abuse.

SYNONYMS

Geriatric abuse
Battered elder syndrome

ICD-9CM CODES
995.81 Adult maltreatment syndrome

EPIDEMIOLOGY & DEMOGRAPHICS

U.S. INCIDENCE & PREVALENCE: Unknown, statistics are thought to underreport the problem significantly. There were estimated to be 1 million victims of elder abuse in 1996; if self-neglect is included, that number increases to more than 2 million (National Center on Elder Abuse).
- Some experts estimate that only 1 of 14 abuse incidents is reported.
- In 1996 there were about 300,000 reports of domestic elder abuse.

- Neglect is the most common form of elder mistreatment.

PREDOMINANT AGE: Risk increases as level of disability increases
PEAK INCIDENCE: >80 yr old
RISK FACTORS: (Victim)
- Poor health
- Impaired cognition
- Social isolation

RISK FACTORS: (Perpetrator)
- Substance abuse
- Mental illness
- Dependence on the victim
- Being an involuntary or ill-equipped caregiver
- History of violence

CLINICAL PRESENTATION

- Physical abuse with multiple injuries at various stages with implausible or inconsistent descriptions of their origins; injuries are usually to head, neck, chest, breast, and abdomen.
- Extreme fear, hypervigilance, or withdrawal.
- Evidence of poor nutrition or hygiene.
- Toxicologic evidence of unprescribed medications.
- Poor adherence, frequent no-shows.

DIAGNOSIS

DIFFERENTIAL DIAGNOSIS

- Advancing dementia
- Depression or other psychiatric disorders
- Malnutrition due to intrinsic causes
- Conscious nonadherence
- Financial hardship
- Falling
- Diogenes syndrome

WORKUP

- Interview patient separately from the suspected abuser.
- Build trust; patients may be reticent.
- Ask direct questions.
- Be aware that physical findings are usually unexplained injuries or burns.
- Pelvic examination if sexual abuse suspected.

LABORATORY TESTS

- If sexual abuse suspected, screening for sexually transmitted diseases
- Toxicology screens or therapeutic drug monitoring

IMAGING STUDIES

X-rays as indicated by physical presentation

TREATMENT

NONPHARMACOLOGIC THERAPY

Reporting abuse to Adult Protective Services is mandatory in most states. This also provides the physician access to specialized personnel who can aid in evaluation and disposition.
- Separate patient and abuser.
- If the burden of care appears to be the major factor in contributing to abuse, referral to respite services, if available, can be useful.

Patient and caregiver may benefit from screening and treatment for depression, substance abuse, anxiety, mental illness, or cognitive impairment.

ACUTE GENERAL Rx

As indicated for injury or pain relief

DISPOSITION

In emergencies, hospitalization may be required. If the patient's level of disability does not allow for independent living, institutionalization may be required. Guidelines vary at the state and county levels regarding guardianship and conservatorship requirements.

REFERRAL

Adult Protective Services (mandatory in most states)

PEARLS & CONSIDERATIONS

COMMENTS

Consider home visit if abuse, neglect, or self-neglect is suspected.

PREVENTION

- Screen for caregiver stress.
- Respite services, if possible.
- Make financial arrangements and arrange durable power of attorney for health care and finances while patient still cognitively intact.

PATIENT/FAMILY EDUCATION

Alzheimer's Association for caregivers of patients with dementia

SUGGESTED READINGS

Fulmer T et al: Progress in elder abuse screening and assessment instruments, *J Am Geriatr Soc* 52(2):297, 2004.
Jogerst GJ et al: Domestic elder abuse and the law, *Am J Public Health* 93:2131, 2003.
Levine JM: Elder neglect and abuse. A primer for primary care physicians, *Geriatrics* 58(10):37,42, 2003.
National Center on Elder Abuse: http://www. elderabusecenter.org.

AUTHORS: **BREE JOHNSTON, M.D., M.P.H.,** and **MIKE HARPER, M.D.**

BASIC INFORMATION

DEFINITION

Although it is impossible to define alcoholism precisely, among the commonly used screening instruments for this disorder are the CAGE questionnaire, short Michigan Alcoholism Screening Test (SMAST), National Council on Alcoholism criteria, and DSM-IV-R criteria. Moderate drinking has been defined as two standard drinks (e.g., 12 oz of beer) per day and one drink per day for women and persons older than 65 years of age.

Although not generally included under the alcoholism topic, hazardous or at-risk drinking should also be considered. For men, *at-risk drinking* is defined as greater than 14 drinks/week or more than 4 drinks/occasion. For women, at-risk drinking is defined as about half that given for men.

The American Psychiatric Association defines diagnostic criteria for *alcohol withdrawal* as follows:

A. Cessation of (or reduction in) alcohol use that has been heavy and prolonged.
B. Two (or more) of the following, developing within several hours to a few days after criterion A:
1. Autonomic hyperactivity (e.g., sweating or pulse rate >100 beats/min)
2. Increased hand tremor
3. Insomnia
4. Nausea and vomiting
5. Transient visual, tactile, or auditory hallucinations or illusions
6. Psychomotor agitation
7. Anxiety
8. Grand mal seizures
C. The symptoms in criterion B cause clinically significant distress or impairment in social, occupational, or other important areas of functioning.
The symptoms are not due to a general medical condition and are not better accounted for by another mental disorder.

SYNONYMS

Alcohol abuse
Substance abuse

ICD-9CM CODES
303.9 Alcoholism

EPIDEMIOLOGY & DEMOGRAPHICS

INCIDENCE (IN U.S.):
- The clinical history suggests alcohol problems in 15% to 20% of patients in primary care and patients that are hospitalized. In the U.S. alcohol abuse generates nearly $185 billion in annual economic costs.
- 20% achieve abstinence without help, 70% achieve sobriety for 1 yr.

PREVALENCE (IN U.S.): 7% of population 18 yr or older
PREDOMINANT SEX:
- Lifetime risk for males 8% to 10%
- Lifetime risk for females 3% to 5%
GENETICS: More common with a family history of alcoholism and in patients of Irish, Scandinavian, and Native American descent

PHYSICAL FINDINGS & CLINICAL PRESENTATION

- Recurring minor trauma
- GI bleeding from gastris and/or varices
- Pancreatitis (acute and chronic)
- Liver disease
- Odor of alcohol on breath
- Tremulousness
- Tachycardia
- Peripheral neuropathy
- Recent memory loss

ETIOLOGY

- Social and genetic factors important
- Risk factors:
1. Broken homes
2. Unemployment
3. Divorce
4. Recurrent depression
5. Addiction to another substance, including tobacco

DIAGNOSIS **Dx**

WORKUP

- Several screening tests (CAGE, AUDIT, SMAST) are available. The four-item CAGE (feeling need to Cut down, Annoyed by criticism, Guilty about drinking, and need for an Eye-opener in the morning) is the most popular screening test in primary care. A positive response should lead to further questioning. The sensitivity of the CAGE ranges from 43% to 94% and its specificity ranges from 70% to 97%. Screening tools are available at the National Institute on Alcohol Abuse and Alcoholism Web site: http://www.niaaa.nih.gov/publications/niaaa-guide.
- Blood studies (see "Laboratory Tests")

LABORATORY TESTS

- γ-Glutamyltransferase (GGTP), generally elevated
- Liver transaminases (ALT, AST), often elevated, may be normal or low in advanced liver disease
- Low albumin level, hypophosphatemia, hypomagnesemia from malnutrition
- CBC reveals elevated mean corpuscular volume (MCV) from toxic effect of alcohol on erythrocyte development on nutritional deficiencies
- Stool for occult blood may be positive secondary to gastritis, or variceal bleeding

IMAGING STUDIES

Indicated only if there is a history of trauma. CT or ultrasound of abdomen may reveal fatty liver or cirrhosis in advanced stages.

TREATMENT

NONPHARMACOLOGIC THERAPY

- Complete abstinence
- Depression, if present, should be treated at same time ETOH is withdrawn

ACUTE GENERAL Rx

Alcohol withdrawal syndrome occurs when a person stops ingesting alcohol after prolonged consumption. It can result in four possible clinical patterns depending on the severity of the patient's alcohol abuse and the time interval from the patient's previous alcohol ingestion. Blood ethanol level decreases by 20 mg/dL/hr in a normal person. Although discussed separately in the text, these alcohol withdrawal states blend together in real life.

1. **Tremulous state:** (early alcohol withdrawal, "impending DTs," "shakes," "jitters")
   a. Time interval: usually occurs 6 to 8 hr after the last drink or 12 to 48 hr after reduction of alcohol intake; becomes most pronounced at 24 to 36 hr
   b. Manifestation: tremors, mild agitation, insomnia, tachycardia; symptoms are relieved by alcohol
   c. Inpatient treatment
      (1) Admit to medical floor (private room); monitor vital signs q4h; institute seizure precautions; maintain adequate sedation.
      (2) Administer lorazepam as follows:
         (a) Day 1: 2 mg PO q4h while awake and not lethargic
         (b) Day 2: 1 mg PO q4h while awake and not lethargic
         (c) Day 3: 0.5 mg PO q4h while awake and not lethargic
         (d) NOTE: Hold sedation for lethargy or abnormal vital or neurologic signs. The preceding doses are only guidelines; it is best to titrate the dose case by case
      (3) In patients with mild to moderate withdrawal and without history of seizures, individualized benzodiazepine administration (rather than a fixed-dose regimen) results in lower benzodiazepine administration and avoids unnecessary sedation. The Clinical Institute Withdrawal Assessment-Alco-

hol (CIWA-A) scale can be used to measure the severity of alcohol withdrawal. It consists of 10 items: nausea; tremor; autonomic hyperactivity; anxiety; agitation; tactile, visual, and auditory disturbances; headache; and disorientation. Each item is assigned a score from 0 to 7. For example in the "agitation" category 0 indicates normal activity, 7 indicates that the patient constantly thrashes about; for the category of "tremor," 0 indicates that tremor is not present, 7 tremor is severe, even with arms not extended. The maximum total score is 67. When the CIWA-A score is ≥8, patients are usually given 2 to 4 mg of lorazepam hourly.

(4) β-Adrenergic blockers: β-blockers are useful for controlling BP and tachyarrhythmias. However, they do not prevent progression to more serious symptoms of withdrawal and if used, should not be administered alone but in conjunction with benzodiazepines. β-Blockers should be avoided in patients with contraindications to their use (e.g., bronchospasm, bradycardia, or severe CHF). Centrally acting α-adrenergic agonists such as clonidine ameliorate symptoms in patients with mild to moderate withdrawal but do not reduce delirium or seizures.

(5) Vitamin replacement: thiamine 100 mg IV or IM for at least 5 days, plus PO multivitamins. The IV administration of glucose can precipitate Wernicke's encephalopathy in alcoholics with thiamine deficiency; therefore thiamine administration should precede IV dextrose

(6) Hydration PO or IV (high-caloric solution): if IV, glucose with Na^+, K^+, Mg^{2+}, and phosphate replacement prn

(7) Laboratory studies
  (a) CBC, platelet count, INR
  (b) Electrolytes, glucose, BUN, creatinine
  (c) GGTP, ALT, AST
  (d) Phosphorus and magnesium
  (e) Serum vitamin B_{12} and folic acid (if megaloblastic features in blood smear)

(8) Diagnostic imaging: generally not necessary; if subdural hematoma is suspected (evidence of trauma, persistent lethargy), a CT scan should be ordered.

(9) Social rehabilitation: group therapy such as Alcoholics Anonymous; identification and treatment of social and family problems should be initiated during the patient's hospital stay.

2. **Alcoholic hallucinosis**
  a. Manifestations: usually hallucinations are auditory, but occasionally hallucinations are visual, tactile, or olfactory; usually there is no clouding of sensorium as in delirium. Disordered perceptions become most pronounced after 24 to 36 hr of abstinence.
  b. Treatment: same as for DTs (see Withdrawal seizures).

3. **Withdrawal seizures** ("rum fits")
  a. Time interval: usually occurs 7 to 30 hr after cessation of drinking, with a peak incidence between 13 and 24 hr.
  b. Manifestations: generalized convulsions with loss of consciousness; focal signs are usually absent; consider further investigation with CT scan of head and EEG if clearly indicated (e.g., presence of focal neurologic deficits, prolonged postictal confusion state). In addition, in a febrile patient who is having a seizure or altered mental state, a lumbar puncture is necessary.
  c. Treatment
    (1) Diazepam 2.5 mg/min IV until seizure is controlled (check for respiratory depression or hypotension) may be beneficial for prolonged seizure activity; IV lorazepam 1 to 2 mg every 2 hr can be used in place of diazepam. Generally withdrawal seizures are self-limited and treatment is not required; the use of phenytoin or other anticonvulsants for short-term treatment of alcohol withdrawal seizures is not recommended.
    (2) Thiamine 100 mg IV, followed by IV dextrose, should also be administered.
    (3) Electrolyte imbalances (↑ Mg^{2+}, ↓ K^+, ↑/↓ Na^+, ↓ PO_4^{-3}) that may exacerbate seizures should be corrected.

4. **DTs:**
  a. Time interval: variable; usually occurs within 1 wk after reduction or cessation of heavy alcohol intake and persists for 1 to 3 days. Peak incidence is 72 hr and 96 hr after the cessation of alcohol consumption.
  b. Manifestations: profound confusion, tremors, vivid visual and tactile hallucinations, autonomic hy-

peractivity; this is the most serious clinical presentation of alcohol withdrawal (mortality is approximately 15% in untreated patients).
  c. Treatment
    (1) Admission to a detoxification unit where patient can be observed closely
    (2) Vital signs q30min (neurologic signs, if necessary)
    (3) Use of lateral decubitus or prone position if restraints are necessary
    (4) NPO: NG tube for abdominal distention may be necessary but should not be routinely used
    (5) Laboratory studies: same as for early alcohol withdrawal
    (6) Vigorous hydration (4-6 L/day): IV with glucose (Na^+, K^+, PO_4^{-3}, and Mg^{2+} replacement)
    (7) Vitamins: thiamine, 100 mg IV qd. The initial dose of thiamine should precede the administration of IV dextrose; multivitamins (may be added to the hydrating solution)
    (8) Sedation: Control of agitation should be achieved using rapid-acting sedative-hypnotic agents in adequate doses to maintain light somnolence for the duration of delirium.
      (a) Initially: lorazepam 2 to 5 mg IM/IV repeated prn
      (b) Maintenance (individualized dosage): chlordiazepoxide, 50 to 100 mg PO q4-6h, lorazepam 2 mg PO q4h, or diazepam 5 to 10 mg PO tid; withhold doses or decrease subsequent doses if signs of oversedation are apparent
      (c) Midazolam is also effective for managing DTs. Its rapid onset (sedation within 2 to 4 min of IV injection) and short duration of action (approximately 30 min) make it an ideal agent for titration in continuous infusion.
    (9) Treatment of seizures (as previously described)
    (10) Diagnosis and treatment of concomitant medical, surgical, or psychiatric conditions

CHRONIC Rx

- See "Referral."
- Pharmacotherapies for alcoholism include the opiate antagonists (naltrexone 50 mg PO qd or nalmefene 10 to 40 mg qd), disulfiram, acamprosate, and SSRIs.

DISPOSITION

See "Referral."

REFERRAL

- To Alcoholics Anonymous or Adult Children of Alcoholics
- Family members to Al-Anon or Al-A-Teen
- Many cities have Salvation Army Adult Rehabilitation centers; all patients accepted, regardless of ability to pay

PEARLS & CONSIDERATIONS

COMMENTS

- Relative indications for inpatient alcohol detoxification are as follows: history of DTs or withdrawal seizures, severe withdrawal symptoms, concomitant psychiatric or medical illness, multiple previous detoxifications, recent high levels of alcohol consumption, and lack of reliable support network.
- The cure rate for alcoholism is very disappointing, regardless of the modality. Only those who want to be helped will be helped. An effective strategy for the primary care physician is a prominently displayed sign in the office that states, "If you think you consume too much alcoholic beverage, please discuss it with me." Those who do open up the discussion can be given the facts in a nonjudgmental way and often can be helped. All too often, problem drinkers lie on the questionnaire until they face a life-threatening health issue—and even then denial often reigns supreme.

SUGGESTED READINGS

Bayard M et al: Alcohol withdrawal syndrome, *Am Fam Physician* 69:1443, 2004.

Daeppen JB et al: Symptom-triggered vs fixed-schedule doses of benzodiazepine for alcohol withdrawal: a randomized treatment trial, *Arch Intern Med* 162:1117, 2002.

Enoch ME, Goldman D: Problem drinking and alcoholism: diagnosis and treatment, *Am Fam Physician* 65:441, 2002.

Fleming MF et al: Brief physician advice for problem drinkers: long-term efficacy and benefit-cost analysis, *Alcohol Clin Exp Res* 26:36, 2002.

Kosten TR, O'Connor PG: Management of drug and alcohol withdrawal, *N Engl J Med* 348:1786, 2003.

Krystal JH et al: Naltrexone in the treatment of alcohol dependence, *N Engl J Med* 345:1734, 2001.

Mayo-Smith MF et al: Management of alcohol withdrawal delirium, *Arch Intern Med* 164:1405, 2004.

Moyer A et al: Brief interventions for alcohol problems: a meta-analytic review of controlled investigations in treatment-seeking populations, *Addiction* 97:279, 2002.

Nicholas JM et al: The effect of controlled drinking in alcoholic cardiomyopathy, *Ann Intern Med* 136:192, 2002.

O'Connor PG, Schotrenfeld RS: Patients with alcohol problems, *N Engl J Med* 9:592, 1998.

Schneekloth TD et al: Point prevalence of alcoholism in hospitalized patients: continuing challenges of detection, assessment, and diagnosis, *Mayo Clin Proc* 76:460, 2001.

U.S. Preventive Services Task Force: Screening and behavioral counseling interventions in primary care to reduce alcohol misuse: recommendation statement, *Ann Intern Med* 140:554, 2004.

White IR et al: Alcohol consumption and mortality: modelling risks for men and women at different ages, *BMJ* 325:191, 2002.

AUTHOR: **FRED F. FERRI, M.D.**

BASIC INFORMATION

DEFINITION

Amyloidosis is a generic term describing the deposition of amyloid fibrils in body tissues. *Amyloid* is an amorphous, eosinophilic material; it is birefringent and usually extracellular. Electron microscopy reveals nonbranching fibrils that are soluble and relatively resistant to proteolytic digestion. There are two major forms of acquired systemic amyloidosis:

- AA, associated with chronic inflammatory diseases (e.g., rheumatoid arthritis) and amyloid deposits in kidneys, liver, and spleen
- AL (formerly known as primary amyloidosis) affecting the kidneys, heart, liver, intestines, skin, peripheral sensory nervous system, spleen, and lungs

ICD-9CM CODES
277.3 Amyloidosis

EPIDEMIOLOGY & DEMOGRAPHICS

- Amyloidosis affects primarily males between the ages of 60 and 70 yr.
- There are between 1500 and 3500 new cases annually in the U.S.
- The most common type in the U.S. is immunoglobulin light chain related (AL) occurring in 5 to 12 persons/yr in the U.S.

PHYSICAL FINDINGS & CLINICAL PRESENTATION

- Findings are variable with organ system involvement. Symmetric polyarthritis, peripheral neuropathy, and carpal tunnel syndrome may be present with joint involvement.
- Signs and symptoms of nephrotic syndrome may be present with renal involvement.
- Fatigue and dyspnea may occur with pulmonary involvement.
- Diarrhea, macroglossia (20% of patients), malabsorption, hepatomegaly, and weight loss may occur with GI involvement.
- Cardiac involvement is common and can lead to predominantly right-sided CHF, JVD, peripheral edema, and hepatomegaly.
- Vascular involvement can result in easy bleeding and periorbital purpura ("raccoon-eyes").

ETIOLOGY

In patients with amyloidosis, a soluble circulating protein (serum amyloid P [SAP]) is deposited in tissues as insoluble β-pleated sheets. The source of amyloid protein is a population of monoclonal plasma cells in the bone marrow. There are several chemically documented amyloidoses that can be principally subdivided into:

1. Acquired systemic amyloidosis (immunoglobulin light chain, multiple myeloma, hemodialysis amyloidosis)
2. Heredofamilial systemic (polyneuropathy, familial Mediterranean fever)
3. Organ-limited (Alzheimer's disease)
4. Localized endocrine (pancreatic islet, medullary thyroid carcinoma)

DIAGNOSIS

DIFFERENTIAL DIAGNOSIS

Variable, depending on the organ involvement:

- Renal involvement (toxin- or drug-induced necrosis, glomerulonephritis, renal vein thrombosis)
- Interstitial lung disease (sarcoidosis, connective tissue disease, infectious etiologies)
- Restrictive cardiac (endomyocardial fibrosis, viral myocarditis)
- Carpal tunnel (rheumatoid arthritis, hypothyroidism, overuse)
- Mental status changes (multiinfarct dementia)
- Peripheral neuropathy (alcohol abuse, vitamin deficiencies, diabetes mellitus)

WORKUP

Diagnostic approach is aimed at demonstration of amyloid deposits in tissues. This may be accomplished with rectal biopsy (positive in >60% of cases). Renal, myocardial, and bone marrow biopsy are other options. Abdominal fat pad biopsy can also be diagnostic; however, its yield is low and it should generally be reserved for evaluation of patients with peripheral neuropathy who also have findings associated with systemic amyloidosis.

LABORATORY TESTS

- Initial laboratory evaluation should include CBC, TSH, renal functions studies, ALT, AST, alkaline phosphatase, bilirubin, urinalysis, and serum and urine protein immunoelectrophoresis.
- Various laboratory abnormalities include proteinuria (found in >70% of cases), anemia, renal insufficiency, liver function abnormalities, hypothyroidism (10% to 20% of patients), and elevated monoclonal proteins. The finding of a monoclonal light chain in the serum or urine is very useful for diagnosis.
- DNA analysis is necessary for the diagnosis of hereditary amyloidosis.

IMAGING STUDIES

- Chest x-ray may reveal hilar adenopathy and mediastinal adenopathy.
- Two-dimensional Doppler echocardiography to study diagnostic filling is useful to evaluate for cardiac involvement.

- Nuclear imaging with technetium-labeled aprotinin may detect cardiac amyloidosis. SAP scintigraphy has high sensitivity for the detection of amyloid deposits in liver, spleen, kidneys, adrenal glands, and bones.

TREATMENT

ACUTE GENERAL Rx

- Therapy is variable, depending on the type of amyloidosis. Amyloidosis associated with plasma cell disorders may be treated with melphalan and prednisone, along with colchicine. Colchicine may also be effective in renal amyloidosis.
- Treatment of AL amyloidosis with high-dose melphalan and stem-cell transplantation may result in hematologic remission and improved 5-yr survival.
- Promising results have been found with the use of a molecule known as CPHPC given IV or SC in amyloidosis. This molecule has been shown effective in reducing circulating levels of SAP.

CHRONIC Rx

Renal transplantation is needed in patients with renal amyloidosis. Peritoneal dialysis in place of hemodialysis in patients with renal failure may improve hemodialysis amyloidosis by clearing β-2 microglobulin.

DISPOSITION

Prognosis is determined primarily by the presence or absence of cardiac involvement and with the form of amyloidosis:

- In reactive amyloidosis, eradication of the predisposing disease slows and can occasionally reverse the progression of amyloid disease. Survival of 5 to 10 yr after diagnosis is not uncommon.
- Patients with familial amyloidotic polyneuropathy generally have a prolonged course lasting 10 to 15 yr.
- Amyloidosis associated with immunocytic processes carries the worst prognosis (life expectancy <1 yr).
- The progression of amyloidosis associated with renal hemodialysis can be improved with newer dialysis membranes that can pass β-2 microglobulin.
- Median survival in patients with overt CHF is approximately 6 mo, 30 mo without CHF.

SUGGESTED READING

Skinner M et al: High-dose melphalan and autologous stem-cell transplantation in patients with AL amyloidosis: an 8-year study, *Ann Intern Med* 140:85, 2004.

AUTHOR: **FRED F. FERRI, M.D.**

BASIC INFORMATION

DEFINITION

Amyotrophic lateral sclerosis (ALS) is a progressive, degenerative neuromuscular condition of undetermined etiology affecting corticospinal tracts and anterior horn cells resulting in dysfunction of both upper motor neurons (UMN) and lower motor neurons (LMN), respectively.

ICD-9CM CODES
335.20 Amyotrophic lateral sclerosis

EPIDEMIOLOGY & DEMOGRAPHICS

INCIDENCE: 0.5 to 2 cases/100,000 persons. Onset is usually between the ages of 50 and 70 years. The male:female ratio is 2:1.
PREVALENCE: 5 in 100,000 persons

PHYSICAL FINDINGS & CLINICAL PRESENTATION

- Lower motor neuron signs (weakness, hypotonia, wasting, fasciculations, hypoflexia or areflexia)
- Upper motor neuron signs (loss of fine motor dexterity, spasticity, extensor plantar responses, hyperreflexia, clonus)
- Early deficits may be asymmetric
- Preservation of extraocular movements, sensation, bowel and bladder function
- Dysarthria, dysphagia, pseudobulbar affect, frontal lobe dysfunction
- ALS comprises approximately 90% of adult-onset motor neuron disease. Other presentations of motor neuron disease include progressive muscular atrophy, primary lateral sclerosis, progressive bulbar palsy, progressive pseudobulbar palsy, and ALS-parkinsonism-dementia complex.

ETIOLOGY

- 90% to 95% of all cases are sporadic; of the familial cases, approximately 20% are associated with a genetic defect in the copper-zinc superoxide dismutase enzyme (SOD1).

DIAGNOSIS

DIFFERENTIAL DIAGNOSIS

- Multifocal motor neuropathy with conduction block (MMN)
- Cervical spondylotic myelopathy with polyradiculopathy
- Spinal stenosis with compression of lumbosacral nerve roots
- Chronic inflammatory demyelinating polyneuropathy with CNS lesions

- Syringomyelia
- Syringobulbia
- Foramen magnum tumor
- Spinal muscular atrophy (SMA)
- Late-onset hexosaminidase A deficiency
- Polyglucosan body disease
- Bulbospinal muscular atrophy (Kennedy's disease)
- Monomyelic amyotrophy
- ALS-like syndromes have been reported in the setting of lead intoxication, HIV, hyperparathyroidism, hyperthyroidism, lymphoma, and B$_{12}$ deficiency

WORKUP

- EMG and nerve conduction studies
- Lumbar puncture to assess protein, serum GM-1 Ab if MMN suspected
- Assessment of respiratory function (FVC, NIF)

LABORATORY TESTS

- B$_{12}$, thyroid function, CPK, PTH, HIV may be considered
- Serum protein and immunofixation electrophoresis
- DNA studies for SMA or bulbospinal atrophy, hexosaminidase levels in pure LMN syndrome
- 24-hour urine for lead if indicated

IMAGING STUDIES

- Craniospinal neuroimaging contingent upon clinical scenario
- Modified barium swallow to evaluate aspiration risk

TREATMENT

NONPHARMACOLOGIC THERAPY

- Noninvasive positive pressure ventilation improves quality of life and increases tracheostomy-free survival
- PEG placement improves caloric and fluid status, eases medication administration, and may prolong life on the order of 1-4 mo
- Nutrition, speech therapy, physical and occupational therapy services
- Suction device for sialorrhea
- Communication may be eased with computerized assistive devices
- Early discussion of living will, recusitation orders, desire for PEG and tracheostomy, potential long-term care options
- Encourage contact with local support groups

ACUTE GENERAL Rx

Riluzole (Rilutek), a glutamate antagonist, is the only medication approved to extend tracheostomy-free survival in pa-

tients with ALS. Dosage is 50 mg q12h, at least 1 hr before or 2 hr after meals. Shown to prolong survival by 2-3 mo. Manufacturer recommends checking ALT at an initial frequency of once a month for 3 months, followed by once every 3 months until the first year of therapy is completed. ALT should be checked periodically thereafter.

CHRONIC Rx

- Glycopyrrolate or amitryptyline to help with sialorrhea (propranolol or metoprolol if secretions are thick in addition to sialorrhea)
- Relief of spasticity with baclofen, tizanadine, clonazepam
- Treatment of pseudobulbar affect with amitriptyline, sertraline (Zoloft), dextromethorphan

DISPOSITION

- Mean duration of symptoms is 3 to 5 yr.
- About 20% of patients survive >5 yr.

REFERRAL

- Referral to a neurologist experienced in neuromuscular disease is recommended to confirm the diagnosis.
- GI referral for PEG placement is recommended while forced vital capacity (FVC) remains >50% to minimize the risks inherent to the procedure.

PEARLS & CONSIDERATIONS

COMMENTS

- Patient education material may be obtained through the following:
ALS Association, 21021 Ventura Boulevard, Suite 321, Woodland Hills, CA 91364, phone: (800) 782-4727; or the Muscular Dystrophy Association, 3561 East Sunrise Drive, Tucson, AZ 85718-3204, phone: (800) 572-1717, www.mdausa.org/.

SUGGESTED READINGS

Bradley WG et al: Current management of ALS: comparison of the ALS CARE Database and the AAN Practice Parameter. The American Academy of Neurology, *Neurology* 57(3):500, 2001.
Miller RG et al: Practice parameter: the care of the patient with amyotrophic lateral sclerosis (an evidence-based review), *Muscle Nerve* 22(8):1104, 1999.
Rowland LP, Shneider NA: Amyotrophic lateral sclerosis, *N Engl J Med* 344:1688, 2001.

AUTHOR: **TAYLOR HARRISON, M.D.**

BASIC INFORMATION

DEFINITION

Iron deficiency anemia is anemia secondary to inadequate iron supplementation or excessive blood loss.

ICD-9CM CODES
280.9 Iron deficiency anemia

EPIDEMIOLOGY & DEMOGRAPHICS

- Iron deficiency is the most common nutritional deficiency worldwide.
- Iron deficiency is never a complete diagnosis. If caused by blood loss, the source of bleeding must be identified.

PHYSICAL FINDINGS & CLINICAL PRESENTATION

- Most patients have a normal examination.
- Skin pallor and conjunctival pallor may be present.

ETIOLOGY

- Blood loss from GI (GU blood loss less often the cause)
- Dietary iron deficiency (common in patient with dementia, depression, and other causes of failure to thrive)
- Poor iron absorption in patients with gastric or small bowel surgery
- Repeated phlebotomy
- Increased requirements
- Other: traumatic hemolysis (abnormally functioning cardiac valves), idiopathic pulmonary hemosiderosis (iron sequestration in pulmonary macrophages), paroxysmal nocturnal hemoglobinuria (intravascular hemolysis)

DIAGNOSIS

DIFFERENTIAL DIAGNOSIS

- Anemia of chronic disease
- Sideroblastic anemia
- Thalassemia trait

WORKUP

Diagnostic workup consists primarily of laboratory evaluation. Most patients with iron deficiency anemia are asymptomatic in the early stages. With progressive anemia, the major complaints are fatigue, dizziness, exertional dyspnea, pagophagia (ice eating), and pica. Patient's history may also suggest GI blood loss (melena, hematochezia, hemoptysis).

LABORATORY TESTS

- Laboratory results vary with the stage of deficiency.
- Absent iron marrow stores and decreased serum ferritin are the initial abnormalities.
- Decreased serum iron and increased TIBC are the next abnormalities.
- Hypochromic microcytic anemia is present with significant iron deficiency.
- Peripheral smear in patients with iron deficiency generally reveals microcytic hypochromic RBCs with a wide area of central pallor, anisocytosis, and poikilocytosis when severe.
- Laboratory abnormalities consistent with iron deficiency are low serum ferritin level, elevated RBC distribution width (RDW) with values generally >15, low MCV, elevated TIBC, and low serum iron.
- The reticulocyte hemoglobin content (CHr) may be a good screening test for iron deficiency. It can be measured on an automated hematology analyzer and represents a relatively inexpensive and fast way to detect iron deficiency.

TREATMENT

NONPHARMACOLOGIC THERAPY

Patients should be instructed to consume foods containing large amounts of iron, such as liver, red meat, and legumes.

ACUTE GENERAL Rx

- Treatment consists of ferrous sulfate 325 mg PO qd for at least 6 mo. Calcium supplements can decrease iron absorption; therefore, these two medications should be staggered.
- Parenteral iron therapy is reserved for patients with poor tolerance, noncompliance with oral preparations, or malabsorption.
- Transfusion of packed RBCs is indicated in patients with severe symptomatic anemia (e.g., angina) or life-threatening anemia.

CHRONIC Rx

Patients should be instructed to continue their iron supplements for at least 6 mo or longer to correct depleted body iron stores.

DISPOSITION

Most patients respond rapidly to iron supplementation with improvement in CBC and general well-being. GI side effects from oral iron therapy are common and may require decreased dose to once every other day.

REFERRAL

GI referral for evaluation of GI malignancy is recommended in all patients with iron deficiency and suspected GI blood loss.

PEARLS & CONSIDERATIONS

COMMENTS

If the diagnosis of iron deficiency anemia is made, it is mandatory to try to locate the suspected site of iron loss.

SUGGESTED READING

Tefferi A: Anemia in adults: a contemporary approach to diagnosis, *Mayo Clin Proc* 78:1274, 2004.

AUTHOR: **FRED F. FERRI, M.D.**

BASIC INFORMATION

DEFINITION

Pernicious anemia is an autoimmune disease resulting from antibodies against intrinsic factor and gastric parietal cells.

SYNONYMS

Megaloblastic anemia resulting from vitamin B_{12} deficiency

ICD-9CM CODES
281.0 Pernicious anemia

EPIDEMIOLOGY & DEMOGRAPHICS

- Increased incidence in females and older adults
- The overall prevalence of undiagnosed PA over age 60 yr is 1.9%
- Prevalence is highest in women (2.7%), particularly in black women (4.3%)
- Increased incidence of autoimmune disease (e.g., type 1 DM, Graves' disease, Addison's disease), *Helicobacter pylori* infection

PHYSICAL FINDINGS & CLINICAL PRESENTATION

- Mucosal pallor, glossitis
- Peripheral sensory neuropathy with paresthesias initially and absent reflexes in advanced cases
- Loss of joint position sense, pyramidal or long track signs
- Possible splenomegaly and mild hepatomegaly
- Generalized weakness and delirium/dementia

ETIOLOGY

- Antigastric parietal cell antibodies in >70% of patients, antiintrinsic factor antibodies in >50% of patients
- Atrophic gastric mucosa

DIAGNOSIS

DIFFERENTIAL DIAGNOSIS

- Nutritional vitamin B_{12} deficiency
- Malabsorption
- Chronic alcoholism (multifactorial)
- Chronic gastritis related to *H. pylori* infection
- Folic acid deficiency
- Myelodysplasia

WORKUP

- The clinical presentation of pernicious anemia varies with the stage. Initially, patients may be asymptomatic. In advanced stages, patients may present with impaired memory, depression, gait disturbances, paresthesias, and complaints of generalized weakness.
- Investigation consists primarily of laboratory evaluation.
- Endoscopy and biopsy for atrophic gastritis may be performed in selected cases.
- Diagnosis is crucial because failure to treat may result in irreversible neurologic deficits.

LABORATORY TESTS

- CBC generally reveals macrocytic anemia and leukopenia with hypersegmented neutrophils.
- MCV is generally significantly elevated in the advanced stages.
- Reticulocyte count is low/normal.
- Falsely low serum cobalamin levels can occur in patients with severe folate deficiency, in patients using high doses of ascorbic acid, and when cobalamin levels are measured following nuclear medicine studies (radioactivity interferes with cobalamin RIA measurement).
- Falsely high normal levels in patients with cobalamin deficiency can occur in severe liver disease or chronic granulocytic leukemia.
- The absence of anemia or macrocytosis does not exclude the diagnosis of cobalamin deficiency. Anemia is absent in 20% of patients with cobalamin deficiency, and macrocytosis is absent in >30% of patients at the time of diagnosis. It can be blocked by concurrent iron deficiency or anemia of chronic disease and may be masked by thalassemia trait.
- Schilling test is abnormal in part I; part II corrects to normal after administration of intrinsic factor.
- Laboratory tests used for detecting cobalamin deficiency in patients with normal vitamin B_{12} levels include serum and urinary methylmalonic acid level (elevated), total homocysteine level (elevated), intrinsic factor antibody (positive).
- An increased concentration of plasma methylmalonic acid (P-MMA) does not predict clinical manifestations of vitamin B_{12} deficiency and should not be used as the only marker for diagnosis of B_{12} deficiency.
- Additional laboratory abnormalities can include elevated LDH, direct hyperbilirubinemia, and decreased haptoglobin.
- Antiparietal antibody test should be positive in pernicious anemia and negative in nutritional vitamin B_{12} deficiency.

TREATMENT

NONPHARMACOLOGIC THERAPY

Avoid folic acid supplementation without proper vitamin B_{12} supplementation.

ACUTE GENERAL Rx

- Traditional therapy of a cobalamin deficiency consists of IM injections of vitamin B_{12} 1000 μg/wk for the initial 4 to 6 wk followed by 1000 μg/mo IM indefinitely. When hematologic parameters have returned to normal range, intranasal cyanocobalamin may be used in place of IM cyanocobalamin. The initial dose of intranasal cyanocobalamin (Nascobal) is one spray (500 μg) in one nostril once per week. Monitor response and increase dose if serum B_{12} levels decline. Consider return to intramuscular vitamin B_{12} supplementation if decline persists.
- Oral vitamin B_{12} replacement is appropriate (1 mg/day) for nutritional vitamin B_{12} deficiency.

CHRONIC Rx

Parenteral vitamin B_{12} 1000 μg/mo or intranasal cyanocobalamin 500 μg/wk (see "Acute General Rx") for the remainder of life

DISPOSITION

Anemia generally resolves with appropriate treatment. Neurologic deficits, if present at diagnosis, may be permanent.

REFERRAL

Consider GI referral for endoscopy upon diagnosis of pernicious anemia and surveillance endoscopy every 5 yr to rule out gastric carcinoma

PEARLS & CONSIDERATIONS

COMMENTS

- Patients must understand that therapy is lifelong.
- Self-injection of vitamin B_{12} may be taught in selected patients.
- Oral cobalamin (1000 μ/day) has been reported as also being effective in mild cases of pernicious anemia because about 1% of an oral dose is absorbed by passive diffusion, a pathway that does not require intrinsic factor.

AUTHORS: **FRED F. FERRI, M.D.,** with revisions by **TOM J. WACHTEL, M.D.**

BASIC INFORMATION   *i*

DEFINITION

An abdominal aortic aneurysm (AAA) is a permanent localized dilation of the abdominal aortic artery to at least 50% when compared with the normal diameter. The normal diameter in men is 2.3 cm, and in women it is 1.9 cm.

> **ICD-9CM CODES**
> 441.3 Ruptured abdominal aortic aneurysm
> 441.4 Aneurysm, abdominal (aorta)

EPIDEMIOLOGY & DEMOGRAPHICS

- The incidence of AAAs has been rising from 12.2 cases/100,000 persons to 36.2 cases/100,000 persons from 1951 to 1980.
- The prevalence ranges from 2% to 5% in men >60 yr.
- AAA is predominantly a disease of the elderly, affecting men >women (4:1).
- Rupture of an AAA is the tenth leading cause of death in men >55 yr (15,000 deaths/yr in the U.S.).

PHYSICAL FINDINGS & CLINICAL PRESENTATION

SYMPTOMS

- Abdominal pain radiating to the back, flank, and groin. The pain is thought to be caused by rapid expansion of the aneurysm as it stretches the overlying peritoneum. AAA should be considered in the differential of anyone presenting with abdominal pain or back pain.
- Early satiety, nausea, and vomiting due to compression of adjacent bowel.

PHYSICAL EXAM

- The exam, although not very sensitive for AAA <5 cm in size, has a sensitivity of 82% for detecting AAA >5 cm.
- Pulsatile epigastric mass that may or may not be tender.
- Venous thrombosis from iliocaval venous compression.
- Discoloration and pain of the feet with distal embolization of the thrombus within the aneurysm.
- Shock, hypoperfusion, abdominal distention if rupture occurs.

Rare presentations include hematemesis or melena with abdominal and back pain in patients with aortoenteric fistulas. Aortocaval fistula produces loud abdominal bruits.

ETIOLOGY

- Atherosclerotic (degenerative or nonspecific)
- Trauma
- Cystic medial necrosis (Marfan's syndrome)
- Arteritis, inflammatory
- Mycotic, infected (septic)
- Syphilis

DIAGNOSIS   **Dx**

WORKUP

- Abdominal ultrasound is nearly 100% accurate in identifying an aneurysm and estimating the size to within 0.3 to 0.4 cm. It is not very good in estimating the proximal extension to the renal arteries or involvement of the iliac arteries.
- CT scan is recommended for preoperative aneurysm imaging and estimating the size to within 0.3 mm. There are no false-negatives, and the CT scan can localize the proximal extent, detect the integrity of the wall, and rule out rupture.
- Angiography gives detailed arterial anatomy, localizing the aneurysm relative to the renal and visceral arteries. This is the definitive preoperative study for surgeons.
- MRI can also be used, but it is more expensive and not as readily available.

TREATMENT   **Rx**

Treatment focuses on risk factor modification (diet and exercise for blood pressure, cholesterol, and diabetes, and abstinence from tobacco) and surgery. Serial studies have shown that expansion rates are faster in current smokers than ex-smokers.

- On diagnosing an AAA, surveillance ultrasound for sizing is safe with very low rates of AAA rupture (<1%) with recommendations for prophylactic surgery for AAA >5.5 cm.
- The most commonly used predictor of rupture is the maximum diameter of the AAA. For AAAs with baseline diameters <3.5 cm, 4.0 cm, 4.5 cm, and 5 cm, the recommending screening intervals can be 36, 24, 12, and 3 months, respectively.
- Recent randomized trials found no reduction in mortality from repairing AAAs smaller than 5.5 cm in patients at low operative risk.
- For aneurysms 5.5 cm or greater, prosthetic graft replacement is recommended, providing there is no contraindication (e.g., MI within 6 mo, refractory CHF, life expectancy <2 yr, severe residual from CVA).
- For the high-risk patient deemed inoperable for such major surgery, endovascular stent-anchored grafts under local anesthesia have provided an alternative approach.

- Abdominal aortic rupture is an emergency. Surgery is the only chance for survival.
- Most AAAs are infrarenal. Surgical risk is increased in patients with coexisting coronary artery disease, pulmonary disease (Pao_2 <50 mm Hg, FEV_1 <11), liver cirrhosis, and chronic renal failure (Cr >3 mg/dl). Cardiac preoperative evaluation with radionuclide perfusion studies for ischemia and aggressive perioperative hemodynamic monitoring help identify high-risk patients and decrease postoperative complications.
- In patients with dementia, postoperative delirium should be anticipated and managed.
- It is estimated that AAAs <5 cm expand at a rate of 0.4 cm/yr.
- The risk of rupture is 0% per year in aneurysms <4 cm, 0.6%-1%/yr in aneurysms 4.0 to 5.5 cm, 4.4%/yr in aneurysms 5.5 to 5.9 cm, 10.2%/yr in aneurysms 6.0 to 6.9 cm, and 32.5%/yr in aneurysms >7 cm.
- Mortality after rupture is >90%. Of those patients who reach the hospital, it is estimated 50% will survive compared with a 4% mortality rate for elective repair of the nonruptured aorta.
- The use of the (β-blocker propranolol has demonstrated a trend toward fewer surgeries in patients with asymptomatic small AAAs (3.0-5.0 cm).

SUGGESTED READINGS

Lederle FA: Ultrasonographic screening for abdominal aortic aneurysm, *Ann Intern Med* 139:516, 2003.

Lederle FA et al: Immediate repair compared with surveillance of small abdominal aortic aneurysms, *N Engl J Med* 346:1437, 2002.

Lederle FA et al: Rupture of large abdominal aortic aneurysms in patients refusing or unfit for elective repair, *JAMA* 287:2968, 2002.

Powell J, Brady A: Detection, management and prospects for medical treatment of small abdominal aortic aneurysms, *Arteroscler Thromb Vasc Biol* 24:241, 2004.

Powell J, Greenhalgh R: Small abdominal aortic aneurysms, *N Engl J Med* 348:1895, 2003.

The Propranolol Aneurysm Trial Investigators: Propranolol for small abdominal aortic aneurysms: results of a randomized trial, *J Vasc Surg* 35:72, 2002.

Sparks AR et al: Imaging of abdominal aortic aneurysms, *Am Fam Physician* 65:1565, 2002.

The United Kingdom Small Aneurysm Trial Participants: Long-term outcomes of immediate repair compared with surveillance of small abdominal aortic aneurysms, *N Engl J Med* 346:1445, 2002.

AUTHORS: **PRANAV M. PATEL, M.D., WEN-CHIH WU, M.D.,** and **TOM J. WACHTEL, M.D.**

BASIC INFORMATION

DEFINITION

Angina pectoris is characterized by discomfort that occurs when myocardial oxygen demand exceeds the supply. Myocardial ischemia can be asymptomatic (silent ischemia), particularly in diabetics. Angina can be classified as follows:

1. CHRONIC (STABLE):
   - Usually follows a precipitating event (e.g., climbing stairs, sexual intercourse, a heavy meal, emotional stress, cold weather)
   - Generally same severity as previous attacks; relieved by the customary dose of nitroglycerin
   - Caused by a fixed coronary artery obstruction secondary to atherosclerosis
2. UNSTABLE (REST OR CRESCENDO, CORONARY SYNDROME):
   - Recent onset
   - Increasing severity, duration, or frequency of chronic angina
   - Occurs at rest or with minimal exertion

FUNCTIONAL CLASSIFICATION

- New York Heart Association Functional Classification of Angina:
  Class I—Angina only with unusually strenuous activity.
  Class II—Angina with slightly more prolonged or rigorous activity than usual.
  Class III—Angina with usual daily activity.
  Class IV—Angina at rest.
- Grading of Angina by the Canadian Cardiovascular Society Classification System:
  Class I—Ordinary physical activity does not cause angina, such as walking, climbing stairs. Angina (occurs) with strenuous, rapid, or prolonged exertion at work or recreation.
  Class II—Slight limitation of ordinary activity. Angina occurs on walking or climbing stairs rapidly; walking uphill; walking or stair climbing after meals, in cold, in wind, or under emotional stress; or only during the few hours after awakening. Angina occurs on walking more than two blocks on the level and climbing more than one flight of ordinary stairs at a normal pace and in normal condition.
  Class III—Marked limitations of ordinary physical activity. Angina occurs on walking one to two blocks on the level and climbing one flight of stairs in normal conditions and at a normal pace.
  Class IV—Inability to carry on any physical activity without discomfort—anginal symptoms may be present at rest.

EPIDEMIOLOGY & DEMOGRAPHICS

- Angina is most common in middle-aged and elderly males.
- Females are usually affected after menopause.
- Within 12 mo of initial diagnosis, 10% to 20% of patients with diagnosis of stable angina progress to MI or unstable angina.

PHYSICAL FINDINGS & CLINICAL PRESENTATION

- Although there is significant individual variation, most patients complain of substernal chest pain (pressure, tightness, heaviness, sharp pain, sensation similar to intestinal gas or dysphagia).
- The pain is of short duration (30 sec to 30 min), nonpleuritic, and often accompanied by shortness of breath, nausea, diaphoresis, and numbness or pain in the left arm, jaw, or shoulder.

ETIOLOGY

UNCONTROLLABLE RISK FACTORS FOR ANGINA:
- Advanced age
- Male sex
- Genetic predisposition
MODIFIABLE RISK FACTORS FOR ANGINA:
- Smoking (risk is almost double)
- Hypertension (risk is double if systolic blood pressure is >180 mm Hg)
- Hyperlipidemia
- Impaired glucose tolerance or diabetes mellitus
- Obesity (weight >30% over ideal)
- Hypothyroidism
- Left ventricular hypertrophy (LVH)
- Sedentary lifestyle
- Low serum folate levels (Folate is required for conversion of homocysteine to methionine. Folate deficiencies are associated with an increased risk of fatal coronary heart disease.)
- Elevated homocysteine levels. Elevated plasma homocysteine level is a strong and independent risk factor for CHD events especially in patients with type 2 DM
- Elevated levels of highly sensitive C-reactive protein (hs-CRP, cardio CRP)
- Elevated levels of lipoprotein-associated phospholipase A2
- Elevated fibrinogen levels
- Depression
- Vasculitis

DIAGNOSIS

DIFFERENTIAL DIAGNOSIS

Noncardiac pain mimicking angina may be caused by:
- Pulmonary diseases (pulmonary hypertension, pulmonary embolism, pleurisy, pneumothorax, pneumonia)
- GI disorders (peptic ulcer disease, pancreatitis, esophageal spasm or spontaneous esophageal muscle contraction, esophageal reflux, cholecystitis, cholelithiasis)
- Musculoskeletal conditions (costochondritis, chest wall trauma, cervical arthritis with radiculopathy, muscle strain, myositis)
- Acute aortic dissection
- Herpes zoster
- Anxiety disorder

WORKUP

- In patients presenting with chest pain, the probability of CAD should be estimated on the basis of patient age, sex, cardiovascular risk factors, and pain characteristics.
- The most important diagnostic factor is the history. Chest pain or left arm pain or discomfort reproducing previously documented angina and a known history of CAD or MI are indicative of high likelihood of actue coronary syndrome.
- The physical examination is of little diagnostic help and may be totally normal in many patients, although the presence of an S_4 gallop is suggestive of ischemic chest pain. Transient mitral regurgitation, hypotension, diaphoresis, and rales indicate a high likelihood of acute coronary syndrome.
- An ECG taken during the acute episode may show transient T-wave inversion or ST-segment depression or elevation, but more than 50% of patients with chronic stable angina have normal results on resting ECG.
- Patients with intermediate or high probability should undergo risk stratification through further testing. Treadmill exercise tolerance test is useful to identify patients with coronary artery disease who would benefit from cardiac catheterization. Stress echocardiogram or radionuclide testing (e.g., thallium, Persantine, dobutamine) are useful and sensitive in the detection of myocardial ischemia.
- Although invasive, coronary angiography remains the gold standard for the identification of clinically significant coronary artery disease. Coronary magnetic resonance angiography can also detect coronary artery disease of the proximal and middle segments. This noninvasive approach, where available, can be used to reliably iden-

tify (or rule out) left main coronary artery or three-vessel disease.

LABORATORY TESTS

- Initial laboratory tests in patients with chronic stable angina should include hemoglobin, fasting glucose, and fasting lipid panel.
- Cardiac isoenzymes (CK-MB q8h × 2) should be obtained to rule out MI in patients presenting with acute chest pain.
- Cardiac troponin I and T are specific markers of myocardial necrosis and are useful in evaluating patients with acute chest pain. Elevation of either of these proteins in the setting of an acute coronary syndrome identifies patients with a several-fold increased risk of death in subsequent weeks. Patients with negative troponin assays on arrival in the ER and repeated 4 hr later are at a low level of risk for cardiac events within the following 30 days, and most of these patients can be safely discharged from the ER. Troponin T tests can be false-positive in patients with renal failure, sepsis, rhabdomyolysis, fibrin clots, and heterophile antibodies. The presence of jaundice or the concurrent use of heparin can result in underestimation of troponin.
- Cardio-CRP (hs-CRP)—elevation of cardio-CRP is a relatively moderate predictor of coronary heart disease and it adds prognostic information to that conveyed by the Framingham risk score. However, based on current data, it may be premature to adapt widespread assessment of cardio-CRP.

IMAGING STUDIES

- Echocardiography is indicated in patients with systolic murmur suggestive of aortic stenosis, mitral valve prolapse, or hypertrophic cardiomyopathy. It is also useful in the detection of ischemia-induced regional wall motion abnormalities or mitral regurgitation. Echocardiography combined with treadmill exercise (stress echo) or pharmacologic stress with dobutamine can be used to detect regional wall abnormalities that occur during myocardial ischemia associated with CAD.
- Coronary angiography is performed to define the location and extent of coronary disease; this is indicated in selected patients who are candidates for CABG surgery or angioplasty.
- Noninvasive methods for assessing myocardial viability to predict which patients will have increased LVEF and improved survival after revascularization include positron-emission tomography, dobutamine echocardiography, and contrast-enhanced MRI. Additional studies are needed to determine the cost effectiveness of these studies in patients with ischemic cardiomyopathy.

TREATMENT

NONPHARMACOLOGIC THERAPY

- Aggressive modification of preventable risk factors (weight reduction in obese patients, regular aerobic exercise program, correction of folate deficiency, low-cholesterol and low-sodium diet, cessation of tobacco use)
- Diets using nonhydrogenated unsaturated fats as the predominant form of dietary fat, whole grains as the main form of carbohydrates, an abundance of fruits and vegetables, and adequate omega-3-fatty acids are optimal for prevention of coronary heart disease
- Correction of possible aggravating factors (e.g., anemia, hypertension, diabetes mellitus, hyperlipidemia, thyrotoxicosis, hypothyroidism)

ACUTE GENERAL Rx

The major classes of antiischemic agents are nitrates, β-adrenergic blockers, calcium channel blockers, aspirin, and heparin; they can be used alone or in combination.

- Nitrates cause venodilation and relaxation of vascular smooth muscle; the decreased venous return from venodilation decreases diastolic ventricular wall tension (preload) and thereby reduces mechanical activity (and myocardial oxygen consumption) during systole. Relaxation of vascular smooth muscle increases coronary blood flow and reduces systemic pressure. Tolerance to nitrates can be minimized by avoiding sustained blood levels with a daily nitrate-free period (e.g., omission of bedtime dose of oral isosorbide dinitrate or 12 hr on/12 hr off transdermal nitroglycerin therapy). Nitrates are relatively contraindicated in patients with hypertrophic obstructive cardiomyopathy, and should also be avoided in patients with severe aortic stenosis.
- β-Adrenergic blockers achieve their major antianginal effect by reducing heart rate and systolic blood pressure. Absent contraindications, they should be regarded as initial therapy for stable angina for all patients. Their dose should generally be adjusted to reduce the resting heart rate to 50-60 beats/min.
- Long-acting calcium channel blockers are usually used as second-line agents. Short-acting calcium channel blockers should be avoided. Calcium channel blockers should generally also be avoided after complicated MI (CHF) and in patients with CHF secondary to systolic dysfunction (unless necessary to control heart rate).
- Aspirin: give initial dose of at least 160 mg/day followed by 81 to 325 mg/day. Aspirin inhibits cyclooxygenics and synthesis of thromboxane A_2 and reduces the risk of adverse cardiovascular events by 33% in patients with unstable angina. Patients intolerant to aspirin can be treated with the antiplatelet agent clopidogrel. Clopidogrel acts by irreversibly blocking the P2Y12 adenosine diphosphate receptor on the platelet surface, thereby interrupting platelet activation and aggregation.
- Heparin is useful in patients with unstable angina and reduces the frequency of MI and refractory angina. Patients with unstable angina treated with aspirin plus heparin have a 32% reduction in the risk of MI and death compared with those treated with aspirin alone; therefore, unless heparin is contraindicated, most hospitalized patients with unstable angina should be treated with both aspirin and heparin. Enoxaparin (low–molecular weight heparin) 1 mg bid SC is as effective as continuous unfractionated heparin in reducing the incidence of unstable angina. It is usually given for 3-8 days, or until coronary revascularization is performed. Longer administration does not provide additional cardiac benefits and may increase risk of hemorrhage.
- Early administration of platelet glycoprotein IIb/IIIa receptor antagonists is useful in addition to aspirin and heparin in patients with unstable angina, in high-risk patients with positive troponin tests, or those undergoing percutaneous revascularization. Abciximab, the first GP IIb/IIa inhibitor, is an important component of percutaneous revascularization. Started in the catheterization lab, it reduces the incidence of ischemic events. Abciximab is contraindicated in patients for whom an early invasive strategy is not planned. Contraindications to the use of GP IIb/IIa inhibitors are: severe hypertension (>180/110), internal bleeding within 30 days, history of intracranial hemorrhage, neoplasm, NVM, aneurysm, CVA within 30 days or history of hemorrhagic CVA, thrombocytopenia (<100 k), acute pericarditis, history or symptoms suggestive of aortic dissection, and major surgical procedures or severe physical trauma within previous month.

CHRONIC Rx

Use of lipid-lowering drugs is recommended in patients with coronary heart disease and in patients with hyperlipidemia refractory to diet and exercise. Among patients who have recently had an acute coronary syndrome, an intensive lipid-lowering statin regimen to reduce LDL cholesterol to <70 mg/dl provides greater protection against death or major cardiovascular events than does a standard regimen. Statins also decrease the level of the inflammatory marker hs-CRP independently of the magnitude of change in lipid parameters.

REFERRAL

Surgical therapy:

CABG surgery is recommended for patients with left main coronary disease, for those with symptomatic three-vessel disease, and for those with left ventricular EF <40% and critical (>70% stenosis) in all three major coronary arteries. Surgical therapy improves prognosis, particularly in diabetic patients with multivessel disease.

Minimally invasive direct coronary artery bypass (MIDCAB) is a variation of CABG for patients in whom sternotomy and cardiopulmonary bypass is either contraindicated or unnecessary. In this procedure the left internal mammary is anastomosed to the LAD through a thoracic incision without cardiopulmonary bypass. This operation is generally performed for patients with only single-vessel CAD.

The Port-Access Procedure is another type of minimally invasive technique.

Angioplasty and coronary stents:

Percutaneous coronary intervention (PCI) should be considered for patients with one- or two-vessel disease that does not involve the main left coronary artery and in whom ventricular function is normal or near normal. Patients selected for PCI should also be candidates for CABG. The types of lesions best suited for angioplasty are proximal lesions, noncalcified, concentric, and preferably shorter than 5 mm (should not exceed 10 mm). Approximately 80% of patients show immediate benefit after PCI. The frequency of abrupt closure postangioplasty can be reduced by pretreatment with IV glycoprotein IIb/IIIa receptor inhibitors, which block the final common pathway of platelet aggregation. In patients with clinically documented acute coronary syndrome who are treated with GP IIb/IIa inhibitors, even small elevations in cTmI and cTmT identify high-risk patients who derive a large clinical benefit from an early invasive strategy. Abciximab (ReoPro) and eptifibatide (Integrilin) are approved for use before and during percutaneous coronary interventions. They are expensive (>$1400 per dose of abciximab) and can cause thrombocytopenia in 0.5% to 1% of patients. Platelet counts should be monitored for 24 hours after starting glycoprotein IIb/IIIa inhibitors. Reversal of thrombocytopenia (e.g., patients undergoing emergency CABG) can be achieved with platelet transfusions.

The development of *coronary stents* has broadened the number of patients who can be treated in the cardiac laboratory. Cardiac stents are currently used in nearly 95% of all percutaneous interventional lesions. The rate of restenosis may be reduced by placing a stent electively in primary atheromatous lesions. In patients with symptomatic isolated stenosis of the proximal left anterior descending artery, stenting has advantages over standard coronary angioplasty in that it is associated with both a lower rate of restenosis and a better clinical outcome. The major limitations of stenting are subacute thrombosis, restenosis within the stent, bleeding complications when anticoagulants are used post-stenting, and higher cost ($1500 average unit price). The combination of aspirin and clopidogrel is effective in preventing coronary stent thrombosis. Vitamin therapy to lower homocysteine levels has been recommended by some for the prevention of restenosis after coronary angioplasty; however, recent reports indicate that the administration of folate, vitamin B_6, and vitamin B_{12} after coronary stenting may increase the risk of in-stent restenosis and the need for target-vessel revascularization. Stents coated with sirolimus have been shown to dramatically reduce the incidence of stent restenosis by inhibiting the growth of endothelium and fibrosis within the lumen of the stent on the short term. Stents coated with paclitaxel, which inhibits cellular replication and reduces proliferation and migration of endothelial smooth muscle cells, are also effective in reducing the incidence of restenosis.

CO_2 laser revascularization:

This operation is performed only in selected centers and consists of placing 1-mm laser channels in the heart muscle. It may be indicated in selected Class III or Class IV angina patients who are failing maximum medical therapy and are not amenable to any other PTCA or coronary bypass surgery.

PEARLS & CONSIDERATIONS ⓘ

COMMENTS

Although nitrate responsiveness is usually an integral part of a diagnostic strategy for chronic stable chest pain, recent reports question its value and conclude that in a general population admitted for chest pain, relief of pain after nitroglycerin treatment does not predict active coronary artery disease and should not be used to guide diagnosis in the acute care setting.

SUGGESTED READINGS

Aviles RJ et al: Troponin T levels in patients with acute coronary syndromes, with or without renal dysfunction, *N Engl J Med* 346:2047, 2002.

Brennan ML et al: Prognostic value of myeloperoxidase in patients with chest pain, *N Engl J Med* 349:1595, 2003.

Buffon A et al: Widespread coronary inflammation in unstable angina, *N Engl J Med* 347:5, 2002.

Henrikson C et al: Chest pain relief by nitroglycerin does not predict active coronary artery disease, *Ann Intern Med* 139:979, 2003.

Hu F, Willet W: Optimal diets for prevention of coronary heart disease, *JAMA* 288:2569, 2002.

Kushner I, Sehgal A: Is high-sensitivity C-Reactive protein an effective screening test for cardiovascular risk? *Arch Intern Med* 162:867, 2002.

Lange H et al: Folate therapy and in-stent restenosis after coronary stenting, *N Engl J Med* 350:2673, 2004.

Levinson SS, Elin RJ: What is C-reactive protein telling us about coronary artery disease, *Arch Intern Med* 162:389, 2002.

Moses JW et al: Sirolimus-eluting stents versus standard stents in patients with stenosis in a native coronary artery, *N Engl J Med* 349:1315, 2003.

Ridker PM et al: Plasma homocysteine concentration, statin therapy, and the risk of first acute coronary events, *Circulation* 105:1776, 2002.

Ridker PM et al: Comparison of C-reactive protein and low-density lipoprotein cholesterol levels in the prediction of first cardiovascular events, *N Engl J Med* 347:1557, 2002.

Serruys PW et al: Fluvastatin for prevention of cardiac events following successful first percutaneous coronary intervention, *JAMA* 287:3215, 2002.

Snow V et al: Evaluation of primary care patients with chronic stable angina: Guidelines from the American College of Physicians, *Ann Intern Med* 141:57 and 562, 2004.

Soinio M et al: Elevated plasma homocysteine level is an independent predictor of coronary artery disease events in patients with type 2 DM, *Ann Intern Med* 140:94, 2004.

Yang EHC et al: Current and future treatment strategies for refractory angina, *Mayo Clin Proc* 79(10):1284, 2004.

AUTHOR: **FRED F. FERRI, M.D.**

BASIC INFORMATION

DEFINITION

GAD is most likely to present in combination with other psychiatric and medical conditions. GAD commonly presents with excessive anxiety, fear, and worry for most of the time, continuously for at least 6 mo. The subjective anxiety must be accompanied by at least three somatic symptoms (e.g., restlessness, irritability, sleep disturbance, muscle tension, difficulty concentrating, or fatigability). Because worry is also a symptom of depression, officially, GAD is not present if there is a concurrent Major Depression. However, the field is recognizing that the two conditions can coexist, and research on the commonalities are being conducted.

SYNONYMS

Anxiety neurosis
Chronic anxiety
GAD

ICD-9CM CODES

F41.1 (DSM-IV Code 300.02)

EPIDEMIOLOGY & DEMOGRAPHICS

INCIDENCE (IN U.S.): 31% in 1 yr
PREVALENCE (IN U.S.):
- In general population: prevalence of 5% lifetime
- In primary care setting: 3% (It is the most common anxiety disorder in this setting.)

PREDOMINANT SEX: Females are more frequently affected (2:1 ratio), but they present for treatment less frequently (3:2 female:male).
PEAK INCIDENCE: Chronic condition with onset in early life
GENETICS: Concordance rates in dizygotic twins and monozygotic twins are not different (0% to 5%), but detailed analysis of 1033 female twin pairs finds that heredity contributes about 30% of the factors that may cause GAD.

PHYSICAL FINDINGS & CLINICAL PRESENTATION

- Report of being "anxious" all of their lives
- Excessive worry, usually regarding family, finances, work, or health
- Sleep disturbance, particularly early insomnia
- Muscle tension (typically in the muscles of neck and shoulders)
- Headaches (muscle tension)
- Difficulty concentrating
- Day form of fatigue
- Gastrointestinal symptoms compatible with IBD (one third of patients)
- Physical consequences of anxiety are the driving force for patients seeking medical attention

- Comorbid psychiatric illness (e.g., dysthymia or major depression) and substance abuse (e.g., alcohol abuse) are frequent

ETIOLOGY

- There is no clear etiology.
- Several hypotheses centering on neurotransmitter (catecholamines, indolamines) and developmental psychology are used as framework for treatment recommendations.
- Risk factors include a family history, increase in stress, history of physical or emotional trauma, and medical illness.

DIAGNOSIS

DIFFERENTIAL DIAGNOSIS

- Wide range of psychiatric and medical conditions; however, for a diagnosis of GAD to be made a person must experience anxiety with coexisting physical symptoms the majority of the time continuously for at least 6 mo
- Cardiovascular and pulmonary disease
- Hyperthyroidism
- Parkinson's disease
- Consequence of recreational drug use (e.g., cocaine, amphetamine, and PCP) or withdrawal (e.g., alcohol or benzodiazepines)

WORKUP

- History: required for diagnosis
- Physical examination: confirm the patient's physical complaints
- Exclusion of organic basis for the complaints possibly requiring additional workup
- Physical cause should be suspected if anxiety follows recent changes in medication

TREATMENT

NONPHARMACOLOGIC THERAPY

- Cognitive-behavioral therapy
- Relaxation training
- Biofeedback
- Psychodynamic psychotherapy

NOTE: Studies directly comparing medications with psychotherapy are not available, but the general clinical impression is that the psychotherapies are probably superior to pharmacotherapies.

ACUTE GENERAL Rx

- Acute treatment is rarely indicated because GAD is a chronic condition.
- Occasionally, patients are in acute distress, requiring physician to respond quickly; benzodiazepines are given under these conditions as drug of choice for both daytime anxiety and initial insomnia.

NOTE: Caution should be taken in prescribing benzodiazepines because of the propensity for misuse and dependence in this population. If provided, the patient should be educated about the use of other medications and the risks in using benzodiazepines.

CHRONIC Rx

- SSRIs and venlafaxine are also effective in generalized anxiety disorders and are typically given as a first line treatment. These are particularly useful if comorbid depression is present.
- If used and prescribed with supervision, benzodiazepines can provide long-term symptom control with only occasional problems with tolerance or abuse; however, tolerance to benzodiazepines is common and for this reason they have fallen from a first line treatment to second line treatment for GAD. Further, the rate of relapse after discontinuation of benzodiazepines may be twice the rate after discontinuation of the available nonbenzodiazepine anxiolytic buspirone. Finally, benzodiazepines can contribute to cognitive impairment in elderly patients, with or without dementia.
- Buspirone is effective without any potential for tolerance or abuse.
- Sedating antidepressants are also useful in ameliorating initial insomnia.

DISPOSITION

- This condition is chronic with periodic exacerbations.
- Treatment is given to provide a significant degree of improvement, but symptoms and dysfunction may persist.
- The risk for suicide is higher than general population.

REFERRAL

- If the symptoms are refractory to treatment
- If the case is complicated with a comorbid psychiatric condition
- If treatment response is suboptimal with residual dysfunction

SUGGESTED READINGS

Fricchione G: Clinical practice. Generalized anxiety disorder, *N Engl J Med* 351(7):675, 2004.
Goodman WK: Selecting pharmacotherapy for generalized anxiety disorder, *J Clin Psychiatry* 65(suppl 13):8, 2004.
Lang AJ: Treating generalized anxiety disorder with cognitive-behavioral therapy, *J Clin Psychiatry* 65(suppl 13):14, 2004.
Rouillon F: Long term therapy of generalized anxiety disorder, *Eur Psychiatry* 19(2):96, 2004.

AUTHORS: **PATRICIA AREAN, PH.D.,** and **MITCHELL D. FELDMAN, M.D., M.PHIL.**

BASIC INFORMATION

DEFINITION

Aortic dissection occurs when an intimal tear allows blood to dissect between medial layers of the aorta.

> **ICD-9CM CODES**
> 441.00 Aortic dissection
> 444.01 Aortic dissection, thoracic

SYNONYMS

Dissecting aortic aneurysm, unspecified site

EPIDEMIOLOGY & DEMOGRAPHICS

PREDOMINANT SEX: Males > females
PEAK INCIDENCE: Ages 60 to 80
RISK FACTORS: Hypertension, atherosclerosis, and family history of aortic aneurysms. Others include inflammatory diseases that cause a vasculitis, disorders of collagen (Marfan syndrome, Ehlers-Danlos syndrome), bicuspid aortic valve, aortic coarctation, Turner's syndrome, crack cocaine, and trauma.

CLASSIFICATION

Based on the fact that the majority of aortic dissections originate in the ascending or descending aorta, three major classifications (Fig. 1-1):
- DeBakey type I ascending and descending aorta, II ascending aorta, III descending aorta
- Stanford type A ascending aorta (proximal), type B descending aorta (distal)

PHYSICAL FINDINGS & CLINICAL PRESENTATION

- Sudden onset of very severe chest pain, at its peak at onset
- Little radiation to neck, shoulder, or arm
- Sharp, tearing or ripping pain
- Ascending aortic dissection with anterior chest pain
- Descending aortic dissection with back pain
- Syncope, abdominal pain, CHF, malperfusion may occur
- Most with severe hypertension, 25% with hypotension (SBP <100), which can indicate bleeding, cardiac tamponade, or severe aortic regurgitation
- Pulse and blood pressure differentials common (38%) caused by partial compression of subclavian arteries
- Cardiac and neurological systems are most commonly involved organ systems
- Aortic regurgitation in 18% to 50% of cases of proximal dissection
- Myocardial ischemia caused by coronary artery compression
- Cerebral ischemia/stroke in 5% to 10% of patients
- Rare cause of pericarditis

ETIOLOGY

- Unknown, risk factors known. Chronic HTN affects arterial wall composition
- Medial degeneration of aorta appears to be the culprit
- Aortic dissection reflects systemic illness of vasculature

DIAGNOSIS

DIFFERENTIAL DIAGNOSIS

- Known as the great imitator: PE, ACS, AS, pericarditis, cholecystitis
- Acute MI needs to be ruled out
- Aortic insufficiency
- Nondissecting aortic aneurysm

LABORATORY TESTS

ECG: Helpful to rule out MI, generally nonspecific findings.
Serum biochemical marker: Smooth muscle myosin heavy chain high first 6 hr after onset.

IMAGING STUDIES

- Chest x-ray may show widened mediastinum (62%) nonspecific, and displacement of aortic intimal calcium.
- Transesophageal echocardiography, sensitivity 97% to 100%, can detect aortic insufficiency and pericardial effusion; study of choice in unstable patients, but operator dependent.
- MRI, sensitivity 90% to 100%, gold standard, but length of test and difficult access not suitable for stable intubated patients. Gives best information for surgeons.
- CT, sensitivity 83% to 100%, involves IV contrast.
- Aortography rarely done now.
- Transthoracic echocardiography, poor sensitivity.

TREATMENT

ACUTE GENERAL Rx

- Admit to ICU for hemodynamic monitoring.
- Propanolol 1 mg every 3-5 minutes or metoprolol 5 mg IV every 5 minutes, followed by nitroprusside 0.3-10 mg/kg/min, with target SBP 100-120.
- Decrease contractility and BP with IV β-blocker, β-blocker is cornerstone of treatment.
- IV labetalol can be used instead, 20 mg IV, then 40-80 mg every 10 min.
- IV calcium channel blockers or ACE inhibitors may be used.
- Proximal dissections require emergent surgery (Type I, II, + A) to prevent rupture or pericardial effusion.
- Distal dissections are treated only medically unless distal organ involvement or impending rupture occurs (Type III + B).
- Endovascular stent placement is a new treatment, especially for older high-risk surgical patients.

CHRONIC Rx

Chronic aortic dissection (>2 wks) followed with aggressive BP control

DISPOSITION

- Natural history of untreated aortic dissection is 85% mortality within 2 wk.
- Proximal aortic dissection is a surgical emergency. Time is critical; mortality is 1% to 3% per hr.
- Patients who are postsurgical repair or have chronic aneurysm should be followed with imaging at 1, 3, 6, 9, and 12 months.
- Overall, in-hospital mortality is 30% in patients with proximal dissections and 10% in patients with distal dissections.

REFERRAL

For ICU management and surgery

SUGGESTED READINGS

Hagan PG et al: The international registry of acute aortic dissection: new insights into an old disease, *JAMA* 283:897, 2000.
Khan IA et al: Clinical, diagnostic, and management perspectives of aortic dissection, *Chest* 122(1):311, 2002.
Moore AG et al: Choice of CT, TEE, MRI and aortography in acute AD: IRAD, *Am J Cardiology* 89:1235, 2002.
Nienaber CA: Aortic dissection: new frontiers in diagnosis and management, Part I and II, *Circulation,* 108(6):772, 2003.

AUTHOR: **LYNN BOWLBY, M.D.**

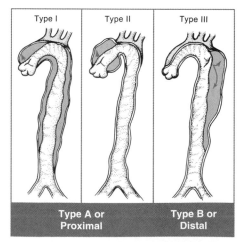

FIGURE 1-1 Classification systems for aortic dissection. (From Isselbacher EM, Eagle KA, DeSanctis RW: Disease of the aorta. In Braunwald E [ed]: *Heart disease: a textbook of cardiovascular medicine,* ed 5, Philadelphia, 1997, WB Saunders.)

BASIC INFORMATION

DEFINITION

Aortic regurgitation is retrograde blood flow into the left ventricle from the aorta secondary to incompetent aortic valve.

SYNONYMS

Aortic insufficiency
AI
AR

ICD-9CM CODES
424.1 Aortic valve disorders

EPIDEMIOLOGY & DEMOGRAPHICS

- The most common cause of isolated severe aortic regurgitation is aortic root dilation.
- Infectious endocarditis is the most frequent cause of acute aortic regurgitation.

PHYSICAL FINDINGS & CLINICAL PRESENTATION

The clinical presentation varies depending on whether aortic insufficiency is acute or chronic. Chronic aortic insufficiency is well tolerated (except when secondary to infective endocarditis), and the patients remain asymptomatic for years. Common manifestations after significant deterioration of left ventricular function are dyspnea on exertion, syncope, chest pain, and CHF. Acute aortic insufficiency manifests primarily with hypotension caused by a sudden fall in cardiac output. A rapid rise in left ventricular diastolic pressure results in a further decrease in coronary blood flow.

Physical findings in chronic aortic insufficiency include the following:
- Widened pulse pressure (markedly increased systolic blood pressure, decreased diastolic blood pressure) is present.
- Bounding pulses, head "bobbing" with each systole (de Musset's sign) are present; "water hammer" or collapsing pulse (Corrigan's pulse) can be palpated at the wrist or on the femoral arteries ("pistol shot" femorals) and is caused by rapid rise and sudden collapse of the arterial pressure during late systole; capillary pulsations (Quincke's pulse) may occur at the base of the nail beds.
- A to-and-fro "double Duroziez" murmur may be heard over femoral arteries with slight compression.
- Popliteal systolic pressure is increased over brachial systolic pressure ≥40 mm Hg (Hill's sign).
- Cardiac auscultation reveals:
  1. Displacement of cardiac impulse downward and to the patient's left
  2. S_3 heard over the apex

  3. Decrescendo, blowing diastolic murmur heard along left sternal border
  4. Low-pitched apical diastolic rumble (Austin-Flint murmur) caused by contrast of the aortic regurgitant jet with the left ventricular wall
  5. Early systolic apical ejection murmur

In patients with acute aortic insufficiency both the wide pulse pressure and the large stroke volume are absent. A short blowing diastolic murmur may be the only finding on physical examination.

ETIOLOGY

- Infective endocarditis
- Rheumatic fibrosis
- Trauma with valvular rupture
- Congenital bicuspid aortic valve
- Myxomatous degeneration
- Syphilitic aortitis
- Rheumatic spondylitis
- SLE
- Aortic dissection
- Fenfluramine, dexfenfluramine
- Takayasu's arteritis, granulomatous arteritis

DIAGNOSIS

DIFFERENTIAL DIAGNOSIS

- Patent ductus arteriosus, pulmonary regurgitation, and other valvular abnormalities
- The differential diagnosis of cardiac murmurs is described in Section II

WORKUP

- Echocardiogram, chest x-ray, ECG, and cardiac catheterization (selected patients)
- Medical history and physical examination focused on the following clinical manifestations:
  1. Dyspnea on exertion
  2. Syncope
  3. Chest pain
  4. CHF

IMAGING STUDIES

- Chest x-ray
  1. Left ventricular hypertrophy (chronic aortic regurgitation)
  2. Aortic dilation
  3. Normal cardiac silhouette with pulmonary edema: possible in patients with acute aortic regurgitation
- ECG: left ventricular hypertrophy
- Echocardiography: coarse diastolic fluttering of the anterior mitral leaflet; LVH in patients with chronic aortic regurgitation
- Cardiac catheterization: assesses degree of left ventricular dysfunction, confirms the presence of a wide pulse pressure, assesses surgical risk, and determines if there is coexistent coronary artery disease

TREATMENT   Rx

NONPHARMACOLOGIC THERAPY

- Avoidance of competitive sports and strenuous activity
- Salt restriction

ACUTE GENERAL Rx

MEDICAL:
- Digitalis, diuretics, ACE inhibitors, and sodium restriction for CHF; nitroprusside in patients with acute aortic regurgitation
- Long-term vasodilator therapy with ACE inhibitors or nifedipine for reducing or delaying the need for aortic valve replacement in asymptomatic patients with severe aortic regurgitation and normal left ventricular function
- Bacterial endocarditis prophylaxis for surgical and dental procedures

SURGICAL: Reserved for:
- Symptomatic patients with chronic aortic regurgitation despite optimal medical therapy
- Patients with acute aortic regurgitation (i.e., infective endocarditis) producing left ventricular failure
- Evidence of systolic failure:
  1. Echocardiographic fractional shortening <25%
  2. Echocardiographic and diastolic dimension >55 mm
  3. Angiographic ejection fraction <50% or end-systolic volume index (ESVI) >60 ml/m2
- Evidence of diastolic failure:
  1. Pulmonary pressure >45 mm Hg systolic
  2. Left ventricular end-diastolic pressure (LVEDP) >15 mm Hg at catheterization
  3. Pulmonary hypertension detected on examination
- In general, the "55 rule" has been used to determine the timing of surgery: surgery should be performed before EF <55% or end-systolic dimension >55 mm.

REFERRAL

Surgical referral (see "Acute General Rx" for indications)

PEARLS & CONSIDERATIONS   !

COMMENTS

The operative mortality rate for aortic regurgitation is 3% to 5%.

AUTHOR: **FRED F. FERRI, M.D.**

BASIC INFORMATION

DEFINITION

Aortic stenosis is obstruction to systolic left ventricular outflow across the aortic valve. Symptoms appear when the valve orifice decreases to <1 cm² (normal orifice is 3 cm²). The stenosis is considered severe when the orifice is <0.5 cm²/m² or the pressure gradient is 50 mm Hg or higher.

SYNONYMS

Aortic valvular stenosis
AS

ICD-9CM CODES
424.1 Aortic valvular stenosis

EPIDEMIOLOGY & DEMOGRAPHICS

- Aortic stenosis is the most common valve lesion in adults in Western countries.
- Calcific stenosis (most common cause in patients >60 yr old) occurs in 75% of patients.

PHYSICAL FINDINGS & CLINICAL PRESENTATION

- Rough, loud systolic diamond-shaped murmur, best heard at base of heart and transmitted into neck vessels; often associated with a thrill or ejection click; may also be heard well at the apex
- Absence or diminished intensity of sound of aortic valve closure (in severe aortic stenosis)
- Late, slow-rising carotid upstroke with decreased amplitude
- Strong apical pulse
- Narrowing of pulse pressure in later stages of aortic stenosis
- Some patients with aortic stenosis experience bleeding into their GI tract or skin. This is caused by an acquired defect in von Willebrand factor. Aortic valve replacement restores normal hemostasis.

ETIOLOGY

- Rheumatic inflammation of aortic valve
- Progressive stenosis of congenital bicuspid valve (found in 1%-2% of population)
- Idiopathic calcification of the aortic valve
- Congenital (major cause of aortic stenosis in patients <30 yr)

DIAGNOSIS

DIFFERENTIAL DIAGNOSIS

- Hypertrophic cardiomyopathy
- Mitral regurgitation
- Ventricular septal defect

- Aortic sclerosis. Aortic stenosis is distinguished from aortic sclerosis by the degree of valve impairment. In aortic sclerosis, the valve leaflets are abnormally thickened but obstruction to outflow is minimal.

WORKUP

- Echocardiography
- Chest x-ray examination, ECG
- Cardiac catheterization in selected patients (see "Imaging Studies")
- Medical history focusing on symptoms and potential complications:
  1. Angina
  2. Syncope (particularly with exertion)
  3. CHF
  4. GI bleeding: in patients with associated hemorrhagic telangiectasia (AVM)

IMAGING STUDIES

- Chest x-ray examination
  1. Poststenotic dilation of the ascending aorta
  2. Calcification of aortic cusps
  3. Pulmonary congestion (in advanced stages of aortic stenosis)
- ECG:
  1. Left ventricular hypertrophy (found in >80% of patients)
  2. ST-T wave changes
  3. Atrial fibrillation: frequent
- Doppler echocardiography: thickening of the left ventricular wall; if the patient has valvular calcifications, multiple echoes may be seen from within the aortic root and there is poor separation of the aortic cusps during systole. Gradient across the valve can be estimated but is less precise than with cardiac catheterization.
- Cardiac catheterization: indicated in symptomatic patients; it confirms the diagnosis and estimates the severity of the disease by measuring the gradient across the valve, allowing calculation of the valve area. It also detects coexisting coronary artery stenosis that may need bypass at the same time as aortic valve replacement.

TREATMENT

NONPHARMACOLOGIC THERAPY

- Strenuous activity should be avoided.
- Sodium restriction if CHF is present.

GENERAL Rx

MEDICAL:
- Diuretics and sodium restriction are needed if CHF is present; digoxin is used only to control rate of atrial fibrillation.
- ACE inhibitors are relatively contraindicated.

- Calcium channel blocker verapamil may be useful only to control rate of atrial fibrillation.
- Antibiotic prophylaxis is necessary for surgical and dental procedures.

SURGICAL:
- Valve replacement is the treatment of choice in symptomatic patients because the 5-yr mortality rate after onset of symptoms is extremely high, even with optimal medical therapy; valve replacement is indicated if cardiac catheterization establishes a pressure gradient >50 mm Hg and valve area <1 cm².
- Balloon aortic valvotomy for adult acquired aortic stenosis is useful only for palliation.

DISPOSITION

- The 5-yr survival rate in adults is 40%.
- The average duration of symptoms before death is as follows: angina, 60 mo; syncope, 36 mo; CHF, 24 mo.
- About 75% of patients with symptomatic aortic stenosis will be dead 3 yr after onset of symptoms unless the aortic valve is replaced.

REFERRAL

- Surgical referral for valve replacement in symptomatic patients. However, the presence of moderate or severe valvular calcification, together with a rapid increase in aortic-jet velocity, identifies patients with a very poor prognosis who should be considered for early valve replacement rather than have surgery delayed until symptoms develop.
- Surgical mortality rate for valve replacement is 3% to 5%; however, it varies with patient's age (>8% in patients >75 yr old).
- Balloon valvuloplasty is useful in poor surgical candidates who do not have calcified valve apparatus; it can be done as an intermediate procedure to stabilize high-risk patients before surgery.
- When performed in adults who have calcified valves, balloon valvuloplasty is useful only for short-term reduction in severity of aortic stenosis when surgery is contraindicated, because restenosis occurs rapidly.

SUGGESTED READINGS

Alpert JS: Aortic stenosis, a new face for an old disease, *Arch Intern Med* 163:1769, 2003.
Carabello BA: Aortic stenosis, *N Engl J Med* 346:677, 2002.
Vincentelli A et al: Acquired von Willebrand syndrome in aortic stenosis, *N Engl J Med* 349:343, 2003.

AUTHOR: **FRED F. FERRI, M.D.**

BASIC INFORMATION

DEFINITION

Rheumatoid arthritis (RA) is a systemic disorder characterized by chronic joint inflammation that most commonly affects peripheral joints. This process results in the development of pannus, a destructive tissue that damages cartilage.

ICD-9CM CODES
714.0 Rheumatoid arthritis

EPIDEMIOLOGY & DEMOGRAPHICS

PREVALENCE: 5 cases/1000 adults
PREDOMINANT SEX:
- Female:male ratio of 3:1
- After age 50 yr, sex difference less marked

PHYSICAL FINDINGS & CLINICAL PRESENTATION

- Usually gradual onset; common prodromal symptoms of weakness, fatigue, and anorexia
- Initial presentation: multiple symmetric joint involvement, most often in the hands and feet, usually MCP, MTP, and PIP joints (Fig. 1-2)
- Joint effusions, tenderness, and restricted motion usually present early in the disease
- Eventual characteristic deformities: subluxations, dislocations, and joint contractures
- Extraarticular findings:
  1. Tendon sheaths and bursae frequently affected by chronic inflammation
  2. Possible tendon rupture
  3. Rheumatoid nodules over bony prominences such as the elbow and shaft of the ulna
  4. Splenomegaly, pericarditis, and vasculitis
  5. Findings of carpal tunnel syndrome resulting from flexor tenosynovitis

ETIOLOGY

Unknown. There is increasing evidence that the inflammation and destruction of bone and cartilage that occur in many rheumatic diseases are the result of the activation by some unknown mechanism of proinflammatory cells that infiltrate the synovium. These cells, in turn, release various substances, such as cytokines and tumor necrosis factor (TNF) alpha, which subsequently cause the pathologic changes typical of this group of diseases. Many of the newer therapeutic agents are directed at the suppression of these final mediators of inflammation.

DIAGNOSIS **Dx**

DIFFERENTIAL DIAGNOSIS

- SLE
- Seronegative spondyloarthropathies
- Polymyalgia rheumatica
- Acute rheumatic fever
- Scleroderma

According to the American College of Rheumatology, RA exists when four of seven criteria are present, with criteria 1 to 4 being present for at least 6 wk.
1. Morning stiffness over 1 hr
2. Arthritis in three or more joints with swelling
3. Arthritis of hand joints with swelling
4. Symmetric arthritis
5. Rheumatoid nodules
6. Roentgenographic changes typical of RA
7. Positive serum rheumatoid factor

LABORATORY TESTS

- Increase in rheumatoid factor in 80% of cases (rheumatoid factor also present in the normal population)
- Possible mild anemia
- Usually, elevated acute phase reactants (ESR, C-reactive protein)
- Possible mild leukocytosis
- Usually, turbid joint fluid, which forms a poor mucin clot; elevated cell count, with an increase in polymorphonuclear leukocytes

IMAGING STUDIES

Plain radiography
- Usually reveals soft-tissue swelling and osteoporosis early (Fig. 1-3)
- Eventually, joint space narrowing, erosion, and deformity visible as a result of continued inflammation and cartilage destruction

TREATMENT **Rx**

NONPHARMACOLOGIC THERAPY

Proper management requires close cooperation among primary physician, therapist, rheumatologist, and orthopedist.
- Patient education is important.
- Rest with proper exercise and splinting can prevent or correct joint deformities.
- Maintain proper diet and control obesity.

CHRONIC Rx

- NSAIDs: commonly used as the initial treatment to relieve inflammation (drug of choice for most patients: aspirin, but other NSAIDs also effective)
- Disease-modifying drugs (DMARDs): are traditionally begun when NSAIDs

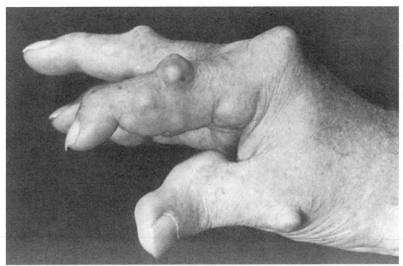

FIGURE 1-2 Rheumatoid arthritis. Hand of a 60-year-old man with seropositive rheumatoid arthritis. There are fixed deformities and gross rheumatoid nodules. (From Canoso JJ: *Rheumatology in primary care,* Philadelphia, 1997, WB Saunders.)

are not effective; current recommendations favor early aggressive treatment with DMARDs, seeking to minimize long-term joint damage. Commonly used agents are methotrexate, cyclosporine, hydroxychloroquine, sulfasalazine, leflunomide, adalimumab and infliximab. Most of these are associated with potential toxicity and require close monitoring. They are also usually slow-acting drugs that require more than 8 wk to become effective.

- Oral prednisone
- Intrasynovial steroid injections
- Etanercept (Enbrel), a tumor necrosis factor α-blocker, is indicated in moderately to severely active RA in patients who respond inadequately to DMARDs. The combination of etanercept and methotrexate has been reported to be effective and promising in the treatment of RA.

DISPOSITION

- Remissions and exacerbations are common, but condition is chronically progressive in the majority of cases.
- Joint degeneration and deformity often lead to disability.
- Early diagnosis and treatment are important and can improve quality of life.

REFERRAL

Early referral to rheumatologist
Orthopedic consultation for corrective surgery

SUGGESTED READINGS

Chen AL, Joseph TN, Zuckerman JD: Rheumatoid arthritis of the shoulder, *J Am Acad Orthop Surg* 11:12, 2003.

Cohen S et al: Treatment of rheumatoid arthritis with anakinra, a recombinant human interleukin-1 receptor antagonist, in combination with methotrexate: results of a twenty-four-week, multicenter, randomized, double-blind, placebo controlled trial, *Arthritis Rheum* 46:614, 2002.

Dayer J-M, Bresnihan B: Targeting interleukin-1 in the treatment of rheumatoid arthritis, *Arthritis Rheum* 46:574, 2002.

Edwards JC, Szczepanski L et al: Efficacy of β-cell-targeted therapy with rituximab in patients with rheumatoid arthritis, *N Engl J Med* 350:2572, 2004.

Gardner GC, Kadel MJ: Ordering and interpreting rheumatologic laboratory tests, *J Am Acad Orthop Surg* 11:60, 2003.

Genovese MC et al: Etanercept versus methotrexate in patients with early rheumatoid arthritis: two-year radiographic and clinical outcomes, *Arthritis Rheum* 46:1443, 2002.

Kremer JM: Rational use of new and existing disease-modifying agents in rheumatoid arthritis, *Ann Intern Med* 134:695, 2001.

Olsen NJ, Stein CM: New drugs for rheumatoid arthritis, *N Engl J Med* 350:2167, 2004.

Maini SR: Infliximab treatment of rheumatoid arthritis, *Rheum Dis Clin North Am* 30:329, 2004.

Smith JB, Haynes MK: Rheumatoid arthritis: a molecular understanding, *Ann Intern Med* 136:908, 2002.

Van Everdingen AA et al: Low dose prednisone therapy for patients with early active rheumatoid arthritis: clinical efficacy, disease-modifying properties, and side effects, *Ann Intern Med* 136:1, 2002.

AUTHOR: **LONNIE R. MERCIER, M.D.**

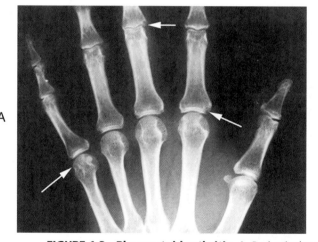 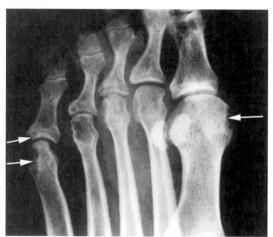

FIGURE 1-3 Rheumatoid arthritis. A, Periarticular osteopenia and marginal erosions in MCPs and a PIP (*arrows*). **B,** In the same patient, marginal erosions at metatarsal heads. (From Canoso JJ [ed]: *Rheumatology in primary care*, Philadelphia, 1997, WB Saunders.)

BASIC INFORMATION

DEFINITION

Cell death in components of bone: hematopoietic fat marrow and mineralized tissue.

SYNONYMS

Osteonecrosis, avascular necrosis

ICD-9CM CODES
733.40 Aseptic necrosis
733.43 Aseptic necrosis of femoral condyle
733.42 Aseptic necrosis of femoral head
733.41 Aseptic necrosis of humeral head
733.44 Aseptic necrosis of talus

EPIDEMIOLOGY & DEMOGRAPHICS

- 15,000 new cases per year in the U.S.
- Associated conditions:
  1. Corticosteroid treatment: 35%
  2. Alcohol abuse: 22%
  3. Idiopathic and other: 43%
- Common sites involved
  1. Femoral head
  2. Femoral condyle
  3. Humeral head
  4. Navicular and lunate wrist bones
  5. Talus

PHYSICAL FINDINGS & CLINICAL PRESENTATION

- May be asymptomatic
- Pain in the involved area exacerbated by movement or weight bearing
- Decreased range of motion as the disease progresses
- Functional limitation

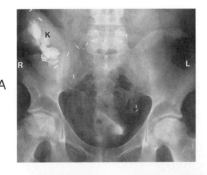

ETIOLOGY

Final common pathway of conditions that lead to impairment of the blood supply to the involved bone.

Stages:

Stage 0
- Asymptomatic
- Normal imaging
- Histologic findings only (i.e., silent osteonecrosis)

Stage 1
- Asymptomatic or symptomatic
- Normal x-ray and CT scan
- Abnormal bone scan and/or MRI

Stage 2
- Abnormal x-rays and/or CT scan including linear sclerosis, focal bead mineralization, cysts; however, the overall architecture of the involved bone is normal

Stage 3
- Early evidence of mechanical bone failure (subchondral fracture), but the overall shape of the bone is still intact

Stage 4
- Flattening or collapse of the bone

Stage 5
- Joint space narrowing

Stage 6
- Extensive joint destruction

DIAGNOSIS **Dx**

DIFFERENTIAL DIAGNOSIS

- None in late stages
- Early: any condition causing focal musculoskeletal pain including arthritis, bursitis, tendinitis, myopathy, neoplastic bone and joint diseases, traumatic injuries, pathologic fractures

IMAGING STUDIES See Fig. 1-4.

1. X-ray: insensitive early in the course. The earliest changes include diffuse osteopenia, areas of radiolucency with sclerotic border, and linear sclerosis. Later a subchondral lucency (crescent sign) indicates subchondral fracture. More advanced cases reveal flattening, collapsed bone and abnormal bone contour. In late disease, osteoarthritic changes are seen.

2. Bone scan:
   - Early: "cold" area
   - Later: increased radionuclide uptake as a result of remodeling
   - Sensitivity in early disease is only 70% and specificity is poor
3. CT scan: may reveal central necrosis and area of collapse before those are visible in x-ray.
4. MRI: the most sensitive technology to diagnose early aseptic necrosis. The first sign is a margin of low signal. An inner border of high signal associated with a low-signal line is specific of aseptic necrosis ("double line sign"). Sensitivity is 75%-100%.

TREATMENT

PREVENTION

- Management of etiologic conditions
- Minimize corticosteroid use

MEDICAL TREATMENT

- Decrease weight bearing of affected area
- Pulsing electromagnetic fields applied externally (still experimental)
- Peripheral vasodilators (e.g., dihydroergotamine) (unproven)

SURGICAL TREATMENT

- Core decompression: effectiveness 35%-95% in early phases
- Bone grafting
- Osteotomies
- Joint replacement

PROGNOSIS

- When diagnosed at an early stage treatment is appropriate in all cases because 85%-90% can be expected to progress to a more advanced stage
- Contralateral joint involvement is common (30%-70%)

SUGGESTED READING

Mazieres R: *Osteonecrosis:* In Klippel JH, Dieppe PA (eds): *Rheumatology,* ed 2, St. Louis, 1998, Mosby.

AUTHOR: **TOM J. WACHTEL, M.D.**

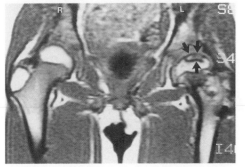

FIGURE 1-4 Aseptic necrosis of the hips. A, Aseptic necrosis can occur from a number of causes, including trauma and steroid use. In this patient, an anteroposterior view of the pelvis shows a transplanted kidney (K) in the right iliac fossa. Use of steroids has caused this patient to have bilateral aseptic necrosis. The femoral heads are somewhat flattened, irregular, and increased in density. **B,** Aseptic necrosis in a different patient is demonstrated on an MRI scan as an area of decreased signal (*arrows*) in the left femoral head. This is the most sensitive method for detection of early aseptic necrosis. (From Mettler FA [ed]: *Primary care radiology,* Philadelphia, 2000, WB Saunders).

BASIC INFORMATION

DEFINITION

The American Thoracic Society defines asthma as a "disease characterized by an increased responsiveness of the trachea and bronchi to various stimuli and manifested by a widespread narrowing of the airways that changes in severity either spontaneously or as a result of treatment." *Status asthmaticus* can be defined as a severe continuous bronchospasm.

SYNONYMS

Bronchospasm
Reactive airways disease
Bronchial asthma

ICD-9CM CODES
493.9 Asthma, unspecified
493.1 Intrinsic asthma
493.0 Extrinsic asthma

EPIDEMIOLOGY & DEMOGRAPHICS

- Asthma affects 5% to 12% of the population and accounts for over 450,000 hospitalizations and nearly 2 million emergency department visits yearly in the U.S.
- Overall asthma mortality in the U.S. is 20 per 1 million persons per year.
- In older individuals, asthma and COPD may overlap.

PHYSICAL FINDINGS & CLINICAL PRESENTATION

Physical examination varies with the stage and severity of asthma and may reveal only an increased expiratory phase of respiration. The triad of typical asthma symptoms includes shortness of breath, wheezing, and cough. The hallmark physical finding in any patient with active asthma is wheezing (expiratory > inspiratory) and a prolonged expiratory phase during lung auscultation.
Physical examination during status asthmaticus may reveal:
- Tachycardia and tachypnea
- Use of accessory respiratory muscles
- Pulsus paradoxus (inspiratory decline in systolic blood pressure >10 mm Hg)
- Wheezing: absence of wheezing (silent chest) or decreased wheezing can indicate worsening obstruction
- Mental status changes: generally secondary to hypoxia and hypercapnia and constitute an indication for urgent intubation
- Paradoxic abdominal and diaphragmatic movement on inspiration (detected by palpation over the upper part of the abdomen in a semirecumbent position): important sign of impending respiratory crisis; indicates diaphragmatic fatigue

- The following abnormalities in vital signs are indicative of severe asthma:
  1. Pulsus paradoxus >18 mm Hg
  2. Respiratory rate >30 breaths/min
  3. Tachycardia with heart rate >120 beats/min

ETIOLOGY

- Intrinsic asthma: occurs in patients who have no history of allergies; may be triggered by upper respiratory infections or psychologic stress
- Extrinsic asthma (allergic asthma): brought on by exposure to allergens (e.g., dust mites, cat allergen, industrial chemicals)
- Exercise-induced asthma: manifests with bronchospasm following initiation of exercise and improves with discontinuation of exercise
- Drug-induced asthma: often associated with use of NSAIDs, beta blockers, sulfites, certain foods and beverages

DIAGNOSIS

DIFFERENTIAL DIAGNOSIS

- CHF
- COPD
- Pulmonary embolism
- Foreign body aspiration
- Pneumonia and other upper respiratory infections
- Rhinitis with postnasal drip
- TB
- Hypersensitivity pneumonitis
- Anxiety disorder
- Wegener's granulomatosis
- Diffuse interstitial lung disease
- GERD

WORKUP

Medical history, physical examination, pulmonary function studies and peak flow meter determination, blood gas analysis and oximetry (during acute bronchospasm), chest radiography if infection is suspected

LABORATORY TESTS

Laboratory tests can be normal if obtained during a stable period. The following laboratory abnormalities may be present during an acute bronchospasm:
- ABGs can be used in staging the severity of an asthmatic attack:
  1. Mild: decreased Pao_2 and $Paco_2$, increased pH
  2. Moderate: decreased Pao_2, normal $Paco_2$, normal pH
  3. Severe: marked decreased Pao_2, increased $Paco_2$, and decreased pH
- CBC, leukocytosis with "left shift" may indicate the existence of bacterial infection.

- Sputum: eosinophils, Charcot-Leyden crystals, PMNs, and bacteria may be found on Gram stain in patients with pneumonia.
- Useful diagnostic tests for asthma:
  1. Pulmonary function studies: during acute severe bronchospasm, FEV_1 is <1 L and peak expiratory flow rate (PEFR) is <80 L/min
  2. Methacholine challenge test
  3. Skin test: to assess the role of atopy (when suspected)

IMAGING STUDIES

- Chest x-ray: usually normal, may show evidence of thoracic hyperinflation (e.g., flattening of the diaphragm, increased volume over the retrosternal air space)
- ECG: tachycardia, nonspecific ST-T wave changes; may also show cor pulmonale, right bundle-branch block, right axial deviation, counter-clockwise rotation

TREATMENT

NONPHARMACOLOGIC THERAPY

- Avoidance of triggering factors (e.g., salicylates, sulfites).
- Encouragement of regular exercise (e.g., swimming).
- Patient education regarding warning signs of an attack and proper use of medications (e.g., correct use of inhalers). Elderly asthmatics must be observed using the handheld inhalers. A spacer may be helpful and should be ordered routinely. If they cannot be taught to use metered-dose inhalers, they should be prescribed nebulizers for routine use at home. Albuterol, ipratropium, and fluticasone are available for nebulizer use.

GENERAL Rx

The Expert Panel of the National Asthma Education and Prevention Program (NAEPP) based on the classification of asthma severity recommends the following stepwise approach in the pharmacologic management of asthma in adults:
STEP 1 (MILD INTERMITTENT ASTHMA): NO DAILY MEDICATIONS ARE NEEDED.
- Short-acting inhaled β_2-agonists as needed (e.g., albuterol).
STEP 2 (MILD PERSISTENT ASTHMA): DAILY TREATMENT MAY BE NEEDED.
- Low-dose inhaled corticosteroid (e.g., beclomethasone [Beclovent, Vanceril], flunisolide [AeroBid], triamcinolone [Azmacort]) or fluticasone (Flovent) can be used.
- Cromolyn (Intal) or nedocromil (Tilade) can also be used.

- Additional considerations for long-term control are the use of the leukotriene receptor antagonist montelukast (Singulair).
- Quick relief of asthma can be achieved with short-acting inhaled β_2-agonists (see Step 1) (often described as "rescue treatment").

STEP 3 (MODERATE PERSISTENT ASTHMA): DAILY MEDICATION IS RECOMMENDED.

- Low-dose or medium-dose inhaled corticosteroids (see Step 2) plus long-acting inhaled β_2-agonist (salmeterol [Serevent]), or long-acting oral β_2-agonists (e.g., albuterol, sustained-release tablets). Salmeterol is also available as a dry powder inhaler (Discus) that does not require a spacer device; the dosage is one puff bid. A salmeterol-fluticasone combination for the Discus inhaler (Advair) is available and simplifies therapy for patients with asthma. It generally should be reserved for patients with at least moderately severe asthma not controlled by an inhaled corticosteroid alone.
- Use short-acting inhaled β_2-agonists on a prn basis for quick relief.

STEP 4 (SEVERE PERSISTENT ASTHMA):

- Daily treatment with high-dose inhaled corticosteroids plus long-acting inhaled β-agonists plus long-acting oral β_2-agonist plus long-term systemic corticosteroids (e.g., methylprednisolone, prednisolone, prednisone) can be used.
- Short-acting β_2-agonists can be used on a prn basis for quick relief.

Treatment of *status asthmaticus* is as follows:

- Oxygen generally started at 2 to 4 L/min via nasal cannula or Venti-Mask at 40% Fio$_2$; further adjustments are made according to the ABGs.
- Bronchodilators: various agents and modalities are available. Inhaled bronchodilators are preferred when they can be administered quickly. Albuterol (Proventil, Ventolin): 0.5 to 1 ml (2.5 to 5 mg) in 3 ml of saline solution tid or qid via nebulizer is effective.

Parenteral administration of sympathomimetics (e.g., SC epinephrine) is not recommended routinely and should always be accompanied by electrocardiographic monitoring.

- Corticosteroids
  1. Early administration is advised, particularly in patients using steroids at home.
  2. Patients may be started on hydrocortisone (Solu-Cortef) 2.5 to 4 mg/kg or methylprednisolone (Solu-Medrol) 0.5 to 1 mg/kg IV loading dose, then q6h prn; higher doses may be necessary in selected patients (particularly those receiving steroids at home); steroids given by inhalation should be (re)initiated after the acute phase, are useful for controlling bronchospasm and tapering oral steroids, and should be used in all patients with severe asthma.
  3. Rapid but judicious tapering of corticosteroids will eliminate serious steroid toxicity; long-term low-dose methotrexate may be an effective means of reducing the systemic corticosteroid requirement in some patients with severe refractory asthma.
  4. The most common errors regarding steroid therapy in acute bronchospasms are the use of "too little, too late" and too rapid tapering with return of bronchospasm.
- IV hydration: judicious use is necessary to avoid CHF in elderly patients.
- IV antibiotics are indicated when there is suspicion of bacterial infection (e.g., infiltrate on chest x-ray, fever, or leukocytosis).
- Intubation and mechanical ventilation are indicated when previous measures fail to produce significant improvement.
- General anesthesia: halothane may reverse bronchospasm in a severe asthmatic who cannot be ventilated adequately by mechanical means.

REFERRAL

Box 1-1 describes indications for referral to an asthma specialist.

COMMENTS

- Inhaled low-dose corticosteroids are the single most effective therapy for adult patients with asthma who require more than an occasional use of short-acting β_2-agonists to control their asthma.
- Leukotriene modifiers/receptor agonists represent a reasonable alternative in adults unable or unwilling to use corticosteroids; however, these agents are less effective than monotherapy with inhaled corticosteroids.
- Patients who remain symptomatic despite inhaled corticosteroids benefit from the addition of long-acting β_2-agonists.
- In patients with allergies and elevated serum IgE levels, use of anti-IgE therapy is beneficial.

SUGGESTED READINGS

Diette GB et al: Asthma in older patients: factors associated with hospitalization, *Arch Intern Med* 162:1123, 2002.

Holgate ST: Therapeutic options for persistent asthma, *JAMA* 285:2637, 2001.

Mintz M: Asthma update: part I. Diagnosis, monitoring, and prevention of disease progression, *Am Fam Physician* 70:893-898, 2004.

National Asthma Education and Prevention Program: *Expert panel report 2: guidelines for diagnosis and management of asthma,* Bethesda, Md, 1997, National Institutes of Health.

Naureckas ET, Solway J: Mild asthma, *N Engl J Med* 345:1257, 2001.

Sin DD et al: Pharmacological management to reduce exacerbations in adults with asthma, *JAMA* 292:367-376, 2004.

AUTHORS: **FRED F. FERRI, M.D.,** with revisions by **TOM J. WACHTEL, M.D.**

BOX 1-1 Possible Indications for Referral to an Asthma Specialist

Severe, acute asthma that has caused loss of consciousness, hypoxia, respiratory failure, convulsions, or near death

Poorly controlled asthma as indicated by admission to a hospital, frequent need for emergency care, need for oral corticosteroids, absence from work, disruption of sleep, interference with quality of life

Severe, persistent asthma requiring step 4 care (consider for patients who require step 3 care)

Requirement for continuous oral corticosteroids or high-dose inhaled corticosteroids or more than two short courses of oral corticosteroids within 1 year

Need for additional diagnostic testing such as allergy skin testing, rhinoscopy, provocative challenge, complete pulmonary function testing, bronchoscopy

Consideration for immunotherapy

Need for additional education regarding asthma, complications of asthma and treatment of asthma, problems with adherence to management recommendations, or allergen avoidance

Uncertainty of diagnosis

Complications of asthma, including sinusitis, nasal polyposis, aspergillosis, severe rhinitis, vocal cord dysfunction, gastroesophageal reflux

Modified from National Asthma Education and Prevention Program, National Heart, Lung, and Blood Institute, Expert Panel Report 2: *Guidelines for the diagnosis and management of asthma.* Washington, DC, NIH Pub No 97-4051, July 1997.

BASIC INFORMATION

DEFINITION

Atrial fibrillation is totally chaotic atrial activity caused by simultaneous discharge of multiple atrial foci.

SYNONYMS

AF
A-fib

ICD-9CM CODES

427.31 Atrial fibrillation

EPIDEMIOLOGY & DEMOGRAPHICS

The prevalence of atrial fibrillation increases with age, from 2% in the general population to 5% in patients older than 60 yr, and 9% of those aged 80 years or older.

PHYSICAL FINDINGS & CLINICAL PRESENTATION

Clinical presentation is variable:
- Asymptomatic patients
- Most common complaint: palpitations
- Fatigue, dizziness, light-headedness in some patients
- CHF
- Cardiac auscultation revealing irregularly irregular rhythm

ETIOLOGY

- Coronary artery disease
- MS, MR, AS, AR
- Thyrotoxicosis
- Pulmonary embolism, COPD
- Pericarditis
- Myocarditis, cardiomyopathy
- Tachycardia-bradycardia syndrome
- Alcohol abuse
- MI
- WPW syndrome
- Other causes: left atrial myxoma, atrial septal defect, carbon monoxide poisoning, pheochromocytoma, idiopathic hypoxia, hypokalemia, sepsis, pneumonia

DIAGNOSIS

DIFFERENTIAL DIAGNOSIS

- Multifocal atrial tachycardia
- Atrial flutter
- Frequent atrial premature beats

WORKUP

New-onset atrial fibrillation: ECG, echocardiogram, Holter monitor (selected patients), and laboratory evaluation

LABORATORY TESTS

- TSH
- CBC, glu, creatinine, sodium, potassium, ALT, alkaline, phosphatase, calcium

IMAGING STUDIES

- ECG
  1. Irregular, nonperiodic wave forms (best seen in V1) reflecting continuous atrial reentry
  2. Absence of P waves
  3. Conducted QRS complexes showing no periodicity
- Echocardiography to evaluate left atrial size and detect valvular disorders in all patients
- Holter monitor: useful only in selected patients to evaluate paroxysmal atrial fibrillation

TREATMENT

NONPHARMACOLOGIC THERAPY

- Avoidance of alcohol in patients with suspected excessive alcohol use
- Avoidance of caffeine and nicotine

ACUTE GENERAL Rx

- New-onset atrial fibrillation:
  1. If the patient is hemodynamically unstable, emergency synchronized cardioversion may be required following immediate conscious sedation with a rapid short-acting sedative (e.g., midazolam).
     - Cardioversion is indicated if the ventricular rate is >140 bpm and the patient is symptomatic (particularly in acute MI, chest pain, dyspnea, CHF) or when there is no conversion to normal sinus rhythm after 3 days of pharmacologic therapy. The likelihood of cardioversion-related clinical thromboembolism is low in patients with atrial fibrillation lasting <48 hr. Patients with atrial fibrillation lasting >2 days have a 5% to 7% risk of clinical thromboembolism if cardioversion is not preceded by several weeks of warfarin therapy. However, if transesophageal echocardiography reveals no atrial thrombus, cardioversion may be performed safely after only a short period of anticoagulant therapy. Anticoagulant therapy should be continued for at least 1 mo after cardioversion to minimize the incidence of adverse thromboembolic events following conversion from atrial fibrillation to sinus rhythm.
  2. If the patient is hemodynamically stable, treatment options include the following in a hospital setting:
     - Diltiazem 0.25 mg/kg given over 2 min followed by a second dose of 0.35 mg/kg 15 min later if the rate is not slowed. May then fol-

low with intravenous infusion 10 mg/hr (range 5-15 mg/hr). Onset of action following IV administration is usually within 3 min, with peak effect most often occurring within 10 min. After the ventricular rate is slowed, the patient can be changed to oral diltiazem 60 to 90 mg q6h.
- Verapamil 2.5 to 5 mg IV initially, then 5 to 10 mg IV 10 min later if the rate is still not slowed. After the ventricular rate is slowed, the patient can be changed to oral verapamil 80 to 120 mg q6-8h.
- Esmolol, metoprolol, atenolol are β-blockers that are available in IV preparations that can be used in atrial fibrillation.
- Other medications useful for converting atrial fibrillation to sinus rhythm are ibutilide, flecainide, propafenone, disopyramide, amiodarone, and quinidine.
- Digoxin is not a very potent AV nodal blocking agent and cannot be relied on for acute control of the ventricular response. When used, give 0.5 mg IV loading dose (slow), then 0.25 mg IV 6 hours later. A third dose may be needed after 6 to 8 h; daily dose varies from 0.125 to 0.25 mg (decrease dosage in patients with renal insufficiency and elderly patients). Digoxin should be avoided in WPW patients with atrial fibrillation. Procainamide is the preferred pharmacologic agent in these patients.
- Loop diuretics and oxygen are used for CHF.
- If the patient is asymptomatic or if the only symptom is palpitation or mild CHF, treatment may be initiated on an outpatient basis with any of the above medications given orally.
- IV heparin or SC low-molecular-weight heparin for hospitalized patients; sometimes omitted for outpatients.
- Anticoagulate with warfarin (unless patient has specific contraindications).
- Long-term anticoagulation with warfarin (adjusted to maintain an INR of 2 to 3) is indicated in all patients with atrial fibrillation; however, the safety of long-term anticoagulation with warfarin in the long-term care setting is not established and should therefore be individualized to the patient and nursing home.
- Aspirin 325 mg/day may be a suitable alternative to warfarin in patients >70 yr with increased risk of bleeding. The efficacy of clopidogrel (Plavix) is not known.

- Medical cardioversion:
  1. Attempts at medical (pharmacologic) intervention should be considered only after proper anticoagulation because cardioversion can lead to systemic emboli. Following successful cardioversion, anticoagulation with warfarin should be continued for 4 wk.
  2. Useful agents for medical cardioversion are quinidine, flecainide, propafenone, amiodarone, ibutilide, sotalol, dofetilide, and procainamide.
  3. Amiodarone appears to be the most effective agent for converting to sinus rhythm in patients who do not respond to other agents. Amiodarone therapy should be considered for patients with recent atrial fibrillation and structural heart disease, particularly those with left ventricular dysfunction. Amiodarone should also be considered for patients with refractory conditions who do not have heart disease, before therapies with irreversible effects such as AV nodal ablation are attempted.

CHRONIC Rx

- Anticoagulation with warfarin (see "Acute General Rx")
- Rate control with digoxin, verapamil, diltiazem, or β-blockers

DISPOSITION

Factors associated with maintenance of sinus rhythm following cardioversion:
- Left atrium diameter <60 mm
- Absence of mitral valve disease
- Short duration of atrial fibrillation

REFERRAL

- Catheter-based radiofrequency ablation procedures designed to eliminate atrial fibrillation represent newer approaches to atrial fibrillation.
- Implantable pacemakers and defibrillators that combine pacing and cardioversion therapies to both prevent and treat atrial defibrillation are likely to have an increasing role in the future management of atrial fibrillation.

PEARLS & CONSIDERATIONS   (!)

COMMENTS

The American Academy of Family Physicians and the American College of Physicians provide the following recommendations for the management of newly detected atrial fibrillation:

1. Rate control with chronic anticoagulation is the recommended strategy for the majority of patients with atrial fibrillation. Rhythm control has not been shown to be superior to rate control (with chronic anticoagulation) in reducing morbidity and mortality and may be inferior in some patient subgroups to rate control. Rhythm control is appropriate when based on other special considerations, such as patient symptoms, exercise tolerance, and patient preference.
2. Patients with atrial fibrillation should receive chronic anticoagulation with adjusted-dose warfarin, unless they are at low risk of stroke or have a specific contraindication to the use of warfarin (thrombocytopenia, recent trauma or surgery, alcoholism).
3. For patients with atrial fibrillation, the following drugs are recommended for their demonstrated efficacy in rate control during exercise and while at rest: atenolol, metoprolol, diltiazem, and verapamil (drugs listed alphabetically by class). Digoxin is only effective for rate control at rest and therefore should only be used as a second line agent for rate control in atrial fibrillation.
4. For those patients who elect to undergo acute cardioversion to achieve sinus rhythm in atrial fibrillation, both direct-current cardioversion and pharmacologic conversion are appropriate options.
5. Both transesophageal echocardiography with short-term prior anticoagulation followed by early acute cardioversion (in absence of intracardiac thrombus) with postcardioversion anticoagulation and delayed cardioversion with pre- and postanticoagulation are appropriate management strategies for those patients who elect to undergo cardioversion.
6. Most patients converted to sinus rhythm from atrial fibrillation should not be placed on rhythm maintenance therapy because the risks outweigh the benefits. In a selected group of patients whose quality of life is compromised by atrial fibrillation, the recommended pharmacologic agents for rhythm maintenance are amiodarone, disopyramide, propafenone, and sotalol (drugs listed in alphabetical order). The choice of agent depends on specific risk of side effects based on patient characteristics.

SUGGESTED READINGS

Cooper JM et al: Implantable devices for the treatment of atrial fibrillation, *N Engl J Med* 346:2062, 2002.

Ezekowitz M, Falk RH: The increasing need for anticoagulation therapy to prevent stroke in patients with atrial fibrillation, *Mayo Clin Proc* 79(7):904-913, 2004.

Hart RG: Atrial fibrillation and stroke prevention, *N Engl J Med* 349:1015, 2003.

Hilek E et al: Effect of intensity of oral anticoagulation on stroke severity and mortality in atrial fibrillation, *N Engl J Med* 349:1019, 2003.

Klein AL et al: Use of transesophageal echocardiography to guide cardioversions in patients with atrial fibrillation, *N Engl J Med* 344:1411, 2001.

Petersen P et al: Ximelagran versus warfarin for stroke prevention in patients with nonvalvular atrial fibrillation. SPORTIF II: A dose-guiding, tolerability, and safety study, *J Am Coll Cardiol* 41:1445, 2003.

Snow V et al: Management of newly detected atrial fibrillation: a clinical practice guideline from the American Academy of Family Physicians and the American College of Physicians, *Ann Intern Med* 139:1009-1017, 2003.

AUTHORS: **FRED F. FERRI, M.D.,** with revisions by **TOM J. WACHTEL, M.D.**

BASIC INFORMATION

DEFINITION

Barrett's esophagus occurs when the squamous lining of the lower esophagus is replaced by metaplastic, intestinalized columnar epithelium. The condition is associated with an increased risk of adenocarcinoma of the esophagus.

SYNONYMS

Intestinal metaplasia of the lower esophagus

ICD-9CM CODES
530.85 Barrett's esophagus

EPIDEMIOLOGY & DEMOGRAPHICS

- Male predominance with a 4:1 ratio of men to women
- Mean age of onset is 40 yr with a mean age of diagnosis of 55 to 60 yr
- Occurs more frequently in Caucasians and Hispanics than in African Americans with a ratio of 10-20:1
- Mean prevalence of 5% to 15% in patients undergoing endoscopy for symptoms of GERD

PHYSICAL FINDINGS & CLINICAL PRESENTATION

Symptoms:
- Typically, chronic (>5 yr) heartburn
- May be an incidental finding in patients undergoing endoscopy for indications unrelated to GERD
- Dysphagia for solid food
- Less frequent: chest pain, hematemesis, or melena

Physical findings:
- Nonspecific
- Ranges from epigastric tenderness on palpation to completely normal

ETIOLOGY

- Metaplasia is thought to result from re-epithelialization of esophageal tissue injured secondary to, and in the background of, chronic gastroesophageal reflux (Fig. 1-5).

- Patients with Barrett's tend to have more severe esophageal motility disturbances (decreased lower esophageal sphincter pressure, ineffective peristalsis) and greater esophageal acid exposure on 24-hour pH monitoring than GERD patients without Barrett's.
- Intraesophageal bile (duodenogastroesophageal) reflux may also play a role in the pathogenesis.
- Familial clustering of GERD and Barrett's suggests a genetic predisposition for the disease.
- The progression from metaplasia to carcinoma is associated with a number of changes in gene structure and expression.

DIAGNOSIS Dx

DIFFERENTIAL DIAGNOSIS

- GERD, uncomplicated
- Erosive esophagitis
- Gastritis
- Peptic ulcer disease
- Angina
- Malignancy
- Stricture or Schatzki's ring

WORKUP

- Endoscopy with biopsy necessary for diagnosis.
- Diagnosis requires the presence of intestinal metaplasia in columnar epithelium displaced proximal to the gastroesophageal junction (see Fig. 1-6). Longer segment Barrett's is more readily diagnosed, but the length of the segment does not define the diagnosis.
- Intestinal metaplasia of the gastric cardia is not considered Barrett's and does not appear to convey the same risk of malignant transformation.
- Imaging studies are nonspecific and insensitive for the diagnosis.
- Screening for *H. pylori* infection in patients with GERD and Barrett's esophagus is not recommended.

TREATMENT Rx

The primary therapeutic goal is to control GERD symptoms and maintain healed mucosa.

NONPHARMACOLOGIC THERAPY

Same as treatment for GERD alone (lifestyle modifications, elevating the head of the bed, avoiding chocolate, tobacco, caffeine, mints, avoiding certain drugs [see Gastroesophageal reflux disease]); however, chronic acid suppression is often necessary to control symptoms and promote healing.

ACUTE GENERAL Rx

- Proton pump inhibitors (PPIs) are most effective at relieving symptoms and healing mucosal injury.
- Adequate control of GERD symptoms in patients with Barrett's esophagus may or may not completely control intraesophageal acid exposure. Some studies have suggested that normalization of intraesophageal acid exposure may lead to either regression of Barrett's or reduce the risk of dysplasia. Large-scale longitudinal studies that would support a general recommendation of aggressive pH control and monitoring have not been performed or reported.
- If asymptomatic and incidentally found to have Barrett's esophagus, medication use may be considered for the above-mentioned reasons.

CHRONIC Rx

- Thermal ablation techniques, photodynamic therapy, and endoscopic mucosal resection have all been suggested as possible approaches in patients with Barrett's and high-grade dysplasia, either in conjunction with aggressive surveillance, or as an alternate to surgery in poor operative candidates. All of these options have significant risks and run the risk of residual intestinal metaplasia.
- Antireflux surgery may be considered for management of GERD and associated sequelae. Surgical resection is offered for multifocal high-grade dysplasia or carcinoma.

SCREENING

- GERD highly prevalent in general population.
- Only 4% to 10% of patients with reflux symptoms develop Barrett's esophagus.
- Patients with chronic GERD symptoms should be considered for a one-time endoscopy to exclude the presence of Barrett's. Because many patients with Barrett's are asymptomatic, some will be missed; however, general population screening is not currently recommended.

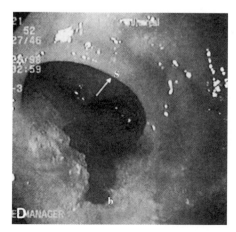

FIGURE 1-5 Endoscopic view of the distal esophagus from a patient with gastroesophageal reflux disease showing a tongue of Barrett's mucosa (*b*) and a Schatzki's ring (*s*) (*arrow*). (From Goldman L, Bennett JC [eds]: *Cecil textbook of medicine,* ed 21, Philadelphia, 2000, WB Saunders.)

DISPOSITION

- Overall, 30 to 50 times increased risk of adenocarcinoma of the esophagus in patients with Barrett's esophagus than in general population
- This risk corresponds to 500 cancers per yr per 100,000 persons with Barrett's esophagus
- Specifics of frequency of monitoring are controversial, no prospective controlled studies to prove that surveillance increases life expectancy
- ACG recommends that patients with Barrett's undergo surveillance endoscopy and systematic 4-quadrant biopsy at intervals determined by the presence and grade of dysplasia. All mucosal abnormalities should be biopsied as well. Patients who have had two endoscopies showing no evidence of dysplasia should have follow-up every 3 years. Patients with low-grade dysplasia should have extensive mucosal sampling, and then follow-up every year. Patients with high-grade dysplasia should have expert confirmation and extensive mucosal sampling. Consideration may be given to intensive surveillance every 3 months for patients with focal high-grade dysplasia. Patients with multifocal high-grade dysplasia or carcinoma should be considered for resection or ablation if not an operative candidate.
- Patients should be treated aggressively for GERD before surveillance.

REFERRAL

- For endoscopy with biopsy in patients with chronic GERD symptomatology who have not had previous endoscopy
- For surveillance in those with a previous biopsy-proven diagnosis of Barrett's esophagus
- For those with high-grade dysplasia, biopsies should be confirmed by an expert pathologist; patients should be offered intensive surveillance or esophageal resection; ablative therapy may be considered either as part of a research protocol, or if not an operative candidate

SUGGESTED READINGS

Bammer T et al: Rationale for surgical therapy of Barrett esophagus, *Mayo Clin Proc* 76:335, 2001.

Cameron A: Management of Barrett's esophagus, *Mayo Clin Proc* 73:5, 1998.

Falk GW: Barret's esophagus, *Gastroenterology* 122:1569, 2002.

Falk GW: Current challenges in Barrett's esophagus, *Cleve Clin J Med* 68:415, 2001.

Hirota WK: Specialized intestinal metaplasia, dysplasia, and cancer of the esophagus: prevalence and clinical date, *Gastroenterology* 116:277, 1999.

Morales TG, Sampliner RE: Barrett's esophagus, *Arch Intern Med* 159:1411, 1999.

Oatu-Lasear R, Fitzgerald RC, Triadafilopoulas G: Differentiation and proliferation in Barrett's esophagus and the effects of acid suppression, *Gastroenterology* 117:327, 1999.

Provenzale D, Schmitt C, Wong JB: Barrett's esophagus: a new look at surveillance based on emerging estimates of cancer risk, *Am J Gastroenterol* 94:2043, 1999.

Rajan E, Burgart LJ, Gostout CJ: Endoscopic and histologic diagnosis of Barrett esophagus, *Mayo Clin Proc* 76:217, 2001.

Samplinear RE and the Practice Parameters Committee of the American College of Gastroenterology: Updated guidelines for the diagnosis, surveillance, and therapy of Barrett's esophagus, *Am J Gastroenterol* 97:1888, 2002.

Shaheen N et al: Gastroesophageal reflux, Barrett esophagus, and esophageal cancer: clinical applications, *JAMA* 287(15):1982, 2002.

Sharma P: Short segment Barrett esophagus and specialized columnar mucosa at the gastroesophageal junction, *Mayo Clin Proc* 76:331, 2001.

Spechler SJ, Barr B: Review article: screening and surveillance of Barrett's esophagus: what is a cost-effective framework? *Aliment Pharmacol Ther* 19(Suppl 1):49, 2004.

Spechler SJ: Barrett's esophagus, *N Engl J Med* 346:836, 2002.

Wang KK, Samplinear RE: Mucosal ablation therapy of Barrett esophagus, *Mayo Clin Proc* 76:433, 2001.

Wijnhoven BPL et al: Molecular biology of Barrett's adenocarcinoma, *Ann Surg* 233:322, 2001.

AUTHOR: **HARLAN G. RICH, M.D.**

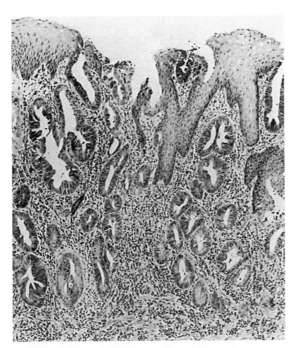

FIGURE 1-6 Epithelial metaplasia (original magnification, x16). The esophageal mucosa consists of columnar epithelium (Barrett's esophagus) intermixed with squamous epithelium. (Photomicrograph courtesy Frank Mitros, M.D., Department of Pathology, University of Iowa. From Stein JH [ed]: *Internal medicine*, ed 5, St Louis, 1998, Mosby.)

BASIC INFORMATION

DEFINITION

Basal cell carcinoma (BCC) is a malignant tumor of the skin arising from basal cells of the lower epidermis and adnexal structures. It may be classified as one of six types (nodular, superficial, pigmented, cystic, sclerosing or morpheaform, and nevoid). The most common type is nodular (21%); the least common is morpheaform (1%); a mixed pattern is present in approximately 40% of cases. Basal cell carcinoma advances by direct expansion and destroys normal tissue.

SYNONYMS

BCC

ICD-9CM CODES
179.9 Basal cell carcinoma, site unspecified
173.3 Basal cell carcinoma, face
173.4 Basal cell carcinoma, neck, scalp
173.5 Basal cell carcinoma, trunk
173.6 Basal cell carcinoma of the limb
173.7 Basal cell carcinoma, lower limb

EPIDEMIOLOGY & DEMOGRAPHICS

- Most common cutaneous neoplasm in humans (>400,000 cases/yr)
- 85% appear on the head and neck region
- Most common site: nose (30%)
- Increased incidence with age >40 yr
- Increased incidence in men
- Risk factors: fair skin, increased sun exposure, use of tanning salons with ultraviolet A or B radiation, history of irradiation (e.g., Hodgkin's disease), personal or family history of skin cancer, impaired immune system

PHYSICAL FINDINGS & CLINICAL PRESENTATION

Variable with the histologic type:
- Nodular: dome-shaped, painless lesion that may become multilobular and frequently ulcerates (rodent ulcer); prominent telangiectatic vessels are noted on the surface; border is translucent, elevated, pearly white (Fig. 1-7);

some nodular basal cell carcinomas may contain pigmentation, giving an appearance similar to a melanoma.
- Superficial: circumscribed scaling black appearance with a thin raised pearly white border; a crust and erosions may be present; occurs most frequently on the trunk and extremities.
- Morpheaform: flat or slightly raised yellowish or white appearance (similar to localized scleroderma); appearance similar to scars, surface has a waxy consistency.

ETIOLOGY

Sun exposure and use of tanning salons with equipment that emits ultraviolet A or B radiation

DIAGNOSIS

DIFFERENTIAL DIAGNOSIS

- Keratoacanthoma
- Melanoma (pigmented basal cell carcinoma)
- Xeroderma pigmentosa
- Basal cell nevus syndrome
- Molluscum contagiosum
- Sebaceous hyperplasia
- Psoriasis

WORKUP

Biopsy to confirm diagnosis

TREATMENT

NONPHARMACOLOGIC THERAPY

Avoidance of excessive tanning, use of sunscreens to prevent damage from excessive sun exposure

ACUTE GENERAL Rx

Variable with tumor size, location, and cell type:
- Excision surgery: preferred method for large tumors with well-defined borders on the legs, cheeks, forehead, and trunk.
- Mohs' micrographic surgery: preferred for lesions in high-risk areas (e.g., nose, eyelid), very large primary tumors, recurrent basal cell carcinomas,

and tumors with poorly defined clinical margins.
- Electrodesiccation and curettage: useful for small (<6 mm) nodular basal cell carcinomas.
- Cryosurgery with liquid nitrogen: useful in basal cell carcinomas of the superficial and nodular types with clearly definable margins; no clear advantages over the other forms of therapy; generally reserved for uncomplicated tumors.
- Radiation therapy: generally used for basal cell carcinomas in areas requiring preservation of normal surrounding tissues for cosmetic reasons (e.g., around lips); also useful in patients who cannot tolerate surgical procedures or for large lesions and surgical failures.
- Photodynamic therapy uses a skin cream (Metvix, known as methyl aminolevulinate cream) and concentrated light to activate the cream, which kills cancer cells. Is used in Europe and Australia but not yet FDA-approved in the U.S.
- Imiquimod (Aldara) 5% cream can be used for treatment of small, superficial BCCs of the trunk and extremities. Efficacy rate is approximately 80%. Its main advantage is lack of scarring, which must be weighed against higher cure rates with surgical intervention.

CHRONIC Rx

Periodic evaluation for at least 5 yr because of increased risk of recurrence of another basal cell carcinoma (>40% risk within 5 yr of treatment)

DISPOSITION

- More than 90% of patients are cured.
- A lesion is considered low risk if it is <1.5 cm in diameter, is nodular or cystic, is not in a difficult-to-treat area (H zone of face), and has not been previously treated.
- Nodular and superficial basal cell carcinomas are the least aggressive.
- Morpheaform lesions have the highest incidence of positive tumor margins (>30%) and the greatest recurrence rate.

AUTHOR: **FRED F. FERRI, M.D.**

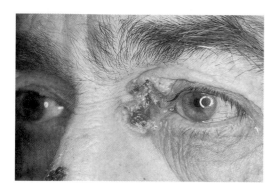

FIGURE 1-7 Basal cell carcinoma. Note rolled translucent border and central ulceration in typical facial location. (From Noble J et al: *Textbook of primary care medicine,* ed 3, St Louis, 2001, Mosby.)

BASIC INFORMATION

DEFINITION

Bell's palsy is an idiopathic, isolated, usually unilateral facial weakness in the distribution of the seventh cranial nerve (<1% of the facial palsies are bilateral)

SYNONYMS

Idiopathic facial paralysis

ICD-9CM CODES
351.0 Bell's palsy

EPIDEMIOLOGY & DEMOGRAPHICS

INCIDENCE: 13-34 cases/100,000 persons
RISK FACTORS:
- Diabetes (present in 5%-10% of patients)
- Travel to area endemic for Lyme disease

PHYSICAL FINDINGS & CLINICAL PRESENTATION

- Unilateral paralysis of the upper and lower facial muscles (asymmetric eye closure, brow, and smile). Upward rolling of eye on attempted eye closure ("Bell's phenomenon")
- Ipsilateral loss of taste
- Ipsilateral ear pain, usually 2-3 days before presentation
- Increased or decreased unilateral eye tearing
- Hyperacusis
- Subjective ipsilateral facial numbness
- In about 8% of cases, other cranial neuropathies may occur

ETIOLOGY

- Most cases are idiopathic.
- The cause is often viral (herpes simplex).
- Herpes zoster can cause Bell's palsy in association with herpetic blisters affecting the outer ear canal or the area behind the ear (Ramsay-Hunt syndrome).
- Bell's palsy can also be one of the manifestations of Lyme disease.

DIAGNOSIS

DIFFERENTIAL DIAGNOSIS

- Neoplasms affecting the base of the skull or the parotid gland
- Bacterial infectious process (meningitis, otitis media, osteomyelitis of the base of the skull)
- Brainstem stroke
- Multiple sclerosis
- Sarcoidosis
- Head trauma with fracture of temporal bone
- Other: Guillain-Barré, carcinomatous or leukemic meningitis, leprosy, Melkersson-Rosenthal syndrome

WORKUP

Bell's palsy is a clinical diagnosis. A focused history and neurologic examination will confirm the diagnosis.

LABORATORY TESTS

- Fasting blood sugar to evaluate for diabetes
- Consider CBC, VDRL, ESR, ACE in selected patients
- Lyme titer in endemic areas

IMAGING STUDIES

- Contrast-enhanced MRI to exclude neoplasms is indicated only in patients with atypical features or course.
- Chest x-ray examination may be useful to exclude sarcoidosis or to rule out TB in selected patients before treating with steroids.

TREATMENT

NONPHARMACOLOGIC THERAPY

- Reassure patient that the disease is most likely a result of a virus attacking the nerve, not a stroke. It is also important to inform the patient that the prognosis is usually good.
- Avoid corneal drying by applying skin tape to the upper lid to keep the palpebral fissure narrowed. Lacri-Lube ophthalmic ointment at night and artificial tears during the day are also useful to prevent excessive drying.

ACUTE GENERAL Rx

- Although the benefits of corticosteroid therapy remain unproven, most practitioners use a brief course of prednisone therapy. Combination therapy with acyclovir and prednisone may possibly be effective in improving clinical recovery.
- If used, prednisone therapy should be started within 24-48 hr of symptom onset.
- Optimal steroid dose is unknown. Prednisone can be given as one 50-mg tablet qd for 7 days without tapering or can be started at 80 mg and tapered by 5 mg/day until finished. A Medrol dose-pack may also be given. A randomized controlled trial of patients treated with high dose IV steroids within 72 hr compared with placebo found a significant improvement in recovery rate and time to return to work but no statistical difference in final outcome.
- There is preliminary evidence for the effectiveness of methylcobalamin (active form of vitamin B_{12}) and hyperbaric oxygen, but these have not yet received widespread acceptance.
- Botulinum toxin may be helpful for the treatment of synkinesis and hemifacial spasm, two of the late sequelae of Bell's palsy.
- Treat Lyme disease if present

CHRONIC Rx

Patients should be monitored for evidence of corneal abrasion and ulceration or hemifacial spasm. Physical therapy including moist heat and massage may be beneficial.

DISPOSITION

- 71% of patients should recover completely. Prognosis is improved for those with clinical improvement within 3 wk and with less severity of symptoms at onset.
- Recovery begins within 3 wk in 85% of patients, with the remainder having some improvement within 3-6 mo.
- Recurrence is experienced in 5% of Bell's palsy cases.

REFERRAL

- Persistent redness or irritation of the eye requires referral to an ophthalmologist.
- Neurology referral is recommended if diagnosis is unclear or if the clinical course is atypical.

SUGGESTED READINGS

Benatar M, Edlow JA: The spectrum of cranial neuropathy in patients with Bell's palsy, *Arch Intern Med* 164:2283, 2004.

Grogan PM: Practice parameter: steroids, acyclovir, and surgery for Bell's palsy (an evidence-based review): report of the Quality Standards Subcommittee of the American Academy of Neurology, *Neurology* 56(7): 830, 2001.

Holland NJ, Weiner GM: Recent developments in Bell's palsy, *Br J Med* 329:553, 2004.

Jabor MA, Gianoli G: Management of Bell's palsy, *J La State Med Soc* 148:279, 1996.

Lagalla G et al: Influence of early high-dose steroid treatment on Bell's palsy evolution, *Neurol Sci* 23:107, 2002.

Mountain RE et al: The Edinburgh facial palsy clinic: a review of three years' activity, *J R Coll Surg Edinb* 39:275, 1994.

Peitersen E: The natural history of Bell's palsy, *Am J Otol* 4:107, 1982.

AUTHOR: **RICHARD S. ISAACSON, M.D.**

BASIC INFORMATION

DEFINITION

Benign prostatic hyperplasia is the benign growth of the prostate, generally originating in the periureteral and transition zones, with subsequent irritative and obstructive voiding symptoms.

SYNONYMS

BPH
Prostatic hypertrophy

ICD-9CM CODES

600 Benign prostatic hyperplasia

EPIDEMIOLOGY & DEMOGRAPHICS

- 80% of men have evidence of benign prostatic hypertrophy by age 80 yr.
- Medical and surgical intervention for problems caused by BPH is required in >20% of males by age 75 yr.
- Transurethral resection of the prostate (TURP) is the tenth most common operative procedure (>400,000/yr in U.S.).
- 10% to 30% of men with BPH have occult prostate cancer.

PHYSICAL FINDINGS & CLINICAL PRESENTATION

- Irritative symptoms are usually the first to manifest. The hallmark is urgency; the patient has progressively less time between the first sensation of bladder fullness and an irresistible urge to void. "When I have to go, I need to go real fast." These symptoms progress in association with reduced urinary flow, especially in the morning. In time, obstructive symptoms take center stage with difficulty initiating flow (hesitancy), dribbling during micturition, incomplete emptying of the bladder resulting in double-voiding (need to urinate again a few minutes after voiding), and postvoid dribbling or incontinence. Eventually, obstructive symptoms can lead to urinary retention.
- Digital rectal examination (DRE) reveals enlargement of the prostate.
- Focal enlargement may be indicative of malignancy.
- Correlation between size of prostate and symptoms is poor (BPH may be asymptomatic if it does not encroach on the urethral lumen).

ETIOLOGY

Multifactorial; a functioning testicle is necessary for development of BPH (as evidenced by the absence of BPH in males who were castrated before puberty).

DIAGNOSIS

Dx

DIFFERENTIAL DIAGNOSIS

- Prostatitis
- Prostate cancer
- Strictures (urethral)
- Medication interfering with the muscle fibers in the prostate and also with bladder function

WORKUP

Symptom assessment as described previously (may use American Urological Association [AUA] or Symptom Index for BPH [Table 1-1]), laboratory tests, and imaging studies

LABORATORY TESTS

- Prostate-specific antigen (PSA) to screen for prostate cancer: protease secreted by epithelial cells of the prostate; elevated in 30% to 50% of patients with BPH; also increases with

TABLE 1-1	International Prostate Symptom Score (I-PSS)						

SCORE

Symptom	Not at All	Less than 1 Time in 5	Less than Half the Time	About Half the Time	More than Half the Time	Almost Always	Total Score
Incomplete emptying: Over the past month, how often have you had a sensation of not emptying your bladder completely after you finished urinating?	0	1	2	3	4	5	
Frequency: Over the past month, how often have you had to urinate again <2 hr after you finished urinating?	0	1	2	3	4	5	
Intermittency: Over the past month, how often have you found you stopped and started again several times when you urinated?	0	1	2	3	4	5	
Urgency: Over the past month, how often have you found it difficult to postpone urination?	0	1	2	3	4	5	
Weak stream: Over the past month, how often have you had a weak urinary stream?	0	1	2	3	4	5	
Straining: Over the past month, how often have you had to push or strain to begin urination?	0	1	2	3	4	5	
	None	1 Time	2 Times	3 Times	4 Times	5 or More Times	
Nocturia: Over the past month, how many times did you most typically get up to urinate from the time you went to bed at night until the time you got up in the morning?	0	1	2	3	4	5	

Total I-PSS score =

age independent of prostate size. Therefore, the PSA test does not discriminate well between patients with BPH and those with prostate cancer, particularly if the cancers are pathologically localized and curable. Nonetheless, testing for PSA increases detection rate for prostate cancer and tends to detect cancer at an earlier stage. PSA testing and digital rectal examination should be offered to any asymptomatic man older than 50 years of age with a life expectancy of 10 years. PSA testing can also be offered at an earlier age in men at higher risk of prostatic cancer (e.g., first-degree relatives with prostate cancer; black men).

- Measurement of "free" PSA is useful to assess the probability of prostate cancer in patients with normal digital rectal examination and total PSA between 4 and 10 ng/ml. In these patients the global risk of prostate cancer is 25%; however, if the free PSA is >25%, the risk of prostate cancer decreases to 8%, whereas if the free PSA is <10%, the risk of cancer increases to 56%. Another approach is to measure "PSA velocity." Repeat PSA measurements are obtained every 3 months to assess the rate of increase. PSA should increase by less than 0.85 ng/ml per year and should take at least 4 years to double.
- Urinalysis, urine C&S to rule out infection (if suspected).
- BUN and creatinine to rule out postrenal insufficiency.

IMAGING STUDIES

- Transrectal ultrasound may be indicated in patients with palpable nodules or significant elevation of PSA. It is also useful to estimate prostate size.
- Uroflowmetry may be used to determine relative impact of obstruction on urine flow (not routine).
- Pressure flow studies, although invasive, are useful in occasional patients for whom a distinction between prostatic obstruction and impaired detrusor contractility may affect the choice of therapy.
- Postvoid residual (PVR) urine measurement may identify patients who should not receive anticholinergic drugs (PVR >100 ml).
- Cystoscopy is an option during later evaluation if invasive treatment is being planned.

TREATMENT

NONPHARMACOLOGIC THERAPY

- Avoidance of caffeine or any other foods that may exacerbate symptoms.
- Avoidance of medications that may exacerbate symptoms (e.g., most cold and allergy remedies). Indeed, anticholinergic drugs (e.g., antihistamines) decrease detrusor contractility, and sympathomimetics (e.g., decongestants) increase bladder outlet pressure. They are relatively contraindicated in anyone with a PVR >100 cc.
- The dietary supplement saw palmetto is effective in relieving BPH symptoms in some patients with mild obstruction.

GENERAL Rx

- Asymptomatic patients with prostate enlargement caused by BPH generally do not require treatment. Patients with mild to moderate symptoms are candidates for pharmacologic treatment (see as follows).

MEDICAL TREATMENT

- α-1 blockers (e.g., tamsulosin, alfuzosin, doxazosin, prazosin, and terazosin) relax smooth muscle of the bladder neck and prostate and can increase urinary flow rate. They have no effect on the size of the prostate. α-1 blockers are useful in symptomatic patients to relieve symptoms of obstruction by causing relaxation of smooth muscle tone in the prostatic capsule and urethra and bladder neck. Tamsulosin and alfuzosin are more specific to bladder α-1 receptors and do not cause much hypotension. Prazosin, doxazosin, and terazosin are nonspecific α-1 blockers and are used to treat hypertension; they can cause (postural) hypotension. α-1 blockers are the most effective medical pharmacologic therapy for BPH-associated lower urinary tract symptoms.
- Hormonal manipulation with finasteride (Proscar) 5 mg qd or dutasteride (Avodart) 0.5 mg qd. Both are 5 α-reductase inhibitors that block conversion of testosterone to dihydrotestosterone; they can reduce the size of the prostate. Treatment requires 6 mo or more for maximal effect.

SURGICAL TREATMENT

- TURP is the most commonly used surgical procedure for BPH. Transurethral incision of the prostate (TUIP), a procedure almost equivalent in efficacy, is limited to patients whose estimated resection tissue weight would be 30 g or less. TUIP can be performed in an ambulatory setting or during a 1-day hospitalization. Open prostatectomy is typically performed on patients with very large prostates. Surgery may result in significant complications (e.g., incontinence, infection).
- Laser therapy for BPH is a less invasive alternative to TURP; however, TURP is moderately more effective than laser therapy in relieving symptoms of BPH.
- Balloon dilation of the prostatic urethra is less effective than surgery for relieving symptoms but is associated with fewer complications. It is a reasonable treatment option for patients with smaller prostates and no middle lobe enlargement.

CHRONIC Rx

- Avoid medications and foods that exacerbate symptoms.
- Symptomatic improvement occurs in >70% of patients with proper treatment.

DISPOSITION

With appropriate therapy, symptoms improve or stabilize in >70% of patients with BPH.

REFERRAL

Urology referral for patients with severe or intolerable symptoms and for any patient suspected of having prostate cancer (10% to 30% of men with BPH)

PEARLS & CONSIDERATIONS

COMMENTS

Emerging technologies for treating BPH include lasers, coils, stents, thermal therapy, and hyperthermia. Laser prostatectomy appears promising; however, long-term effectiveness has not yet been demonstrated.

- The increase in the use of pharmacologic management has resulted in over 30% reduction in the total number of transurethral resections of the prostate.
- Caution: 5 α-reductase inhibitors cut PSA levels in half. Therefore, the PSA should be doubled to interpret the result in a patient using such treatment.

SUGGESTED READINGS

Dull P et al: Managing benign prostatic hyperplasia, *Am Fam Physician* 66:77, 2002.

AUTHORS: **FRED F. FERRI, M.D.,** and **TOM J. WACHTEL, M.D.**

BASIC INFORMATION

DEFINITION

Bladder cancer is a heterogeneous spectrum of neoplasms ranging from non–life-threatening, low-grade, superficial papillary lesions to high-grade invasive tumors, which often have metastasized at the time of presentation. It is a field change disease in which the entire urothelium from the renal pelvis to the urethra may be susceptible to malignant transformation. *Types:* Transitional cell carcinoma (TCCa), squamous cell carcinoma, and adenocarcinoma.

ICD-9CM CODES
Primary: 188.9
Secondary: 198.1
CIS: 233.7
Benign: 223.3
Uncertain behavior: 236.7
Unspecified: 239.4

EPIDEMIOLOGY & DEMOGRAPHICS

Each year approximately 54,000 new cases are diagnosed and more than 12,000 deaths are attributed to bladder cancer.

Until 1990, the incidence of bladder cancer in the U.S. was rising. Since 1990, the incidence of bladder cancer is decreasing at a rate of 0.8% per year (1.2% among men and 0.4% among women).

PREDOMINANT SEX: In males, it is the fourth most common cancer; it accounts for 10% of all cancers. In females, it is the eighth most common cancer; it accounts for 4% of all cancers.

RISK: The lifetime risk of developing bladder cancer is 2.8% in white males, 0.9% in black males, 1% in white females, and 0.6% in black females.
Smoking:
- Users of "black" tobacco in place of "blond" tobacco have a twofold to threefold increase in developing bladder cancer.
- Smoking risk is based on consumption:

With a twofold to threefold increase for subjects smoking at least 10 cigarettes per day
The risk increases again when the daily consumption rises above 40-60 cigarettes per day
- Smokers of low-tar and nicotine cigarettes have a lower risk when compared with higher tar and nicotine cigarettes.
- Unfiltered cigarettes have a 50% increased risk of bladder cancer compared with those who smoke filtered cigarettes.
- Pipe smokers have a lower risk of bladder cancer compared with cigarette smokers.

- Cigar smoking, snuff, and chewing tobacco, although implicated in nonurologic cancers, are not believed to influence bladder cancer risk.
Diet:
- Diets rich in beef, pork, and animal fat consumption increase risk of bladder cancer.
- There is no indication that consumption of nonbeer alcoholic drinks contributes to bladder cancer development.
- Beer consumption has been linked to bladder cancer development as a result of the presence of nitrosamines in the beer. Similarly, these nitrosamines have been implicated in the development of rectal cancer.
- Drinking coffee is not believed to contribute to bladder cancer risk. There is additional evidence that coffee consumption is protective for colorectal cancers, possibly by diminishing fecal transit time.

PEAK INCIDENCE: Incidence increases with age, high >60 yr, uncommon <40 yr.

GENETICS: It is thought to be multifactorial in etiology, involving both genetic and environmental interactions. Overall, it is estimated that approximately 20% to 25% of the male population in the U.S. with bladder cancer has the disease as a result of occupational exposure.

DISTRIBUTION: In North America, transitional cell carcinomas comprise 93%, squamous cell carcinomas comprise 6%, and adenocarcinomas account for 1% of bladder cancers.

PATHOGENESIS: Two pathways exist for bladder cancer (TCCa):
1. Papillary superficial disease occasionally leading to invasive cancer (75%)
2. Carcinoma-in-situ (CIS) and solid invasive cancer with high risk of disease progression (25%)

Two distinct forms of "Superficial Cancer" exist:
T_a Papillary low-grade tumor. High rate of recurrence. Disease progression occurs 5%
T_1 Higher-grade papillary tumors that infiltrate the lamina propria. Often associated with flat CIS that may involve the urothelium diffusely. Disease progression occurs between 30% and 50%
Subdivided into:
T_{1a} Penetration of tumor up to the muscularis mucosae. Disease progression 5.3%
T_{1b} Penetration of tumor through the muscularis mucosae. Disease progression 53%
Flat CIS:
Entirely different and separate pathway of cancer development whose mechanism is manifested by dyspla-

sia, which leads to the occurrence of poorly differentiated malignant cells that replace or undermine the normal urothelium and extend along the plane of the bladder wall. It penetrates the basement membrane and lamina propria in 20% to 30% of the cases and is associated with the development of solid tumor growth. A defect in chromosome 17p53 occurs in 50% of the cases.

At presentation, 72% of cancers are localized to the bladder, 20% of the cancers extend to the regional lymph nodes, and 3% present with distant metastases. 80% of superficial TCCa recur with up to 30% progressing to a higher stage or grade. Younger patients most commonly develop low-grade papillary noninvasive TCCa and are less likely to have recurrences when compared with older patients with similar lesions. Involvement of the upper tracts with tumor occurs in 25% to 50% of the cases.

STAGING (BASED ON THE TNM SYSTEM):

T_0 No tumor in specimen
T_{is} CIS
T_a Papillary TCCa noninvasive
T_1 Papillary TCCa into lamina propria
T_2 TCCa invasive of superficial ms
T_{3a} Invasive of deep ms
T_{3b} Invasive of perivesical fat
T_{4a} Invasive of adjacent pelvic organ
T_{4b} Invasive of pelvic wall with fixation
Invasive of nodal status:
N_0 No nodal involvement
N_{1-3} Pelvic nodes
N_4 Nodes above bifurcation
N_x Unknown
Invasive of metastatic status:
M_0 No distant metastases
M_1 Distant metastases
M_x Unknown

MOLECULAR EPIDEMIOLOGY: TCCa is usually a field change disease with tumors arising at different times and sites in the urothelium, suggesting a polyclonal etiology of bladder cancer. Bladder cancers have been associated with abnormalities on chromosomes 1, 4, 11, 5, 7, 3, 9, 21, 18, 13, 8; with alterations in suppressor genes P53, retinoblastoma gene, and P16; and with alterations in oncogenes H-ras and epidermal growth factor receptor.

PHYSICAL FINDINGS

- Gross painless hematuria
- Microhematuria
- Frequency, urgency, occasional dysuria

With locally invasive to distant metastatic disease, the presentation can include:
- Abdominal pain
- Flank pain

- Lymphedema
- Renal failure
- Anorexia
- Bone pain

ETIOLOGY

Bladder cancer is a potentially preventable disease associated with specific etiologic factors:

- Cigarette smoking is associated with 25% to 65% of the cases. The risk of developing a TCCa is 2 to 4 times higher in smokers than in nonsmokers, and that risk persists for many years, being equal to nonsmokers only after 12 to 15 yr of smoking abstinence. Smoking tobacco is associated with tumors that are characterized by higher histologic grade, increased tumor stage, increase in the numbers of tumors present, and increased tumor size.
- Occupational exposures: dye workers, textile workers, tire and rubber workers, petroleum workers
- Chemical exposure: O-toluidine, 2-naphthylamine, benzidine, 4-aminobiphenyl, and nitrosamines
- Exposure to HPV type 16

Squamous carcinomas are associated with:

- Schistosomiasis
- Urinary calculi
- Indwelling catheters
- Bladder diverticula

Miscellaneous causes:

- Phenacetin abuse
- Cyclophosphamide
- Pelvic irradiation
- Tuberculosis

Adenocarcinomas are associated with:

- Exstrophy
- Endometriosis
- Neurogenic bladder
- Urachal abnormalities
- As a secondary site for distant metastases from other organs (i.e., colon cancer)

DIAGNOSIS

- History and physical examination
- Urinalysis
- Cystoscopy with bladder barbotage and biopsy
- Transurethral resection of bladder tumor(s)
- There is insufficient evidence to determine whether a decrease in mortality from bladder cancer occurs with hematuria testing, urinary cytology, or a variety of other tests on exfoliated urinary cells or other substances.
- In addition to urinary cytologies and bladder barbotage, BTA, NMP22, and Fibrin Degradation Products (FDP) have been approved by the FDA as bladder cancer tumor markers. No marker has general, widespread acceptance because the results are affected by the presence of stents, recent urologic manipulation, stones, infection, bowel interposition, and prostatitis creating false-positive results.

DIFFERENTIAL DIAGNOSIS

- Urinary tract infection
- Frequency-urgency syndrome
- Interstitial cystitis
- Stone disease
- Endometriosis
- Neurogenic bladder

LABORATORY TESTS

RADIOLOGIC TESTS:

- IVP, renal ultrasound, retrograde pyelography, CT scan, and MRI.
- One or a combination of studies can be used. In the absence of skeletal symptoms, bone scan is not recommended.

TREATMENT

NONPHARMACOLOGIC THERAPY

- Initially, transurethral resection of bladder tumor (TURBT)
- Loop biopsy of the prostatic urethra if high-grade TCCa is suspected
- If superficial disease, follow-up protocol with repeat TURBT and/or the use of intravesical agents is recommended
- For advanced bladder cancer, radical cystectomy with urethrectomy (unless orthotopic diversion is planned) and either ileal loop conduit or orthotopic diversion

BLADDER PRESERVATION APPROACHES: Following cystectomy for muscle invasive disease, 50% or more of the patients will develop metastases. Most patients develop metastases at distant sites, a third relapse locally. Bladder preservation management is offered in those individuals who refuse surgery or who might not be suitable radical cystectomy patients. Bladder-sparing protocols include extensive TURBT or partial cystectomy with external beam or interstitial radiotherapy and systemic chemotherapy. Radiotherapy as a single treatment modality is not effective. The best predictor of successful bladder preservation is a complete response following the combination of initial TURBT and two cycles of CMV (cisplatin, methotrexate, vinblastine) chemotherapy seen with stages T2-T3a.

INDICATIONS FOR PARTIAL CYSTECTOMY:

- Tumor within a bladder diverticulum
- Solitary, primary, and muscle-invasive or high-grade lesion of a region of the bladder that allows complete excision with adequate surgical margins
- Inability to adequately resect tumor by TURBT alone because of size or location
- Tumor overlying a ureteral orifice requiring ureteral reimplantation
- Biopsy of a radiation-induced ulceration
- Palliation of severe local symptoms
- Patient refusal of urinary diversion
- Poor-risk patient who is not a diversion candidate

Contraindications:

- Multiple tumors
- CIS
- Cellular atypia on biopsy
- Prostatic invasion
- Invasion of the trigone
- Inability to achieve adequate surgical margins
- Prior radiotherapy
- Inability to maintain adequate bladder volume after resection
- Evidence of extravesical tumor extension
- Poor surgical risk

ACUTE GENERAL Rx

INDICATIONS FOR INTRAVESICAL CHEMOTHERAPY:

- High-grade tumor
- Tumor size >5 cm
- Tumor multiplicity
- Presence of CIS
- Positive urinary cytologies following a resection
- Incomplete tumor resection

Intravesical agents: thiotepa, Adriamycin, mitomycin C, AD-32, BCG, interferon, bropirimine, interleukin-2, and keyhole-limpet hemocyanin. Photodynamic therapy with hematoporphyrin derivatives has also been used.

INDICATIONS FOR CYSTECTOMY:

- Large tumors not amenable to complete TURBT
- High-grade tumor
- Multiple tumors with frequent recurrences
- Diffuse CIS not responsive to intravesical chemotherapy
- Prostatic urethra involvement
- Irritative bladder symptoms with upper tract deterioration
- Muscle-invasive disease
- Disease outside of the bladder

SYSTEMIC CHEMOTHERAPY: Used as neoadjuvant and adjuvant therapy for systemic disease. The most effective agents are cisplatin, methotrexate, vinblastine, Adriamycin (MVAC). Other agents include mitoxantrone, vincristine, etoposide (VP16), 5FU, ifosfamide, Taxol, gemcitabine, piritrexim, and gallium nitrate. Chemotherapy in combination can provide palliation and modest survival benefit.

RADIOTHERAPY: Conflicting reports suggest that superficial bladder cancer is more sensitive to radiotherapy. Squamous changes within the tumor and secretion of human chorionic gonadotropin by the lesion are associated with poor response to radiotherapy. Only 20% to 30% of patients with invasive bladder cancer can be cured by external beam radiation therapy alone. It is used in combination with surgery or with systemic agents to treat bladder cancer primarily in those patients who are not surgical candidates or who refuse surgery.

CHRONIC Rx

FOLLOW-UP RECOMMENDATIONS FOR SUPERFICIAL BLADDER CANCER:
- Cystoscopy, bladder barbotage, and bimanual examination every 3 mo for 2 yr, then every 6 mo for 2 yr, and annually thereafter.

- Upper tract studies are based on the risk of upper tract tumor development, generally every 2 to 5 yr.

FOLLOW-UP RECOMMENDATIONS FOR ADVANCED DISEASE:

Bladder Preservation:
- Cystoscopy, barbotage, bimanual examination, biopsy (when indicated), every 3 mo for 2 yr, then every 6 mo for 2 yr, yearly thereafter.
- CT scan of abdomen and pelvis every 6 mo for 2 yr in addition to chest x-ray examination, liver function testing, and serum creatinine.

Cystectomy with Ileal Loop/Orthotopic Bladder:
- Neobladder endoscopy and IVP yearly.
- CT scan of abdomen and pelvis every 6 mo for 2 yr in addition to chest x-ray examination, liver function tests, and serum creatinine.
- Loopogram every 6 mo for 2 yr, then yearly.

PEARLS & CONSIDERATIONS

COMMENTS
- The most useful prognostic parameters for bladder tumor recurrence and subsequent cancer progression are tumor grade, depth of tumor penetration, multifocal tumors, frequency of recurrence, tumor size, CIS, lymphatic invasion, papillary or solid tumor configuration.
- Box 1-2 describes the American Urological Association Guideline Recommendations for bladder cancer.

SUGGESTED READINGS
Lamm DL et al: Megadose vitamins in bladder cancer: a double-blind clinical trial, *J Urol* 151:21, 1994.

Messing EM: In Walsh PC et al. (eds): *Campbell's urology*, ed 8, Philadelphia, 2002, WB Saunders.

AUTHOR: **PHILIP J. ALIOTTA, M.D., M.S.H.A.**

BOX 1-2 American Urological Association Guideline Recommendations

1. Undiagnosed bladder tumor: obtain a histologic diagnosis of the tumor: Transurethral resection of the tumor is the most common method.
2. Stage Ta or T1 cancer: Complete surgical eradication of all visible tumors. The lesion can be treated with electrocautery resection, fulguration, or laser ablation. Adjuvant intravesical therapy is recommended for patients with carcinoma-in-situ, T1, or high-grade Ta tumors. The agent recommended is BCG or mitomycin C. Cystectomy is an option for this set of tumors because of risk of progression to muscle-invasive disease even after intravesical chemotherapy.
   An increased risk of disease progression is associated with large tumor, high-grade tumor, location of the tumor in a site that is poorly accessible to complete resection, diffuse disease, infiltration of lymphatic or vascular spaces, and prostatic urethral involvement.
3. Carcinoma-in-situ or high-grade T1 cancer and prior intravesical chemotherapy: Cystectomy is the recommendation based on the panel's expert opinion rather than evidence from outcomes data. The data show a substantial risk of progression to muscle-invasive cancer in patients with diffuse carcinoma-in-situ and high-grade T1 tumors. The response to intravesical chemotherapy in terms of altering this disease progression is unknown, and as a result of this, cystectomy is an option for the afflicted patient.

American Urological Association, Guideline Division, 1120 North Charles Street, Baltimore, MD 21201.

BASIC INFORMATION

DEFINITION

The term *breast cancer* refers to invasive carcinoma of the breast, whether ductal or lobular.

SYNONYMS

Carcinoma of the breast

ICD-9CM CODES
174.9 Malignant neoplasm female breast

EPIDEMIOLOGY & DEMOGRAPHICS

- Nearly exclusively the disease of women, with only 1% of breast cancers in males
- Steady increase in its incidence in the U.S., with 205,000 new patients annually
- Annual mortality of 40,000
- Risk steadily increases with age
- Genetically defined group of women with BRCA-1 or BRCA-2 identified to carry lifetime risk as high as 85%

PHYSICAL FINDINGS & CLINICAL PRESENTATION

- Increasing number of small breast cancers found by mammograms
- Patients usually completely free of physical findings
- Palpable tumors possibly as small as 1 cm or even smaller
- Size of the mass and its location measured and documented
- Skin or nipple retraction and skin edema/erythema/ulcer/satellite nodule
- Nodal enlargement in axilla and supraclavicular areas
- Advanced disease: clinical signs of pleural effusion or hepatomegaly
- Rare instances: clear, serous, bloody discharge, or eczematous dermatitis of nipple could be Paget's disease of the breast

ETIOLOGY

- Precise mechanism of carcinogenesis not understood
- Possibly interaction of ovarian estrogen, nonovarian estrogen, estrogens of exogenous origin with breast tissue of varied carcinogenic susceptibility to develop cancer
- Other known or suspected variables: childbearing, breast-feeding practice, diet, physical activities, body mass, alcohol intake
- Have identified families with known high risk

DIAGNOSIS

DIFFERENTIAL DIAGNOSIS

The following nonmalignant breast lesions can simulate breast cancer on both physical and mammogram examinations:
1. Fibrocystic changes
2. Fibroadenoma
3. Hamartoma
4. Mastitis
5. Hematoma
6. Duct ectasia

IMAGING STUDIES

Mammograms: 30% to 50% of breast cancers detected by screening mammograms only as a spiculated mass, a mass with or without microcalcifications, or a cluster of microcalcifications (Fig. 1-8)

WORKUP

- Physical examination:
  1. Mass detected by patient or medical professional: workup required
  2. Negative mammogram: breast cancer not ruled out
  3. Sonogram: to demonstrate mass to be cyst (not common in elderly); usually eliminating need for further workup
- To establish diagnosis:
  1. Positive aspiration cytology on a clinically and mammographically malignant mass—highly accurate but still requires open biopsy confirmation
  2. Stereotactic core needle biopsy diagnosis: reliable with invasive carcinoma identified, but negative or equivocal results require careful evaluation
  3. Atypical hyperplasia or in situ carcinoma found by core needle biopsy: open surgical biopsy confirmation still required
  4. Excisional or incisional biopsy: establishes diagnosis
- Note: Do not rely on negative mammogram or negative aspiration cytology to exclude malignancy. Make appropriate referral. Obtain imaging studies such as bone scan, chest x-ray examination, CT scan of abdomen, or CT scan of liver.

TREATMENT

NONPHARMACOLOGIC THERAPY

- Early breast cancer: primarily surgical or surgical and radiotherapeutic.
- Choice in 60% to 70% of women between modified mastectomy and breast-conserving treatment, which consists of lumpectomy, axillary staging with sentinel node biopsy or axillary dissection, and breast irradiation.
- In elderly women lumpectomy without radiation therapy constitutes adequate primary breast treatment in many cases.

ACUTE GENERAL Rx

- May require adjuvant chemotherapy or endocrine therapy depending on receptor status of cancer cells for estrogen and progesterone
- Evaluation and treatment by medical oncologist

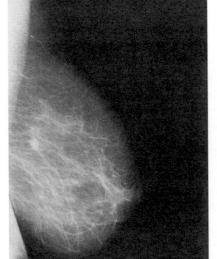
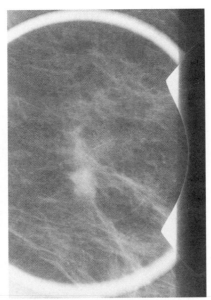

FIGURE 1-8 **A,** Right mediolateral and, **B,** spot magnification view from routine screening mammography demonstrates a small, ill-defined mass with minimal spiculation. This was nonpalpable, and biopsy demonstrated infiltrating ductal carcinoma. (From Specht N [ed]: *Practical guide to diagnostic imaging,* St Louis, 1998, Mosby.)

CHRONIC Rx

Follow-up required after proper treatment of primary breast cancer includes:
1. Periodic clinical evaluations
2. Annual mammograms
3. Other tests as indicated
4. Patient instruction in monthly breast self-examination technique

DISPOSITION

- Prognosis after curative therapy: depends on size of tumor, extent of nodal metastasis, and pathologic grade of tumor
  1. Patient with 1-cm tumor with no axillary node metastasis: 10-yr disease-free survival rate of 90%
  2. Patient with 3-cm tumor with metastasis in four nodes: 10-yr disease-free survival rate of 15% if no systemic adjuvant therapy given
  3. Outlook for most patients between these extremes
- Systemic adjuvant therapy: improves prognosis significantly

REFERRAL

Referral is necessary as soon as breast cancer is even remotely suspected.

PEARLS & CONSIDERATIONS

SCREENING

- Breast self-exam monthly not proven effective but recommended nonetheless.
- Breast exam by physician yearly.
- Screening mammography yearly beginning at age 40, with no specific upper age limit. So long as a woman is a candidate for lumpectomy, she is also a candidate for screening.

Ductal carcinoma in situ (DCIS, intraductal carcinoma):
1. "New" disease mostly found by mammogram as cluster of microcalcification or density
2. Less often, presents as palpable mass or nipple discharge
3. Before mammogram screening, DCIS accounted for 1% of all breast cancers
4. Now, 15% to 20% or even higher proportion present with DCIS
5. Formerly treated with mastectomy, now lumpectomy
6. Cure rates 98% to 99%
7. No axillary dissection required
8. With radiation, breast recurrences reduced
9. Mastectomy possibly required with extensive or high-grade DCIS
10. Systemic adjuvant treatment is not indicated

Inflammatory carcinoma:
1. Rare but rapidly progressive and often lethal form of breast cancer
2. Presents as erythematous and edematous breast resembling mastitis
3. Biopsy required, including skin
4. Treatment with combination chemotherapy followed by surgery and radiation therapy
5. Prognosis once dismal, now 5-yr disease-free survival in 50% of patients

COMMENTS

- Patient education material can be obtained from the following:
  1. SHARE: Self-Help for Women with Breast Cancer, 19 W 44th Street, No. 415, New York, NY 10036-5902.
  2. Y-ME National Organization of Breast Cancer Information and Support, 18220 Harwood Avenue, Homewood, IL 80430.

- Breast radiologic evaluation, evaluation of nipple discharge, and evaluation of palpable mass are described in Section III.

SUGGESTED READINGS

The ATAC Trialists' Group: Anastrozole alone or in combination with tamoxifen versus tamoxifen alone for adjuvant treatment of postmenopausal women with early breast cancer: first results of the ATAC randomized trial, *Lancet* 359:2131, 2002.

Boyd NF et al: Heritability of mammographic density, a risk factor for breast cancer, *N Engl J Med* 347:886, 2002.

Hughes K et al: Post lumpectomy radiation not necessary for all elderly women, *N Engl J Med* 351:971-977, 2004.

Hellekson KL: NIH statement on adjuvant therapy for breast cancer, *Am Fam Physician* 63:1857, 2001.

Humphrey LL et al: Breast cancer screening: a summary of the evidence for the U.S. Preventive Services Task Force, *Ann Intern Med* 137:347, 2002.

Marchbanks PA et al: Oral contraceptives and the risk of breast cancer, *N Engl J Med* 346:2025, 2002.

Miller AB et al: The Canadian National Breast Screening Study—1: breast cancer mortality after 11 to 16 years of follow-up, *Ann Intern Med* 137:305, 2002.

Pruthi S: Detection and evaluation of palpable breast mass, *Mayo Clin Proc* 76:641, 2001.

Rebbeck TR et al: Prophylactic oophorectomy the risk of ovarian and breast cancer in carriers of BRCA1 or BRCA2 mutations, *N Engl J Med* 346:1616, 2002.

U.S. Preventive Services Task Force: Chemoprevention of breast cancer. Recommendations and rationale, *Ann Intern Med* 137:56, 2002.

AUTHORS: **TAKUMA NEMOTO, M.D.,** with revisions by **TOM J. WACHTEL, M.D.**

BASIC INFORMATION

DEFINITION

Bursitis is an inflammation of a bursa and is usually aseptic. A *bursa* is a closed sac lined with a synovial-like membrane that sometimes contains fluid that is found or that develops in an area subject to pressure or friction.

SYNONYMS

Housemaid's knee (prepatellar bursitis)
Weaver's bottom (ischial gluteal bursitis)
Baker's cyst (gastrocnemius-semimembranosus bursa)

ICD-9CM CODES

726.19 Subacromial bursitis
726.33 Olecranon bursitis
726.5 Ischiogluteal bursitis (hip)
726.5 Iliopsoas bursitis (hip)
726.61 Anserine bursitis
726.5 Trochanteric bursitis
726.65 Prepatellar bursitis
727.51 Baker's cyst
726.79 Retrocalcaneal bursitis

PHYSICAL FINDINGS & CLINICAL PRESENTATION

- Swelling, especially if bursa is superficial (olecranon, prepatellar)
- Local tenderness with pain on pressure against bursa
- Pain with joint movement
- Referred pain
- Palpable occasional fibrocartilaginous bodies (most common in olecranon and prepatellar bursae)

ETIOLOGY

- Acute trauma
- Repetitive trauma
- Sepsis
- Crystalline deposit disease
- Rheumatoid arthritis

DIAGNOSIS

DIFFERENTIAL DIAGNOSIS

- Degenerative joint disease
- Tendinitis (sometimes occurs in conjunction with bursitis)
- Cellulitis (if bursitis is septic)
- Infectious arthritis

WORKUP

Aspiration with Gram stain and C&S

IMAGING STUDIES

- Plain radiography to rule out other potential or coexisting bone or joint problems (Fig. 1-9)
- MRI

TREATMENT

NONPHARMACOLOGIC THERAPY

- If chronic, elimination of cause of pressure or irritation
- Use of relief pads, avoidance of direct pressure
- Rest
- Elevation
- Ice for acute trauma

ACUTE GENERAL Rx

- Septic:
  1. Appropriate antibiotic coverage and drainage
  2. Aspiration of purulent fluid with a large-bore needle (if there is no rapid clinical response, incision and drainage are indicated)
- Nonseptic:
  1. Aspiration of blood from acute trauma
  2. Application of compression dressing

CHRONIC Rx

- Aspiration if excessive fluid volume present, followed by application of compression dressing to prevent fluid reaccumulation (repeat aspiration may be required)
- Steroid injection into bursa (1 ml of triamcinolone, 40 mg, mixed with 1 to 3 cc of Xylocaine depending on size of bursa)
- NSAIDs

DISPOSITION

- Many bursal sacs "dry up" eventually.
- Nonsurgical treatment is effective in most cases.

REFERRAL

For orthopedic consultation to assist in treatment of sepsis or for excision of chronic enlarged bursa when indicated

PEARLS & CONSIDERATIONS

COMMENTS

- Injection of trochanteric bursa may require spinal needle in large patient.
- Sterile bursae should not be incised and drained because a chronic draining sinus tract may develop.
- Involvement of the iliopsoas bursa may cause groin pain, although the diagnosis is difficult to make because of the inaccessibility of the area to direct examination. (This also makes steroid injection impossible even if the diagnosis could be established.)

SUGGESTED READINGS

Floemer F, Morrison WB et al: MRI characteristics of olecranon bursitis, *Am J Roentgenol* 183:29, 2004.
Sofka CM, Adler RS: Sonography of cubital bursitis, *Am J Roengenal* 183:51, 2004.
Tortolani PJ, Carbone JJ, Quartaro LG: Greater trochantoric pain syndrome in patients referred to orthopedic spine specialists, *Spine* 2:251, 2002.
Van Mieghem IM, Boets A et al: Ischiogluteal bursitis: an uncommon type of bursitis, *Skeletal Radiol* 33:413, 2004.
Webner D, Drezner JA: Lesser trochanteric bursitis: a rare cause of anterior hip pain, *Clin J Sport Med* 14:242, 2004.

AUTHOR: **LONNIE R. MERCIER, M.D.**

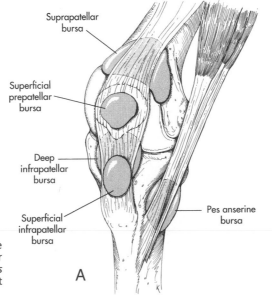

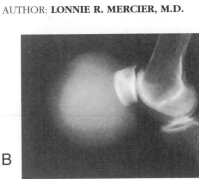

FIGURE 1-9 A, Bursae around the knee. **B,** Markedly swollen prepatellar bursa. (From Scudieri G [ed]: *Sports medicine principles of primary care,* St Louis, 1997, Mosby.)

Suprapatellar bursa

Superficial prepatellar bursa

Deep infrapatellar bursa

Superficial infrapatellar bursa

Pes anserine bursa

A

B

BASIC INFORMATION

DEFINITION

Pes anserinus "goose foot" is the insertion of the conjoined tendons into the antero-medial proximal tibia. From anterior to posterior, pes anserinus is made up of the tendons of the sartorius, gracilis, and semitendinosus muscles.

Anserine bursitis describes inflammation of the pes anserine bursa underlying the conjoined tendons of the gracilis and semitendinosus muscles and separating them from the head of the tibia.

SYNONYMS

Pes anserinus bursitis
Anserine tendinitis

ICD-9CM CODES
726.61

EPIDEMIOLOGY & DEMOGRAPHICS

- Age: common in patients 50 to 80 yr old who suffer from osteoarthritis of the knees
- Sex: incidence also higher among obese, elderly women with or without associated knee osteoarthritis, perhaps because of broader female pelvis and greater angulation of the legs at the knees, placing additional stresses on these structures
- Association with diabetes even after adjusting to weight
- The presence of underlying knee os-teoarthritis should not dissuade clini-cians from diagnosing anserine bursitis as a potential cause for knee pain

PHYSICAL FINDINGS & CLINICAL PRESENTATION

SYMPTOMS

- Pain involves the distal inner knee on ascending or descending stairs.
- Pain (same location) occurs when aris-ing from a seated position or at night. Patients usually do not experience pain with walking on level surfaces.
- Pain may be acute or chronic.
- Intensity of the pain is variable but can be severe, unrelenting, and disabling.
- Symptoms of anserine bursitis may be associated with certain athletic activi-ties such as running, tennis, or breast-stroke swimming.

PHYSICAL FINDINGS

- Hallmark is tenderness over the proxi-mal medial tibia at the insertion of the conjoined tendons of the pes anserinus, approximately 2 to 3 cm below the an-teromedial joint margin of the knee, and no tenderness at the joint line itself unless other conditions are present.
- Local swelling may be noted but the bursa is not palpable unless effusion and thickening are present.

- Palpable crepitus is occasionally ob-served.
- Anserine bursitis occurs more fre-quently on the right side than the left, and one third of patients have bilateral involvement.
- If swelling or tenderness can be pal-pated more proximally along the pes anserinus tendons, tendinitis may be present.

ETIOLOGY

- Anserine bursitis is an inflammatory condition of the medial knee resulting from trauma, overuse, or degenerative processes and often coexists with other knee disorders.
- The sartorius, gracilis, and semitendi-nosus muscles are primary flexors of the knee. These three muscles also pro-tect the knee against rotary and valgus strain. Bursitis may result from stress to this area such as when an obese indi-vidual with anatomic deformity from arthritis ascends or descends stairs.
- Degenerative joint disease (DJD) of the knee is often associated with bursitis. Up to 75% of patients with DJD may have symptoms of anserine bursitis.
- Obesity is associated with anserine bur-sitis, most notably in elderly women.
- Flat feet may predispose patients to anserine bursitis.

DIAGNOSIS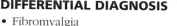

DIFFERENTIAL DIAGNOSIS

- Fibromyalgia
- Hamstring strain
- Medial collateral and lateral collateral ligament injury
- Osteoarthritis of the knee
- Patellofemoral syndrome
- Prepatellar bursitis and inflammation of other knee bursae
- Medial meniscus injury or degenera-tive tear
- Inflammatory arthritis involving the knee
- Sarcomas and other tumors involving the knee structures
- Painful neuropathies

WORKUP

- Usually the diagnosis is based on his-tory and physical exam. Response to treatment (e.g., bursa injection) is also helpful.
- Rarely, bursa aspiration may be indi-cated if infection or crystal-induced in-flammation is suspected. When done, the aspirate should be analyzed for cell count, culture and sensitivity, and crys-tals. In this scenario, it may be appro-priate also to perform a CBC and ESR.

IMAGING STUDIES

- Imaging is rarely indicated.

- X-ray may show osteoarthritis. This finding does not make the diagnosis of anserine bursitis any more or less likely.

TREATMENT

NONPHARMACOLOGIC THERAPY

- Physical therapy
  - Stretching and strengthening of the adductor and quadriceps muscles and stretching of the hamstrings
- Rest but avoid disuse atrophy
- Weight loss if overweight
- Ice massage for 10 minutes three times daily
- Ultrasound therapy
- Cushion between thighs or knee at night if nocturnal pain

PHARMACOLOGIC THERAPY

- Nonsteroidal antiinflammatory drugs are not very effective.
- Topical capsaicin may be applied (use 0.075% strength tid).
- Intrabursal injection of an anesthetic (e.g., 1 to 2 cc lidocaine 1% or 2%) combined with a corticosteroid (e.g., 1 to 2 cc of triamcinolone 20 to 40 mg) using a 22- or 23-gauge needle is ef-fective in confirming the diagnosis (pain relief occurs in less than 5 min-utes if the diagnosis is correct and the medication is injected in the bursa). The injection site is usually the area of maximum tenderness, but it should be located 1 to 2 inches below the an-teromedial proximal end of the tibia to be consistent with the location of the anserine bursa. Some clinicians limit the number of intrabursal steroid in-jections to three or four per year, but this is based on recommendations that apply to intraarticular injection. A suc-cessful injection provides 3 to 4 weeks of symptom relief and may be re-peated when symptoms recur.

REFERRAL

- Referral to orthopedic surgeon in case of medical treatment failure. Surgery for bursectomy or removal of exos-toses is rarely necessary.
- Prognosis remissions and recurrences are common and often parallel the progression of the underlying os-teoarthritis.

SUGGESTED READINGS

Fireman HH: Don't forget anserine bursitis, *CMAJ* 165(10):1300, 2001.
Gnanadesigan N, Smith RL: Knee pain: os-teoarthritis or anserine bursitis? *J Am Med Dir Assoc* 4(3):164-166, 2003.

AUTHOR: **TOM J. WACHTEL, M.D.**

BASIC INFORMATION

DEFINITION

Carpal tunnel syndrome is an entrapment neuropathy involving the median nerve at the wrist (Fig. 1-10). It is the most common entrapment neuropathy in the upper extremity.

ICD-9CM CODES
354.0 Carpal tunnel syndrome

EPIDEMIOLOGY & DEMOGRAPHICS

PREVALENT AGE: Any age (bilateral up to 50%)
PREVALENT SEX: Females are affected two to five times as often as males

PHYSICAL FINDINGS & CLINICAL PRESENTATION

- Nocturnal pain
- Occasional median nerve sensory impairment (often only index and long fingers)
- Positive Tinel's sign at wrist (tapping over the median nerve on the flexor surface of the wrist produces a tingling sensation radiating from the wrist to the hand)
- Positive Phalen's test (reproduction of symptoms after 1 min of gentle, unforced wrist flexion)
- Carpal compression test: Pressure with the examiner's thumb over the patient's carpal tunnel for 30 sec elicits symptoms
- Thenar atrophy in long-standing cases

ETIOLOGY

- Idiopathic in most cases
- Space-occupying lesions in carpal tunnel (tenosynovitis, ganglia, aberrant muscles)
- Job-related mechanical overuse may be a risk factor
- Traumatic injuries to wrist

DIAGNOSIS

DIFFERENTIAL DIAGNOSIS

- Cervical radiculopathy
- Chronic tendinitis
- Vascular occlusion
- Reflex sympathetic dystrophy
- Osteoarthritis
- Other arthritides
- Other entrapment neuropathies

IMAGING STUDIES

Routine roentgenograms may be helpful in establishing cause or ruling out other conditions.

ELECTRODIAGNOSTIC STUDIES

Nerve conduction velocity tests and electromyography are useful in establishing the diagnosis and ruling out other syndromes.

TREATMENT

ACUTE GENERAL Rx

- Elimination of repetitive trauma
- Occupational splints or braces
- NSAIDs
- Injection of carpal canal on ulnar side of palmaris longus tendon at wrist flexor crease (avoiding median nerve)
- Low-dose oral corticosteroids (e.g., prednisolone 20 mg qd for 2 wk, followed by 10 mg qd for 2 more wk) are also effective for symptom relief in selected patients
- Stretching exercises

DISPOSITION

Prognosis is variable. Some cases resolve spontaneously. Relief from local injection appears transient and symptoms recur in the majority of cases following injection.

REFERRAL

Surgical referral in cases of failed medical management or signs of motor weakness. Results of surgery usually excellent with return to full activity in 4-6 weeks.

SUGGESTED READINGS

Dias JJ, Burke FD et al: Carpal tunnel syndrome and work, *J Hand Surg* 29:329, 2004.
Geoghegan JM, Clark DI et al: Risk factors in carpal tunnel syndrome, *J Hand Surg* 29:315, 2004.
Gerritsen AM et al: Splinting vs surgery in the treatment of carpal tunnel syndrome, *JAMA* 288:1245, 2002.
Goodyear-Smith F, Arroll B: What can family physicians offer patients with carpal tunnel syndrome other than surgery? A systematic review of nonsurgical management, *Ann Fam Med* 2:267, 2004.
Hui AC, Wong SM et al: Long-term outcome of carpal tunnel syndrome after conservative treatment, *Int J Clin Pract* 58:337, 2004.
Katz JN, Simmons BP: Carpal tunnel syndrome, *N Engl J Med* 346:1807, 2002.
Lee DH, Claussen GC, Oh S: Clinical nerve conduction and needle electromyography studies, *J Am Acad Orthop Surg* 12:276, 2004.
Shum C et al: The role of flexor tenosynovectomy in the operative treatment of carpal tunnel syndrome, *J Bone Joint Surg* 84(A):221, 2002.
Vjera AJ: Management of carpal tunnel syndrome, *Am Fam Physician* 68:265, 2003.

AUTHOR: **LONNIE R. MERCIER, M.D.**

CARPAL TUNNEL SYNDROME

Median nerve in carpal tunnel

Tapping produces paresthesias (Tinel's sign)

FIGURE 1-10
Distribution of pain and/or paresthesias (dark-shaded area) when the median nerve is compressed by swelling in the wrist (carpal tunnel). (From Arnett FC: Rheumatoid arthritis. In Andreoli TE [ed]: *Cecil essentials of medicine,* ed 4, Philadelphia, 1997, WB Saunders.)

BASIC INFORMATION

DEFINITION

Cataracts are the clouding and opacification of the normally clear crystalline lens of the eye. The opacity may occur in the cortex, the nucleus of the lens, or the posterior subcapsular region, but it is usually in a combination of areas.

SYNONYMS

Congenital cataracts (e.g., from rubella)
Metabolic cataracts (e.g., caused by diabetes)
Collagen vascular disease cataracts (caused by lupus)
Hereditary cataracts
Age-related senile cataracts
Traumatic cataracts
Toxic or drug-induced cataracts (e.g., caused by steroids)

ICD-9CM CODES
366 Cataract

EPIDEMIOLOGY & DEMOGRAPHICS

INCIDENCE (IN U.S.): Highest cause of treatable blindness; cataract removal is the most frequent surgical procedure in patients >65 yr old (1.3 million operations/yr, with an annual cost of approximately $3 billion). By year 2020 expect over 30 million Americans to have cataracts. Of Americans >40, 20.5 million (17.2%) have cataracts. Of these, 5% have had surgery.
PREDOMINANT AGE: Elderly; some stage of cataract development is present in >50% of persons 65 to 74 yr old and 65% of those >75 yr old. Lens clouding begins at 39 to 40 yr old and then usually progresses either slowly or rapidly depending upon individual and health.
GENETICS: Hereditary with such syndromes as homocystinuria, diabetes, myotonic dystrophy

PHYSICAL FINDINGS & CLINICAL PRESENTATION

Cloudiness and opacification of the crystalline lens of the eye (Fig. 1-11)

ETIOLOGY

- Heredity
- Trauma
- Toxins
- Age-related
- Drug-related
- Congenital
- Inflammatory
- Diabetes
- Collagen vascular disease

DIAGNOSIS   **Dx**

DIFFERENTIAL DIAGNOSIS

- Corneal lesions
- Retinal lesions, detached retina, tumors
- Vitreous disease, chronic inflammation

WORKUP

- Complete eye examination, including slit lamp examination, funduscopic examination, and brightness acuity testing
- Complete physical exam for other underlying causes

LABORATORY TESTS

- Fasting glucose
- Consider Collagen vascular and other metabolic diseases in selected cases

TREATMENT   **Rx**

There is no evidence that antioxidants or drugs will slow down or help cataracts.

NONPHARMACOLOGIC THERAPY

- Wait until vision is compromised before doing surgery.
- Surgery is indicated when corrected visual acuity in the affected eye is >20/30 in the absence of other ocular disease; however, surgery may be justified when visual acuity is better in specific situations (especially disabling glare, monocular diplopia). Surgery indicated when vision in one eye is greatly different from other and affects patient's life.

ACUTE GENERAL Rx

None necessary except when acute glaucoma or inflammation occurs.

CHRONIC Rx

- Change glasses as cataracts develop.
- Myopia is common, and glasses can be adjusted until surgery is contemplated.

DISPOSITION

Refer if sight compromised or inflamed red eye.

REFERRAL

Refer to ophthalmologist for evaluation extraction when vision is compromised (see Nonpharmacologic Therapy).

PEARLS & CONSIDERATIONS   **!**

Patients want to know five things about cataracts:
1. chance for vision improvement
2. when will vision improve
3. risk from surgery
4. effect of surgery
5. types of complications

COMMENTS

Success rate with surgery is 95% to 98%.

SUGGESTED READINGS

Congdon N et al: Prevalence of cataract and pseudophakia/aphakia among adults in the US, *Arch Ophthalmol* 122(4)487, 2004.
Consultation section: Cataract surgical problem, *J Cataract Refract Surg* 28:577, 2002.
Solomon R, Donninfeld ED: Recent advances and future frontiers in treating age-related cataracts, *JAMA* 290:248, 2003.
Wong TY et al: Relation of ocular trauma to cortical, nuclear and posterior subcapsular cataracts, *Br J Ophthalmol* 86:152, 2002.

AUTHOR: **MELVYN KOBY, M.D.**

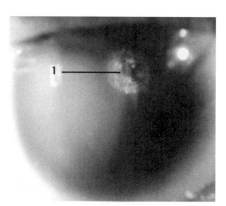

FIGURE 1-11 The central location of a posterior subcapsular cataract *(1).* (From Palay D [ed]: *Ophthalmology for the primary care physician,* St Louis, 1997, Mosby.)

BASIC INFORMATION

DEFINITION

Cellulitis is a superficial inflammatory condition of the skin. It is characterized by erythema, warmth, and tenderness of the area involved.

SYNONYMS

Erysipelas (cellulitis generally secondary to group A β-hemolytic streptococci)

ICD-9CM CODES
682.9 Cellulitis

EPIDEMIOLOGY & DEMOGRAPHICS

- Occurs most frequently in diabetics, immunocompromised hosts, and patients with venous and lymphatic compromise.
- Frequently found near skin breaks (trauma, surgical wounds, ulcerations, tinea infections). Edema, animal or human bites, subadjacent osteomyelitis, and bacteremia are potential sources of cellulitis

PHYSICAL FINDINGS & CLINICAL PRESENTATION

Variable with the causative organism
- Erysipelas: superficial-spreading, warm, erythematous lesion distinguished by its indurated and elevated margin; lymphatic involvement and vesicle formation are common.
- Staphylococcal cellulitis: area involved is erythematous, hot, and swollen; differentiated from erysipelas by nonelevated, poorly demarcated margin; local tenderness and regional adenopathy are common; up to 85% of cases occur on the legs and feet.
- *Vibrio vulnificus:* larger hemorrhagic bullae, cellulitis, lymphadenitis, myositis; often found in critically ill patients in septic shock.

ETIOLOGY

- Group A β-hemolytic streptococci (may follow a streptococcal infection of the upper respiratory tract)
- Staphylococcal cellulitis
- *Vibrio vulnificus:* higher incidence in patients with liver disease (75%) and in immunocompromised hosts (corticosteroid use, diabetes mellitus, leukemia, renal failure)
- *Erysipelothrix rhusiopathiae:* common in people handling poultry, fish, or meat
- *Aeromonas hydrophila:* generally occurring in contaminated open wound in fresh water
- Fungi *(Cryptococcus neoformans):* immunocompromised granulopenic patients

- Gram-negative rods *(Serratia, Enterobacter, Proteus, Pseudomonas):* immunocompromised or granulopenic patients

DIAGNOSIS **Dx**

DIFFERENTIAL DIAGNOSIS

- Angiodema
- Necrotizing fasciitis
- DVT
- Peripheral vascular insufficiency
- Paget's disease of the breast
- Thrombophlebitis
- Acute gout
- Psoriasis
- Candida intertrigo
- Pseudogout
- Osteomyelitis
- Insect bite
- Fixed drug eruption

WORKUP

Physical examination and laboratory evaluation

LABORATORY TESTS

- Gram stain and culture (aerobic and anaerobic)
  1. Aspirated material from:
     a. Advancing edge of cellulitis
     b. Any vesicles
  2. Swab of any drainage material
  3. Punch biopsy (in selected patients)
- Blood cultures in hospitalized patients, in patients who have cellulitis superimposed on lymphedema, in patients with buccal or periorbital cellulitis, and in patients suspected of having a salt-water or fresh-water source of infection. Bacteremia is uncommon in cellulitis (positive blood cultures in only 4% of patients)

Despite the previous measures, the cause of cellulitis remains unidentified in most patients.

IMAGING STUDIES

Radiologic examination is unnecessary in most cases of cellulitis. CT or MRI in patients with suspected necrotizing fasciitis (deep-seated infection of the subcutaneous tissue that results in the progressive destruction of fascia and fat).

TREATMENT **Rx**

NONPHARMACOLOGIC THERAPY

Immobilization and elevation of the involved limb. Cool sterile saline dressings to remove purulence from any open lesion. Support stockings in patients with peripheral edema.

ACUTE GENERAL Rx

Erysipelas
- PO: dicloxacillin 500 mg PO q6h
- IV: cefazolin 1 g q6-8h or nafcillin 1.0 or 1.5 g IV q4-6h

NOTE: Use erythromycin, cephalosporins, clindamycin, or vancomycin in patients allergic to penicillin.

Staphylococcus cellulitis
- PO: dicloxacillin 250 to 500 mg qid
- IV: nafcillin, 1 to 2 g q4-6h
- Cephalosporins (cephalothin, cephalexin, cephradine) also provide adequate antistaphylococcal coverage except for MRSA
- Use vancomycin 1.0-2.0 g IV qd or linezolid 0.6 g IV q12h in patients allergic to penicillin or cephalosporins and in patients with methicillin-resistant *S. aureus* (MRSA). Daptomycin (Cubicin), a cyclic lipopeptide can be used as an alternative to vancomycin for complicated skin and skin structure infections. Usual dose is 4 mg/kg IV given over 30 min every 24 hr. Linezolide (Zyvox) can also be used (400 mg PO bid for 10 days).

Vibrio vulnificus
- Doxycycline 100 mg IV or PO bid +/− third-generation cephalosporin. Ciprofloxacin is an alternative antibiotic
- IV support and admission into ICU (mortality rate >50% in septic shock)

Erysipelothrix
- Penicillin

Aeromonas hydrophila
- Aminoglycosides
- Chloramphenicol
- Complicated skin and skin structure infections in hospitalized patients can be treated with daptomycin (Cubicin) 4 mg/kg IV every 24 hr

DISPOSITION

Prognosis is good with prompt treatment.

REFERRAL

For surgical debridement in addition to antibiotics in patients with suspected necrotizing fasciitis

PEARLS & CONSIDERATIONS

Bilateral distal leg erythema is more likely venous insufficiency and stasis dermatitis than cellulitis.

SUGGESTED READING

Swartz MN: Cellulitis, *N Engl J Med* 350:904, 2004.

AUTHOR: **FRED F. FERRI, M.D.**

BASIC INFORMATION

DEFINITION

Cholelithiasis is the presence of stones in the gallbladder.

SYNONYMS

Gallstones

ICD-9CM CODES
574.2 Calculus of the gallbladder without mention of cholecystitis
574.0 Calculus of the gallbladder with acute cholecystitis

EPIDEMIOLOGY & DEMOGRAPHICS

- Gallstone disease can be found in 20 million Americans. Of these, 2% to 3% (500,000 to 600,000) are treated with cholecystectomies each year.
- Annual medical expenditures for gallbladder surgeries in the U.S. exceed $5 billion.
- Incidence of gallbladder disease increases with age. Highest incidence is in the fifth and sixth decades. Predisposing factors for gallstones are female sex, family history of gallstones, obesity, ileal disease, diabetes mellitus, rapid weight loss, estrogen replacement therapy.
- Patients with gallstones have a 20% chance of developing biliary colic or its complications at the end of a 20-yr period.

PHYSICAL FINDINGS & CLINICAL PRESENTATION

- Physical examination is entirely normal unless patient is having a biliary colic; 80% of gallstones are asymptomatic.
- Typical symptoms of obstruction of the cystic duct include intermittent, severe, cramping pain affecting the RUQ.
- Pain occurs mostly at night and may radiate to the back or right shoulder. It can last from a few minutes to several hours.

ETIOLOGY

- 75% of gallstones contain cholesterol and are usually associated with obesity, female sex, diabetes mellitus; mixed stones are most common (80%), pure cholesterol stones account for only 10% of stones.
- 25% of gallstones are pigment stones (bilirubin, calcium, and variable organic material) associated with hemolysis and cirrhosis. These tend to be black pigment stones that are refractory to medical therapy.
- 50% of mixed-type stones are radiopaque.

DIAGNOSIS

DIFFERENTIAL DIAGNOSIS

- PUD
- GERD
- IBD
- Pancreatitis
- Neoplasms
- Nonulcer dyspepsia
- Functional bowel disease

LABORATORY TESTS

Generally normal unless patient has biliary obstruction (elevated alkaline phosphatase, bilirubin).

IMAGING STUDIES

- Ultrasound of the gallbladder will detect small stones and biliary sludge (sensitivity, 95%; specificity, 90%); the presence of dilated gallbladder with thickened wall is suggestive of acute cholecystitis.
- Nuclear imaging (HIDA scan) can confirm acute cholecystitis (>90% accuracy) if gallbladder does not visualize within 4 hr of injection and the radioisotope is excreted in the common bile duct.

TREATMENT

NONPHARMACOLOGIC THERAPY

Lifestyle changes (avoidance of diets high in polyunsaturated fats, weight loss in obese patients—however, avoid rapid weight loss)

ACUTE GENERAL Rx

- The management of gallstones is affected by the clinical presentation.
- Asymptomatic patients do not require therapeutic intervention.
- Surgical intervention is generally the ideal approach for symptomatic patients. Laparoscopic cholecystectomy is generally preferred over open cholecystectomy because of the shorter recovery period.
- Laparoscopic cholecystectomy after endoscopic sphincterectomy is recommended for patients with common bile duct stones and residual gallbladder stones. Where possible, single-stage laparoscopic treatments with removal of duct stones and cholecystectomy during the same procedure are preferable.
- Patients who are not appropriate candidates for surgery because of coexisting illness or patients who refuse surgery can be treated with oral bile salts: ursodiol (Actigall) 8 to 10 mg/kg/day

in two to three divided doses for 16 to 20 mo, or chenodiol (Chenix) 250 mg bid initially, increasing gradually to a dose of 60 mg/kg/day. Candidates for oral bile salts are patients with cholesterol stones (radiolucent, noncalcified stones), with a diameter of ≤15 mm and having three or fewer stones. Candidates for medical therapy must have a functioning gallbladder and must have absence of calcifications on CT scans.

- Direct solvent dissolution with methyl *tert*-butyl ether (MTBE) can be used in patients with multiple stones with diameter ≥3 cm; this method should be used only by physicians experienced with contact dissolution. Administration of the solvent is either through percutaneous transhepatic placement of a catheter into the gallbladder or endoscopic retrograde catheter placement with subsequent continuous infusion and aspiration of the solvent either manually or by automatic pump system. MTBE is a powerful cholesterol solvent and can dissolve stones in a few hours (>90% dissolution over a 2-hr infusion).
- Extracorporeal shock wave lithotripsy (ESWL) is another form of medical therapy. It can be used in patients with stone diameter of ≤3 cm and having three or fewer stones.

DISPOSITION

- Recurrence rate after bile acid treatment is approximately 50% in 5 yr. Periodic ultrasound is necessary to assess the effectiveness of treatment.
- Gallstones recur after dissolution therapy with MTBE in >40% of patients within 5 yr.
- Following extracorporeal shock wave lithotripsy, stones recur in approximately 20% of patients after 4 yr.
- Patients with at least one gallstone <5 mm in diameter have a greater than fourfold increased risk of presenting with acute biliary pancreatitis. A policy of watchful waiting in such cases is generally unwarranted.
- A potential serious complication of gallstones is acute cholangitis. ERCP and endoscopic sphincterectomy (EC) followed by interval laparoscopic cholecystectomy is effective in acute cholangitis.
- Patients with functional bowel disease and co-existing gall stones may continue to have symptoms after cholecystectomy.

AUTHOR: **FRED F. FERRI, M.D.**

BASIC INFORMATION

DEFINITION

Chronic obstructive pulmonary disease (COPD) is a disorder characterized by the presence of airflow limitation that is not fully reversible. COPD includes emphysema, characterized by loss of lung elasticity and destruction of lung parenchyma with enlargement of air spaces, and chronic bronchitis, characterized by obstruction of small airways and productive cough greater than 3 months' duration for more than 2 successive years. Patients with COPD are classically subdivided in two major groups based on their appearance:

1. *Blue bloaters* are patients with chronic bronchitis; the name is derived from the bluish tinge of the skin (secondary to chronic hypoxemia); chronic cough with production of large amounts of sputum is characteristic.
2. *Pink puffers* are patients with emphysema; they are often cachectic and have pink skin color (adequate oxygen saturation); shortness of breath may be manifested by pursed-lip breathing and use of accessory muscles of respiration.

Both may cause hypercapnia and both often coexist.

SYNONYMS

COPD
Emphysema
Chronic bronchitis

ICD-9CM CODES
496 COPD
492.8 Emphysema

EPIDEMIOLOGY & DEMOGRAPHICS

- COPD affects 16 million Americans and is responsible for >80,000 deaths/yr.
- COPD is the fourth leading cause of death in the U.S. and is expected to become the third leading cause of death by 2020.
- Highest incidence is in males >40 yr.
- 16 million office visits, 500,000 hospitalizations, and >$18 billion in direct health care costs annually can be attributed to COPD.

PHYSICAL FINDINGS & CLINICAL PRESENTATION

- Blue bloaters (chronic bronchitis): peripheral cyanosis, productive cough, tachypnea, tachycardia
- Pink puffers (emphysema): dyspnea, pursed-lip breathing with use of accessory muscles for respiration, decreased breath sounds
- Possible wheezing in both patients with chronic bronchitis and emphysema

- Features of both chronic bronchitis and emphysema in many patients with COPD
- Acute exacerbation of COPD is mainly a clinical diagnosis and generally manifests with worsening dyspnea, increase in sputum purulence, and increase in sputum volume
- Complications often involve right-sided heart failure (cor pulmonale), sometimes precipitated by arrhythmias such as atrial fibrillation or multifocal atrial tachycardia

ETIOLOGY

- Tobacco exposure
- Occupational exposure to pulmonary toxins (e.g., cadmium)
- Atmospheric pollution
- α-1 antitrypsin deficiency (rare; <1% of COPD patients)

DIAGNOSIS

DIFFERENTIAL DIAGNOSIS

- CHF
- Asthma
- Respiratory infections
- Bronchiectasis
- Pulmonary embolism
- Sleep apnea, obstructive
- Pulmonary fibrosis
- Other restrictive lung diseases
- Anxiety disorders

WORKUP

Chest x-ray examination, pulmonary function testing, blood gases

LABORATORY TESTS

- CBC may reveal leukocytosis with "shift to the left" during acute exacerbation.
- Sputum may be purulent with bacterial respiratory tract infections. Sputum staining and cultures are usually reserved for cases that are refractory to antibiotic therapy.
- ABGs: hypercapnia and hypoxemia may be present.
- Pulmonary function testing (PFT): the primary physiologic abnormality in COPD is an accelerated decline in forced expiratory volume in one second (FEV_1) from the normal rate in adults over 30 yr of age of approximately 30 ml/yr to nearly 60 ml/yr. PFT results in COPD reveal abnormal diffusing capacity, increased total lung capacity or residual volume, and fixed reduction in FEV_1 in patients with emphysema and normal diffusing capacity and reduced FEV_1 in patients with chronic bronchitis. Patients with COPD can generally be distinguished from asthmatics by their incomplete response to albuterol (change in FEV_1 <200 ml and 12%) and absence of an

abnormal bronchoconstrictor response to methacholine or other stimuli. However, nearly 40% of patients with COPD respond to bronchodilators.

IMAGING STUDIES

Chest x-ray examination:
- Hyperinflation with flattened diaphragm, tending of the diaphragm at the rib, and increased retrosternal chest space
- Decreased vascular markings and bullae in patients with emphysema
- Thickened bronchial markings and enlarged right side of the heart in patients with chronic bronchitis

ECG and echocardiogram may be appropriate to diagnose associated heart disease (also caused by smoking).

TREATMENT

NONPHARMACOLOGIC THERAPY

- Weight loss in patients who are obese
- Avoidance of tobacco use and elimination of air pollutants
- Supplemental oxygen, usually through a nasal cannula, to ensure oxygen saturation >90% measured by pulse oximetry

ACUTE EXACERBATION

- Acute exacerbation of COPD can be treated with:
  1. Pulmonary toilet: careful nasotracheal suction is indicated in patients with excessive secretions and inability to expectorate. Mechanical percussion of the chest as applied by a physical or respiratory therapist is ineffective with acute exacerbations of COPD.
  2. Aerosolized β-agonists (e.g., albuterol nebulizer solution 5% 0.3 ml or albuterol nebulized 5% solution 2.5 to 5 mg).
  3. Anticholinergic agents, which have equivalent efficacy to inhaled β-adrenergic agonists. Inhalant solution of ipratropium bromide 0.5 mg can be administered every 4 to 8 hours. Tiotropium bromide (Spiriva) has a much longer duration of action than ipratropium and produces a more sustained response over time than long-acting β_2-agonists. Usual dose is inhalation of one capsule daily with a breath-activated dry powder inhalation device (Handi-Haler).
  4. Short courses of systemic corticosteroids, which have been shown to improve spirometric and clinical outcomes. In the hospital setting give IV methylprednisolone 50- to 100-mg bolus, then q6-8h; taper as soon as possible. In the outpatient

setting, oral prednisone 40 mg/day initially, decreasing the dose by 10 mg every other day is generally effective.

5. Judicious oxygen administration (hypercapnia and further respiratory compromise may occur after high-flow oxygen therapy). Use of a Venturi-type mask delivering an inspired oxygen fraction of 24% to 28% is preferred to nasal cannula.

6. Noninvasive positive pressure ventilation, which when delivered by a facial or nasal mask may obviate the need for intratracheal intubation.

7. Inhaled corticosteroids, whose role in COPD is controversial. Although some trials have demonstrated mild improvement in patients' symptoms and decreased frequency of exacerbations, most pulmonologists believe that these drugs are ineffective in most patients with COPD but should be considered for patients with moderate to severe airflow limitation who have persistent symptoms despite optimal bronchodilator therapy.

8. IV aminophylline administration, which is controversial. When used, serum levels should be closely monitored to minimize risks of tachyarrhythmias.

- Cor pulmonale or comorbid heart failure may be exacerbated by hypoxia and must be treated along with the pulmonary management (see Heart Failure, Congestive in Section I).
- Antibiotics are indicated in suspected respiratory infection (e.g., increased purulence and volume of phlegm).
  1. *Haemophilus influenzae* and *Streptococcus pneumoniae* are frequent causes of acute bronchitis.
  2. Oral antibiotics of choice are azithromycin, levofloxacin, amoxicillin-clavulanate, and cefuroxime.
  3. The use of antibiotics is beneficial in exacerbations of COPD presenting with increased dyspnea and sputum purulence (especially if the patient is febrile).
- Guaifenesin may improve cough symptoms and mucus clearance; however, mucolytic medications are generally ineffective. Their benefits may be greatest in patients with more advanced disease.
- Intubation and mechanical ventilation may be necessary if above measures fail to provide improvement.

CHRONIC Rx

- Inhaled β-agonists, short-acting agents such as albuterol can be used on a schedule (e.g., two to four puffs q4-6h).
- Inhaled β-agonists, long-acting agents such as salmeterol (Serevent) can be given twice daily.
- Anticholinergic short-acting agent such as ipratropium (Atrovent) can be used on a schedule or prn, alone, or in combination with the β-agonist albuterol (Combivent).
- Anticholinergic long-acting agent tiotropium (Spiriva): one inhalation (18 μg dry powder) qd may be more effective than ipratropium.
- An inhaled glucocorticoid drug such as fluticasone is given twice daily alone or in combination with β-agonists or anticholinergic drugs (e.g., Advair combines fluticasone and salmeterol).
- Elderly patients may be unable to coordinate their breathing and hand motion or may otherwise be unable to operate a handheld metered dose inhaler. If such treatment is prescribed, the physician must educate and observe the patient using this therapy. A spacer may be helpful and should be prescribed routinely. Elderly patients often do better with a nebulizer than with a handheld aerosol delivery system.
- Pulmonary rehabilitation may improve exercise capacity, reduce dyspnea, reduce hospitalizations, and enhance quality of life.
- Lung-volume-reduction surgery in patients with severe upper-lobe emphysema can improve exercise capacity, pulmonary function, and quality of life but not overall survival.

DISPOSITION

- Following the initial episode of respiratory failure, 5-yr survival is approximately 25%.
- Development of cor pulmonale or hypercapnia and persistent tachycardia are poor prognostic indicators.

PEARLS & CONSIDERATIONS

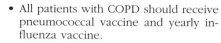

COMMENTS

- All patients with COPD should receive pneumococcal vaccine and yearly influenza vaccine.

- In assessing the severity of COPD, the FEV_1 is limited by the fact that it does not take into account the systemic manifestations of COPD. The BODE index (body-mass index [B], degree of obstruction [O], dyspnea [D], and exercise capacity [E]) has been proposed as a multidimensional scale to better assess the morbidity and mortality associated with COPD. It is better than the FEV_1 at predicting the risk of death from any cause and from respiratory causes among patients with COPD.
- Osteoporosis is often associated with COPD; consider DXA.

SUGGESTED READINGS

Aaron SD et al: Outpatient oral prednisone after emergency treatment of chronic obstructive pulmonary disease, *N Engl J Med* 348:2618, 2003.

Anthonisen NR et al: Smoking and lung function of Lung Health Study participants after 11 years, *Am J Resp Crit Care Med* 166:675-679, 2002.

Celli B et al: The body-mass index, airflow obstruction, dyspnea, and exercise capacity index in chronic obstructive pulmonary disease, *N Engl J Med* 350:1005-1012, 2004.

Hogg JC et al: The nature of small-airway obstruction in chronic obstructive pulmonary disease, *N Engl J Med* 350:2645-2653, 2004.

Man PS et al: Contemporary management of chronic obstructive pulmonary disease, clinical applications, *JAMA* 290:2313, 2003.

National Emphysema Treatment Trial Research Group: a randomized trial comparing lung-volume-reduction surgery with medical therapy for severe emphysema, *N Engl J Med* 348:2059-2073, 2003.

Sethi S et al: New strains of bacteria and exacerbations of chronic obstructive pulmonary disease, *N Engl J Med* 347:465, 2002.

Sin DD et al: Contemporary management of chronic obstructive pulmonary disease, a scientific review, *JAMA* 290:2301, 2003.

Stoller JK: Acute exacerbations of chronic obstructive pulmonary disease, *N Engl J Med* 346:988, 2002.

Sutherland ER, Cherniak RM: Management of chronic obstructive pulmonary disease, *N Engl J Med* 350:2689-2697, 2004.

Vincken W et al: Improved health outcomes in patients with COPD during 1 year's treatment with tiotropium, *Eur Respir J* 19:209-216, 2002.

AUTHORS: **FRED F. FERRI, M.D.,** and **TOM J. WACHTEL, M.D.**

BASIC INFORMATION

DEFINITION

Cirrhosis is defined histologically as the presence of fibrosis and regenerative nodules in the liver. It can be classified as micronodular, macronodular, and mixed; however, each form may be seen in the same patient at different stages of the disease. Cirrhosis manifests clinically with portal hypertension, hepatic encephalopathy, and variceal bleeding.

ICD-9CM CODES
571.5 Cirrhosis of the liver
571.2 Cirrhosis of the liver secondary to alcohol

EPIDEMIOLOGY & DEMOGRAPHICS

- Cirrhosis is the eleventh leading cause of death in the U.S. (death rate 9 deaths/100,000 persons/yr).
- Alcohol abuse and viral hepatitis are the major causes of cirrhosis in the U.S.
- Nonalcoholic fatty liver disease (NAFLD) is becoming recognized as an important cause of cirrhosis, and its prevalence is increasing.

PHYSICAL FINDINGS & CLINICAL PRESENTATION

SKIN: Jaundice, palmar erythema (alcohol abuse), spider angiomata, ecchymosis (thrombocytopenia or coagulation factor deficiency), dilated superficial periumbilical vein (caput medusae), increased pigmentation (hemochromatosis), xanthomas (primary biliary cirrhosis), needle tracks (viral hepatitis)
EYES: Kayser-Fleischer rings (corneal copper deposition seen in Wilson's disease; best diagnosed with slit lamp examination), scleral icterus
BREATH: Fetor hepaticus (musty odor of breath and urine found in cirrhosis with hepatic failure)
CHEST: Possible gynecomastia in men
ABDOMEN: Tender hepatomegaly (congestive hepatomegaly), small, nodular liver (cirrhosis), palpable, nontender gallbladder (neoplastic extrahepatic biliary obstruction), palpable spleen (portal hypertension), venous hum auscultated over periumbilical veins (portal hypertension), ascites (portal hypertension, hypoalbuminemia)
RECTAL EXAMINATION: Hemorrhoids (portal hypertension), guaiac-positive stools (alcoholic gastritis, bleeding esophageal varices, PUD, bleeding hemorrhoids)
GENITALIA: Testicular atrophy in males (chronic liver disease, hemochromatosis)
EXTREMITIES: Pedal edema (hypoalbuminemia, failure of right side of the heart), arthropathy (hemochromatosis)

NEUROLOGIC: Flapping tremor, asterixis (hepatic encephalopathy), choreoathetosis, dysarthria (Wilson's disease)

ETIOLOGY

- Alcohol abuse
- Nonalcoholic steatohepatitis (NASH)
- Secondary biliary cirrhosis, obstruction of the common bile duct (stone, stricture, pancreatitis, neoplasm, sclerosing cholangitis)
- Drugs (e.g., acetaminophen, isoniazid, methotrexate, methyldopa)
- Hepatic congestion (e.g., CHF, constrictive pericarditis, tricuspid insufficiency, thrombosis of the hepatic vein, obstruction of the vena cava)
- Primary biliary cirrhosis
- Hemochromatosis
- Chronic hepatitis B or C
- Wilson's disease
- α-1 antitrypsin deficiency
- Infiltrative diseases (amyloidosis, glycogen storage diseases, hemochromatosis)
- Nutritional: jejunoileal bypass
- Others: parasitic infections (schistosomiasis), idiopathic portal hypertension, congenital hepatic fibrosis, systemic mastocytosis, autoimmune hepatitis, hepatic steatosis, IBD

DIAGNOSIS

WORKUP

In addition to an assessment of liver function, the evaluation of patients with cirrhosis should also include an assessment of renal and circulatory function. Diagnostic workup is aimed primarily at identifying the most likely cause of cirrhosis. The history is extremely important:
- Alcohol abuse: alcoholic liver disease
- History of hepatitis B (chronic active hepatitis, primary hepatic neoplasm, or hepatitis C)
- History of IBD (primary sclerosing cholangitis)
- History of pruritus, hyperlipoproteinemia, and xanthomas in an elderly female (primary biliary cirrhosis)
- Impotence, diabetes mellitus, hyperpigmentation, arthritis (hemochromatosis)
- Neurologic disturbances (Wilson's disease, hepatolenticular degeneration)
- Family history of "liver disease" (hemochromatosis [positive family history in 25% of patients], α-1 antitrypsin deficiency)
- History of recurrent episodes of RUQ pain (biliary tract disease)
- History of blood transfusions, IV drug abuse (hepatitis C)
- History of hepatotoxic drug exposure
- Coexistence of other diseases with immune or autoimmune features (ITP, myasthenia gravis, thyroiditis, autoimmune hepatitis)

- Existence of the metabolic syndrome (obesity, hyperlipidemia, diabetes)

LABORATORY TESTS

- Decreased Hgb and Hct, elevated MCV, increased BUN and creatinine (the BUN may also be "normal" or low if the patient has severely diminished liver function), decreased sodium (dilutional hyponatremia), decreased potassium (as a result of secondary aldosteronism or urinary losses). Evaluation of renal function should also include measurement of urinary sodium and urinary protein from a 24-hr urine collection.
- Decreased glucose in a patient with liver disease indicating severe liver damage
- Other laboratory abnormalities:
  1. Alcoholic hepatitis and cirrhosis: there may be mild elevation of ALT and AST, usually <500 IU; AST > ALT (ratio >2:3).
  2. Extrahepatic obstruction: there may be moderate elevations of ALT and AST to levels <500 IU.
  3. Viral, toxic, or ischemic hepatitis: there are extreme elevations (>500 IU) of ALT and AST.
  4. Transaminases may be normal despite significant liver disease in patients with jejunoileal bypass operations or hemochromatosis or after methotrexate administration.
  5. Alkaline phosphatase elevation can occur with extrahepatic obstruction, primary biliary cirrhosis, and primary sclerosing cholangitis.
  6. Serum LDH is significantly elevated in metastatic disease of the liver; lesser elevations are seen with hepatitis, cirrhosis, extrahepatic obstruction, and congestive hepatomegaly.
  7. Serum γ-glutamyl transpeptidase (GGTP) is elevated in alcoholic liver disease and may also be elevated with cholestatic disease (primary biliary cirrhosis, primary sclerosing cholangitis).
  8. Serum bilirubin may be elevated; urinary bilirubin can be present in hepatitis, hepatocellular jaundice, and biliary obstruction.
  9. Serum albumin: significant liver disease results in hypoalbuminemia.
  10. Prothrombin time: an elevated PT in patients with liver disease indicates severe liver damage and poor prognosis.
  11. Presence of hepatitis B surface antigen implies acute or chronic hepatitis B.
  12. Presence of antimitochondrial antibody suggests primary biliary cirrhosis, chronic hepatitis.

13. Elevated serum copper, decreased serum ceruloplasmin, and elevated 24-hr urine may be diagnostic of Wilson's disease.
14. Protein immunoelectrophoresis may reveal decreased α-1 globulins (α-1 antitrypsin deficiency), increased IgA (alcoholic cirrhosis), increased IgM (primary biliary cirrhosis), increased IgG (chronic hepatitis, cryptogenic cirrhosis).
15. An elevated serum ferritin and increased transferrin saturation are suggestive of hemochromatosis.
16. An elevated blood ammonia suggests hepatocellular dysfunction; serial values, however, are generally not useful in following patients with hepatic encephalopathy because there is poor correlation between blood ammonia level and degree of hepatic encephalopathy.
17. Serum cholesterol is elevated in cholestatic disorders.
18. Antinuclear antibodies (ANA) may be found in autoimmune hepatitis.
19. Alpha fetoprotein: levels >1000 pg/ml are highly suggestive of primary liver cell carcinoma.
20. Hepatitis C viral testing identifies patients with chronic hepatitis C infection.
21. Elevated level of serum globulin (especially γ-globulins), positive ANA test may occur with autoimmune hepatitis.

IMAGING STUDIES

- Ultrasonography is the procedure of choice for detection of gallstones, fatty liver, and dilation of common bile ducts.
- CT scan is useful for detecting mass lesions in liver and pancreas, assessing hepatic fat content, identifying idiopathic hemochromatosis, early diagnosing of Budd-Chiari syndrome, dilation of intrahepatic bile ducts, and detection of varices and splenomegaly.
- Technetium-99m sulfur colloid scanning is occasionally useful for diagnosing cirrhosis (there is a shift of colloid uptake to the spleen, bone marrow), identifying hepatic adenomas (cold defect is noted), diagnosing Budd-Chiari syndrome (there is increased uptake by the caudate lobe).
- ERCP is the procedure of choice for diagnosing periampullary carcinoma, common duct stones; it is also useful in diagnosing primary sclerosing cholangitis.
- Percutaneous transhepatic cholangiography (PTC) is useful when evaluating patients with cholestatic jaundice and dilated intrahepatic ducts by ultrasonography; presence of intrahepatic strictures and focal dilation is suggestive of PSC.
- Percutaneous liver biopsy is useful in evaluating hepatic filling defects, diagnosing hepatocellular disease or hepatomegaly, evaluating persistently abnormal liver function tests, and diagnosing hemachromatosis, primary biliary cirrhosis, Wilson's disease, glycogen storage diseases, chronic hepatitis, autoimmune hepatitis, infiltrative diseases, alcoholic liver disease, NASH, drug-induced liver disease, primary or secondary carcinoma, and gauging the severity of fibrosis.

TREATMENT

Rx

NONPHARMACOLOGIC THERAPY

Avoid any hepatotoxins (e.g., ethanol, acetaminophen); improve nutritional status.

GENERAL Rx

- Correct any mechanical obstruction to bile flow (e.g., calculi, strictures).
- Provide therapy for underlying cardiovascular disorders in patients with cardiac cirrhosis.
- Remove excess body iron with phlebotomy and deferoxamine in patients with hemochromatosis.
- Remove copper deposits with D-penicillamine in patients with Wilson's disease.
- Long-term ursodiol therapy will slow the progression of primary biliary cirrhosis. It is, however, ineffective in primary sclerosing cholangitis.
- Glucocorticoids (prednisone 20 to 30 mg/day initially or combination therapy or prednisone and azathioprine) are useful in autoimmune hepatitis.
- Treatment of complications of portal hypertension (ascites, esophagogastric varices, hepatic encephalopathy, and hepatorenal syndrome).

DISPOSITION

- Prognosis varies with the etiology of the patient's cirrhosis and whether there is ongoing hepatic injury. Mortality rate exceeds 80% in patients with hepatorenal syndrome.
- Two markers of portal hypertension, thrombocytopenia and splenomegaly, moderately increase the likelihood of large esophageal varices.
- If advanced cirrhosis is present and transplantation is not feasible, survival is 1 to 2 yr.

REFERRAL

- Hospital admission for bleeding varices, hepatic encephalopathy, or onset of hepatorenal syndrome
- Liver transplantation in suitable candidates is the only effective long-term treatment of complications resulting from cirrhosis

PEARLS & CONSIDERATIONS

!

COMMENTS

Thrombocytopenia and advanced Child-Pugh cases are associated with the presence of varices. These factors are useful to identify cirrhotic patients who benefit most from referral for endoscopic screening for varices.

SUGGESTED READINGS

Gines P et al: Management of cirrhosis and ascites, *N Engl J Med* 350:1645, 2004.
Ong JP et al: Correlation between ammonia levels and the severity of hepatic encephalopathy, *Am J Med* 114:189, 2003.

AUTHORS: **FRED F. FERRI, M.D.,** with revisions by **TOM J. WACHTEL, M.D.**

BASIC INFORMATION

DEFINITION

Colorectal cancer is a neoplasm arising from the luminal surface of the large bowel: descending colon (40% to 42%), rectosigmoid and rectum (30% to 33%), cecum and ascending colon (25% to 30%), transverse colon (10% to 13%).

ICD-9CM CODES
154.0 Colorectal cancer

EPIDEMIOLOGY & DEMOGRAPHICS

- Colorectal cancer is the second leading cause of cancer deaths in the U.S. (>135,000 new cases and >50,000 deaths/yr).
- Peak incidence is in the seventh decade of life.
- 50% of rectal cancers are within reach of the examiner's finger, 50% of colon cancers are within reach of the flexible sigmoidoscope.
- Colorectal cancer accounts for 14% of all cases of cancer (excluding skin malignancies) and 14% of all yearly cancer deaths.
- Risk factors:
  1. Hereditary polyposis syndromes
     a. Familial polyposis (high risk)
     b. Gardner's syndrome (high risk)
     c. Turcot's syndrome (high risk)
     d. Peutz-Jeghers syndrome (low to moderate risk)
  2. IBD, both ulcerative colitis and Crohn's disease
  3. Family history of "cancer family syndrome"
  4. Heredofamilial breast cancer and colon carcinoma
  5. History of previous colorectal carcinoma
  6. Women undergoing irradiation for gynecologic cancer
  7. First-degree relatives with colorectal carcinoma
  8. Age >40 yr
  9. Possible dietary factors (diet high in fat or meat, beer drinking, reduced vegetable consumption)
  10. Hereditary nonpolyposis colon cancer (HNPCC): autosomal-dominant disorder characterized by early age of onset (mean age of 44 yr) and right-sided or proximal colon cancers, synchronous and metachronous colon cancers, mucinous and poorly differentiated colon cancers; it accounts for 1% to 5% of all cases of colorectal cancer
  11. Previous endometrial or ovarian cancer, particularly when diagnosed at an early age

PHYSICAL FINDINGS & CLINICAL PRESENTATION

- Physical examination may be completely unremarkable.
- Digital rectal examination can detect approximately 50% of rectal cancers.
- Palpable abdominal masses may indicate metastasis or complications of colorectal carcinoma (abscess, intussusception, volvulus).
- Abdominal distention and tenderness are suggestive of colonic obstruction.
- Hepatomegaly may be indicative of hepatic metastasis.

ETIOLOGY

Colorectal cancer can arise through two mutational pathways: microsatellite instability or chromosomal instability. Germline genetic mutations are the basis of inherited colon cancer syndromes; an accumulation of somatic mutations in a cell is the basis of sporadic colon cancer.

DIAGNOSIS (Dx)

DIFFERENTIAL DIAGNOSIS

- Diverticular disease
- Strictures
- IBD
- Infectious or inflammatory lesions
- Adhesions
- Arteriovenous malformations
- Metastatic carcinoma (prostate, sarcoma)
- Extrinsic masses (cysts, abscesses)

WORKUP

- The clinical presentation of colorectal malignancies is initially vague and nonspecific (weight loss, anorexia, malaise). It is useful to divide colon cancer symptoms into those usually associated with right side of colon and those commonly associated with left side of colon, because the clinical presentation varies with the location of the carcinoma.
  1. Right side of colon
     a. Anemia (iron deficiency secondary to chronic blood loss)
     b. Dull, vague, and uncharacteristic abdominal pain may be present or patient may be completely asymptomatic
     c. Rectal bleeding is often missed because blood is mixed with feces
     d. Obstruction and constipation are unusual because of large lumen and more liquid stools
  2. Left side of colon
     a. Change in bowel habits (constipation, diarrhea, tenesmus, pencil-thin stools)
     b. Rectal bleeding (bright red blood coating the surface of the stool)
     c. Intestinal obstruction is frequent because of small lumen

- Early diagnosis of patients with surgically curable disease (Dukes' A, B) is necessary, because survival time is directly related to the stage of the carcinoma at the time of diagnosis. Appropriate screening recommendations are discussed in Section V.

CLASSIFICATION

Dukes' and UICC classification for colorectal cancer:
A Confined to the mucosa-submucosa (I)
B Invasion of muscularis propria (II)
C Local node involvement (III)
D Distant metastasis (IV)

LABORATORY TESTS

- Positive fecal occult blood test
- Newer modalities for early detection of colorectal neoplasms include the detection of mutations in the adenomatous polyposis coli (APC) gene from stool samples
- Microcytic anemia
- Elevated plasma carcinoembryonic antigen (CEA). CEA should not be used as a screening test for colorectal cancer because it can be elevated in patients with many other conditions (smoking, IBD, alcoholic liver disease). A normal CEA does not exclude the diagnosis of colorectal cancer
- Liver function tests

IMAGING STUDIES

- Colonoscopy with biopsy (primary assessment tool)
- CT scan of abdomen to assist in preoperative staging
- Chest x-ray examination to look for evidence of metastatic disease
- Air-contrast barium enema only in patients refusing colonoscopy or unable to tolerate colonoscopy

TREATMENT (Rx)

GENERAL Rx

- Surgical resection: 70% of colorectal cancers are resectable for cure at presentation; 45% of patients are cured by primary resection.
- Radiation therapy is a useful adjunct to fluorouracil and levamisole therapy for stage II or III rectal cancers.
- Adjuvant chemotherapy with combination of 5-fluorouracil (5-FU) and levamisole substantially increases cure rates for patients with stage III colon cancer and should be considered standard treatment for all such patients and selected patients with high-risk stage II colon cancer.
- Leucovorin (folinic acid) enhances the effect of fluorouracil and is given together with it (FL). When given as adjuvant therapy after a complete resection in stage III disease, FL increases overall

5-year survival from 51% to 64%. The use of adjuvant FL in stage II disease (no involvement of regional nodes) is controversial because 5-yr overall survival is 80% for treated or untreated patients and the addition of FL only increases the probability of 5-yr disease-free interval from 72% to 76%. For patients with standard-risk stage III tumors (e.g., involvement of one to three regional lymph nodes), FL alone or FL with oxaliplatin (Eloxatin, an inhibitor of DNA synthesis) are both reasonable choices. Generally reversible peripheral neuropathy is the main side effect of FL plus oxaliplatin.

- Irinotecan (Camptosar), a potent inhibitor of topoisomerase I, a nuclear enzyme involved in the unwinding of DNA during replication, can be used to treat metastatic colorectal cancer refractory to other drugs, including 5-FU; it may offer a few months of palliation but is expensive and associated with significant toxicity.
- Oxaliplatin can be used in combination with fluorouracil and leucovorin (FL) for patients with metastatic colorectal cancer whose disease has recurred or progressed despite treatment with fluorouracil/leucovorin plus irinotecan. FL plus oxaliplatin should be considered for high-risk patients with stage III cancers (e.g., >3 involved regional nodes [N2] or tumor invasion beyond the serosa [T4 lesion]).
- The monoclonal antibodies cetuximab (Erbitux) and bevacizumab (Avastatin) have also been approved by the FDA for advanced colorectal cancer. Bevacizumab is an angiogenesis inhibitor that binds and inhibits the activity of human vascular endothelial growth factor (VEGF). Cetuximab is an epidermal growth factor receptor (EGFR) blocker that inhibits the growth and survival of tumor cells that overexpress EGFR. Cetuximab has synergism with irinotecan and its addition to irinotecan in patients with advanced disease resistant to irinotecan increases response rate from 10% when cetuximab is used alone to 22% with combination of cetuximab and irinotecan. The addition of bevacizumab to FL in patients with advanced colorectal cancer has been reported to increase the response rate from 17% to 40%.
- In patients who undergo resection of liver metastases from colorectal cancer, postoperative treatment with a combination of hepatic arterial infusion of floxuridine and IV fluorouracil improves the outcome at 2 yr.

CHRONIC Rx

Follow-up is indicated with:
- Physician visits with a focus on the clinical and disease-related history, directed physical examination guided by this history, coordination of follow-up, and counseling every 3 to 6 mo for the first 3 yr, then decreased frequency thereafter for 2 yr
- Colonoscopy yearly for the initial 2 yr, then every 3 yr
- CEA level should be obtained baseline; if elevated, it can be used postoperatively as a measure of completeness of tumor resection or to monitor tumor recurrence; if used to monitor tumor recurrence, CEA should be obtained every 3 to 6 mo for up to 5 yr. The role of CEA for monitoring patients with resected colon cancer has been questioned because of the small number of cures attributed to CEA monitoring despite the substantial cost in dollars and physical and emotional stress associated with monitoring

DISPOSITION

- The 5-yr survival varies with the stage of the carcinoma:
  1. Dukes' A 5-yr survival, >80%
  2. Dukes' B 5-yr survival, 60%
  3. Dukes' C 5-yr survival, 20%
  4. Dukes' D 5-yr survival, 3%
- Overall 5-yr disease-free survival is approximately 50% for colon cancer.
- High-frequency microsatellite instability in colorectal cancer is independently predictive of a relatively favorable outcome and, in addition, reduces the likelihood of metastases.
- In patients with Dukes' C (stage III) colorectal cancer there is improved 5-yr survival among women treated with adjuvant chemotherapy (53% with chemotherapy vs. 33% without) and among patients with right-sided tumors treated with adjuvant chemotherapy.
- Retention of 18q alleles in microsatellite-stable cancers and mutation of the gene for the type I receptor for TGF-B1 in cancers with high levels of microsatellite instability point to a favorable outcome after adjuvant chemotherapy with fluorouracil-based regimens for stage II colon cancer.

REFERRAL

- Surgical referral for resection
- Oncology referral for adjuvant chemotherapy in selected patients
- Radiation oncology referral for patients with stage II or III rectal cancers

PEARLS & CONSIDERATIONS

COMMENTS

- Decreased fat intake to 30% of total energy intake, increased fiber, and fruit and vegetable consumption may lower colorectal cancer risk. Recent literature reports, however, do not support a protective effect from dietary fiber against colorectal cancer in women.
- Chemoprophylaxis with aspirin (81 mg/day) reduces the incidence of colorectal adenomas in persons at risk.
- The National Cancer Institute has published consensus guidelines for universal screening for hereditary nonpolyposis colon cancer (HNPCC) in patients with newly diagnosed colorectal cancer. Tumors in mutation carriers of HNPCC typically exhibit microsatellite instability, a characteristic phenotype that is caused by expansions or contractions of short nucleotide repeat sequences. These guidelines (Bethesda Guidelines) are useful for selective patients for microsatellite instability testing. Screening patients with newly diagnosed colorectal cancer for HNPCC is cost effective, especially if the benefits to their immediate relatives are considered.
- Expression of guanylyl cyclase C mRNA in lymph nodes is associated with recurrence of colorectal cancer in patients with stage II disease. Analysis of guanylyl cyclase mRNA expression by RT-PCR may be useful for colorectal cancer staging.
- The use of either annual or biennial fecal occult-blood testing significantly reduces the incidence of colorectal cancer. In addition, screening should include a yearly rectal exam and a colonoscopy every 10 years. There is no evidence-based information to provide an upper age limit for screening.
- The detection of mutations in the adenomatous polyposis coli (APC) gene from stool samples is a promising new modality for early detection of colorectal neoplasms.

SUGGESTED READINGS

Andre T et al: Oxaliplatin, fluorouracil, and leucovorin as adjuvant treatment for colon cancer, *N Engl J Med* 350:2343, 2004.

Baron JA et al: A randomized trial of aspirin to prevent colorectal adenomas, *N Engl J Med* 348:891, 2003.

Cunningham D et al: Cetuximab monotherapy and cetuximab plus irinotecan in irinotecan-refractory metastatic colon cancer, *N Engl J Med* 351:337, 2004.

Hurwitz H et al: Bevacizumab plus irinotecan, fluorouracil, and leucovorin for metastatic colon cancer, *N Engl J Med* 350:2335, 2004.

Mayer R: Two steps forward in the treatment of colorectal cancer, *N Engl J Med* 350:2406, 2004.

Pfister D et al: Surveillance strategies after curative treatment of colorectal cancer, *N Engl J Med* 350:2375, 2004.

AUTHOR: **FRED F. FERRI, M.D.**

BASIC INFORMATION

DEFINITION

The term *conjunctivitis* refers to an inflammation of the conjunctiva resulting from a variety of causes, including allergies and bacterial, viral, and chlamydial infections.

SYNONYMS

"Red eye"/"Pink eye"
Acute conjunctivitis
Subacute conjunctivitis
Chronic conjunctivitis
Purulent conjunctivitis
Pseudomembranous conjunctivitis
Papillary conjunctivitis
Follicular conjunctivitis

ICD-9CM CODES
372.30 Conjunctivitis, unspecified

EPIDEMIOLOGY & DEMOGRAPHICS

PREVALENCE (IN U.S.):
- Very common
- Often seasonal and can be extremely contagious

PREDOMINANT AGE: Occurs at any age
PEAK INCIDENCE: More common in the fall when viral infections and pollens increase

PHYSICAL FINDINGS & CLINICAL PRESENTATION

- Injection and chemosis of conjunctivae with discharge (Fig. 1-12)
- Cornea clear
- Vision often normal

ETIOLOGY

- Bacterial
- Viral
- Chlamydial
- Allergic
- Traumatic

DIAGNOSIS

DIFFERENTIAL DIAGNOSIS

- Acute glaucoma
- Corneal lesions
- Acute iritis
- Episcleritis
- Scleritis
- Uveitis
- Blepharitis
- Canalicular obstruction
- The differential diagnosis of red eye is described in Section II

WORKUP

- History and physical examination
- Reports of itching, pain, visual changes

LABORATORY TESTS

Cultures are useful if not successfully treated with antibiotic medications; initial culture is usually not necessary.

TREATMENT

NONPHARMACOLOGIC THERAPY

- Warm compresses if infective conjunctivitis
- Cold compresses in irritative or allergic conjunctivitis

ACUTE GENERAL Rx

- Antibiotic drops (e.g., levofloxacin, ofloxin, ciprofloxacin, tobramycin, gentamicin ophthalmic solution one or two drops q2-4h)
- Caution: be careful with corticosteroid treatment and avoid unless sure of diagnosis; corticosteroids can exacerbate infections
- Povidine-iodine (Betadine) eyedrops when available

CHRONIC Rx

- Depends on cause
- If allergic, nonsteroidals such as Voltaren ophthalmic solution, mast cell stabilizers such as Alocril, Patanol, Zaditor are useful
- If infectious, antibiotic drops (see Acute General Rx)
- Dry eyes need artificial tears, ristasis, lacrimal duct plugs when indicated

DISPOSITION

Follow carefully for the first 2 wk to make sure secondary complications do not occur.

REFERRAL

To ophthalmologist if symptoms refractory to initial treatment

PEARLS & CONSIDERATIONS

COMMENTS

- Red eyes are not just conjunctivitis when there is significant pain or loss of sight. However, it is usually safe to treat pain-free eyes and the normal seeing red eye with lid hygene and topical treatment.
- Beware of patients wearing soft contact lenses and the elderly.
- Do not use steroids indiscriminately; use only when the diagnosis is certain.

SUGGESTED READINGS

Bennett C: Treatment of viral conjunctivitis in children, *Am Fam Physician* 67(9):1873, 2003.
Fischer PR et al: Route of antibiotic administration for conjunctivitis, *Pediatr Infect Dis J* 21(10):989, 2002.
Nichols GR: The red eye, *N Engl J Med* 343(21):1577, 2000.
Sheikh A, Hurwitz B: Topical antibiotics for acute bacterial conjunctivitis: a systematic review, *Br J Gen Pract* 51:473, 2001.

AUTHOR: **MELVYN KOBY, M.D.**

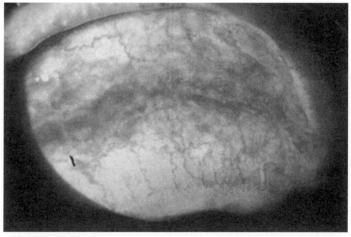

FIGURE 1-12　Conjunctival infection from viral conjunctivitis. (From Marx JA [ed]: *Rosen's emergency medicine,* ed 5, St Louis, 2002, Mosby.)

BASIC INFORMATION

DEFINITION

A recent consensus panel defined constipation as at least 12 weeks, not necessarily consecutive, within the previous 12 months of two or more of the following: straining, lumpy/hard stools, sensation of incomplete evacuation, sensation of anorectal obstruction, manual maneuvers to facilitate stooling, or less than three defecations per week. The patient should be devoid of loose stools and not meet criteria for irritable bowel syndrome. More commonly, constipation is present when a patient has two or less bowel movements per week or the patient complains of straining with defecation.

ICD-9CM CODES
594.0

EPIDEMIOLOGY & DEMOGRAPHICS

PREVALENCE (IN U.S.): The literature estimates the prevalence to be between 2% and 28%. An inconsistent definition of constipation has resulted in the variation of these findings.
PREDOMINANT SEX: Women
PREDOMINANT AGE: Prevalence increases with age.

PHYSICAL FINDINGS & CLINICAL PRESENTATION

On rectal exam the physician should evaluate for the presence of rectal tone, anorectal masses, stricture, fecal impaction, consistency of the rectal wall. A pelvic exam should be performed as pelvic floor dysfunction or a rectocele can lead to alteration in bowel movements.

ETIOLOGY

Behavioral:
- Inactivity, poor bowel habits are common causes of constipation in the older population.

Medications:
- Most commonly anticholinergics and opiates; however, other drugs including calcium channel blockers, iron supplements, chronic laxative abuse, NSAIDs, sucralfate, cholestyramine, and diuretics can lead to constipation.

Dietary:
- Dehydration whether by decreased fluid consumption, aggressive diuresis, or other insensible fluid losses can result in constipation. No study has shown that low fiber intake results in constipation; yet, increasing a person's fiber intake can effectively treat constipation.

Structural:
- Colonic lesions—stricture, mass, ulcer
- Anorectal lesions—prolapse, stricture, fissure, ulcer, mass

Systemic disease:
- Endocrine—hypothyroidism, hyperparathyroidism, diabetes mellitus
- Metabolic—hypokalemia, hypercalcemia, uremia, porphyria

Neurologic disorders
- Parkinson's disease, multiple sclerosis, damage to the sacral nerve, autonomic dysfunction

Pelvic floor dysfunction
Irritable bowel syndrome

DIAGNOSIS

WORKUP

The first step is to identify that the patient meets the definition of constipation. Physicians should ascertain what is most distressing to the patient and request a journal of diet regimen and bowel patterns. The majority of elderly patients have constipation symptoms due to poor eating habits, immobility, and medications. A review of all medications, including over-the-counter medications, is imperative because alteration in bowel habits is a side effect of a variety of medications. All patients with new-onset constipation, thinning of stools, weight loss, hematochezia/melena should have an evaluation for abnormality of colonic or anorectal structures (e.g., rule out colon cancer).

LABORATORY TESTS

A patient's history will direct laboratory testing—potassium, calcium, blood glucose, TSH.

IMAGING STUDIES

Anatomic lesions can be visualized with colonoscopy, barium enema, or virtual colonoscopy.

TREATMENT

GENERAL Rx

Interestingly, although immobility is a risk factor of constipation, exercise has not been shown to be an effective treatment for constipation.

PHARMACOLOGIC MANAGEMENT (TABLE 1-2)

The patient should gradually increase fiber supplementation every 7 to 10 days and, if necessary, advance to saline agents like milk of magnesia or Epsom salts. A patient could alternatively be prescribed a stool softener. Patients can increase the dose of stool softener with the goal of attaining soft, not liquid, stools. If the previous measures fail, then the physician should add a stimulant or an osmotic agent.

REFERRAL

A gastroenterologist should be consulted when a colonoscopy is appropriate, when the primary physician has not identified the culprit condition causing symptoms of constipation, or when fiber supplementation/laxatives/stool softener have failed to alleviate the constipation.

PEARLS & CONSIDERATIONS

- Pelvic floor dysfunction and irritable bowel syndrome should be considered in patients in whom pharmacologic management fails to control the symptoms of constipation.
- All patients on narcotics should also be on a combination drug regimen including a stimulant and stool softener.

SUGGESTED READINGS

Locke III GR, Pemberton JH, Phillips SF: American Gastroenterological Association practice technical review on constipation, *Gastroenterology* 119:1161-1178, 2000.
Rao SSC: Constipation: evaluation and treatment, *Gastroenterol Clin North Am* 32:659-683, 2003.

AUTHOR: **MICHAEL P. GERARDO, D.O., M.P.H.**

TABLE 1-2 Pharmacologic Management of Constipation

Type	Dosage	Onset of Action	Side Effects
Fiber		12-24 hr	Bloating and flatulence
Bran	1-4 tsp daily		
Psyllium	1 tsp twice daily		
Methylcellulose	1 tsp twice daily		
Calcium polycarbophil	1-2 tablets twice daily		
Stool Softener		12-72 hr	
Docusate sodium	100 mg twice daily		
Osmotic Agents			Cramping, bloating, flatulence
Sorbitol	15-16 mL three times daily	24-48 hr	
Lactulose	15-60 mL three times daily	24-48 hr	
Polyethylene glycol (PEG)	17 gm in 8 oz liquid once or twice daily	0.5-1 hr	
Magnesium hydroxide, magnesium sulfate	15-30 mL twice daily	3-12 hr	
Stimulants			Cramping, bloating, flatulence
Bisacodyl	5-15 mL twice daily	6-8 hr	
Senna	2-4 tabs bid	8-12 hr	
Cascara	5-15 mL prn	8-12 hr	
Lubricants			Malabsorption of fat-soluble vitamins
Mineral oils	15-45 mL twice daily	1-6 hr	
Enemas			Trauma, hyperphosphatemia
Tap water	500 mL per rectum	5-15 min	
Mineral oils	100-250 mL per rectum	1-6 hr	
Phosphate	120 mL per rectum	5-15 min	
Soap suds	up to 1500 mL per rectum	5-15 min	

BASIC INFORMATION

DEFINITION

Delirium is an acute change in mental status that is not otherwise explained by an underlying psychiatric illness such as dementia. It is often a harbinger of a serious medical illness in older persons and may be the only presenting sign of an occult illness.

SYNONYMS

Acute change in mental status
Acute confusion
Acute brain failure
Delirium tremens—associated with alcohol withdrawal

ICD-9CM CODES

290.11 Presenile dementia with delirium
290.3 Senile dementia with delirium
290.41 Multi-infarct dementia with delirium
291.0 Alcohol withdrawal delirium
292.81 Drug-induced delirium
293.0 Acute delirium
293.1 Subacute delirium
293.81 Delirium, transient organic with delusions
293.82 Delirium, transient organic with hallucinations
296.0 Mania with delirium

EPIDEMIOLOGY & DEMOGRAPHICS

Delirium may arise at any point during the course of a medical illness but is most common in the hospital setting. Prevalence rates range from 10% to 40% on admission to the hospital with another 25% to 50% developing delirium during the course of hospitalization. Postoperative and intensive care patients are at much greater risk of delirium with rates of 10% to 60% and 70% to 87%, respectively. There is no gender difference with delirium.

- Delirium is a multifactorial syndrome and is thus caused by multiple interrelated factors. Essentially any medical condition may precipitate a delirium but older persons have identifiable risk factors that increase their risk of delirium and contribute to the development and severity of delirium. These are often divided into baseline or predisposing risk factors and hospital-related or predisposing risk factors.
- Common predisposing risk factors are:
  ○ Medications (anticholinergic medications)
  ○ Comorbid conditions
  ○ Sensory impairment
  ○ Malnutrition
  ○ Preexisting cognitive impairment

- Common precipitating risk factors include:
  ○ Medications (narcotics or sedatives)
  ○ Immobilization
  ○ Restraints
  ○ Dehydration
  ○ Indwelling catheters
  ○ Infection
  ○ Metabolic abnormalities (e.g., hypoxia, hypoglycemia)

PHYSICAL FINDINGS & CLINICAL PRESENTATION

- Delirium must occur in the context of a medical illness, metabolic derangement, drug toxicity, or drug withdrawal. The symptoms cannot be explained by an underlying dementia.
- Symptoms and signs:
  ○ Acute change in mental status
  ○ Fluctuating course
  ○ Inattention
  ○ Disorganized thinking
  ○ Altered level of consciousness (hypoactive/lethargic or hypervigilant and agitated)
  ○ Altered perceptions (illusions, hallucinations)
  ○ Decreased function
- Review history, establish baseline cognitive and functional status, and look for symptoms of occult infection/illness.
- Review medications (new, omitted, withdrawn, interactions, herbal therapies, OTC).
- Full set of vital signs.
- Complete physical exam.
- Neurologic exam (new focal deficits).

ETIOLOGY

The etiology of delirium is unknown. Increasing evidence points to the suppression of the cholinergic nervous system as a strong contributor.

DIAGNOSIS

DIFFERENTIAL DIAGNOSIS

- Dementia
- Depression
- Acute psychotic illness

WORKUP

The initial diagnosis of delirium must include a thorough assessment of baseline cognitive function in older persons, especially for those with potential preexisting cognitive impairment. Often, caregivers and family members can provide valuable information concerning baseline functional and cognitive status. According to the Confusion Assessment Method (CAM), a screening test for detecting delirium, the diagnosis of delirium is made if the following have been met:
1. There is an acute change in cognition based on an objective cognitive assessment and a fluctuating course.

2. Inattention is present; that is, difficulty focusing on the task at hand or easily distracted.
3. Disorganized thinking is present, including decreased memory, disorientation, altered visual perceptions.
4. Altered level of consciousness is present, which can be present as either agitation or hypervigilance, or lethargy and hypoactive state.

Criteria 1 and 2 must be present and either 3 or 4 to screen positive for delirium.

LABORATORY TESTS

- No specific test exists to screen for or diagnose delirium. Refer to algorithm for details.
- Complete blood count, electrolytes including calcium, glucose, kidney function, urinalysis, urine culture.
- Consider, blood culture, TSH, ABG, cortisol, vitamin B_{12} level, toxic screen, drug levels if applicable, or lumbar puncture with CSF analysis (for fever of unknown origin).

IMAGING STUDIES

- CXR to rule out occult pneumonia, CHF
- Brain imaging—with focal neurologic signs and symptoms

TREATMENT Rx

NONPHARMACOLOGIC THERAPY

Treatment involves both the identification and reduction of any potential risk factors and the treatment of acute agitation simultaneously.
Identification of risk factors:
- It is important to identify all contributing risk factors and try to eliminate or reduce any risk factors that can be changed. For example, reorientation, assistance with nutrition and fluid intake, or elimination of medications with deliriogenic or anticholinergic properties. Removal of restraints and prevention of bed rest with frequent ambulation in the hallway will prevent delirium and help reduce symptoms.
- Other nonpharmacologic strategies include increasing the family presence to reduce anxiety, transferring to a quiet room, and correcting sensory deficits (using glasses for vision loss and hearing amplifier devices for hearing loss).
- Use of a nonpharmacologic sleep protocol (which includes a backrub, warm drink, relaxing music, and uninterrupted sleep) has been validated as an important method to avoid sleep medications and prevent delirium.

ACUTE GENERAL Rx

- Medications to treat delirium should only be used in severely agitated individuals whose behavior threatens to interrupt medical care or if a safety hazard for patients or staff exists.
- Doses should be started at the lowest dose and for a limited time. Often standing low doses of antipsychotics may help manage symptoms with minimal side effects. Recommendations are largely based on empiric evidence; little research on treatment of delirium exists.
- Types of medications:
  - Haloperidol 0.25 to 1.0 mg may be repeated every 30 minutes until the patient is calm and alert. Maximum 24-hour dose should be limited to 5 mg.
  - Atypical antipsychotics including risperidone, olanzapine, and quetiapine can also be used with the same principles.
  - Benzodiazepines, especially lorazepam, are the drugs of choice for alcohol or sedative withdrawal but should be limited to third line therapy for agitation.

CHRONIC Rx

- Minimize medications that can contribute to delirium.
- Minimize risk factors.
- Avoid hospitalization if possible.
- Discontinue or wean off antipsychotic or anxiolytic medications that were begun for acute management of agitation and delirium. These medications are often continued indefinitely for no definite reason and result in significant side effects.

DISPOSITION

- Older persons with delirium are at higher risk of dying or being transferred to a skilled nursing facility where the symptoms of delirium can persist for up to 6 months. Delirium is also associated with an increased hospital and postacute cost of care.

REFERRAL

- Consider referral to a geriatrician or geriatric psychiatrist for complicated delirium or for patients with agitation that is difficult to manage.

PEARLS & CONSIDERATIONS

COMMENTS

- Delirium is common in the elderly and associated with negative outcomes.
- Delirium is often the only sign of a life-threatening medical illness.
- Delirium is a multifactorial syndrome often precipitated by multiple predisposing and precipitating risk factors.
- Older persons with dementia are at much higher risk of developing delirium and are more likely not to be recognized as having a delirium.
- Recognition of delirium can be enhanced by using tools such as the Confusion Assessment Method.

- Treatment of delirium should include both the reduction of risk factors and the treatment of agitation.

PREVENTION

- Identification of high-risk patients and implementing nonpharmacologic strategies can help reduce the rate of delirium by 33%. Avoidance of medications highly associated with delirium can also prevent the development of delirium.

PATIENT/FAMILY EDUCATION

- Patients and families should be educated on delirium if it occurs to improve understanding of the changes and that most of the changes are reversible.

SUGGESTED READINGS

Hospital Elder Life Program: http://elderlife.med.yale.edu/public/public-main.php

Inouye SK et al: A multicomponent intervention to prevent delirium in hospitalized older patients, *New Engl J Med* 340:669, 1999.

Marcantonio ER et al: Reducing delirium after hip fracture: a randomized trial, *J Am Geriatr Soc* 49:516, 2001.

McCusker J et al: Delirium predicts 12-month mortality, *Arch Intern Med* 162:457, 2002.

McDowell JA et al: A non-pharmacological sleep protocol for hospitalised older persons, *J Am Geriatr Soc* 46:700, 1998.

AUTHOR: **LYNN MCNICOLL, M.D.**

BASIC INFORMATION

DEFINITION

Dementia means loss of mental functions. It is a syndrome of acquired and persistent cognitive deficits that includes memory impairment in association with impairments in abstract thinking, judgment, or other disturbances of higher cortical function (e.g., aphasia, apraxia, agnosia, executive functioning) or personality change. The disturbances are severe enough to interfere significantly with work, usual social activities, or relationships with others. Dementia is not diagnosed if the symptoms occur exclusively in the context of delirium. It must be an acquired loss of function, and hence is distinguished from developmental disorders such as mental retardation. Dementia can have many etiologies, as will be noted. (Adapted from DSM-III-R and DSM-IV.)

ICD-9CM CODES

290.0 Senile dementia, uncomplicated
      DSM-IV: Dementia of the Alzheimer's type, late onset
290.1 Presenile dementia
      DSM-IV: Dementia of the Alzheimer's type, early onset, uncomplicated
290.4 Arteriosclerotic dementia
      DSM-IV: Vascular dementia
294.1 Dementia in conditions classified elsewhere (code first underlying physical condition, e.g., listed as follows)
      DSM-IV: Dementia due to:
      331.0 Alzheimer's disease
      331.82 Dementia with Lewy bodies
      331.19 Frontotemporal dementia
      310.1 Mild memory disturbances, not amounting to dementia, associated with senile brain disease
294.9 Unspecified organic brain syndrome (chronic)
      DSM-IV: Cognitive Disorder NOS

SYNONYMS

Senile dementia
Presenile dementia
Senile psychosis

EPIDEMIOLOGY & DEMOGRAPHICS

INCIDENCE: Annual dementia incidence rate approximately doubles every 5 years after age 65; approximately 7 to 9 per 1000 at age 65-69 and 85 to 118 per 1000 at age 85 and older.

PREVALENCE: Approximately 8% to 10% of U.S. population (4 million to 6 million) above age 65 have dementia; prevalence approximately doubles every 5 years after age 65; prevalence is ap-

proximately 2% at age 65 and 34% to 68% at age 85 and older.

PREDOMINANT ETIOLOGY: Alzheimer's disease (AD) is by far the most common cause of dementia. Approximately 55% to 70% of all dementias have a significant contribution from Alzheimer's pathology and approximately 35% of all dementias may be attributable to pure AD. Vascular dementia and dementia with Lewy bodies are thought to be the next most common etiologies. Prevalence rates of dementia etiologies vary across ethnic groups.

PREDOMINANT SEX: Varies by dementia diagnosis; AD is more common in females; vascular dementia and dementia with Lewy bodies is more common in males; frontotemporal dementia appears to occur equally in males and females.

PREDOMINANT AGE: Incidence and prevalence increase over age 65 and are highest at age 85 and older; average age of onset is younger in frontotemporal dementia and some relatively rare, familial subtypes of AD (see as follows).

PEAK INCIDENCE AND PREVALENCE: Age 85 and older.

GENETICS: First-degree relatives may be at increased risk for certain types of dementia (e.g., AD, frontotemporal dementia); apolipoprotein ε4 allele is a genetic risk factor for AD but is not diagnostic. Genetic disorders causing dementia include Huntington's disease, CADASIL (cerebral autosomal dominant arteriopathy with subcortical infarcts and leukoencephalopathy), and early-onset familial AD. Some forms of frontotemporal dementia have genetic linkages.

PHYSICAL FINDINGS & CLINICAL PRESENTATION

See Fig. 1-13.
Physical findings and clinical presentation differ across dementia etiologies.

ETIOLOGY

ALZHEIMER'S DISEASE

Prevalence: AD is the most common cause of dementia; contributes to dementia in approximately 55% to 70% of all cases; pure AD accounts for approximately 35% of all cases.

Core features:
- Gradually progressive memory impairment with insidious onset.
- Impairment in executive function, spatial abilities, and language follow later.
- Behavioral dysregulation may also occur later.

Pathology:
- Extraneuronal plaques (protein: β amyloid-42).
- Intraneuronal neurofibrillary tangles (protein: hyperphosphorylated form of tau).
- Definitive diagnosis requires clinicopathologic correlation.

Genetics and family history:
- Risk of AD is about four times greater in patients with a first-degree relative with AD.
- ApoE ε4 allele on chromosome 19 increases risk of AD and shifts age of onset 3 to 7 years earlier than in those with sporadic onset who do not have an ε4 allele; risk is further increased in presence of first-degree relative with AD.
- Approximately 2% of AD cases are early-onset familial AD related to mutations in either chromosome 14 (presenilin 1), 1 (presenilin 2), or 21 (amyloid precursor protein).
- Almost all patients with Down syndrome will develop AD pathology after age 40.

Key cognitive features:
- Memory impairment is cardinal feature; impairment in language, visuoconstructional ability, executive functioning, and other cognitive domains follows.
- Motor and sensory function generally intact until late stages.

Neurologic features:
- Normal exam early.
- Later stages can be associated with extrapyramidal or parkinsonian features.
- Impairment in gait, speech, urinary and fecal continence, and reemergence of primitive reflexes may occur in final stages.

Key neuroimaging features:
- Useful for ruling out alternate (e.g., neoplasm, hydrocephalus) or concomitant (e.g., vascular lesions) causes of dementia.
- MRI may reveal diffuse cortical atrophy with ex vacuo ventricular enlargement particularly in temporal horns of lateral ventricle due to hippocampal volume loss; severity of imaging findings generally increases with severity of dementia.
- Temporoparietal hypometabolism on SPECT or PET.
- Neuroimaging is not diagnostic.

Course:
- Insidious onset with gradual progression; memory is usually first symptom.
- Average survival is about 8 years depending on age at diagnosis and concomitant medical conditions; survival may be up to 20 years.

VASCULAR DEMENTIA (VAD)

Prevalence: VaD is the second or third most common cause of dementia, accounting for about 10% to 30% of all dementia cases; prevalence increases with age; more common in men.

Core features:
- Focal neurologic signs/symptoms.
- Neuroimaging evidence of cerebrovascular disease.

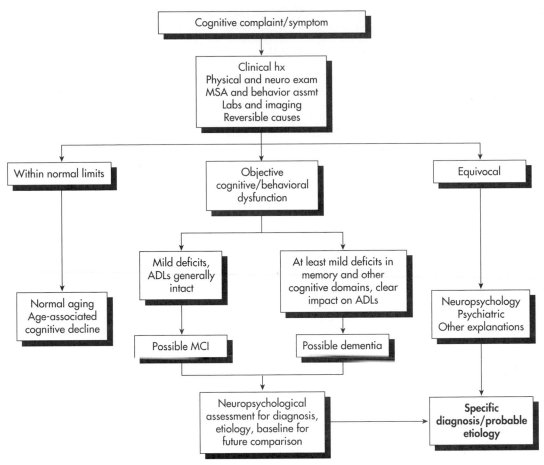

FIGURE 1-13 Evaluation of dementia. *ADLs,* Activities of daily living

- Impairment in executive functioning, speed of mental processing, with relatively mild memory deficits in most cases (particularly true for VaD due to microvascular disease).
- Apathy may be prominent.

Pathology: VaD can result from large-vessel or small-vessel disease or a combination of the two. Most VaD cases are caused by small-vessel disease. Mendez and Cummings (2003) identify three main pathologic mechanisms of VaD:

- Large-vessel (macrovascular) VaD typically arises from multiple bilateral thromboembolic infarctions; involvement of cortical regions.
- Small-vessel (microvascular) VaD typically arises from arteriosclerotic changes in subcortical arteries causing injury to periventricular and deep white matter and to subcortical grey nuclei (e.g., caudate, putamen, and thalamus). The injuries include complete infarction (i.e., lacunar infarction) and incomplete infarction that appear as diffuse white matter lesions on neuroimaging (i.e., hyperintense on T2 MRI sequences; hypodense on CT). In some cases, a single strategic small-vessel infarction in a critical circuit (e.g., left thalamus) may cause multiple cognitive deficits of sufficient

severity to warrant a diagnosis of dementia. Diffuse white matter lesions may also cause dementia, if sufficiently extensive (i.e., involves ≧25% of white matter).
- Episodes of hypoperfusion hypoxia.

Genetics and family history:
- Increased risk with family history of stroke.
- Genetic causes are relatively rare; CADASIL is one cause of dementia due to microvascular disease; it is autosomal dominant and linked to mutation in the notch3 gene on chromosome 19.

Key cognitive features:
- When due to multiple cortical infarcts, the pattern of cognitive impairment may vary depending on location of infarcts (e.g., language deficits from left hemisphere lesion, spatial deficits from right hemisphere lesion).
- Subcortical ischemic vascular disease is characterized by deficits in psychomotor processing speed, mental flexibility, executive function, and memory retrieval.
- Single subcortical strategic infarct (i.e., anterior thalamus) may be sufficient to cause widespread cognitive dysfunction and dementia.
- Apathy may be prominent.

Neurologic features:
- Focal neurologic signs or symptoms (e.g., exaggerated deep tendon reflexes, extensor plantar response, spastic limb weakness) that vary with location and size of lesions.

Key neuroimaging features:
- Evidence of cortical or subcortical infarction.
- Diffuse areas of high signal on T2-weighted MRI (low signal on CT), particularly in periventricular and deep white matter regions.
- Clinical or radiologic evidence of cerebrovascular disease required for diagnosis.
- Absence of cortical or hippocampal atrophy adds confidence to differential diagnosis of VaD vs. AD.

Course:
- Difficult to predict.
- May have abrupt onset with stepwise course.
- Onset and course may be more gradual, especially when due to subcortical small-vessel disease.
- Onset and progression may be gradual with punctuated declines associated with discrete cerebrovascular events.
- High mortality rate and lower life expectancy than AD; 50% survival rate from symptom onset is about 6.7

years; heart disease or stroke is common cause of death.

DEMENTIA WITH LEWY BODIES (DLB)

Prevalence: Second or third most common cause of dementia; accounts for approximately 14% to 20% of all dementia cases.

- Almost two thirds are male.
- Majority do not have pure DLB but also have concomitant AD pathology.

Core features:
- Parkinsonism
- Cognitive fluctuations
- Visual hallucinations (occur in 40% to 70% of cases)
  - Usually vivid, well-formed of humans or animals
- Dementia plus two core features are needed for diagnosis of *probable* DLB; one core feature is needed for *possible* DLB.
- Other supportive features:
  - Repeated falls
  - Syncope; transient loss of consciousness
  - Delusions
  - Rapid eye movement (REM) sleep behavior disorder
  - Neuroleptic sensitivity

Pathology: Lewy body inclusions (protein: mainly α-synuclein, but ubiquitin and tau are also present) in diffuse brain regions including cortical neurons.

Genetics and family history:
- No genes identified in sporadic DLB cases.
- A rare autosomal dominant form exists related to mutations in α-synuclein gene on chromosome 4.

Key cognitive features:
- Marked attentional fluctuations.
- Frontal-executive dysfunction.
- Prominent visuospatial impairment.
- Deficits occur in memory, confrontational naming, and praxis; may not be as severe as in AD.

Neurologic features:
- Extrapyramidal signs present in 25% to 50% at diagnosis and most develop it over disease course.
- Up to 25% of autopsy-confirmed cases may not have report of extrapyramidal symptoms.
- Axial bias to symptoms; i.e., greater postural instability, gait impairment, and facial impassivity and relatively less tremor than in Parkinson's disease.

Key neuroimaging features:
- Less pronounced hippocampal/medial temporal lobe atrophy compared with AD.
- Quantitative volumetric measurements may show atrophy of putamen.
- Neuroimaging not diagnostic.

Course:
- Initial symptoms could be parkinsonism followed by cognitive impairment or the opposite: cognitive symptoms followed by parkinsonism.

- Shorter survival times than AD; about 7.7 ± 3.0 years from onset of cognitive symptoms.

FRONTOTEMPORAL DEMENTIA (FTD)

Prevalence:
- Accounts for approximately 2% to 5% of all dementia cases.
- Accounts for 20% of neurodegenerative dementias in people under 65 years old.
- Average age of onset is 57 years with a typical range of 51 to 63.

Core features:
- Personality changes are most prominent symptom and typically precede cognitive changes:
  - Decline in social comportment
  - Impaired regulation of personal conduct
  - May become disinhibited but are more likely to display apathy
  - Lack of attention to personal hygiene can be supportive of diagnosis

Pathology:
- FTD is the main syndrome of frontotemporal lobar degeneration (FTLD)—a spectrum of dementing disorders involving degeneration of the frontal and anterior temporal lobes.
- Mendez and Cummings (2003) describe three main pathologic variants of FTD:
  - Lacking distinctive histology (FTLD-ldh): neuronal loss, astrogliosis with spongiosis in frontotemporal cortex
  - Pick bodies (FTLD-Pick): severe frontal atrophy ("knife-like" gyri); enlarged neurons called Pick cells and neuronal Pick body inclusions (tau-positive, ubiquitin-positive); FTLD-Pick is diagnosed when Pick bodies are present irrespective of presence of Pick cells
  - Motor neuron disease (MND): involvement of anterior horn cells with or without ubiquitin inclusions

Genetics and family history:
- 38% to 50% of cases have positive history of similar dementia in first-degree family member.
- Several mutations in tau gene have been found in familial FTD.
- Some cases associated with mutations on chromosome 17; linkage to chromosome 3 in some families; presenilin 1 may be involved in some phenotypes.

Key cognitive and behavioral features:
- Early blunting of emotional responsiveness; loss of basic emotions.
- Executive cognitive impairment prominent.
- Compulsive behaviors are common:
  - Klüver-Bucy syndrome may occur: emotional blunting, reduction or loss of fear responding, oral exploration of the environment with dietary preference alterations, hypermetamorphosis (exploration of environmental stimuli as soon as noticed), sensory agnosia, altered sexual behavior.
- Reduction of verbal output.
- Pattern of memory deficits suggests retrieval impairment rather than storage impairment characteristic of AD.

Neurologic features:
- Neurologic features may be absent early with exception of primitive ("frontal release") reflexes (grasp, snout, suck).
- Parkinsonism may be present; may precede dementia and may resemble progressive supranuclear gaze palsy; fasciculations may occur.
- Urinary or fecal incontinence may occur later.

Key imaging features:
- MRI might not be sensitive to early changes; the majority of patients will eventually show anterior-posterior asymmetry of cortical atrophy, being greater in frontal and anterior temporal lobe regions than in posterior brain regions.
- SPECT reveals frontotemporal hypometabolism
- Neuroimaging not diagnostic by itself.

Course:
- Initial and most prominent symptoms are usually changes in personality, social awareness, and behavior, especially disinhibition or apathy.
- Mean age of onset is 57 years with a range of 51 to 63 years.
- Duration is typically 8 to 11 years; may be shorter in MND variant.

MISCELLANEOUS CAUSES OF DEMENTIA

Toxic-metabolic etiologies (4%, including alcohol, recreational drugs, medications); infectious (3%); other movement disorders (6%, e.g., Parkinson's disease, progressive supranuclear palsy, Huntington's disease, corticobasal degeneration); normal pressure hydrocephalus (2.5%); other psychiatric (4%); and miscellaneous (<1%, e.g., dementia due to AIDS, head trauma)

POTENTIALLY REVERSIBLE CAUSES OF DEMENTIA

Medication toxicity/drug interactions; hydrocephalus; brain tumor; infection; electrolyte imbalance; malnutrition; metabolic (i.e., B_{12} deficiency, hepatic encephalopathy); and endocrine disorders (i.e., hypothyroidism)

COGNITIVE CHANGES IN NORMAL AGING

- General slowing of mentation and physical responses; declines occur in complex and divided attention, ability to recall names, executive and visuospatial functions; reduced efficiency in learning and spontaneous recall of new information but memory storage is maintained.

- Terms used to describe cognitive changes in aging: *normal aging, age-associated cognitive decline, age-associated memory impairment.*

MILD COGNITIVE IMPAIRMENT (MCI)

- MCI is a syndrome (not an etiology) defined by subjective and objective impairment in memory or other cognitive domains that represents a decline and is greater than expected for age, but is of insufficient severity to significantly affect activities of daily living or to warrant a diagnosis of dementia.
- The term *mild cognitive impairment* is often used to describe this period, but the term is not universally accepted and alternatives have been proposed (e.g., *cognitive impairment no dementia*).
- Diagnostic criteria for MCI were developed based on those at high risk for AD. Criteria include subjective memory complaint, objective memory impairment for age/education on formal testing; generally intact global cognitive functioning; generally persevered daily functioning; and no dementia.
  - These criteria are now thought to describe *amnestic MCI*—a group with an approximately 12% annual rate of conversion to AD (vs. 1% to 2% for normal elderly).
  - Current MCI conceptualization includes other subtypes that might go on to develop different types of dementia.

DIAGNOSIS

- Two-step process:
  1. Is dementia present? and if so
  2. What is the most likely etiology?
- No definitive test or algorithm for determining the presence or absence of dementia exists; differentiating normal aging from MCI and MCI from mild dementia is difficult.

DIFFERENTIAL DIAGNOSIS

- Determining etiology requires careful assessment of cognitive and behavioral symptoms, neurologic features, and the onset and temporal course of illness along with laboratory and neuroimaging assessments.
- Determining etiology requires differentiating non-AD dementia from AD.

DEMENTIA VS. AMNESIA

- Amnesia is isolated and profound memory impairment; dementia involves multiple cognitive domains.

DEMENTIA VS. APHASIA

- Difficult because many cognitive tests require a strong language component.
- Nonverbal testing may reveal intact non-language-based cognitive functions.

- Patients with aphasia are more likely than dementia patients to recognize and respond to what is happening around them; and to remember people, places, and routines.

DEMENTIA VS. DEPRESSION

- Depression with cognitive impairment is common in the elderly and may be a risk factor for dementia. Moreover, depression occurs in 12% to 20% of patients with dementia.
- Cognitive deficits: attention, psychomotor processing speed, executive functioning, and memory retrieval; may reflect reduced concentration, loss of interest, and motivation.
- Neuropsychologic testing may be helpful. Depressed patients are likely to benefit from cueing and recognition formats during memory testing, whereas AD patients do not.
- Follow-up assessment after a period of treatment may be needed to rule out dementia.

DEMENTIA VS. DELIRIUM

- Delirium generally has a more rapid onset than dementia.
- Marked attentional disturbances/fluctuations are more common in delirium.
- Delirium can be superimposed on a preexisting dementia or mild cognitive impairment.

NORMAL AGING VS. MCI

- The key judgments are whether the complaints and severity of cognitive impairment represent a decline that exceeds normal aging; the extent to which the impairments disrupt normal functioning; and whether they are better explained by psychiatric disorder, substance abuse, medication effects, situational stressors, or other nonneurodegenerative etiologies.
- Neuropsychologic testing may be very helpful.

MCI VS. MILD DEMENTIA

- The key judgments are the scope and severity and stability of cognitive or behavioral impairment and the degree to which they affect daily functioning.
- Neuropsychologic testing may be very helpful.

WORKUP

CLINICAL HISTORY

- Key symptoms; onset and progression; impact on activities of daily living.
- Obtain information from a reliable informant.
- Obtain a medication history and identify those that can disrupt cognition.
- Screen for depression.
- Family history of dementia.
- Review of systems.

PHYSICAL AND NEUROLOGIC EXAM

- General health
- Focal neurologic signs

- Frontal release signs
- Apraxias

MENTAL STATUS ASSESSMENT (MSA)

- Evaluate arousal, orientation, attention/mental control, memory, language, conceptual or semantic knowledge, praxis (ability to perform skilled movements, e.g., ask the patient to pretend to light a cigarette), mental calculations, visuoconstructional abilities, executive functions, and behavior.
- Mini Mental State Exam (MMSE): the most commonly administered formal mental status test; takes 5 to 10 minutes (see Appendix 2); can be supplemented with assessment of executive functions and abstract reasoning.
  - Executive function
    1. *Alternating figures:* copy and continue producing alternating figures (e.g., ++O ++O). Look for loss of sequence or perseverations.
    2. *Alternating movements:* place both hands on a table, one in a fist, one palm down; then alternate repeatedly. Demonstrate briefly and then have the patient continue independently. Look for loss of sequence.
  - Abstract conceptualization: similarities (e.g., "How are an apple and a banana alike?" include more than one similarity pair e.g., boat-car, watch-ruler, desk-bookcase). Look for concrete responses; differences instead of similarities. Responses can be influenced by educational and intellectual background.
- Mini-Cog exam consists of a 3-item memory test and clock drawing; it takes 2 to 3 minutes to administer. It may be as accurate as the MMSE in a primary care setting.
- Behavior: appearance; mood and affect; level of insight; thought content and process; psychosis; anxiety disorders; sleep and appetite.

LABORATORY TESTS

- Blood
  - Thyroid panel or thyroid stimulating hormone
  - Complete blood count, vitamin B_{12}, folate
  - Electrolytes, BUN, creatinine
  - Liver function tests
  - Glucose
  - Syphilis or AIDS if high clinical suspicion
  - Other tests directed by differential diagnosis
- Urinalysis
- Lumbar puncture: optional; if suspicion of cancer, infectious process, atypical presentation (e.g., rapid progression)
- EEG: if history of seizures, rapid decline, suspicion of Creutzfeldt-Jacob disease

- Neuroimaging: CT or MRI of the head is appropriate to rule out hydrocephalus, mass lesions, and subdural hematomas and to assess for extent of cortical and subcortical atrophy, and cerebrovascular lesion load; SPECT or PET for cerebral metabolism may be helpful, especially for FTD

TREATMENT

NONPHARMACOLOGIC THERAPY

- Ensure patient safety: e.g., driving, wandering, cooking, ironing, tool use, medication management, nutrition, hygiene and grooming, financial management.
- Establish routines, avoid chaotic or overstimulating environments.
- Family education.
- Caregiver support/respite: support groups, daycare, sharing caregiving with other family members.
- Cerebrovascular risk factor control includes adequate treatment of hypertension, hypercholesterolemia, and diabetes.

PHARMACOLOGIC THERAPY

- Cognitive impairment:
  - Acetylcholinesterase inhibitors (i.e., donepezil, galantamine, rivastigmine) approved for AD; they slow the course of cognitive decline, not disease modifying. May also be useful for vascular dementia.
  - Memantine (NMDA receptor antagonist) for moderate to severe AD.
  - For dementias other than AD, there are few pharmacologic options.
- Agitation and psychosis:
  - Atypical antipsychotics including risperidone and olanzapine are widely used but not FDA approved.

Use lowest dose needed and try to wean off as soon as possible. Potential increased risk of cerebrovascular accidents. Avoid use of antipsychotics in patients with diffuse Lewy body dementia.
  - Benzodiazepines can occasionally be useful usually as second line therapy.
- Depression: selective serotonin reuptake inhibitors can be effective for the treatment of coexisting depression among those with dementia.

DISPOSITION

- Deterioration over time is a common feature of most dementias.
- Goals of currently available treatments are to slow course and maximize functioning.
- Transition to assisted living facilities may be helpful as dementia worsens; nursing home placement may follow.

REFERRAL

- Neuropsychologic assessment can help determine presence/absence of dementia and the pattern of cognitive impairment may help identify etiology.
- Geriatric psychiatry if depression or other psychiatric disturbance is prominent.
- Neurology referral is necessary to assess general neurologic status, especially if motor, sensory, or gait disturbance is present.

PEARLS & CONSIDERATIONS

- Search for and treat potentially reversible causes of dementia.
- Treat psychiatric disturbances (e.g., depression, agitation, psychosis, but be careful with antipsychotics in DLB).

- Reduce/control risk factors for cognitive impairment: cerebrovascular risk; medications that may contribute to cognitive impairment; alcohol; depression.

PREVENTION

- Reduction of cardiovascular risk factors including treatment of hypertension, hypercholesterolemia, and diabetes.
- Promoting cognitive exercises and mental activity can help ward off progression.
- Maintaining a healthy social life.

PATIENT/FAMILY EDUCATION

- Alzheimer's Association local support groups can offer useful education for families and caregivers.

SUGGESTED READINGS

Knopman DS et al: Practice parameter: diagnosis of dementia (an evidence-based review). Report of the quality standards subcommittee of the American Academy of Neurology, *Neurology* 56:1143-1153, 2001.

McKeith I et al: Dementia with Lewy bodies, *Lancet Neurol* 3:19-28, 2004.

Mendez MF, Cummings JL: *Dementia: A Clinical Approach,* ed 3, Philadelphia, 2003, Butterworth Heinemann.

Petersen RC: Mild cognitive impairment as a diagnostic entity, *J Intern Med* 256:183-194, 2004.

Roman GC: Vascular dementia revisited: diagnosis, pathogenesis, treatment, and prevention, *Med Clin North Am* 86:477-499, 2002.

Rosenstein LD: Differential diagnosis of the major progressive dementias and depression in middle and late adulthood: a summary of the literature of the early 1990s, *Neuropsychol Rev* 8:109-167, 1998.

Strub RL, Black FW: *The Mental Status Examination in Neurology,* ed 4, Philadelphia, 2000, FA Davis.

AUTHORS: **STEPHEN CORREIA, PH.D.,** and **LYNN MCNICOLL, M.D.**

BASIC INFORMATION

DEFINITION

Major depressive disorder (MDD) is defined as having one or more major depressive episodes (MDE). According to the *Diagnostic and Statistical Manual of Mental Disorders* (DSM-IV-TR), an MDE is defined as at least 2 weeks of depressed mood or loss of interest, accompanied by four or more of the following symptoms: change in appetite or weight, sleep disturbance, psychomotor agitation or slowing, fatigue or loss of energy, worthlessness or guilt, poor concentration or indecisiveness, and thoughts of suicide or death.

RELATED DISORDERS

- Bipolar disorder includes MDEs and manic episodes.
- Minor depressive disorder is defined as 2 weeks of two to four of the MDE criteria.
- Dysthymic disorder is a low-grade chronic condition that entails depressed mood most days for 2 years without ever experiencing an MDE.
- Psychotic depression is a severe form of MDD in which the criteria for an MDE are met and delusions or hallucinations are also present.
- There are additional mood and anxiety disorders that include symptoms of depression.
- In the context of bereavement or reactions to stress, consider the diagnosis of MDD if significant symptoms exist or if social or occupational functioning is impaired.
- In the elderly, "depression" may encompass more than just MDD because some people experience severe depressive symptoms that do not meet diagnostic criteria for MDD.

ICD-9CM CODES

296.2 Major depressive disorder, single episode
296.3 Major depressive disorder, recurrent episode
296.1 Manic disorder, recurrent episode
298.0 Depressive type psychosis
300.4 Neurotic depression
311 Depressive disorder, not elsewhere classified

EPIDEMIOLOGY & DEMOGRAPHICS

PREVALENCE: Studies suggest that the point prevalence of MDD in elderly community-dwelling individuals is about 1%. In addition, 3% to 4% of community elderly report symptoms consistent with dysthymia and 8% to 15% have clinically significant depressive symptoms. Among nursing home residents, major depression is present in 10% to 15% and depressive symptoms in another 18%. Among persons with dementia, depression rates can range from 15% to 25%.
PREDOMINANT SEX: Female > male, approximately 2:1. The highest risk for suicide is in older Caucasian men.
PREDOMINANT AGE: Studies suggest that depressive symptoms peak in midlife; however, older patients may underreport their symptoms.
PEAK INCIDENCE: For people over age 65, the highest rates are in the oldest old and in medical settings.
GENETICS: First-degree relatives may have increased risk. The apolipoprotein E4 allele may be associated with the onset of depressive symptoms in late life.

PHYSICAL FINDINGS & CLINICAL PRESENTATION

- Older depressed patients sometimes focus on somatic complaints.
- Any symptoms of an MDE could be the chief complaint, including paranoid thinking.
- Carefully distinguish between psychomotor slowing and parkinsonism.
- Additional symptoms include anhedonia, guilt feelings, frequent crying episodes, and a sense of helplessness and worthlessness.
- Severe concentration disturbance in a depressed older person can mimic early dementia.
- History of the depressive illness should include the following:
  ○ Past history of psychiatric symptoms (i.e., MDEs, manic symptoms, psychotic symptoms, substance abuse, dangerous behavior or emergency evaluation or inpatient treatment)
  ○ Targeted review of medical symptoms (i.e., fever, fatigue, weight loss, decreased exercise tolerance)
  ○ Assessment of situational factors (i.e., social support, financial strain, recent losses)
- Physical examination should include a complete neurologic examination.

ETIOLOGY

- Depression is likely the result of complex interactions between genetic predisposition, neurochemical and endocrine status, stressful psychosocial circumstances, and dysfunctional patterns of thinking.
- Some depressive syndromes in late life may be due, in part, to frontostriatal and limbic system dysfunction.
- Stroke is a risk factor for depression.
- Subcortical atrophy may correlate with depressive symptoms in late life.

DIAGNOSIS

DIFFERENTIAL DIAGNOSIS

- Hypothyroidism
- Anemia
- Vascular disease
- Major organ system impairment (i.e., lymphoma, congestive heart failure, renal failure)
- Treatment side effect (i.e., antihypertensives, chemotherapy)
- Parkinson's disease
- Dementia
- Consider other late-life mood or anxiety disorders
- Consider a primary sleep disorder if insomnia is prominent

WORKUP

- Mental Status Examination, including assessment of appearance, alertness, orientation, speech/language function, reported mood, observed affect, thought content (with particular attention to the presence or absence of (1) suicidal thoughts, (2) homicidal thoughts, or (3) delusions), thought process (i.e., logical vs. disorganized), perception (if auditory hallucinations exist, check to see if the "voices" command or instruct the patient, and what the specific instructions entail), attention, memory, insight, and judgment.
- Consider using the Geriatric Depression Scale (GDS) to quantify the intensity of depressive symptoms; and if significant concentration or attention disturbance exists, conduct a structured cognitive assessment such as the Mini Mental State Examination (MMSE). See Appendix 2 for scales.
- If allowable, elicit additional behavioral information from family or well-informed others (such as nursing home staff).
- Risk assessment (see Pearls & Considerations).

LABORATORY TESTS

- Thyroid panel or thyroid stimulating hormone
- Complete blood count, vitamin B_{12}, and folate
- Electrolytes, blood urea nitrogen, creatinine
- Additional tests as directed by the differential diagnosis

NEUROIMAGING & OTHER STUDIES

- Neuropsychologic testing can help distinguish depression from dementia.
- If significantly disrupted sleep or signs and symptoms of apnea are present, obtain a formal sleep study including electroencephalogram.
- Brain MRI may be helpful in cases of known vascular disease.

TREATMENT

NONPHARMACOLOGIC THERAPY

- In the community, the first step in treating depression is to help the family and patient recognize and understand the problem.
- Interpersonal therapy (IPT) and cognitive behavioral therapy (CBT) may be useful for elderly outpatients with depression.
- Electroconvulsive therapy (ECT) is effective and should be considered in cases of severe depression.
- Exercise or bright light treatment can be considered for mild depressive symptoms, depression with a seasonal pattern, or as augmentation of psychotherapy or pharmacologic treatment.

PHARMACOLOGIC THERAPY

- Several algorithms for the treatment of depression have been studied and psychiatric practice guidelines have been published.
- Many depressed geriatric patients prefer to receive treatment in the primary care setting, which has led to investigations toward improving this care.
- Treatment algorithms often begin with the use of an antidepressant medication.
- When choosing a medication, first consider comorbid medical conditions. Avoid agents contraindicated for specific conditions (e.g., do not use bupropion for patients with a history of seizure).
- Selective serotonin reuptake inhibitors (SSRIs) are generally used first line for geriatric patients. Some of the SSRIs have fewer cytochrome P450 hepatic enzyme system interactions (citalopram, escitalopram, and sertraline). Use caution and watch for SSRI-induced hyponatremia.
- Tricyclic antidepressants (TCAs) are used less frequently in the elderly due to potential anticholinergic and cardiac effects.
- A medication's side effect profile can occasionally be of benefit. For example, mirtazapine can be sedating and may also increase appetite, making it a logical choice for depressive symptoms associated with prominent anorexia and insomnia.
- Monoamine oxidase inhibitors (MAOIs) are used only in severely treatment-refractory cases.
- Lithium can be considered for the treatment of an MDE if the patient has a history of bipolar disorder; however use caution due to the potential for drug-induced delirium. Use low doses and target lower serum concentrations for older patients.

- In the outpatient setting, start antidepressants at half the general adult starting dose. Reassess regularly and titrate the dosage for maximum benefit.
- If side effects persist and prevent use of a medication beyond the lowest starting dose, switch to another agent. Otherwise, attempt to complete an adequate trial. For example, reassess depressive symptoms, medical comorbidity, drug dose, and side effects every 2 to 4 weeks during acute outpatient treatment and gradually increase the medication to the highest tolerated dose, up to 50% of the maximum recommended dose, and maintain this for 4 to 6 weeks. If inadequate response persists, refer to psychiatry.

COMBINED TREATMENTS

- For geriatric depression, combined treatment with medication and IPT may be more effective than either treatment alone.
- Combined treatment is preferred for moderate to severe nonpsychotic depression. For mild cases of depression, either medication or psychotherapy alone may be adequate.
- For psychotic depression, patients should be treated by a psychiatrist in an inpatient setting. Treatment with both antidepressant and antipsychotic medication is recommended. ECT is an alternative.

COMPLEMENTARY & ALTERNATIVE TREATMENT

- St. John's wort (Hypericum) is used in Europe as a pharmacologic treatment for depression. It can be purchased over-the-counter in the U.S. but is not approved by the FDA as a treatment for depression. People taking St. John's wort should be advised of potential drug interactions with other antidepressants.

DISPOSITION

- The goals of treatment are to promote remission and decrease the risk of recurrence.
- Continued treatment after remission decreases the likelihood of relapse. For patients who experience their first episode of depression in late life, the general recommendation is at least 1 year symptom free on medication, then reassess. Inform patients of the increased risk for relapse if medication is discontinued. If a decision is made to discontinue treatment, then wean off slowly to prevent withdrawal symptoms and complete a risk assessment in association with each dose reduction.
- The time to recurrence may be shorter in the elderly.

- Patients with a history of more than one MDE should remain on antidepressant treatment.
- Patients with significant cognitive impairment should receive a comprehensive neuropsychologic assessment.

REFERRAL

- Medical inpatients with undertreated depression can benefit from psychiatric consultation.
- Psychologists or care managers can augment pharmacologic treatment provided by a primary care clinician.
- Patients should be seen by a psychiatrist if severe symptoms are present or initial adequate treatment is not effective.
- If significant suicidal thoughts are reported or suspected, an urgent or emergent psychiatric evaluation should be obtained. If necessary, most states allow facilities to hold a patient involuntarily until a thorough examination can be conducted.

PEARLS & CONSIDERATIONS

CAUTION

- Any mention of suicidal thoughts should prompt immediate careful assessment.
- Risk assessment:
  ○ Assess risk factors for dangerous behavior, including:
    1. Current suicidal or homicidal thoughts and any specific plans
    2. Psychotic symptoms or disorganized thinking
    3. Personal or family history of self-injury, violence, psychiatric illness, or substance abuse
    4. Comorbid medical illness
    5. Hopelessness
    6. Access to weapons
    7. Social isolation
  ○ Conduct this assessment in the following circumstances:
    1. When depression is first evaluated
    2. When medications are adjusted or treatment is changed
    3. At any follow-up when an acute worsening or suicidal thoughts are noted
- Additional treatment recommendations and results of the NIH Consensus Development Conference on Depression in Late Life can be found in Alexopoulos (2004).

PATIENT/FAMILY EDUCATION

- Community programs can help elders understand how to recognize depression.
- Support groups and other resources for both patients and family caregivers

may improve the clinical outcome of depression.

SUGGESTED READINGS

Alexopoulos GS: Late-life mood disorders. In Sadavoy J et al. (eds): *Comprehensive Textbook of Geriatric Psychiatry*, New York, 2004, WW Norton, pp 609-654.

American Psychiatric Association, Practice Guidelines: www.psych.org/psych_pract/treatg/pg/prac_guide.cfm

Bruce ML et al: Reducing suicidal ideation and depressive symptoms in depressed older primary care patients: a randomized controlled trial, *JAMA* 291:1081-1091, 2004.

Colenda CC et al: Comparing clinical practice with guideline recommendations for the treatment of depression in geriatric patients: findings from the APA practice research network, *Am J Geriatr Psychiatry* 11:448-457, 2003.

Jacobson SA, Pies RW, Greenblatt DJ: *Handbook of Geriatric Psychopharmacology*, Washington, DC, 2002, American Psychiatric Publishing.

Koenig HG, Blazer DG: Mood disorders. In Blazer DG, Steffens DC, Busse EW (eds): *The American Psychiatric Publishing Textbook of Geriatric Psychiatry*, Washington, DC, 2004, American Psychiatric Publishing, 241-268.

Mueller TI et al: The course of depression in elderly patients, *Am J Geriatr Psychiatry* 12:22-29, 2004.

AUTHOR: **GARY EPSTEIN-LUBOW, M.D.**

BASIC INFORMATION

DEFINITION

- Diabetes mellitus (DM) refers to a syndrome of hyperglycemia resulting from many different causes (see "Etiology"). It can be classified into type 1 (insulin-dependent) and type 2 (non-insulin-dependent) DM. When a type 2 diabetic person needs insulin, she becomes classified as type 2 insulin requiring. Table 1-3 provides a general comparison of the two most common types of diabetes mellitus.
- The American Diabetes Association (ADA) defines DM as (1) a fasting plasma glucose ≥126 mg/dl or (2) a nonfasting plasma glucose ≥200 mg/dl or (3) an oral glucose tolerance test (OGTT) ≥200 mg/dl in the 2-hr sample. Furthermore, the ADA also defines a value of 110 mg/dl on fasting blood sugar as the upper limit of normal for glucose. A fasting glucose between 110 mg/dl and 126 mg/dl is classified as "impaired fasting glucose" (IFG).

SYNONYMS

IDDM (insulin-dependent diabetes mellitus)

NIDDM (non-insulin-dependent diabetes mellitus)

Type 1 diabetes mellitus (insulin-dependent diabetes mellitus)

Type 2 diabetes mellitus (non-insulin-dependent diabetes mellitus)

ICD-9CM CODES

250.0 Diabetes mellitus (NIDDM)
250.1 Insulin-dependent diabetes mellitus without complication (IDDM)

EPIDEMIOLOGY & DEMOGRAPHICS

- DM affects 5% to 7% of the U.S. population. Prevalence in Pima Indians is 35%.
- The vast majority of DM in geriatric patients is type 2.
- Incidence increases with age, with 2% in persons ages 20 to 44 yr to 18% in persons 65 to 74 yr of age.
- Diagnosis is delayed in many patients with type 2 DM.
- Diabetes accounts for 8% of all blindness and is the leading cause of end-stage renal disease in the U.S.
- Patients with diabetes are twice as likely as nondiabetic patients to develop cardiovascular disease.

PHYSICAL FINDINGS & CLINICAL PRESENTATION

1. Symptoms of hyperglycemia: polyuria, thirst, blurred vision.
2. Physical examination varies with the presence of complications and may be normal in early stages.
3. Diabetic retinopathy:
   a. Nonproliferative (background diabetic retinopathy):
      (1) Initially: microaneurysms, capillary dilation, waxy or hard exudates, dot and flame hemorrhages, AV shunts
      (2) Advanced stage: microinfarcts with cotton wool exudates, macular edema
   b. Proliferative retinopathy: characterized by formation of new vessels, vitreal hemorrhages, fibrous scarring, and retinal detachment
4. Cataracts and glaucoma occur with increased frequency in diabetics.
5. Peripheral neuropathy: patients often complain of paresthesias of extremities (feet more than hands); the symptoms are symmetric, bilateral, and associated with intense burning pain (particularly during the night).
   a. Mononeuropathies involving cranial nerves III, IV, and VI; intercostal nerves; and femoral nerves are also common.
   b. Physical examination may reveal:
      (1) Decreased pinprick sensation, sensation to light touch, and pain sensation.
      (2) Decreased vibration sense.
      (3) Loss of proprioception (leading to ataxia).
      (4) Motor disturbances (decreased DTR, weakness and atrophy of interossei muscles); when the hands are affected, the patient has trouble picking up small objects, dressing, and turning pages in a book.
      (5) Diplopia, abnormalities of visual fields.

TABLE 1-3   General Comparison of the Two Most Common Types of Diabetes Mellitus

	Type 1	Type 2
Previous terminology	Insulin-dependent diabetes mellitus (IDDM), type I, juvenile-onset diabetes	Non–insulin-dependent diabetes mellitus, type II, adult-onset diabetes
Age of onset	Usually <30 yr, particularly childhood and adolescence, but any age	Usually >40 yr, but any age
Genetic predisposition	Moderate; environmental factors required for expression; 35%-50% concordance in monozygotic twins; several candidate genes proposed	Strong; 60%-90% concordance in monozygotic twins; many candidate genes proposed; some genes identified in maturity-onset diabetes of the young
Human leukocyte antigen associations	Linkage to DQA and DQB, influenced by DRB (3 and 4) [DR2 protective]	None known
Other associations	Autoimmune; Graves' disease, Hashimoto's thyroiditis, vitiligo, Addison's disease, pernicious anemia	Heterogenous group, ongoing subclassification based on identification of specific pathogenic processes and genetic defects
Precipitating and risk factors	Largely unknown; microbial, chemical, dietary, other	Age, obesity (central), sedentary lifestyle, previous gestational diabetes
Findings at diagnosis	85%-90% of patients have one and usually more autoantibodies to ICA512/IA-2/IA-2β, GAD$_{65}$, insulin (IAA)	Possibly complications (microvascular and macrovascular) caused by significant preceeding asymptomatic period
Endogenous insulin levels	Low or absent	Usually present (relative deficiency), early hyperinsulinemia
Insulin resistance	Only with hyperglycemia	Mostly present
Prolonged fast	Hyperglycemia, ketoacidosis	Euglycemia
Stress, withdrawal of insulin	Ketoacidosis	Nonketotic hyperglycemia, occasionally ketoacidosis

From Andreoli TE (ed): *Cecil essentials of medicine*, ed 5, Philadelphia, 2001, WB Saunders.
GAD, Glutamic acid decarboxylase; *IA-2/IA-2β*, tyrosine phosphatases; *IAA*, insulin autoantibodies; *ICA*, islet cell antibody; *ICA512*, islet cell autoantigen 512 (fragment of IA-2).

6. Autonomic neuropathy:
   a. GI disturbances: esophageal motility abnormalities, gastroparesis, diarrhea (usually nocturnal).
   b. GU disturbances: neurogenic bladder (hesitancy, weak stream, and dribbling), impotence.
   c. Orthostatic hypotension: postural syncope, dizziness, light-headedness
7. Nephropathy: pedal edema, pallor, weakness, uremic appearance. Neuropathy can be detected with a simple exam of the lower extremities using a 10-g monofilament to test sensation.
8. Foot ulcers: occur frequently and are usually secondary to peripheral vascular insufficiency, repeated trauma (unrecognized because of sensory loss), and superimposed infections. If a diabetic foot ulcer has been present for weeks and foot pulses are palpable, neuropathy should be considered a major cause.
9. Neuropathic arthropathy (Charcot's joints). bone or joint deformities from repeated trauma (secondary to peripheral neuropathy).
10. Necrobiosis lipoidica diabeticorum: plaquelike reddened areas with a central area that fades to white-yellow found on the anterior surfaces of the legs; in these areas the skin becomes very thin and can ulcerate readily.
11. May be diagnosed as a result of screening or incidentally.

ETIOLOGY

IDIOPATHIC DIABETES
Type 1 DM
- Hereditary factors:
  1. Islet cell antibodies (found in 90% of patients within the first year of diagnosis)
  2. Higher incidence of HLA types DR3, DR4
  3. 50% concordance in identical twins
- Environmental factors: viral infection (possibly coxsackie virus, mumps virus)
Type 2 DM
- Hereditary factors: 90% concordance in identical twins
- Environmental factor: obesity

DIABETES SECONDARY TO OTHER FACTORS
- Hormonal excess: Cushing's syndrome, acromegaly, glucagonoma, pheochromocytoma
- Drugs: glucocorticoids, diuretics
- Insulin receptor unavailability (with or without circulating antibodies)
- Pancreatic disease: pancreatitis, pancreatectomy, hemochromatosis
- Genetic syndromes: hyperlipidemias, myotonic dystrophy, lipoatrophy
- Gestational diabetes
- Polycystic ovary syndrome

DIAGNOSIS (Dx)

Diagnosis is made on the basis of the following tests and should be confirmed by repeated testing on a different day:
1. Fasting glucose ≥126 mg/dl (ADA criteria)
2. Nonfasting plasma glucose ≥200 mg/dl
- Use of glycosylated hemoglobin (Hb A1c) level is not recommended for diagnosis at this time by the ADA because of lack of standardization of hemoglobin A1c values and the imperfect correlation between HbA1c and fasting plasma glucose levels. However, some physicians use this test to make the diagnosis of diabetes mellitus if the random plasma glucose is >200 mg/dl and the hemoglobin A1c level is ≥2 standard deviations above the laboratory mean.
- Creatinine, urine microalbumin, and lipids should be monitored yearly.
- TSH should be checked from time to time (perhaps less than yearly).

DIFFERENTIAL DIAGNOSIS
- Diabetes insipidus
- Stress hyperglycemia
- Diabetes secondary to hormonal excess, drugs, pancreatic disease

TREATMENT (Rx)

NONPHARMACOLOGIC THERAPY
1. Diet
   a. Calories
      (1) The diabetic patient can be started on 15 calories/lb of ideal body weight; this number can be increased to 20 calories/lb for an active person and 25 calories/lb if the patient does heavy physical labor.
      (2) The calories should be distributed as 55% to 60% carbohydrates, 25% to 35% fat, and 15% to 20% protein.
      (3) The emphasis should be on complex carbohydrates rather than simple and refined starches and on polyunsaturated instead of saturated fats in a ratio of 2:1.
   b. Seven food groups
      (1) The exchange diet of the ADA includes protein, bread, fruit, milk, and low- and intermediate-carbohydrate vegetables.
      (2) The name of each exchange is meant to be all inclusive (e.g., cereal, muffins, spaghetti, potatoes, rice are in the bread group; meats, fish, eggs, cheese, peanut butter are in the protein group).
      (3) The glycemic index compares the rise in blood sugar after the ingestion of simple sugars and complex carbohydrates with the rise that occurs after the absorption of glucose; equal amounts of starches do not give the same rise in plasma glucose (pasta equal in calories to a baked potato causes less of a rise than the potato): thus, it is helpful to know the glycemic index of a particular food product.
      (4) Fiber: insoluble fiber (bran, celery) and soluble globular fiber (pectin in fruit) delay glucose absorption and attenuate the postprandial serum glucose peak; they also appear to lower the elevated triglyceride level often present in uncontrolled diabetics.
2. Exercise increases the cellular glucose uptake by increasing the number of cell receptors. The following points must be considered.
   a. Exercise program must be individualized and built up slowly.
   b. Insulin is more rapidly absorbed when injected into a limb that is then exercised, and this can result in hypoglycemia.
3. Weight loss: to ideal body weight if the patient is overweight. This is the single most important goal of the nonpharmacologic arm of management.

PHARMACOLOGIC THERAPY
- When the previous measures fail to normalize the serum glucose, oral hypoglycemic agents (e.g., metformin, glitazones, or a sulfonylurea) should be added to the regimen in type 2 DM. Table 1-4 describes commonly used oral hypoglycemic agents. The sulfonamides and the biguanide metformin are the oldest and most commonly used classes of hypoglycemic drugs.
- The goal of treatment is to achieve a stable Hb A1c under 6.5%.
- Metformin's primary mechanism is to decrease hepatic glucose output. Because metformin does not produce hypoglycemia when used as a monotherapy, it is preferred for most patients. It is contraindicated in patients with renal insufficiency and used with caution in patients with chronic liver disease or CHF.
- Pioglitazone and rosiglitazone increase insulin sensitivity and are useful as single agents or in addition to other agents in type 2 diabetics whose hyperglycemia is inadequately controlled. Serum transaminase levels should be obtained before starting therapy and monitored periodically. Edema is a common complication.

TABLE 1-4 Oral Antidiabetic Agents as Monotherapy

	Sulfonylureas	Biguanides	α-Glucosidase inhibitors	Thiazolidinediones	Meglitinides
Generic name	Glimepiride, glyburide, glipizide, chlorpropamide, tolbutamide	Metformin	Acarbose, miglitol	Rosiglitazone, pioglitazone	Repaglinide, nateglinide
Mode of action	↑↑ Pancreatic insulin secretion chronically	↓↓ HGP; ↓ peripheral IR; ↓ intestinal glucose absorption	Delays PP digestion of carbohydrates and absorption of glucose	↓↓ Peripheral IR; ↑↑ glucose disposal; ↓ HGP	↑↑ Pancreatic insulin secretion acutely
Preferred patient type	Diagnosis age >30 yr, lean, diabetes <5 yr, insulinopenic	Overweight, IR, fasting hyperglycemia, dyslipidemia	PP hyperglycemia	Overweight, IR, dyslipidemia, renal dysfunction	PP hyperglycemia, insulinopenic
Therapeutic effects					
↓ HBA$_{1c}$* (%)	1-2	1-2	0.5-1	0.8-1	1-2
↓ FPG* (mg/dl)	50-70	50-80	15-30	25-50	40-80
↓ PPG* (mg/dl)	~90	80	40-50	—	30
Insulin levels	↑	—	—	—	↑
Weight	↑	−/↓	—	−/↑	↑
Lipids	—	↓ LDL ↓↓ TG	—	↑ Large "fluffy" LDL ↓↓ TG ↑ HDL	—
Side effects	Hypoglycemia	Diarrhea, lactic acidosis	Abdominal pain, flatulence, diarrhea	Edema	Hypoglycemia (low-risk)
Dose(s)/day	1-3	2-3	1-3	1	1-4+
Maximum daily dose (mg)	Depends on agent	2550	150 (<60-kg bw) 300 (>60-kg bw)	Depends on agent	16 (repaglinide), 360 (nateglinide)
Range/dose (mg)	Depends on agent	500-1000	25-50 (<60-kg bw) 25-100 (>60-kg bw)	Depends on agent	0.5-4 (repaglinide), 60, 120 (nateglinide)
Optimal administration time	~30 min premeal (some with food, others on empty stomach)	With meal	With first bite of meal	With meal (breakfast)	Preferably <15 (0-30 min) premeals (omit if no meal)
Main site of metabolism/ excretion	Hepatic/renal, fecal	Not metabolized/ renal	Only 2% absorbed/fecal	Hepatic/fecal	Hepatic/fecal

Modified from Andreoli TE (ed): *Cecil essentials of medicine*, ed 5, Philadelphia, 2001, WB Saunders.

↑, Increased; ↓, decreased; —, unchanged; *bw*, body weight; *FPG*, fasting plasma glucose; *HDL*, high-density lipoprotein; *HGP*, hepatic glucose production; *IR*, insulin resistance; *LDL*, low-density lipoprotein; *PP*, postprandial; *PPG*, postprandial plasma glucose; *TG*, triglyceride.

*Values combined from numerous studies; values are also dose dependent.

- Sulfonylureas and meglitinides are insulin secretagogues. The latter work best when given before meals because they increase the postprandial output of insulin from the pancreas. All sulfonylureas are relatively contraindicated in patients allergic to sulfa.
- Acarbose and miglitol work by competitively inhibiting pancreatic amylase and small intestinal glucosidases delay gastrointestinal absorption of carbohydrates, thereby reducing alimentary hyperglycemia. The major side effects are flatulence, diarrhea, and abdominal cramps.
- Insulin is indicated for the treatment of all type 1 and type 2 DM patients whose diabetes cannot be adequately controlled with diet and oral agents. Table 1-5 describes commonly used types of insulin. The risks of insulin therapy include weight gain, hypoglycemia, and, in rare cases, allergic or cutaneous reactions. Replacement insulin therapy should mimic normal release patterns. Approximately 50% to 60% of daily insulin should be a basal type consisting of a long-acting insulin (NPH, Ultralente, glargine) injected once or twice daily; the remaining 40% to 50% should be short-acting or rapid-acting insulin (regular, aspart, lispro) to cover mealtime carbohydrates and correct elevated current glucose levels. Among long-acting insulins, once-daily bedtime insulin glargine is as effective as once- or twice-daily NPH but has a lower risk of nocturnal hypoglycemia and less weight gain. When using short-acting insulins, insulin aspart and insulin lispro are more effective in lowering postprandial glucose levels than regular insulin.
- Combination therapy of various hypoglycemic agents is commonly used when monotherapy results in inadequate glycemic control.
- Continuous subcutaneous insulin infusion (CSII, or insulin pump) provides better glycemic control than does conventional therapy and comparable to or slightly better control than multiple daily injections.
- Low-dose ASA to decrease the risk of cerebrovascular disease is beneficial for diabetics over age 30 with other risk factors (hypertension, dyslipidemia, smoking, obesity).
- A fasting serum lipid panel should be obtained yearly on all adult diabetic

TABLE 1-5 Types of Insulin

Insulin type	Generic name	Preprandial injection timing* (hr)	Onset* (hr)	Peak* (hr)	Duration* (hr)	Blood glucose (BG) nadir* (hr)
Rapid acting	Lispro†	0-0.2	0.2-0.5	0.5-2	<5	2-4
Short acting	Regular	0.5-(1)	0.3-1	2-6	4-8 (≤16)	3-7 (Pre-next meal)
	Lente		1-2	4-12		
Intermediate acting	NPH	0.5-(1)	1-3	6-15	16-26	6-13
Long acting‡	Ultralente	0.5-(1)	4-6	8-30	24-36	10-28
Mixed, short/intermediate acting	70/30					
	50/50	0.5-(1)	0.5-1	3-12	16-24	3-12

From Andreoli TE (ed): *Cecil essentials of medicine,* ed 5, Philadelphia, 2001, WB Saunders.
70/30, 70% NPH, 30% regular; *50/50,* 50% NPH, 50% regular; *NPH,* neutral protamine Hagedorn.
*Times depend on several factors including dose, anatomic site of injection, method (SQ, IM, IV), duration of diabetes, degree of insulin resistance, level of activity, and body temperature. Some time ranges are wide to include data from several separate studies. Preprandial injection depends on premeal BG values as well as insulin type. If BG is low, may need to inject insulin and eat immediately (carbohydrate portion of meal first). If BG is high, may delay meal after insulin injection and eat carbohydrate portion last.
†Insulin analogue with reversal of lysine and proline at positions 28 and 29 on the β chain.
‡Insulin glargine [rDNA origin] is a newer, once-daily insulin analog (Lantus) that provides 24-hour basal glucose-lowering with once-a-day bedtime dosing. Onset of action is 2-3 hr, duration of action is 24+ hr.

patients. Strict lipid control (LDL <70 mg/dl) is indicated in all diabetics. Use of statins is often necessary to achieve therapeutic goals.

DISPOSITION

The Diabetes Control and Complications Trial (DCCT) proved that intensive treatment decreases the development and progression of complications of DM. In this trial, the risks of retinopathy, nephropathy, and neuropathy were decreased by 35% to 90%. Each patient should be made aware of these findings. The United Kingdom Prospective Diabetes Study (UKPDS) confirmed the benefit of tight glycemic control, but also demonstrated that blood pressure control in patients with DM is as important as glycemic control. Target BP control in patients with DM is 130/80 or lower.

- Retinopathy occurs in approximately 15% of diabetic patients after 15 yr and increases 1%/yr after diagnosis.
- The frequency of neuropathy in type 2 diabetics approaches 70% to 80%. Gabapentin (900-3600 mg/day) is effective for the symptomatic treatment of peripheral neuropathic pain. Amitriptyline, duloxetine, and carbamazepine can also be effective.
- Nephropathy occurs in 35% to 45% of patients with type 1 DM and in 20% of type 2 DM. The first sign of renal involvement in patients with DM is most often microalbuminuria, which is classified as incipient nephropathy. ACE inhibitors are effective in slowing the progression of renal disease in both type 1 and type 2 DM, independently of their reduction in blood pressure. ARBs and nondihydropyridine calcium channel blockers are also effective in protecting against the progression of

nephropathy in diabetics, especially in type 2 DM.
- Infections are generally more common in diabetics because of multiple factors, such as impaired leukocyte function, decreased tissue perfusion secondary to vascular disease, repeated trauma because of loss of sensation, and urinary retention secondary to neuropathy.
- Hyperosmolar coma is described in detail in Section I.

REFERRAL

- Diabetic patients should be advised to have annual ophthalmologic examination. In type 1 DM, ophthalmologic visits should begin within 3 to 5 years, whereas type 2 DM patients should be seen from disease onset.
- Podiatric care can significantly reduce the rate of foot infections and amputations in patients with DM. Noninfected neuropathic foot ulcers require debridement and reduction of pressure.

PEARLS & CONSIDERATIONS

COMMENTS

- Because normalization of serum glucose level is the ultimate goal, all patients should measure their blood glucose unless contraindicated by senility or blindness.
- For blood glucose monitoring, glucose oxidase strips are used in conjunction with a meter to give a digital reading. The testing can be done once-a-day, but the time should be varied each day so that over a period of time the serum glucose level before meals and at bedtime can be assessed frequently without pricking the patient's fingers four times daily.

- Glycosylated hemoglobin should be measured at least twice yearly; measurement of microalbumin in the urine on a yearly basis is also recommended.

SUGGESTED READINGS

American Diabetes Association: Position statement: standards of medical care for patients with diabetes mellitus, *Diabetes Care* 25:S33, 2002.

Barr RG et al: Tests of glycemia for the diagnosis of type 2 diabetes mellitus, *Ann Intern Med* 137:263, 2002.

Beckman JA et al: Diabetes and atherosclerosis, *JAMA* 287:2570, 2002.

Boulton AJM et al: Neuropathic diabetic foot ulcers, *N Engl J Med* 351:48-55, 2004.

DeWitt DE, Hirsch IB: Outpatient insulin therapy in type 1 and type 2 DM, *JAMA* 289:2254, 2003.

Holmboe ES: Oral antihyperglycemic therapy for type 2 diabetes, *JAMA* 287:373, 2002.

Mayfield J, White R: Insulin therapy for type 2 DM: rescue, augmentation, and replacement of beta cell function, *Am Fam Physician* 70:489-512, 2004.

Nathan DM: Initial management of glycemia in type 2 diabetes mellitus, *N Engl J Med* 347:1342, 2002.

Remuzzi G et al: Nephropathy in patients with type 2 diabetes, *N Engl J Med* 346:1145, 2002.

Stern MP et al: Identification of persons at high risk for type 2 diabetes mellitus: do we need the oral glucose tolerance test? *Ann Intern Med* 136:575, 2002.

U.S. Preventive Services Task Force: Screening for type 2 DM in adults: recommendations and rationale, *Ann Intern Med* 138:212, 2003.

Zandbergen AM et al: Effect of losartan on microalbuminuria in normotensive patients with type 2 DM, *Ann Intern Med* 139:90, 2003.

AUTHORS: **FRED F. FERRI, M.D.,** with revisions by **TOM J. WACHTEL, M.D.**

BASIC INFORMATION

DEFINITION

- Colonic diverticula are herniations of mucosa and submucosa through the muscularis. They are generally found along the colon's mesenteric border at the site where the vasa recta penetrates the muscle wall (anatomic weak point).
- *Diverticulosis* is the asymptomatic presence of multiple colonic diverticula.
- *Diverticulitis* is an inflammatory process or localized perforation of diverticulum.

ICD-9CM CODES
562.10 Diverticulosis of colon
562.11 Diverticulitis of colon

EPIDEMIOLOGY & DEMOGRAPHICS

- Incidence of diverticulosis in the general population is 35% to 50%.
- Diverticulosis is more common in Western countries, affecting >30% of people >40 yr and >50% of people >70 yr.

PHYSICAL FINDINGS & CLINICAL PRESENTATION

- Physical examination in patients with diverticulosis is generally normal.
- Painful diverticular disease can present with LLQ pain, often relieved by defecation; location of pain may be anywhere in the lower abdomen because of the redundancy of the sigmoid colon.
- Diverticulitis can cause muscle spasm, guarding, and rebound tenderness predominantly affecting the LLQ.

ETIOLOGY

- Diverticular disease is believed to be secondary to low intake of dietary fiber.

DIAGNOSIS

DIFFERENTIAL DIAGNOSIS

- Irritable bowel syndrome
- IBD
- Carcinoma of colon
- Endometriosis
- Ischemic colitis
- Infections (pseudomembranous colitis, appendicitis, pyelonephritis, PID)
- Lactose intolerance

LABORATORY TESTS

- WBC count in diverticulitis reveals leukocytosis with left shift.
- Microcytic anemia can be present in patients with chronic bleeding from diverticular disease. MCV may be ele-vated in acute bleeding secondary to reticulocytosis.

IMAGING STUDIES

- Barium enema will demonstrate multiple diverticula and muscle spasm ("sawtooth" appearance of the lumen) in patients with painful diverticular disease. Barium enema can be hazardous and should not be performed in the acute stage of diverticulitis because it may produce free perforation.
- A CT scan of the abdomen can be used to diagnose acute diverticulitis; typical findings are thickening of the bowel wall, fistulas, or abscess formation.
- Evaluation of suspected diverticular bleeding:
  1. Arteriography if the bleeding is faster than 1 ml/min (advantage: the possible infusion of vasopressin directly into the arteries supplying the bleeding, as well as selective arterial embolization; disadvantages: its cost and invasive nature)
  2. Technetium-99m sulfa colloid
  3. Technetium-99m labeled RBC (can detect bleeding rates as low as 0.12 to 5 ml/min)

TREATMENT

NONPHARMACOLOGIC THERAPY

- Increase in dietary fiber intake and regular exercise to improve bowel function
- NPO and IV hydration in severe diverticulitis; NG suction if ileus or small bowel obstruction is present

ACUTE GENERAL Rx
TREATMENT OF DIVERTICULITIS:

- Mild case: broad-spectrum PO antibiotics (e.g., ciprofloxacin 500 mg bid to cover aerobic component of colonic flora and metronidazole 500 mg q6h for anaerobes) and liquid diet for 7 to 10 days
- Severe case: NPO and IV antibiotic therapy
  a. Ampicillin-sulbactam (Unasyn) 3 g IV q6h *or*
  b. Piperacillin-tazobactam (Zosyn) 4.5 g IV q8h *or*
  c. Ciprofloxacin 400 mg IV q12h plus metronidazole 500 mg IV q6h *or*
  d. Cefoxitin 2 g IV q8h plus metronidazole 500 mg IV q6h
- Life-threatening case: Imipenem 500 mg IV q6h *or* meropenem 1 g IV q8h
- Surgical treatment consisting of resection of involved areas and reanastomosis (if feasible); otherwise a diverting colostomy with reanastomosis performed when infection has been controlled; surgery should be considered in patients with:
  1. Repeated episodes of diverticulitis (two or more)
  2. Poor response to appropriate medical therapy (failure of conservative management)
  3. Abscess or fistula formation
  4. Obstruction
  5. Peritonitis
  6. Immunocompromised patients, first episode in young patient (<40 yr old)
  7. Inability to exclude carcinoma (10% to 20% of patients diagnosed with diverticulosis on clinical grounds are subsequently found to have carcinoma of the colon)

DIVERTICULAR HEMORRHAGE: 70% of diverticular bleeding occurs in the right colon.

1. Bleeding is painless and stops spontaneously in the majority of patients (60%); it is usually caused by erosion of a blood vessel by a fecalith present within the diverticular sac.
2. Medical therapy consists of blood replacement and correction of volume and any clotting abnormalities.
3. Colonoscopic treatment with epinephrine injections, bipolar coagulation, or both may prevent recurrent bleeding and decrease the need for surgery.
4. Surgical resection is necessary if bleeding does not stop spontaneously after administration of 4 to 5 U of PRBCs or recurs with severity within a few days; if attempts at localization are unsuccessful, total abdominal colectomy with ileoproctostomy may be indicated (high incidence of rebleeding if segmental resection is performed without adequate localization).

CHRONIC Rx

Asymptomatic patients with diverticulosis can be treated with a high-fiber diet or fiber supplements.

DISPOSITION

- Most patients with diverticulitis respond well to antibiotic management and bowel rest. Up to 30% of patients with diverticulitis will eventually require surgical management.
- Diverticular bleeding can recur in 15% to 20% of patients within 5 yr.

REFERRAL

Surgical referral when considering resection (see Acute General Rx)

AUTHOR: **FRED F. FERRI, M.D.**

BASIC INFORMATION

DEFINITION

Dupuytren's contracture is a disease of the palmar fascia characterized by nodular fibroblastic proliferation that often results in progressive contractures of the fascia and flexion deformity of the fingers.

ICD-9CM CODES
728.6 Dupuytren's contracture

EPIDEMIOLOGY & DEMOGRAPHICS

PREVALENCE: Varies depending on nationality (see Pearls & Considerations)
PREVALENT AGE: Fifth decade and up
PREVALENT SEX: Male:female ratio of 10:1

PHYSICAL FINDINGS & CLINICAL PRESENTATION

- Usually asymptomatic
- Most common complaints: deformity and interference with the use of the hand by the flexed, contracted fingers (Fig. 1-14)
- Process usually begins in the ulnar side of the hand, often starting at the ring finger
- Isolated painless nodules that eventually harden and mature into a longitudinal cord that extends into the finger
- Lesion often begins in the distal palmar crease
- Overlying skin adherent to the fascia
- Later stages: fibrous cord begins to contract and pull the finger into flexion
- Possible involvement of other fingers, particularly small finger

ETIOLOGY
Unknown

DIAGNOSIS **Dx**

DIFFERENTIAL DIAGNOSIS

- Soft tissue tumor, tendon cyst
- Trigger finger

TREATMENT **Rx**

NONPHARMACOLOGIC THERAPY

- Stretching exercises
- Local heat

DISPOSITION
Rate of development is variable.

REFERRAL

- If joint contracture begins to develop
- For excision of rare nodule that is painful (at any stage)

PEARLS & CONSIDERATIONS

COMMENTS

- Dupuytren's contracture develops earlier and more often in certain families.
- The disorder is more common in Scandinavians, and some Northern Europeans have a 25% prevalence over age 60 yr.
- About 5% of patients develop a similar condition elsewhere, such as Peyronie's disease or Ledderhose disease (involvement of the plantar fascia).
- Soft tissue "pads" in the knuckles may also be present.
- Individuals with these additional findings are considered to have Dupuytren's diathesis, and their disease is generally more severe and recurrent.

SUGGESTED READINGS

Frank PL: An update on Dupuytren's contracture, *Hosp Med* 62:678, 2001.
Khan AA et al: The role of manual occupation in the aetiology of Dupuytren's disease in men in England and Wales, *J Hand Surg* 299(1):12, 2004.
McFarlane RM: On the origin and spread of Dupuytren's disease, *J Hand Surg* 27:385, 2002.
Ragsowansi RH, Britto JA: Genetic and epigenetic influence on the pathogenesis of Dupuytren's disease, *J Hand Surg* 26:1157, 2001.
Thurston AJ: Dupuytren's disease, *J Bone Joint Surg Br* 85(4):469, 2003.

AUTHOR: **LONNIE R. MERCIER, M.D.**

FIGURE 1-14 Dupuytren's contracture. A flexion deformity of the finger is present, with nodular thickening of the fascia to the ring finger.

BASIC INFORMATION

DEFINITION

Dysphagia is defined as difficulty in swallowing either from problems in transferring the food bolus from the oropharynx to the upper esophagus or impairment in transport of the bolus through the body of the esophagus.

SYNONYMS

Oropharyngeal dysphagia
Esophageal dysphagia

ICD-9CM CODES
787.2 Dysphagia
438.82 Dysphagia, late effects CVA
530.3 Esophageal stricture/stenosis
787.2 Dysphagia
530.0 Achalasia

EPIDEMIOLOGY & DEMOGRAPHICS

INCIDENCE
- 7% to 10% people over age 50.
- 30% to 40% of nursing home patients experience some amount of dysphagia.
- 25% of hospitalized patients experience problems swallowing.

PHYSICAL FINDINGS & CLINICAL PRESENTATION

HISTORY: A thorough history often gives clues to the site of the lesion and nature of the problem:
- Are symptoms progressive or intermittent in nature?
- What is the duration and course of the dysphagia?
- What type of food causes dysphagia?
- Describe the symptom; patients often report food "sticking" after swallowing or have to repeat swallows to relieve the dysphagia.
- Is there any substernal pain or heartburn on swallowing?
- Odynophagia—painful swallowing associated with sharp substernal pain
- Medication history.
- Are there any associated symptoms (e.g., aspiration, weight loss, nasal regurgitation, unilateral wheezing, chest pain)?

PHYSICAL EXAMINATION
- Skin for signs of collagen vascular disease such as scleroderma
- Oral cavity and pharynx for lesions causing obstruction or painful swallowing (mucositis)
- Neck and axilla for thyroid swelling, lymph nodes, or tumor
- Pulmonary for unilateral wheezing, aspiration pneumonia, foreign body, mass
- Neurologic for signs of a neuromuscular disease, cerebrovascular accident, Parkinson's disease, or tardive dyskinesia
- Abdomen for liver and other organomegaly or masses

ETIOLOGY

- Oropharyngeal dysphasia: may be due to a variety of mechanical and neuromuscular conditions.
- Esophageal dysphagia: may be due to mechanical lesions or motility disorders.

DIAGNOSIS

DIFFERENTIAL DIAGNOSIS

- Causes of oropharyngeal dysphagia:
  - Neurologic disorders—ALS, dementia, MS, Parkinson's disease, cerebrovascular accident, tardive dyskinesia, Huntington's disease
  - Muscular and rheumatologic disorders—myopathies, polymyositis, Sjögren's syndrome
  - Metabolic disorders—thyrotoxicosis, Cushing's, amyloidosis
  - Medication side effects—anticholinergics, metoclopramide, amiodarone, HMG COA reductase inhibitors, phenothiazines, over-the-counter medications, bisphosphonates
  - Infectious disease—mucositis (Candida, herpes)
  - Structural disorders—Zenker's diverticulum, esophageal tumors, postsurgical or radiation changes, cervical osteoarthritis and osteophytic impingement, pill-induced injury
- Causes of esophageal dysphagia:
  - Mechanical lesions—intrinsic narrowing, a very large food bolus, or compression from an extrinsic source
    1. Malignant stricture
    2. Peptic stricture
    3. Schatzki's ring
  - Motility disorders—dysphagia equally for both solids and liquids, episodic, usually nonprogressive
    1. Achalasia
    2. Diffuse esophageal spasm
    3. Scleroderma
- Other causes:
  - Globus hystericus—a sensation of a "ball" in the throat, often underlying psychiatric causes. No abnormality in swallowing exists.

WORKUP

- Swallowing evaluation by speech therapist, particularly when there is a risk of aspiration (e.g., in the context of aspiration pneumonia)

LABORATORY TESTS

- Necessary in some cases of metabolic disorders (thyrotoxicosis, Cushing's)
- To identify infections (candida, herpes)

IMAGING STUDIES

- Oropharyngeal dysphagia
  - Barium esophagography.
- Esophageal dysphagia:
  - Upper endoscopy procedure of choice. Barium swallow an alternative.
  - Esophageal manometry and pH.

TREATMENT

ACUTE GENERAL Rx

- Oropharyngeal dysphagia:
  - Treat the underlying neuromuscular or metabolic disorder.
  - Adjust diet as tolerated.
  - Swallowing techniques designed to strengthen muscles used in swallowing.
  - Eliminate medications known to cause or worsen dysphagia (NSAIDs, potassium tablets, doxycycline, bisphosphonates).
  - Gastrostomy tubes—unproven if this reduces the risk of aspiration pneumonia.
- Esophageal dysphagia:
  - Radical surgery
  - Motility disorders can be treated with balloon dilators for the lower esophageal sphincters or injections of botulinum toxin.
  - Dilation of benign strictures or rings.
- Esophageal cancer:
  - Symptomatic relief with stents or dilation.
  - Ablation of tumors with laser or cautery.
- Diffuse esophageal spasm:
  - Supportive care
  - Empirical trial of smooth muscle relaxants (i.e., isosorbide dinitrate, nifedipine)
  - Empirical trial of an antidepressant (i.e., trazodone or amitriptyline)

REFERRAL

- Gastroenterology

PEARLS & CONSIDERATIONS

COMMENTS

- Dysphagia, heartburn, and odynophagia symptoms always indicate a primary esophageal disorder.
- Persistent symptoms should be investigated by an upper endoscopy.
- Consider risk of aspiration; when present, request a swallowing evaluation by a speech therapist and implement recommendations for special textured diets.

SUGGESTED READINGS
American Gastroenterological Association: Medical position statement on management of oropharyngeal dysphagia, *Gastroenterology* 116:452, 1999.
Spieker MR: Evaluating dysphagia, *Am Fam Physician* 61:3639, 2000.

AUTHORS: **SUSAN BERNER, M.D.,** and **ARVIND MODAWAL, M.D., M.P.H., M.R.C.G.P.**

BASIC INFORMATION

DEFINITION

Dystonia is characterized by involuntary muscle contractions (sustained or spasmodic) that lead to abnormal body movements or postures. Dystonia can be generalized or focal.

SYNONYMS

Blepharospasm
Oromandibular dystonia
Torticollis
Writer's cramp

ICD-9CM CODES
333.6 Dystonia musculorum deformans
335.7 Dystonia caused by drugs
333.7 Dystonia, torsion, symptomatic

EPIDEMIOLOGY & DEMOGRAPHICS

PREVALENCE: Estimated at 1 in 3000 persons.
PREDOMINANT SEX: Cervical dystonia has a 3:2 female preponderance.
PREDOMINANT AGE
- Focal cervical dystonia usually has its onset in the fifth decade.
- Hereditary forms may have an onset in childhood or adulthood.
GENETICS: Autosomal dominant, autosomal recessive, and X-linked forms of dystonia have been identified.

PHYSICAL FINDINGS & CLINICAL PRESENTATION

Focal dystonias produce abnormal sustained muscle contractions in an area of the body:
- Neck (torticollis): most commonly affected site with a tendency for the head to turn to one side
- Eyelids (blepharospasm): involuntary closure of the eyelids
- Mouth (oromandibular dystonia): involuntary contraction of muscles of the mouth, tongue, or face
- Hand (writer's cramp) (Fig. 1-15)
Generalized dystonia affects multiple areas of the body and can lead to marked joint deformities.

ETIOLOGY

- Exact pathophysiology is unknown; thought to involve abnormalities of basal ganglia.
- Hereditary forms have been described, including the severe progressive form, dystonia musculorum deformans.

- Sporadic or idiopathic forms occur.
- Dystonia can occur secondary to other diseases such as CNS disease, hypoxia, kernicterus, Huntington's disease, Wilson's disease, Parkinson syndrome, lysosomal storage diseases.
- Acute dystonia can occur following treatment with drugs that block dopamine receptors, such as phenothiazines or butyrophenones.
- Tardive dyskinesia or dystonia can result from long-term treatment with antipsychotic drugs such as phenothiazines or butyrophenones.

DIAGNOSIS

DIFFERENTIAL DIAGNOSIS

- Parkinson's disease
- Progressive supranuclear palsy
- Wilson's disease
- Huntington's disease
- Drug effects

WORKUP

History (including family history, birth history, medication use) and physical examination

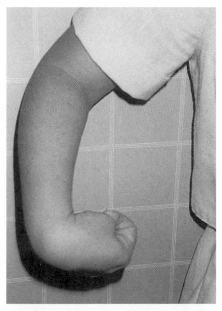

FIGURE 1-15 Focal dystonia of the distal right arm. (From Goldman L, Bennett JC [eds]: *Cecil textbook of medicine,* ed 21, Philadelphia, 2000, WB Saunders.)

LABORATORY TESTS

- Usually not helpful for establishing diagnosis
- Serum ceruloplasmin if Wilson's disease is suspected

IMAGING STUDIES

CT scan or MRI of brain if a CNS lesion is suspected

TREATMENT

NONPHARMACOLOGIC THERAPY

- Heat, massage, physical therapy to relieve pain
- Splints to prevent contractures

ACUTE Rx

For acute dystonic reactions to phenothiazines or butyrophenones use diphenhydramine 50 mg IV or benztropine 2 mg IV.

CHRONIC Rx

- Treatment is often ineffective.
- Slowly withdraw potentially offending agents.
- Diazepam, baclofen, or carbamazepine may be helpful.
- Trihexyphenidyl may be helpful in tardive dyskinesia or dystonia.
- Injections of botulinum toxin into the affected muscles can be used for refractory cases of focal dystonias.
- Surgical procedures including myectomy, rhizotomy, or thalamotomy may be helpful for severe, refractory cases.

DISPOSITION

Spontaneous remission of focal cervical dystonia can occur, but dystonia is generally progressive and pharmacologic therapy is often ineffective.

REFERRAL

To neurologist for severe or refractory cases

SUGGESTED READINGS

Tan N-C et al: Hemifacial spasm and involuntary facial movements, *QJM* 95(8):493, 2002.

AUTHOR: **MARK J. FAGAN, M.D.**

BASIC INFORMATION

DEFINITION

Endometrial cancer is a malignant transformation of endometrial stroma or glands typified by irregular nuclear membranes, nuclear atypia, mitotic activity, loss of glandular pattern, irregular cell size (Fig. 1-16).

SYNONYMS

Uterine cancer (some forms)

ICD-9CM CODES
182 Malignant neoplasm of body of uterus

EPIDEMIOLOGY & DEMOGRAPHICS

INCIDENCE: 21.2 cases/100,000 persons; approximately 30,000 new cases annually
PREDOMINANCE: Median age at onset: 60 yr
RISK FACTORS: Obesity, diabetes, nulliparity, early menarche and late menopause, unopposed estrogen therapy, tamoxifen use, endometrial atypical hyperplasia

PHYSICAL FINDINGS & CLINICAL PRESENTATION

- Abnormal uterine bleeding or postmenopausal bleeding in 90%
- Pyometra or hematometra
- Abnormal Pap smear
- Enlarged uterus

ETIOLOGY

Endogenous or exogenous chronic unopposed estrogen stimulation of the endometrium

DIAGNOSIS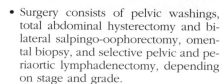

DIFFERENTIAL DIAGNOSIS

- Atypical hyperplasia
- Other genital tract malignancy
- Polyps
- Atrophic vaginitis
- Granuloma cell tumor
- Fibroid uterus

WORKUP

- Complete history and physical examination including pelvic exam to assess uterine size
- Endometrial biopsy or dilation and curettage
- Assessment of operative risk

LABORATORY TESTS

- CBC
- Chemistry profile including liver function tests
- Consider CA-125 level

IMAGING STUDIES

- Chest x-ray examination
- Possible CT scan, BE, or pelvic ultrasound
  - Pelvic ultrasound to assess endometrial thickness may complement a pelvic examination.
- Endovaginal ultrasound in postmenopausal women with vaginal bleeding

TREATMENT

NONPHARMACOLOGIC THERAPY

- Surgery is the mainstay of treatment, with or without radiation, depending on tumor stage and grade.

- Surgery consists of pelvic washings, total abdominal hysterectomy and bilateral salpingo-oophorectomy, omental biopsy, and selective pelvic and periaortic lymphadenectomy, depending on stage and grade.
- Brachytherapy or teletherapy are added in an advanced stage.

ACUTE GENERAL Rx

- Chemotherapy (cisplatin, Adriamycin) or tamoxifen may also be used.

CHRONIC Rx

- Physical and pelvic examination every 3 mo for 2 yr, then every 6 mo for 2 yr, annually thereafter.
- Yearly Pap smear.
- Hormone replacement can be considered in low-risk patients (stage I or early stage II) only to manage bothersome menopausal symptoms that fail to respond to other treatment modalities.

DISPOSITION

The majority of cases present early, where the 5-yr survival is generally good:

Stage I	75% to 100%
Stage II	60%
Stage III	50%
Stage IV	20%

Some histologic types (clear cell, serous papillary) have poorer survival rates.

REFERRAL

A gynecologist may manage early-stage disease; otherwise refer to a gynecologic oncologist.

PEARLS & CONSIDERATIONS

- Any vaginal bleeding in a postmenopausal woman requires ruling out endometrial cancer.
- Pap smear is not a proven method to screen for endometrial cancer.

SUGGESTED READINGS

Smith-Bindman R et al: Endovaginal ultrasound to exclude endometrial cancer and other endometrial abnormalities, *JAMA* 280:1510, 1998.
Suriano KA et al: Estrogen replacement therapy in endometrial cancer patients, *Obstet Gynecol* 97:555, 2001.
Tabor A et al: Endometrial thickness as a test for endometrial cancer in women with postmenopausal vaginal bleeding, *Obstet Gynecol* 99:529, 2002.

AUTHORS: **GIL FARKASH, M.D.,** with revisions by **TOM J. WACHTEL, M.D.**

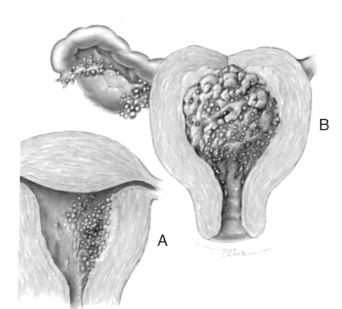

FIGURE 1-16 Carcinoma of the endometrium. A, Stage I. **B,** Stage III, myometrial invasion. (From Sabiston D: *Textbook of surgery,* ed 15, Philadelphia, 1997, WB Saunders.)

BASIC INFORMATION

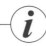

DEFINITION

Erectile dysfunction (ED) is the inability to achieve or sustain a penile erection of adequate rigidity to make intercourse possible.

SYNONYMS

Impotence
Male erectile disorder
Sexual dysfunction (a nonspecific term)

ICD-9CM CODES
F52.2 Male erectile disorder
   DSM-IV Code: 302.72 Male
   erectile disorder

EPIDEMIOLOGY & DEMOGRAPHICS

PREVALENCE (IN U.S.)
- Increases with age.
- 25% for men in their 60s, 80% for men in their 80s.
- The Massachusetts Male Aging Study reports a 1989 prevalence as 52%, with 9.6% of respondents with complete erectile dysfunction; in 2000, the prevalence was 44%.
- Likely underestimated because of social stigma.

PEAK INCIDENCE: Over 70 yr old

CLINICAL PRESENTATION

- Psychogenic impotence: inability to obtain erection, inability to obtain or maintain an adequate erection, or the loss of erection before completion of sexual intercourse; nocturnal penile tumescence usually normal.
- Organic impotence: inability to obtain an erection or inability to obtain an adequate erection; nocturnal penile tumescence usually abnormal.
- Loss of libido suggests hypogonadism.

ETIOLOGY

- Psychogenic erectile dysfunction resulting from a wide range of experiential, historical, or psychological processes.
- Mental health disorders, particularly depression, widower syndrome, and performance anxiety are known psychogenic contributors.
- Organic impotence resulting from a wide variety of insults to neurologic, hormonal, or vascular structures. In approximately 40% of men >50 years of age, the primary cause of ED is related to atherosclerotic disease.
- Medications (antihypertensives, antidepressants, antipsychotics, histamine blockers, nicotine, alcohol, and others) are commonly causative.
- Endocrinopathies such as diabetes, hypogonadism, hypothyroidism or hyperthyroidism, and hyperprolactinemia.

- Neurogenic causes including spinal cord lesions, cortical lesions, and peripheral neuropathies.

DIAGNOSIS

DIFFERENTIAL DIAGNOSIS

- Psychogenic dysfunction distinguished from organic.
- Etiology of organic dysfunction to be determined.
- Erectile dysfunction possible in the setting of another psychiatric condition.

WORKUP

- History (often including partner report) with a focus on risk factors (e.g., smoking, alcohol)
- Report of nocturnal erections
- Physical examination to rule out neuronal damage, direct penile damage (e.g., Peyronie's fibrosis), or testicular atrophy

LABORATORY TESTS

Evaluate for endocrine abnormalities with morning serum testosterone (total and free), FSH, LH, TSH, prolactin, HbA1c or fasting glucose, and lipid panel.

OTHER STUDIES IN SELECTED CASES

- Nocturnal penile tumescence very specific for distinguishing psychogenic versus organic causes.
- Vascular etiologies screened by the penile-brachial pressure index (measures the loss of systolic blood pressure between the arm and penis) or with Doppler studies.
- Neurogenic etiologies examined by the bulbocavernosus reflex or the pudendal-evoked response.
- Intracorporeal injection of prostaglandin E1 to distinguish vascular and nonvascular etiologies (erection is achieved in patients with nonvascular etiologies).

TREATMENT

NONPHARMACOLOGIC THERAPY

- Various psychotherapeutic approaches; success rates decrease with advancing age and duration of symptoms.
- Sex therapy and couples' therapy are used to address technical or social issues that contribute to impotence.
- Vacuum devices (70% to 90% effective) work for many men, but they are difficult to use and cumbersome.

ACUTE GENERAL Rx

- Phosphodiesterase type 5 inhibitors: Sildenafil (Viagra) 50 to 100 mg, or vardenafil (Levitra) 10 to 20 mg before sexual activity, or tadalafil (Cialis) 5 to 20 mg qd prn (effective for 36 hours);

avoid concomitant use of nitrates and α-1 blockers.
- Intracavernosal injections of vasodilators (e.g., papaverine, alprostadil, or prostaglandin E1 pellet).
- Oral medications such as pentoxifylline and yohimbine (limited success).

CHRONIC Rx

- Psychogenic impotence: relatively uncommon and characterized objectively by nocturnal and morning erections and otherwise negative test results. PDE5 inhibitors effective in patients with depression because tissues, nerves, hormones, and vasculature normal. Full psychologic evaluation recommended before starting treatment so underlying problem is addressed.
- For men failing other approaches: penile prosthesis.
- Testosterone therapy in elderly hypogonadal males.

DISPOSITION

- When erectile dysfunction is secondary to an organic cause, it does not remit unless the organic cause is corrected; therefore, it is usually a chronic condition.
- Psychogenic acquired erectile dysfunction will remit spontaneously in 15% to 30% of the cases.

REFERRAL

If psychotherapy, sex therapy, or invasive organic treatment required

PEARLS & CONSIDERATIONS

- Although erectile dysfunction is not part of normal aging, both libido and quality of erection diminish with age. This can lead to performance anxiety, which sometimes can be alleviated with a short-term course of a phosphodiesterase type 5 inhibitor, which can restore ("jump-start") sexual function particularly in older men who have been sexually inactive for a period for a variety of reasons.
- It is often a good idea to involve both partners in a discussion of therapies for ED.
- ED and BPH with lower urinary tract symptoms are often associated. The presence of either should prompt the clinician to inquire about the other.

SUGGESTED READINGS

Fazio L et al: Erectile dysfunction: management update, *Can Med Assoc Jour* 170:1429, 2004.
Fink HA et al: Sildenafil for male erectile dysfunction, *Arch Intern Med* 162:1349, 2002.
Miller TA: Diagnostic evaluation of erectile dysfunction, *Am Fam Physician* 61:95, 2000.

AUTHORS: **AMAR DESAI, M.D., M.P.H.,** with revisions by **TOM J. WACHTEL, M.D.**

BASIC INFORMATION

DEFINITION

Esophageal tumors are defined as benign and malignant tumors arising from the esophagus. Approximately 15% of esophageal cancers arise in the cervical esophagus, 50% in the middle third of the esophagus, and 35% in the lower third. Eighty-five percent of esophageal tumors are squamous cell carcinoma (arising from squamous epithelium). Adenocarcinomas arise from columnar epithelium in the distal esophagus, which have become dysplastic secondary to chronic gastric reflux.

ICD-9CM CODES
150.8 Esophageal cancer, NEC
150.9 Esophageal cancer, NOS
230.1 Carcinoma of esophagus, in situ

EPIDEMIOLOGY & DEMOGRAPHICS

Carcinomas of the esophageal epithelium, both squamous cell and adenocarcinoma, are by far the most common and important tumors of the esophagus. Benign neoplasms are much less common and include leiomyoma, papilloma, and fibrovascular polyps. Prevalence of esophageal carcinoma varies widely in different parts of world, from 7.6 cases per 100,000 persons in the U.S. to 130 cases per 100,000 persons in China. It occurs frequently within the so-called Asian "esophageal cancer belt," extending from the southern shore of the Caspian Sea to northern China, with certain high-incidence pockets in Finland, Ireland, SE Africa, and NW France. In the U.S., 13,900 new cases and 13,000 deaths occur per year, making it the seventh leading cause of death by cancer among men. Esophageal cancer is more common among blacks than whites and has a high male:female ratio of 3:1. It usually develops in the seventh and eighth decades of life and is an illness associated with lower socioeconomic status. More than 50% of patients are diagnosed with esophageal cancer at an advanced stage (unresectable or metastatic disease).

PHYSICAL FINDINGS & CLINICAL PRESENTATION

Symptoms and signs:
- Dysphagia: initially occurs with solid foods and gradually progresses to include semisolids and liquids; later signs usually indicate incurable disease with tumor involving more than 60% of the esophageal circumference, and occurs in 74% of patients.
- Weight loss: more than many of patients present with weight loss usually of short duration. Weight loss >10% of body mass is an independent predictor of poor prognosis.
- Hoarseness: suggests recurrent laryngeal nerve involvement
- Odynophagia: an unusual symptom
- Cervical adenopathy: usually involving supraclavicular lymph nodes
- Dry cough: suggests tracheal involvement
- Aspiration pneumonia: may signal development of a fistula between the esophagus and trachea
- Massive hemoptysis or hematemesis: results from the invasion of vascular structures
- Advanced disease spreads to liver, lungs, and pleura
- Hypercalcemia: usually associated with squamous cell carcinoma because of the secretion of a tumor peptide similar to the parathyroid hormone

ETIOLOGY

Pathogenesis of esophageal cancers is felt to be due to chronic recurrent oxidative damage from any of the following etiological agents listed below, which cause inflammation, esophagitis, increased cell turnover and ultimately, initiation of the carcinogenic process.
Etiologic Agents:
- Excess alcohol consumption: accounts for 80% to 90% of esophageal cancer in the U.S., with whiskey being associated with a higher incidence than wine or beer
- Cigarette smoking: alcohol and tobacco use combined increase the risk substantially
- Other ingested carcinogens:
  Nitrates (converted to nitrites): South Asia, China
  Smoked opiates: Northern Iran
  Fungal toxins in pickled vegetables
- Mucosal damage:
  Long-term exposure to extremely hot tea
  Lye ingestion
- Radiation-induced strictures
- Chronic achalasia: incidence is seven times higher
- Host susceptibility secondary to precancerous lesions:
  Plummer-Vinson syndrome (Paterson-Kelly): glossitis with iron deficiency
  Congenital hyperkeratosis and pitting of palms and soles
- Chronic GERD leading to Barrett's esophagus and adenocarcinoma (whites are affected more than blacks)
- Possible association with celiac sprue or dietary deficiencies of molybdenum, zinc, vitamin A

DIAGNOSIS

DIFFERENTIAL DIAGNOSIS
- Achalasia of the esophagus
- Scleroderma of the esophagus
- Diffuse esophageal spasm
- Esophageal rings and webs

PHYSICAL EXAMINATION
- Monitor weight
- Findings are often limited to cervical and supraclavicular lymph nodes
- Signs of lung consolidation from aspiration pneumonia

LABORATORY TESTS

Complete blood cell count, chemistries, liver enzymes

IMAGING STUDIES
- Double contrast esophagogram effectively identifies large esophageal lesions (Fig. 1-17).
- In contrast to benign esophageal leiomyomata, which cause esophageal narrowing with preservation of normal mucosal pattern, esophageal carcinomas cause ragged ulcerating changes in the mucosa in association with deeper infiltration.
- Smaller tumors can be missed by esophagogram, therefore esophagoscopy is recommended.
- Esophagoscopy is performed to visualize tumor and obtain histopathologic confirmation. In conjunction, an endoscopic ultrasonogram is often performed to determine the depth of tumor invasion.
- This population is also at risk for cancers of head, neck, and lung; therefore endoscopic inspection of larynx, trachea, and bronchi should also be considered.
- Endoscopic biopsies fail to recover malignant tissue one third of the time, thus cytologic examination of tumor brushings should be routinely performed.
- Examination of the fundus of the stomach via retroflexion of the endoscope is also imperative.
- Chest and abdominal CT scan should be performed to determine the extent of tumor spread to mediastinum, paraaortic lymph nodes, and liver.

TREATMENT ℞

ACUTE GENERAL Rx
SURGICAL RESECTION:
- Surgical resection of squamous cell and adenocarcinoma of the lower third of the esophagus is done in most centers if there is no widespread metastasis.
- Less than 20% of patients who survive a total resection can be expected to survive after 5 yr. Usually stomach or colon is used for esophageal replacement.

POSSIBLE COMPLICATIONS OF SURGERY: Anatomic fistula (usually with colon interposition, subphrenic abscesses); respiratory complications are less common as a result of advances in surgical techniques, respiratory therapy, hyperalimentation, and anesthetic support during surgery. Cardiovascular complications are by far the most common including MI, CVA, and PE.

RADIATION THERAPY:

- Squamous cell carcinomas are more radiosensitive than adenocarcinoma, and radiation achieves good local control and is an excellent palliative modality for obstructive symptoms. Usually employed for tumors in upper third of esophagus, often for middle third tumors as well.
- About 40% of tumors cannot be destroyed even after 6000 rads.
- Palliative radiation therapy for bone metastasis is also effective.

COMPLICATIONS OF RADIATION THERAPY:

- Esophageal stricture, radiation-induced pulmonary fibrosis, transverse myelitis are the most feared complications.
- Radiation-induced cardiomyopathy and skin changes occur less frequently given modern techniques.
- Mucositis, GI toxicity, and myelosuppression occur frequently.
- Nephrotoxicity, ototoxicity, and neurotoxicity can develop with cisplatin.

CHEMOTHERAPY:

- Single agent resulted in significant tumor regression in 15% to 25% of patients and combination chemotherapy including cisplatin achieved significant tumor reduction in 30% to 60% of patients.

COMBINATION CHEMOTHERAPY, RADIATION Rx, AND SURGICAL Rx:

- Combination therapy has not been found to be associated with improved survival, however, many centers are using preoperative chemotherapy for many patients with esophageal cancer.
- Palliative procedures such as repeated endoscopic dilation, surgical placement of feeding tube, or polyvinyl prosthesis to bypass tumors have been used for surgically unresectable patients.

DISPOSITION

- Surgery: 5-yr survival rate is 48% in stages I and II, 20% in advanced stages.
- Radiation therapy: 5-yr survival rate is between 6% and 20%.
- Chemotherapy: Single agent response rate 15% to 38%; combination response rate 80%.
- Combined modality: 18% response rate.
- Patients with stage IV disease receive palliative chemotherapy with a median survival of less than 1 year.

SUGGESTED READINGS

Enzinger PC, Mayer RJ: Esophageal cancer, *N Engl J Med* 349:2241, 2003.

Shaheen N et al: Gastroesophageal reflux, Barrett esophagus, and esophageal cancer: clinical applications, *JAMA* 287(15):1982, 2002.

AUTHORS: **LYNN MCNICOLL, M.D.,** and **MADHAVI YERNENI, M.D.**

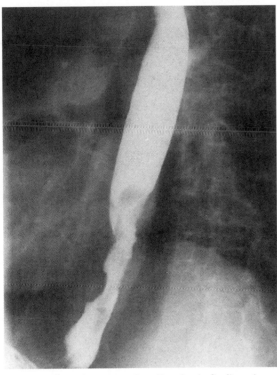

FIGURE 1-17 Barium swallow demonstrating the classic findings in cancer of the distal third of the esophagus. (From Nobel J [ed]: *Primary care medicine,* ed 2, St Louis, 1996, Mosby.)

BASIC INFORMATION

DEFINITION

A predominantly postural and action tremor that is bilateral and tends to progress slowly over the years in the absence of other neurological abnormalities.

ICD-9CM CODES
333.1 Essential tremor

EPIDEMIOLOGY & DEMOGRAPHICS

About 415/100,000 in persons over 40 yr. No gender or racial predominance.

PHYSICAL FINDINGS & CLINICAL PRESENTATION

- Patients complain of tremor that is most bothersome when writing or holding something, such as a newspaper, or trying to drink from a cup. Worsens under emotional duress and drinking liquids
- Tremor, 4 to 12 Hz, bilateral postural and action tremor of the upper extremities. May also affect the head, voice, trunk, and legs. Typically is the same amplitude throughout the action, such as bringing a cup to the mouth. No other neurologic abnormalities on examination. Patients often note improvement with small amount of alcohol.

ETIOLOGY

Often an inherited disease, autosomal dominant; sporadic cases without a family history are frequently encountered

DIAGNOSIS

DIFFERENTIAL DIAGNOSIS

- Parkinson's disease—tremor is usually asymmetric, especially early on in the disease, and is predominantly a resting tremor. Patients with Parkinson's disease will also have increased tone, decreased facial expression, slowness of movement, and shuffling gait.

- Cerebellar tremor—an intention tremor that increases at the end of a goal-directed movement (such as finger to nose testing). Other associated neurologic abnormalities include ataxia, dysarthria, and difficulty with tandem gait.
- Drug-induced—there are many drugs that enhance normal, physiologic tremor. These include caffeine, nicotine, lithium, levothyroxine, β-adrenergic bronchodilators, valproate, and SSRIs.
- Wilson's Disease—wing-beating tremor that is most pronounced with shoulders abducted, elbows flexed, and fingers pointing towards each other. Usually there are other neurologic abnormalities including dysarthria, dystonia, and Kayser-Fleischer rings on ophthalmologic examination.

WORKUP

- All imaging studies normal (MRI, CT) and are usually unnecessary unless there are other associated neurologic abnormalities
- Check TSH

TREATMENT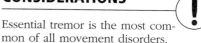

Do not need to treat essential tremor unless it is functionally impairing. Patients need to understand that treatments are only 40%-70% effective.

NONPHARMACOLOGIC THERAPY

Reduction of stress. Minimize use of caffeine. Small quantities of alcohol at social functions tend to be beneficial.

ACUTE GENERAL Rx

Can take a dose of propranolol (20-40 mg) in preparation for specific event.

CHRONIC Rx

First-line agents
- Propranolol: Usual starting dose is 30 mg. Usual therapeutic dose is 160-320 mg. Must be used with caution in those with asthma, depression, cardiac disease, and diabetes.

- Primidone: Usual starting dose is 12.5 to 25 mg hs. Usual therapeutic dose is between 62.5 and 750 mg daily. Sedation and nausea when first beginning medication are biggest side effects.

Other agents
- Neurontin: 400 mg qhs, usual therapeutic dose is 1200-3600 mg
- Topamax: 25 mg qhs, may titrate up to about 400 mg
- Alprazolam: 0.75-2.75 mg

SURGICAL Rx

Thalamic deep brain stimulation contralateral to side of tremor

DISPOSITION

Patients should be reassured that the condition is not associated with other neurologic disabilities; however, it can become quite functionally disabling over time.

REFERRAL

This is a condition that usually can be treated by the primary care physician; however, if patient fails first-line therapies then patient should be referred to specialists for other drug trials and other possible surgical options.

PEARLS & CONSIDERATIONS

Essential tremor is the most common of all movement disorders.

SUGGESTED READINGS

Deuschel G, Volkmann J: Tremors: Differential diagnosis, pathophysiology, and therapy. In Jankovic J, Tolosa E (eds): *Parkinson's disease and movement disorders*, ed 4, 2002, pp. 270-291.

Louis ED: Essential tremor, *N Engl J Med* 345(12):887, 2001.

Zesiewicz TA et al: Phenomenology and treatment of tremor disorders. In Hurtig H, Stern M (eds): *Neurologic clinics: Movement disorders* 19:3, 2001, pp. 651-680.

AUTHOR: **CINDY ZADIKOFF, M.D.**

BASIC INFORMATION

DEFINITION

Failure to thrive is a state of decline in an older person that is multifactorial, manifested by weight loss, decreased appetite, poor nutrition, and inactivity, often accompanied by dehydration, depressive symptoms, impaired immune function, and low cholesterol.

SYNONYMS

Frailty, which could be considered a precursor or potential cause of failure to thrive, is a physiologic state of increased vulnerability to stressors, resulting from decreased physiologic reserves or dysregulation of multiple physiologic systems, clinically characterized by the presence of multiple characteristics, including weight loss, fatigue, weakness, low activity levels, slow motor performance, and balance or gait abnormalities. Sarcopenia, a decrease in muscle mass, is a common component of both failure to thrive and frailty.

ICD-9CM CODES

No specific codes for frailty or failure to thrive, but codes available for some of the symptoms and characteristics:
783.21 Weight loss
780.79 Fatigue
781.2 Gait abnormality
311 Depressive disorders

EPIDEMIOLOGY & DEMOGRAPHICS

Because studies have not used standard definitions of either failure to thrive or frailty, estimations of incidence and prevalence are approximate and tentative. Failure to thrive affects 5% to 35% of community-dwelling older adults and 25% to 40% of nursing home residents. One study of frailty found a prevalence of 6.9% among community-dwelling older persons aged 65 years or greater, with a 4-yr incidence of 7.2%. Prevalence of both frailty and failure to thrive increases with age, and may also be higher among women than men. Although there is likely some genetic component to frailty and failure to thrive, no definitive genetic risk factors have been identified. Other potential risk factors for frailty include lower education, lower income, greater number of chronic diseases, cognitive impairment, and depression.

PHYSICAL FINDINGS & CLINICAL PRESENTATION

Criteria for failure to thrive include some combination of:
- Impaired functional status
- Depressive symptoms
- Cognitive impairment
- Poor nutrition or weight loss

Multiple sets of criteria have been proposed for defining frailty, including:
- Low physical activity levels with weight loss
- Three or more of the following: unintentional weight loss, fatigue/exhaustion, weak grip strength, slow gait speed, low physical activity

Elements of the history consistent with failure to thrive or frailty:
- Fatigue or generalized weakness
- Weight loss
- Falls
- Low levels of physical activity
- Depressive symptoms
- Functional decline or impairment in I/ADLs

Physical findings consistent with failure to thrive or frailty:
- Slow gait speed (<1 m/sec)
- Abnormalities of gait or balance
- Weakness (poor grip strength)
- Low BMI (e.g., <22)
- Cognitive impairment
- Decubitus ulcers

ETIOLOGY

Potential underlying causes of failure to thrive and frailty include:
- Cognitive impairment
- Depression
- Effects of chronic or undiagnosed conditions
- Sarcopenia (the loss of muscle mass and strength with age)
- Immune dysregulation with a low level of chronic inflammation
- Neuroendocrine dysregulation
- Nutritional deficits
- Elevated allostatic load (the wear and tear that occurs in an organism over time in the effort to maintain homeostasis)

DIAGNOSIS

DIFFERENTIAL DIAGNOSIS

Although multiple morbidity and disability often occur in persons with frailty or failure to thrive, there is evidence that these are distinct entities. Failure to thrive is a clinical syndrome, and there is no general differential diagnosis. However, it is important to evaluate for remedial causes of the components of failure to thrive (see Section II).

WORKUP

Important components of the assessment of failure to thrive include:
- Cognitive evaluation (e.g., MMSE)
- Depressive symptoms (e.g., Geriatric Depression Scale)
- Function status, including ADLs and IADLs
- Nutritional status
- Medication review (medications that can contribute to failure to thrive include anticholinergics, antiepileptics, digoxin, β-blockers, benzodiazepines, neuroleptics, antidepressants, and glucocorticoids)
- Evaluation of chronic diseases that contribute to failure to thrive (e.g., cancer, chronic lung disease, heart failure, diabetes, recurrent infections, rheumatologic diseases, dementia, stroke, TB, and other systemic infections)

There are no specific laboratory tests or imaging studies generally indicated for evaluation of frailty or failure to thrive. Some basic tests that may be considered to rule out potentially reversible conditions that may contribute to these syndromes are listed below. This list is not exhaustive, and evaluation should be guided by the findings on history and physical.

LABORATORY TESTS
- CBC to rule out anemia or infection
- Albumin and cholesterol to evaluate nutritional status
- TSH to rule out hypothyroidism
- Basic chemistries to evaluate electrolyte balance, renal function, and liver function
- PPD to rule out tuberculosis
- ESR to rule out systemic inflammatory conditions
- Evaluation for potential drug toxicities or interactions (e.g., digoxin, valproic acid, Tegretol)

IMAGING STUDIES
- Evaluations to rule out cancer as indicated by history and physical exam

TREATMENT

There are no specific treatments for the frailty syndrome. Frail older persons may benefit from comprehensive geriatric evaluation. There are specific treatments for different components of the frailty phenotype, which are listed as follows.

NONPHARMACOLOGIC THERAPY

Malnutrition:
- Speech therapy evaluation and treatment as indicated
- Dental evaluation and treatment
- Dietary evaluation
- Review and minimize dietary restrictions
- Assistance with cooking or feeding

Depression:
- Psychotherapy
- Increased socialization

Functional impairment:
- Resistance training (improve muscle mass and strength)
- Physical therapy (improve gait and balance)
- Occupational therapy (improve ADLs)
- Increased physical activity

ACUTE GENERAL Rx

- Failure to thrive and frailty are chronic conditions, with no acute treatments.

CHRONIC Rx

- Depression: antidepressants
- Cognitive impairment: cholinesterase inhibitors, memantine
- Malnutrition: nutritional supplements, can consider appetite-augmenting medications such as mirtazapine, megestrol, or marinol

DISPOSITION

- Older persons with frailty or failure to thrive are at high risk for adverse events such as further functional decline and death, as well as high health care utilization and costs and need for services such as home health care, assisted living, or skilled nursing facilities.

REFERRAL

- Referral for comprehensive geriatrics assessment, physical therapy, occupational therapy, dietary evaluation, or speech therapy is often appropriate.

- Social work referral for assistance accessing various community services can be beneficial, especially when disability is present.

PEARLS & CONSIDERATIONS

COMMENTS

- Failure to thrive and frailty are concepts under development, with no standard definitions.
- Research into the underlying mechanisms and potential interventions for failure to thrive and frailty is ongoing.

PREVENTION

- Early diagnosis and treatment of depression, cognitive impairment, and malnutrition may help prevent or delay failure to thrive.
- Although there are currently no preventive interventions for frailty with a strong evidence base, there is fair evidence that increased physical activity, particularly with a component of resistance training, can improve or prevent some of the characteristics associated with frailty and potentially decrease functional decline.

PATIENT/FAMILY EDUCATION

- Frail older adults and their caregivers can benefit from referral to community services as appropriate.

- Failure to thrive is often a prelude to death in older persons, and presence of failure to thrive should trigger discussions of goals of care and advanced directives with the patient and family.
- If evaluation and treatment of the components of failure to thrive does not improve the patient's condition, the options of hospice or palliative care should be discussed.
- There is no evidence that artificial feeding or hydration prolong life or relieve suffering in the setting of failure to thrive.

SUGGESTED READINGS

Ferrucci L et al: Designing randomized, controlled trials aimed at preventing or delaying functional decline and disability in frail, older persons: a consensus report, *J Am Geriatr Soc* 52:625-634, 2004.

Fried LP et al: Frailty in older adults: evidence for a phenotype, *J Gerontol A Biol Sci Med Sci* 56:M146-M157, 2001.

Fried LP et al: Untangling the concepts of disability, frailty, and comorbidity: implications for improved targeting and care, *J Gerontol A Biol Sci Med Sci* 59:M255-M263, 2004.

Hogan DB et al: Models, definitions, and criteria of frailty, *Aging Clin Exp Res* 15(suppl 3):1-29, 2003.

Robertson RG, Montagni M: Geriatric failure to thrive, *Am Fam Physician* 70(2):343-350, 2004.

Sarkisian CA, Lachs MS: "Failure to thrive" in older adults, *Ann Int Med* 124(12):1072-1078, 1996.

AUTHOR: **SUSAN E. HARDY, M.D., PH.D.**

BASIC INFORMATION

DEFINITION

A fall is defined as an unintentional change in position resulting in an individual coming to rest at a lower level. They typically result from multiple risk factors, changes in gait and balance, and chronic disease in elders.

ICD-9CM CODES

E880.1 Accidental fall on or from sidewalk
E880.9 Accidental fall on or from other stairs or steps
E885.9 Fall from other slipping, tripping, or stumbling, fall on moving sidewalk
E888.1 Fall resulting in striking against other object
E888.8 Other fall
E888.9 Unspecified fall
781.2 Abnormality of gait: ataxic, paralytic, spastic, staggering

EPIDEMIOLOGY & DEMOGRAPHICS

INCIDENCE: Estimated at one in three people aged 65 or older, living in the community. One in two nursing home dwelling elders. The national nursing home fall rate is 1.6 per bed per year. One in 10 falls results in a serious injury.
RISK FACTORS: Independent risk factors for falls include:
- Arthritis
- Depressive symptoms
- Orthostasis
- Impairment in cognition, vision, balance, gait, or muscle strength
- Use of four or more prescription medications
RECURRENCE RATE: Approximately 50% in a given year

PHYSICAL FINDINGS & CLINICAL PRESENTATION

May present to the emergency department with injury.
Falls may not be a presenting complaint in the geriatrics population; however, due to the frequency of falls in elders, an assessment of fall risk should be integrated into the history and physical examination in all geriatrics patients regardless of whether they are seen for falls or not.
History:
- History of prior falls
  ○ Frequency/pattern of falls
- Cause of the fall
  ○ Activity at the time of the fall
  ○ Environment surrounding the fall (e.g., obstacles, uneven/slippery surface)
- Symptoms preceding the fall
  ○ Weakness, dizziness, palpitations, loss of consciousness

- Symptoms following the fall
  ○ Injury
  ○ Unable to stand without assistance (long lie)
- Use of walking aids—cane/walker
- Detailed medical history
  ○ Current medical diagnoses
  ○ Medication use
  ○ Alcohol consumption
- Home environment—lighting, stairs, loose rugs, bathroom, showers, etc.
- Inquire into fear of falling and restrictions in daily activities due to fear of falling
Physical examination:
- Assessment of vision
- Measurement of postural blood pressure
- Neurologic examination for proprioception, muscle strength
- Assessment of cognitive function
- Musculoskeletal examination of the legs and feet
- Cardiovascular examination for dysrhythmia and potential syncope
- Examine for gait and balance disorders. The Get Up and Go test:
  ○ Rise from a straight-backed chair.
  ○ Walk 10 feet, using usual walking aid (cane, walker, etc.).
  ○ Turn.
  ○ Return to the chair and sit down.
  ○ Observe for:
    1. Balance with sitting and upon standing
    2. Pace and stability with walking
    3. Ability to turn without staggering
    4. Time to complete task

ETIOLOGY

The causes of falls are complex but typically involve the interaction between the environment and multiple predisposing factors that increase in prevalence with age such as:
- Changes that affect gait and balance:
  ○ Decreased proprioception
  ○ Increased postural sway
  ○ Orthostatic hypotension
  ○ Slower righting reflexes
- Medical conditions that can affect stability of gait:
  ○ Osteoarthritis
  ○ Stroke
  ○ Peripheral neuropathy
- Sensory impairment in vision and hearing.
- Medications associated with falls are cardiovascular medications that cause orthostatic hypotension, sedatives, or psychoactive medications that can affect gait and balance.

DIAGNOSIS

DIFFERENTIAL DIAGNOSIS

- Near fall
- Syncope

LABORATORY TESTS

- As dictated by history and physical examination
- Drug levels to diagnose specific medication toxicities where suspected

IMAGING STUDIES

- For the diagnosis or exclusion of fracture
- Neuroimaging to rule out intracranial process if focal neurologic findings present on physical examination

TREATMENT

ACUTE GENERAL Rx

- Treatment of injury resulting from the fall

CHRONIC Rx

Interventions to reduce future falls:
- Optimization of chronic conditions that may have contributed to the fall
- Reduction of medications with potential sedative and orthostatic effects
- Reduction of home environmental hazards
- Minimization of activities with high risk for injury
- Appropriate footwear with low heel and thin sole to maximize proprioceptive input
- Teach compensatory strategies for postural hypotension
- Assess for need of an assist device (cane, walker, etc.) for ambulation
- Physical therapy for strengthening, range of motion, gait and balance training
Interventions to reduce injurious falls:
- Assess for coexistent osteoporosis and treat to ensure proper bone health.
- Consider hip protectors in motivated individuals.

DISPOSITION

- Due to the high recurrence rate of falls, older adults with a history of falls require longitudinal assessments with regular re-evaluation.

REFERRAL

- Where abnormalities of strength, gait, or balance are detected, referral to physical therapy for gait, balance, and strength training
- To home health agency for home environmental hazard assessment
- In frail elders or in recurrent falls, referral for a comprehensive geriatrics assessment

PEARLS & CONSIDERATIONS

COMMENTS

- Although common in older adults, gait instability and falls are not a part of normal aging.
- Falls are typically a manifestation of underlying comorbidity and frailty and it is these underlying causes that need to be addressed to prevent future adverse health outcomes.

PREVENTION

- Early identification of high-risk individuals offers greatest promise for fall prevention.

- Due to the frequency of falls, an assessment of fall risk should be integrated into the evaluation of all geriatrics patients regardless of whether they are seen for falls or not.
- Intervention should be directed at the identified underlying cause.

PATIENT/FAMILY EDUCATION

- Falls are not a manifestation of normal aging.
- It is possible to decrease fall risk with a multifaceted intervention; however, an elder who has fallen will remain at risk for future falls.

SUGGESTED READINGS

Bloem BR et al: Falls in the elderly I. Identification of risk factors. *Wien Klin Wochenschr* 113(10):352-362, 2001.
Boers I et al: Falls in the elderly II. Strategies for prevention. *Wien Klin Wochenschr* 113(11-12):398-407, 2001.
Tinetti ME: Preventing falls in elderly persons, *N Engl J Med* 348(1):42-48, 2003.

AUTHOR: **RAM MILLER, M.D.C.M., M.S., F.R.C.P.C.**

BASIC INFORMATION

DEFINITION

A femoral neck fracture occurs within the capsule of the hip joint between the base of the head and the intertrochanteric line.

SYNONYMS

Intracapsular fracture
Subcapital fracture

ICD-9CM CODES
820.8 Femoral neck fracture

EPIDEMIOLOGY & DEMOGRAPHICS

PREVALENCE: Lifetime risk in women approximately 16%
PREVALENT SEX: Female:male ratio of 3:1
PREVALENT AGE: 90% over age 60

PHYSICAL FINDINGS & CLINICAL PRESENTATION

- A hip or groin pain
- Affected limb usually shortened and externally rotated in displaced fractures
- Impacted fractures: possibly no deformity and only mild pain with hip motion
- Mild external bruising

ETIOLOGY

- Trauma
- Age-related bone weakness, usually caused by osteoporosis
- Increased risk of fractures in elderly (decline in muscle function, use of psychotropic medication, etc.)

DIAGNOSIS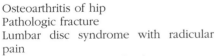

DIFFERENTIAL DIAGNOSIS

Osteoarthritis of hip
Pathologic fracture
Lumbar disc syndrome with radicular pain
Insufficiency fracture of pelvis

WORKUP

Diagnosis usually obvious based on clinical and radiographic findings

IMAGING STUDIES

- Standard roentgenograms consisting of an AP of the pelvis and a cross-table lateral of the hip to confirm the diagnosis (Fig. 1-18)
- If initial roentgenograms negative and diagnosis of an occult femoral neck fracture suspected, hospital admission and further radiographic assessment with either bone scanning or MRI
- Bone scanning most sensitive after 48 to 72 hr.

TREATMENT **Rx**

- Orthopedic consultation
- Surgery indicated in most cases, usually within 24 hr
- DVT prophylaxis

DISPOSITION

- Mortality rate within 1 yr in elderly patients is 25% to 30%.
- Dementia is a particularly poor prognostic sign.

PEARLS & CONSIDERATIONS **!**

COMMENTS

- Complications: nonunion and avascular necrosis
- Intracapsular fractures: occasionally occur in nonambulatory patients
  1. Usually treated nonsurgically, especially in the patient with dementia and limited pain perception
  2. Early bed-to-chair mobilization and vigilant nursing care to avoid skin breakdown
  3. Fracture usually pain free in a short time even if solid bony healing does not occur
- As a result of the increasing life span of the female population, femoral neck fractures are becoming more common. The initial physical examination and roentgenographic studies may be completely negative. Groin pain, sometimes quite severe, may be the only early clue to the diagnosis.

- The rate of hip fracture could be reduced by:
  1. Elimination of environmental hazards (poor lighting, loose rugs)
  2. Regular exercise for balance and strength
  3. Patient education about fall prevention
  4. Medication review to minimize side effects
  5. Prevention and treatment of osteoporosis

SUGGESTED READINGS

Bettelli G et al: Relationship between mortality and proximal femur fractures in the elderly, *Orthopedics* 26:1045, 2003.
Feldstein AC et al: Older women with fractures: patients falling through the cracks of guideline recommended osteoporosis screening and treatment, *J Bone Joint Surg* 85A:2294, 2003.
Jain R et al: Comparison of early and delayed fixation of subcapital hip fractures in patients sixty years of age or less, *Bone Joint Surg* 84(A):1605, 2002.
Kaufman JD et al: Barriers and solutions to osteoporosis care in patients with a hip fracture, *J Bone Joint Surg* 85A:1837, 2003.
Lawrence VA et al: Medical complications and outcomes after hip fracture repair, *Ann Intern Med* 162:2053, 2003.
McClung MR et al: Effect of risedronate on the risk of hip fracture in elderly women. Hip Intervention Program Study Group, *N Engl J Med* 344(5):333, 2001.
McKinley JC, Robinson CM: Treatment of displaced intracapsular fractures with total hip arthroplasty, *J Bone Joint Surg* 84(A):2010, 2002.
Schoofs MW et al: Thiazide diuretics and the risk for hip fractures, *Ann Intern Med* 139:476, 2003.
Stevens JA, Olson S: Reducing falls and resulting hip fractures among older women, *Home Care Prov* 5(4):134, 2000.

AUTHOR: **LONNIE R. MERCIER, M.D.**

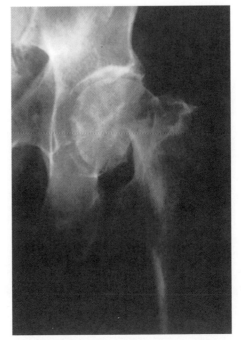

FIGURE 1-18 Femoral neck fracture. (From Scudieri G [ed]: *Sports medicine: principles of primary care*, St Louis, 1997, Mosby.)

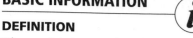

BASIC INFORMATION

DEFINITION

Fibromyalgia is a poorly defined disorder characterized by multiple trigger points and referred pain.

SYNONYMS

Myofascial pain syndrome
Fibrositis
Psychogenic rheumatism
Nonarticular rheumatism
Fibromyalgia syndrome (FS)

ICD-9CM CODES

729.0 Rheumatism, unspecified and fibrositis
729.1 Myalgia and myositis, unspecified

EPIDEMIOLOGY & DEMOGRAPHICS

PREVALENCE: 1% to 2% of the general population
PREVALENT SEX: Female:male ratio of 9:1

PHYSICAL FINDINGS

Tender "nodules" and tender points (Fig. 1-19)

ETIOLOGY

- Unknown
- Pain magnification may play a role
- Associated mood disorder is common

DIAGNOSIS

DIFFERENTIAL DIAGNOSIS

- Polymyalgia rheumatica
- Referred discogenic spine pain
- Rheumatoid arthritis
- Localized tendinitis
- Connective tissue disease
- Osteoarthritis
- Thyroid disease
- Spondyloarthropathies

WORKUP

- Subsets of this disorder are often described:
  1. If symptoms develop in conjunction with other conditions (rheumatoid disease or acute stress)
  2. If findings are more regionally distributed, such as those in the neck following motor vehicle accidents
- The primary condition is often suggested by the following criteria from the American College of Rheumatology:
  1. History of widespread pain
  2. Pain in 11 of 18 selected tender spots on digital palpation (mainly in the spine, elbows, and knees)

LABORATORY TESTS

There are no abnormalities in fibromyalgia, but laboratory assessment may be required to rule out other conditions and may include:
- CBC, ESR, rheumatoid factor, ANA
- CPK, T_4
- 25-hydroxyvitamin D

TREATMENT

ACUTE GENERAL Rx

- Self-management
- Explanation, reassurance
- Vit D replacement in vit D deficient patients
- Aerobic and stretching exercise, particularly swimming
- Mild analgesics; avoidance of chronic narcotic use
- Trigger point injections
- Physical therapy
- SSRIs if associated depression

DISPOSITION

- Prognosis is uncertain.
- Symptoms come and go for years in spite of an aggressive multifaceted approach to treatment.

PEARLS & CONSIDERATIONS

COMMENTS

- Before making this diagnosis, all other more likely disorders should be ruled out.
- The term "fibrositis" is often used, but no inflammation has ever been found.
- The number of trigger points needed to establish the diagnosis is debated.

SUGGESTED READINGS

Clauw DJ: Elusive syndromes: treating the biologic basis of fibromyalgia and related syndromes, *Cleve Clin J Med* 68:830, 2001.

Crofford LJ: Pharmaceutical treatment options for fibromyalgia, *Curr Rheumatol Rep* 6:274, 2004.

Gracely RH et al: Functional magnetic resonance imaging evidence of augmented pain processing in fibromyalgia, *Arthritis Rheum* 46:1333, 2002.

Hakkinen A et al: Strength training induced adaptations in neuromuscular function of premenopausal women with fibromyalgia: comparison with healthy women, *Ann Rheum Dis* 60:21, 2001.

Richards SCM, Scott DL: Prescribed exercise in people with fibromyalgia: parallel group randomized controlled trial, *BMJ* 325:185, 2002.

Robinson RL et al: Depression and fibromyalgia: treatment and cost when diagnosed separately or concurrently, *J Rheumatol* 31:1621, 2004.

Worrel LM et al: Treating fibromyalgia with a brief interdisciplinary program: initial outcomes and predictors of response, *Mayo Clin Proc* 76:381, 2001.

AUTHOR: **LONNIE R. MERCIER, M.D.**

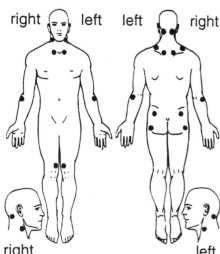

1. Occiput
2. Low cervical
3. Trapezius
4. Supraspinatus
5. Second rib
6. Lateral epicondyle
7. Gluteal
8. Greater trochanter
9. Knees

FIGURE 1-19 The sites of the 18 tender points of the 1990 ACR criteria for the classification of fibromyalgia. (From Conn R: *Current Diagnosis,* ed 9, Philadelphia, 1997, WB Saunders.)

BASIC INFORMATION

DEFINITION

Gastric cancer is an adenocarcinoma arising from the stomach.

SYNONYMS

Stomach cancer
Linitis plastica

ICD-9CM CODES
451 Malignant neoplasm of stomach

EPIDEMIOLOGY & DEMOGRAPHICS

- Annual incidence of gastric cancer in the U.S. is 7 cases/100,000 persons. The incidence is much higher in Japan, with rates as high as 80 cases/100,000 persons.
- Most gastric cancers arise in the antrum (35%).
- The incidence of distal stomach tumors has greatly declined whereas that of proximal tumors of the cardia and fundus is on the rise.
- Gastric cancer occurs most commonly in male patients >65 yr (70% of patients are >50 yr).
- Incidence of gastric cancer has been declining over the past 30 yr.
- Male:female ratio is 3:2.
- Familial diffuse gastric cancer is a disease with autosomal dominant inheritance in which gastric cancer develops at a young age. Germ-line truncating mutations in the E-cadherin gene (CDH1) is found in these families.

PHYSICAL FINDINGS & CLINICAL PRESENTATION

- Medical history may reveal complaints of postprandial fullness with significant weight loss (70% to 80%), nausea/emesis (20% to 40%), dysphagia (20%), and dyspepsia, usually unrelieved by antacids; epigastric discomfort, usually lessened by fasting and exacerbated by food intake, is also common.
- Epigastric or abdominal mass (30% to 50%), epigastric pain.
- Skin pallor secondary to anemia.
- Hard, nodular liver: generally indicates metastatic disease to the liver.
- Hemoccult-positive stools.
- Ascites, lymphadenopathy, or pleural effusions: may indicate metastasis.

ETIOLOGY

Risk factors:
- Chronic *H. pylori* gastritis. Gastric cancer develops in persons infected with *H. pylori*. Those with histologic findings of severe gastric atrophy, corpus-predominant gastritis, or intestinal metaplasia are at increased risk. Persons with *H. pylori* infection and duodenal ulcer are not at risk, whereas those with gastric ulcers, nonulcer dyspepsia, and gastric hyperplastic polyps are.
- Tobacco abuse, alcohol consumption
- Food additives (nitrosamines), smoked foods, occupational exposure to heavy metals, rubber, asbestos
- Chronic atrophic gastritis with intestinal metaplasia, hypertrophic gastritis, and pernicious anemia

DIAGNOSIS

DIFFERENTIAL DIAGNOSIS

- Gastric lymphoma (5% of gastric malignancies)
- Hypertrophic gastritis
- Peptic ulcer
- Reflux esophagitis

WORKUP

Upper endoscopy with biopsy will confirm diagnosis. Endoscopic ultrasonography in combination with CT scanning and operative lymph node dissection can be used in staging of the tumor.

LABORATORY TESTS

- Microcytic anemia
- Hemoccult-positive stools
- Hypoalbuminemia
- Abnormal liver enzymes in patients with metastasis to the liver
- Mutation-specific predictive genetic testing by PCR amplification followed by restriction—enzyme digestion and DNA sequencing for truncating mutations in the E-cadherin gene (CDH1) is recommended in families of patients with familial diffuse cancer because gastric cancer develops in three of every four carriers of a mutant CDH1 gene.

IMAGING STUDIES

- Upper GI series with air contrast (90% accurate) should be considered only if endoscopy is not readily available
- Abdominal CT scan to evaluate for metastasis (70% accurate for regional node metastases)

TREATMENT

ACUTE GENERAL Rx

- Gastrectomy with regional lymphadenectomy is performed in patients with curative potential (<30% of patients at time of diagnosis). Post-op adjuvant chemoradiotherapy using 5-fluorouracil and leucovorin is now the standard of care for resected patients able to tolerate such treatment. Postoperative chemotherapy and radiotherapy, compared with surgical resection alone, can extend the survival of patients with gastric cancer in those who are able to complete adjuvant therapy.
- When surgical cure is not possible, palliative resection may prolong duration and quality of life.
- Chemotherapy (FAM: 5-fluorouracil, Adriamycin, and mitomycin C) may provide some palliation; however, it generally does not prolong survival. Chemotherapy with docetaxel, cisplatin, and 5-fluorouracil can be used for chemotherapy-naive patients with metastatic or locally recurrent gastric cancer.

DISPOSITION

- 5-yr survival rate of gastric carcinoma is 12% overall.
- 5-yr survival for early gastric cancers (usually detected incidentally with endoscopy in populations where screening is recommended) is >35%.

REFERRAL

Surgical referral for resection

PEARLS & CONSIDERATIONS

COMMENTS

- Gastrectomy patients will need vitamin B_{12} replacement. They are also at risk for dumping syndrome and should be advised to ingest frequent, small meals.
- Prophylactic gastrectomy should be considered in young asymptomatic carriers of germ-line truncating CDH1 mutations who belong to families with highly penetrant heredity diffuse gastric cancer.

SUGGESTED READINGS

Layke J, Lopez P: Gastric cancer: Diagnosis and treatment options, *Am Fam Physician* 69:1133, 2004.
McDonald JS: Chemotherapy in the management of gastric cancer, *JCO* 21:2768, 2003.

AUTHOR: **FRED F. FERRI, M.D.**

BASIC INFORMATION

DEFINITION

Gastroesophageal reflux disease (GERD) is a motility disorder characterized primarily by heartburn and caused by the reflux of gastric contents into the esophagus.

SYNONYMS

Reflux esophagitis
GERD

ICD-9CM CODES
530.81 Gastroesophageal reflux disease
530.1 Esophagitis
787.1 Heartburn

EPIDEMIOLOGY & DEMOGRAPHICS

GERD is one of the most prevalent GI disorders. Nearly 7% of persons in the U.S. experience heartburn daily, 20% experience it monthly, and 60% experience it intermittently. Nearly 20% of adults use antacids or OTC H_2-blockers at least once a week for relief of heartburn.

PHYSICAL FINDINGS & CLINICAL PRESENTATION

- Physical examination: generally unremarkable
- Clinical signs and symptoms: heartburn, dysphagia, sour taste, regurgitation of gastric contents into the mouth
- Chronic cough and bronchospasm
- Chest pain, laryngitis, early satiety, abdominal fullness, and bloating with belching

ETIOLOGY

- Incompetent lower esophageal sphincter (LES)
- Medications that lower LES pressure (calcium channel blockers, β-adrenergic blockers, theophylline, anticholinergics)
- Foods that lower LES pressure (chocolate, yellow onions, peppermint)
- Tobacco abuse, alcohol, coffee
- Obesity
- Gastric acid hypersecretion
- Hiatal hernia (controversial) present in >70% of patients with GERD; however, most patients with hiatal hernia are asymptomatic

DIAGNOSIS

DIFFERENTIAL DIAGNOSIS

- Peptic ulcer disease
- Angina
- Esophagitis (from infections such as herpes, *Candida*), medication induced (doxycycline, potassium chloride)
- Esophageal spasm (nutcracker esophagus)
- Cancer of esophagus

WORKUP

Aimed at eliminating the conditions noted in the differential diagnosis and documenting the type and extent of tissue damage

LABORATORY TESTS

- 24-hr esophageal pH monitoring and Bernstein test are sensitive diagnostic tests. They are useful in patients with atypical manifestations of GERD, such as chest pain or chronic cough.
- Esophageal manometry is indicated in patients with refractory reflux in whom surgical therapy is planned.
- Upper GI endoscopy (EGD) is useful to document the type and extent of tissue damage in GERD and to exclude Barrett's esophagus. The American College of Gastroenterology recommends endoscopy to screen for Barrett's esophagus in patients who have chronic GERD symptoms. Barrett's esophagus is a precursor to esophageal cancer. Once diagnosed, yearly surveillance (EGD) is appropriate. Once excluded, EGD need not be repeated unless new symptoms develop (e.g., dysphagia).

IMAGING STUDIES

- Upper GI series can identify ulcerations and strictures; however, it may miss mucosal abnormalities. Only one third of patients with GERD have radiographic signs of esophagitis.

TREATMENT

NONPHARMACOLOGIC THERAPY

- Lifestyle modifications with avoidance of foods (citrus- and tomato-based products, chocolate) and drugs that exacerbate reflux (e.g., caffeine, β-blockers, calcium channel blockers, alpha-adrenergic agonists, theophylline)
- Avoidance of tobacco and alcohol use
- Elevation of head of bed 4 to 8 inches using blocks
- Avoidance of lying down directly after late or large evening meals
- Weight reduction, decreased fat intake
- Avoid clothing tight around the waist

ACUTE GENERAL Rx

- Proton pump inhibitors (PPIs) (esomeprazole 40 mg qd, omeprazole 20 mg qd, lansoprazole 30 mg qd, rabeprazole 20 mg qd, or pantoprazole 40 mg qd) are safe, tolerated, and very effective in most patients.
- H_2-blockers (nizatidine 300 mg qhs, famotidine 40 mg qhs, ranitidine 300 mg qhs, or cimetidine 800 mg qhs) can be used but are generally much less effective than PPIs.
- Antacids (may be useful for relief of mild symptoms; however, they are generally ineffective in severe cases of reflux).
- Prokinetic agents (metoclopramide) are indicated only when PPIs are not fully effective. They can be used in combination therapy; however, side effects limit their use.
- For refractory cases: surgery with Nissen fundoplication. Potential surgical candidates should have reflux esophagitis documented by EGD and normal esophageal motility as evaluated by manometry. Surgery generally consists of reduction of hiatal hernia when present and placement of a gastric wrap around the GE junction (fundoplication). Although laparoscopic fundoplication is now widely used, surgery should not be advised with the expectation that patients with GERD will no longer need to take antisecretory medications or that the procedure will prevent esophageal cancer among those with GERD and Barrett's esophagus.
- Endoscopic radiofrequency heating of the GE junction (Stretta procedure) is a newer treatment modality for GERD patients unresponsive to traditional therapy. Endoscopic gastroplasty (EndoCinch procedure) also aims at treating GERD.

DISPOSITION

- The majority of the patients respond well to therapy.
- Recurrence of reflux is common if treatment is discontinued.
- Postsurgical complications occur in nearly 20% of patients (dysphagia, gas bloating, diarrhea, nausea). Long-term follow-up studies also reveal that within 3 to 5 years 52% of patients who had undergone antireflux surgery are taking antireflux medications again.

REFERRAL

- GI referral for upper endoscopy is needed when there are concerns about associated PUD, Barrett's esophagus, or esophageal cancer.
- Patients with Barrett's esophagus should undergo surveillance endoscopy with mucosal biopsy every 2 yr or less because the risk of developing adenocarcinoma of esophagus is at least 30 times greater than that of the general population.

SUGGESTED READINGS

Heidelbaugh JL et al: Management of gastroesophageal reflux disease, *Am Fam Physician* 68:1311, 2003.
Shaheen N, Ransohoff DF: Gastroesophageal reflux, Barrett esophagus, and esophageal cancer, *JAMA* 287:1972, 2002.

AUTHORS: **FRED F. FERRI, M.D.**, with revisions by **TOM J. WACHTEL, M.D.**

BASIC INFORMATION

DEFINITION

Giant cell arteritis (GCA) is a segmental systemic granulomatous arteritis affecting medium- and large-sized arteries in individuals >50 years. Inflammation primarily targets extracranial blood vessels, and although the carotid system is usually affected, pathology in posterior cerebral artery has been reported.

SYNONYMS

Temporal arteritis
Cranial arteritis
Horton's disease

ICD-9CM CODES
446.5 Temporal arteritis

EPIDEMIOLOGY & DEMOGRAPHICS

PREVALENCE: 200 cases/100,000 persons; female-to-male predominance of two- to four-fold
INCIDENCE: 17 to 23.3 new cases/100,000 persons >50 yr

CLINICAL PRESENTATION & PHYSICAL FINDINGS

GCA can present with the following clinical manifestations:
• Headache, often associated with marked scalp tenderness
• Constitutional symptoms (fever, weight loss, anorexia, fatigue)
• Polymyalgia syndrome (aching and stiffness of the trunk and proximal muscle groups)
• Visual disturbances (transient or permanent monocular visual loss)
• Intermittent claudication of jaw and tongue on mastication
Important physical findings in GCA:
• Vascular examination: Tenderness, decreased pulsation, and nodulation of temporal arteries; diminished or absent pulses in upper extremities

ETIOLOGY

Vasculitis of unknown etiology

DIAGNOSIS

Clinical history and vascular examination are cornerstones of diagnosis. The presence of any three of the following five items allows the diagnosis of GCA with a sensitivity of 94% and a specificity of 91%:
• Age of onset >50 yr
• New-onset or new type of headache
• Temporal artery tenderness or decreased pulsation on physical examination
• Westergren ESR >50 mm/hr

• Temporal artery biopsy with vasculitis and mononuclear cell infiltrate or granulomatous changes

DIFFERENTIAL DIAGNOSIS

• Other vasculitic syndromes
• Nonarteritic Anterior Ischemic Optic Neuropathy (AION)
• Primary amyloidosis
• TIA, stroke
• Infections
• Occult neoplasm, multiple myeloma

WORKUP

LABORATORY TESTS

• ESR >50 mm/hr; however, up to 22.5% patients with GCA have normal ESR before treatment
• C-reactive protein is typically included in lab investigation; it has greater sensitivity than ESR
• Mild to moderate normochromic normocytic anemia, elevated platelet count
• IL-6 levels hold promise for a more sensitive modality, but at this stage remains experimental

IMAGING STUDIES

• Reliability of color duplex ultrasonography of temporal artery is controversial as it is thought that it does not improve diagnostic accuracy over careful physical examination
• Fluorescein angiogram of ophthalmic vessels may be warranted to differentiate between arteritic AION (i.e., GCA) and nonarteritic AION

TREATMENT

ACUTE GENERAL Rx

• Intravenous methylprednisolone (500-1000 mg qd for 3-5 days) is indicated in those with significant clinical manifestations (e.g., visual loss).
• Oral prednisone (1 mg/kg/day) may be used under less urgent circumstances or following the initial period of treatment with intravenous methylprednisolone. High-dose oral regimen should be continued at least until symptoms resolve and ESR returns to normal.
• Prednisone should be tapered gradually (~5 mg every other wk) initially and subsequently even more slowly (2.5 mg every 2-4 wk). Steroid treatment is usually required for at least 6 mo, and sometimes as much as 2 yr.
• Methotrexate or azathioprine may be added to the steroid regimen for their steroid-sparing effect, but efficacy is unproven.

DISPOSITION

If steroid therapy is initiated early, GCA has excellent prognosis; however, 20% of patients have permanent partial or complete loss of vision. Once there is visual loss, improvement is dismal: in one study, only 4% of eyes improved in both visual acuity and central visual field.

REFERRAL

• Surgical referral for biopsy of temporal artery
• Ophthalmology referral in patients with visual disturbances and following initiation of corticosteroid therapy
• Rheumatology referral for difficult cases

PEARLS & CONSIDERATIONS

COMMENTS

• The relationship between polymyalgia rheumatica and GCA is unclear, but the two may frequently coexist.
• Clinical picture rather than ESR should be the prime yardstick for continuing prednisone therapy.
• A rising ESR in a clinically asymptomatic patient with normal hematocrit should raise suspicion for alternate explanations (e.g., infections, neoplasms).
• Although pathologic findings on temporal artery biopsy are the gold standard for the diagnosis of GCA, the false-negative rate is around 9% (the false-negative rate may be lower in the hands of an experienced surgeon); in some cases, a second biopsy from the contralateral side may be required.
• GCA is associated with a markedly increased risk for the development of aortic aneurysm, which is often a late complication and may cause death. Annual chest radiograph in chronic CGA patients has been suggested, as well as emergent chest CT or MRI for clinical suspicion.

SUGGESTED READINGS

Please refer to references within these papers as well as associated 'Letters to the Editor' for further details.

Gold R et al: Therapy of neurological disorders in systemic vasculitis, *Sem Neurol* 23(2):207, 2003.
Hayreh SR et al: Visual improvement with corticosteroid therapy in giant cell arteritis. Report of large study and review of the literature, *Acta Ophthalmol Scand* 80:355, 2002.
Hoffman GS et al: A multicenter, randomized, double-blind, placebo-controlled trial of adjuvant methotrexate for giant-cell arteritis, *Arthritis and Rheum* 46(5):1309, 2002.
Norborg E, Norborg C: Giant cell arteritis: epidemiological clues to its pathogenesis and an update on its treatment, *Rheumatol* 42:413, 2003.
Salvarani C et al: Polymyalgia rheumatica and giant-cell arteritis, *N Engl J Med* 347(4):261, 2002.
Smetana GW, Shmerling RH: Does this patient have temporal arteritis? *JAMA* 287:92, 2002.

AUTHOR: **U. SHIVRAJ SOHUR, M.D, PH.D.**

BASIC INFORMATION

DEFINITION

Chronic open-angle glaucoma refers to optic nerve damage often associated with elevated intraocular pressure; it is a chronic, slowly progressive, usually bilateral disorder associated with visual loss, eye pain, and optic nerve damage. Now felt to be a primary disease of the optic nerve with high pressure a high risk factor for glaucoma.

SYNONYM

Chronic simple glaucoma

ICD-9CM CODES
365.1 Open-angle glaucoma

EPIDEMIOLOGY & DEMOGRAPHICS

INCIDENCE (IN U.S.): Third most common cause of visual loss (75% to 95% of all glaucomas are open angle.)

PREVALENCE (IN U.S.):
- Overall prevalence in U.S. population >40 yr of age is estimated to be 1.86%, with 1.57 million white and 398,000 black patients affected.
- 150,000 patients suffer bilateral blindness.
- Disease occurs in 2% of people >40 yr old.
- Prevalence is higher in diabetics, with high myopia, and among older persons.
- More common in blacks (3 × the age-adjusted prevalence than whites).

PREDOMINANT AGE:
- Persons >50 yr old

PEAK INCIDENCE:
- Increases after 40 yr
- Because of rapid aging of the U.S. population, expect 3 million cases by year 2020.

GENETICS:
- Four to six times higher incidence in blacks than whites
- No clear-cut hereditary patterns but a strong hereditary tendency

PHYSICAL FINDINGS

- High intraocular pressures and large optic nerve cup (Ocular Hypertension Treatment Study—very important)
- Cornea thickens faster in vision loss
- Abnormal visual fields
- Open-angle gonioscopy
- `Red eye
- Restricted vision and field

ETIOLOGY

- Uncertain hereditary tendency
- Topical steroids
- Trauma
- Inflammatory
- High-dose oral corticosteroids taken for prolonged periods

DIAGNOSIS **Dx**

DIFFERENTIAL DIAGNOSIS

- Other optic neuropathies
- Secondary glaucoma from inflammation and steroid therapy
- Red eye differential
- Trauma
- Contact lens injury

WORKUP

- Intraocular pressure
- Slit lamp examination
- Visual fields
- Gonioscopy
- Nerve fiber analysis—GDx
- Corneal thickness—very important in prognosis

LABORATORY TESTS

Blood sugar

IMAGING STUDIES

- Optic nerve photography—stereo photographs
- Visual field testing
- GDx (laser scan of nerve fiber layer)

TREATMENT **Rx**

ACUTE GENERAL Rx

- β-Blockers (Timolol) qd to bid depending on individual response to drug
- Diamox 250 mg qid or pilocarpine
- Hyperosmotic agents (mannitol) in acute treatment
- Prostaglandins
- Laser trabeculoplasty (SLT) as needed
- Pilocarpine qid

CHRONIC Rx

- At least biannual checks of intraocular pressure and adjustment of medication
- Poor control = frequent examinations; good control = drugs
- Trabectalectomy
- Filter valves

DISPOSITION

Must be followed by ophthalmologist

REFERRAL

Immediately to ophthalmologist

PEARLS & CONSIDERATIONS **!**

COMMENTS

- Glaucoma is a serious blinding disease. Must be followed professionally by an ophthalmologist.
- Early diagnosis and treatment may minimize visual loss.
- Glaucoma is not solely caused by increased intraocular pressure, because approximately 20% of patients with glaucoma have normal intraocular pressure, but high pressure is definitely a risk factor to be considered.

SUGGESTED READINGS

Gordon MO et al: Baseline factors that predict the onset of primary open-angle glaucoma, *Arch Ophthalmol* 120:714, 2002.

Heijl A et al: Reduction of intraocular pressure and glaucoma progression: Results from the early manifest glaucoma trial, *Arch Ophthalmol* 120:1268, 2002.

Higginbotham EJ et al: The Ocular Hypertension Treatment Study: topical medication delays or prevents primary open-angle glaucoma in African American individuals, *Arch Ophthalmol* 122(6):813, 2004.

Rezaie T et al: Adult-onset primary open-angle glaucoma caused by mutations in optineurin, *Science* 295:1077, 2002.

AUTHOR: **MELVYN KOBY, M.D.**

BASIC INFORMATION

DEFINITION

Primary closed-angle glaucoma occurs when elevated intraocular pressure is associated with closure of the filtration angle or obstruction in the circulating pathway of the aqueous humor.

SYNONYMS

Acute glaucoma
Pupillary block glaucoma
Narrow-angle glaucoma

ICD-9CM CODES

365.2 Primary angle-closure glaucoma

EPIDEMIOLOGY & DEMOGRAPHICS

INCIDENCE (IN U.S.):

- In 2% to 8% of all patients with glaucoma
- Higher incidence among those with hyperopia, small eyes, dense cataracts, shallow anterior chambers

PREDOMINANT SEX: Females > males

PREDOMINANT AGE: 50 to 60 yr

PEAK INCIDENCE: Greater after 50 yr of age; high association with hypopia, cataracts, and eye trauma

GENETICS: High family history

PHYSICAL FINDINGS & CLINICAL FINDINGS

- Hazy cornea (Fig. 1-20)
- Narrow angle
- Red eyes
- Pain
- Injection of conjunctiva
- Shallow anterior chamber
- Thick cataract

- Old trauma
- Chronic eye infections

ETIOLOGY

- Narrow angles with acute closure—blockage of circulatory path of the aqueous humor causing increase in interior ocular pressure

DIAGNOSIS

DIFFERENTIAL DIAGNOSIS

- High pressure
- Optic nerve cupping
- Field loss
- Shallow chamber
- Open-angle glaucoma
- Conjunctivitis
- Corneal disease-keratitis
- Uveitis
- Scleritis
- Allergies
- Contact lens wearing with irritation

WORKUP

- Intraocular pressure
- Gonioscopy
- Slit lamp examination
- Visual field examination
- GDx examination (laser scan of nerve fiber layer)
- Optic nerve evaluation
- Anterior chamber depth
- Cataract evaluation
- High hyperopia

LABORATORY TESTS

- Blood sugar and CBC (if diabetes or inflammatory disease is suspected)
- Visual field
- GDx nerve fiber analysis

IMAGING STUDIES

- Fundus photography
- Fluorescein angiography for neurovascular disease

TREATMENT

The goal of treatment is to acutely lower pressure on eye and keep it down.

NONPHARMACOLOGIC THERAPY

Laser iridotomy early in disease process

ACUTE GENERAL Rx

- IV mannitol
- Pilocarpine
- β-Blockers
- Diamox
- Laser iridotomy
- Anterior chamber paracentesis (as emergency treatment)

CHRONIC Rx

- Iridotomy
- Trabeculectomy
- Filter valves
- Other laser procedures

DISPOSITION

Refer to ophthalmologist immediately.

REFERRAL

This is an emergency—refer immediately to an ophthalmologist.

PEARLS & CONSIDERATIONS

COMMENTS

- Do not use antihistamines or vasodilators with narrow-angle glaucoma.
- After iridotomy, the majority of patients will be totally cured and will need no further medication and have no visual loss.
- Lower socioeconomic status and higher levels of social deprivation are risk factors for delayed detection and probable worse outcomes in glaucoma.

SUGGESTED READINGS

Foster PJ et al: Defining "occludable" angles in population surveys: drainage angle width, peripheral anterior synechiae, and glaucomatous optic neuropathy in East Asian people, *Br J Ophthalmol* 88(4):486, 2004.

Fraser S et al: Deprivation and late presentation of glaucoma: case control study, *BMJ* 322:638, 2001.

Gazzard G et al: Intraocular pressure and visual field loss in primary angle closure and primary open angle glaucomas, *Br J Ophthalmol* 87(6):720, 2003.

Kapur SB: The lens and angle-closure glaucoma, *J Cataract Refract Surg* 27(2):176, 2001.

Lam DS et al: Angle-closure glaucoma, *Ophthalmology* 109:1, 2002.

AUTHOR: **MELVYN KOBY, M.D.**

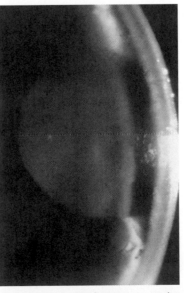

A   B

FIGURE 1-20 Acute angle-closure glaucoma. A, Acutely elevated pressure produces an inflamed eye with corneal edema (note fragmented light reflex) and a middilated pupil. **B,** Slit lamp examination shows a very shallow central anterior chamber (space between cornea and iris) and no peripheral chamber. (From Palay D [ed]: *Ophthalmology for the primary care physician,* St Louis, 1997, Mosby.)

BASIC INFORMATION

DEFINITION

Gout is a clinical disorder in which crystals of monosodium urate become deposited in tissue as a result of hyperuricemia. Gout and hyperuricemia can be classified as either primary or secondary if resulting from another disorder.

ICD-9CM CODES
274.9 Gout

EPIDEMIOLOGY & DEMOGRAPHICS

PREVALENCE: 3 cases/1000 persons
PREDOMINANT SEX: 95% males, rare in females before menopause

PHYSICAL FINDINGS & CLINICAL PRESENTATION

- Usually, initial attack in a single joint or an area of tenosynovium
- Mainly a disease of the lower extremities
- First site of involvement: classically, MP joint of the great toe
- Another common site of acute attack: extensor tenosynovium on the dorsum of the midfoot
- Severe pain and inflammation, which may be precipitated by exercise, dietary indiscretions, and physical or emotional stress
- Attacks following illness or surgery
- Presence of swelling, heat, redness, and other signs of inflammation (the physical findings simulating cellulitis)
- Exquisite soft tissue tenderness
- Fever, tachycardia, and other constitutional symptoms
- Eventually, deposits of urate crystals (tophi) in the subcutaneous tissue

ETIOLOGY

- Hyperuricemia and gout develop from excessive uric acid production, a decrease in the renal excretion of uric acid, or both.
- Primary gout results from an inborn error of metabolism and may be attributed to several biochemical defects.
- Secondary hyperuricemia may develop as a complication of acquired disorders (e.g., leukemia) or as a result of the use of certain drugs (e.g., diuretics).

DIAGNOSIS

DIFFERENTIAL DIAGNOSIS

- Pseudogout
- Rheumatoid arthritis
- Osteoarthritis
- Cellulitis
- Infectious arthritis

Section II describes the differential diagnosis of acute monoarticular and oligoarticular arthritis.

WORKUP

Hyperuricemia accompanying a typical history of monoarticular acute arthritis is usually sufficient to establish the diagnosis.

LABORATORY TESTS

- Mild leukocytosis
- Elevated ESR
- Hyperuricemia
- Synovial aspirate: usually cloudy and markedly inflammatory in nature; urate crystals in fluid: needle-shaped and birefringent under polarized light

IMAGING STUDIES

- Plain radiography to rule out other disorders
- No typical findings in early gouty arthritis but late disease possibly associated with characteristic punched-out lesions and joint destruction

TREATMENT

NONPHARMACOLOGIC THERAPY

- Modification of diet (avoidance of foods high in purines [e.g., anchovies, organ meat, liver, spinach, mushrooms, asparagus, oatmeal, cocoa, sweetbreads]) and lifestyle
- Treatment for obesity
- Moderation in alcohol intake, no more than two drinks per day
- Hypertension and its management requiring careful assessment and possibly nondiuretic drugs

ACUTE GENERAL Rx

- Quick-acting NSAIDs such as ibuprofen
- Colchicine (given PO or IV)
- Corticosteroids or ACTH for those who are intolerant of NSAIDs or colchicine
- Intraarticular cortisone when oral medication cannot be given
- General measures, such as rest, elevation, and analgesics as needed until acute pain subsides.
- Table 1-6 describes treatment options for gout

CHRONIC Rx

- Prevention is achieved through normalization of serum urate concentration.
- Uricosuric agents (e.g., probenecid) or xanthine oxidase inhibitors (allopurinol) are used in patients with recurrent attacks despite adequate dietary restrictions.

- A 24-hr urine collection is useful in deciding which antihyperuricemic agent is indicated. Allopurinol is generally used if the uric acid output is >900 mg/day on a regular diet. However, hyperuricemic therapy should not be started for at least 2 wk after the acute attack has resolved because it may prolong the acute attack and it can also precipitate new attacks by rapidly lowering the serum uric acid level.
- Urinary uric acid hypoexcretors (<700 mg/day) can be given probenecid (250 mg bid for 1 wk, then increased to 500 mg bid) to block absorption of uric acid. Probenecid should be started only after the acute attack of gout has completely subsided.
- Colchicine 0.6 mg bid is indicated for acute gout prophylaxis before starting hyperuricemic therapy. It is generally discontinued 6 to 8 wk after normalization of serum urate levels. Long-term colchicine therapy (0.6 mg qd or bid) may be necessary in patients with frequent gout attacks despite the use of uricosuric agents.
- Surgery usually limited to excision of large tophi and, occasionally, arthroplasty.

DISPOSITION

- Musculoskeletal complications are usually limited to joint disease.
- Surgical intervention may occasionally be indicated.
- Renal disease is the most frequent complication of gout after arthritis; most gouty patients develop renal disease as a result of parenchymal urate deposition but the involvement is only slowly progressive and often has no effect on life expectancy.
- Incidence of urolithiasis is increased, with 80% of calculi being uric acid stones.

REFERRAL

For orthopedic consultation when joint destruction has occurred

PEARLS & CONSIDERATIONS

COMMENTS

- No significant correlation between coronary artery disease and gout
- No indication to treat asymptomatic hyperuricemia
- Acute attacks of gout occasionally associated with normal levels of uric acid
- The main indication for prophylaxis is recurrent attacks of gouty joint inflammation, 3 or more per year

SUGGESTED READINGS

Agudelo CA, Wise CM: Gout: diagnosis, pathogenesis, and clinical manifestations, *Curr Opin Rheumatol* 13:234, 2001.

Riedel AA et al: Compliance with allopurinol therapy among managed care enrollees with gout: a retrospective analysis of administrative claims, *J Rheumatol* 31(8):1575, 2004.

Schlesinger N, Schumacher HR: Gout: can management be improved? *Curr Opin Rheumatol* 13:240, 2001.

Terkeltaub RA: Gout, *N Engl J Med* 349:1647, 2003.

Velilla-Moliner J et al: Podagra, is it always gout? *Am J Emerg Med* 22(4):320, 2004.

Wallace KL et al: Increasing prevalence of gout and hyperuricemia over 10 years among older adults in a managed care population, *J Rheumatol* 31(8):1582, 2004.

AUTHOR: **LONNIE R. MERCIER, M.D.**

TABLE 1-6 Treatment of Gout

Acute gout	Interval gout	Long-term treatment
Therapeutic goal: Terminate acute inflammatory attack.	**Therapeutic goal:** Prevent recurrent attacks.	**Therapeutic goals:** Prevent attacks, resolve tophi, maintain serum urate at ≤6 mg/dl.
NSAIDs *(preferred):* Indomethacin, 50 mg qid, or ibuprofen, 800 mg tid (or other NSAIDs in full doses) *(lower dose in renal insufficiency; contraindicated with peptic ulcer disease).*	**Colchicine, oral:** 0.6-1.2 mg daily as prophylaxis against recurrent attacks.	**Colchicine, oral:** 0.6-1.2 mg daily for 1-2 wk before initiating hypouricemic therapy and for several months afterward to prevent recurrent attacks during initial period of hypouricemic therapy.
OR		**Allopurinol:** Dose variable; usually 300 mg once daily, but up to 900 mg may be needed in occasional patient; dose should be reduced to 100 mg daily or every other day in patients with renal insufficiency.
Colchicine, oral *(used infrequently):* 0.6-1.2 mg (1-2 tablets), then 0.6 mg (1 tablet) q1-2h until attack subsides or until nausea, diarrhea, or GI cramping develops. Maximum total dose, 4-6 mg. If ineffective in 48 hr, do not repeat.	**Hypouricemic agent:** Start only if indicated by frequent attacks, severe hyperuricemia, presence of tophi, urolithiasis, or urate overexcretion.	
Colchicine, IV *(only if oral medication is precluded):* 1-2 mg in 20 ml 0.9% saline infused slowly *(extravasation causes tissue necrosis);* dose may be repeated once in 6 hr. Few GI symptoms with IV use. Maximum total dose, 4 mg per attack. Monitor blood counts	**Other:** Diet—moderate protein, low fat; avoid excessive alcohol. Treat hypertension if present. High fluid intake to promote uric acid excretion in a dilute urine (for uric acid overexcretors).	***OR***
Steroids *(if NSAIDs or colchicines are contraindicated or if oral medication is precluded, e.g., postoperatively):* Triamcinolone acetonide, 60 mg IM, *or* ACTH, 40 U IM *or* 25 U by slow IV infusion, *or* prednisone, 20-40 mg daily. Intra-articular steroids may be used to treat a single inflamed joint: triamcinolone hexacetonide, 5-20 mg, or dexamethasone phosphate, 1-6 mg.		**Uricosuric agent** *(reduced efficacy if creatinine clearance <80 ml; ineffective if <30 ml):* Probenecid, 0.5-1 g bid, or sulfinpyrazone, 100 mg tid or qid; usually well tolerated, but may cause headache, GI upset, rash.
Hypouricemic agents: Of no benefit for inflammatory attack and may initiate recurrent attack. Should not be started until attack has resolved, but *ongoing use should not be interrupted during an attack.*		**Other:** Diet—moderate protein, low fat; avoid excessive alcohol. Treat hypertension if present. For uric acid overexcretors or when initiating uricosuric agent: high fluid intake, particularly at night, to promote uric acid excretion in a dilute urine. Acetazolamide, 250 mg at bedtime, may be used to keep urine pH >6.

From Goldman L, Ausiello D (eds): *Cecil textbook of medicine*, ed 22, Philadelphia, 2004, WB Saunders.
ACTH, Adrenocorticotropic hormone; *bid,* twice daily; *GI,* gastrointestinal; *IM,* intramuscularly; *IV,* intravenously; *NSAIDs,* nonsteroidal antiinflammatory drugs; *q1-2h,* every 1 to 2 hours; *qid,* four times daily; *tid,* three times daily.

BASIC INFORMATION

DEFINITION

Guillain-Barré syndrome (GBS) is an acute immune-mediated polyradiculo-neuropathy (affects nerve roots and peripheral nerves), with predominant motor involvement. Maximal clinical weakness occurs within 4 wk of disease onset.

SYNONYMS

Acute polyneuropathy
Ascending paralysis
Postinfectious polyneuritis

ICD-9CM CODES
357.0 Guillain-Barré

EPIDEMIOLOGY & DEMOGRAPHICS

INCIDENCE: 0.6-1.9 cases/100,000 persons annually without geographical variation. Incidence increases with age. A slight male preponderance (1.25:1) also exists.
PREDISPOSING FACTORS: Viral (HIV, CMV, EBV, influenza) and bacterial (*Campylobacter jejuni, Mycoplasma pneumonia*) infections; systemic illness (Hodgkin's lymphoma, immunizations)

PHYSICAL FINDINGS & CLINICAL PRESENTATION

- Symmetric weakness, initially involving proximal muscles, subsequently involving both proximal and distal muscles; difficulty in ambulating, getting up from a chair, or climbing stairs
- Depressed or absent reflexes bilaterally
- Minimal to moderate glove and stocking paresthesias/dysesthesia/anesthesia and/or back pain
- Pain (caused by involvement of posterior nerve roots) may be prominent
- Autonomic abnormalities (brady- or tachyarrhythmias, hypo- or hypertension)
- Respiratory insufficiency (caused by weakness of bulbar/intercostal muscles)
- Facial paresis, ophthalmoparesis, dysphagia (secondary to cranial nerve involvement)

ETIOLOGY

Unknown. Preceding infectious illness 1-4 wk before disease onset in 66% of patients. Humoral and cell-mediated immune attack of peripheral nerve myelin, Schwann cells; sometimes with axonal involvement

DIAGNOSIS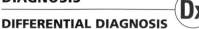

DIFFERENTIAL DIAGNOSIS

- Toxic peripheral neuropathies: heavy metal poisoning (lead, thallium, arsenic), medications (vincristine, disul-firam), organophosphate poisoning, hexacarbon (glue sniffer's neuropathy)
- Nontoxic peripheral neuropathies: acute intermittent porphyria, vasculitic polyneuropathy, infectious (poliomyelitis, diphtheria, Lyme disease); tick paralysis
- Neuromuscular junction disorders: myasthenia gravis, botulism, snake envenomations
- Myopathies; such as polymyositis, acute necrotizing myopathies caused by drugs
- Metabolic derangements such as hypermagnesemia, hypokalemia, hypophosphatemia, thyrotoxicosis
- Acute central nervous system disorders such as basilar artery thrombosis with brainstem infarction, brainstem encephalomyelitis, transverse myelitis, or spinal cord compression
- Hysterical paralysis or malingering

WORKUP

1. Exclude other causes based on clinical history, examination, and laboratory tests.
2. Lumbar puncture (may be normal in the first 1-2 wk of the illness)
   - Typical findings include elevated CSF protein with few mononuclear leukocytes (albuminocytologic dissociation) in 80%-90% of patients. Elevated CSF cell counts is an expected feature in cases associated with HIV seroconversion.
3. EMG/NCS: May be normal in the first 10-14 days of the disease. The earliest electrodiagnostic abnormality is prolongation or absence of H-reflexes.

LABORATORY TESTS

- CBC may reveal early leukocytosis with left shift. Electrolytes to exclude metabolic causes
- Heavy metal testing, urine porphyria screen, creatine kinase, HIV titers, neuroimaging of the brain and spinal cord if diagnosis uncertain

TREATMENT

NONPHARMACOLOGIC THERAPY

- Close monitoring of respiratory function (frequent measurements of vital capacity, negative inspiratory force and pulmonary toilet), because respiratory failure is the major complication in GBS
- Frequent repositioning of patient to minimize formation of pressure sores
- Prevention of thromboembolism with antithrombotic stockings and SC heparin (5000 U q12h) in nonambulatory patients
- Emotional support and social counseling

ACUTE GENERAL Rx

- Infusion of IV immunoglobulins (IVIg; 0.4 g/kg/day for 5 days). Always check serum IgA levels before infusion to prevent anaphylaxis in deficient patients.
- Early therapeutic plasma exchange (TPE or plasmapheresis: 200-250 ml/kg over 5 sessions qod), started within 7 days of onset of symptoms, is beneficial in preventing paralytic complications in patients with rapidly progressive disease. It is contraindicated in patients with cardiovascular disease (recent MI, unstable angina), active sepsis, and autonomic dysfunction.
- Mechanical ventilation may be needed if FVC is <12 to 15 ml/kg, vital capacity is rapidly decreasing or is <1000 ml, negative inspiratory force < −20 cm H_2O, PaO_2 is <70, the patient is having significant difficulty clearing secretions or is aspirating.

CHRONIC Rx

- Ventilatory support: may be necessary in 10% to 20% of patients. Adequate fluid/electrolyte support and nutrition necessary, especially in patients with dysautonomia or bulbar dysfunction
- Aggressive nursing care to prevent decubiti, infections, fecal impactions, and pressure nerve palsies
- Monitoring and treatment of autonomic dysfunction (bradyarrhythmias or tachyarrhythmias, orthostatic hypotension, systemic hypertension, altered sweating)
- Treatment of back pain and dysesthesia with low-dose tricyclics, gabapentin, etc.
- Stress ulcer prevention in patients receiving ventilator support
- Physical and occupational therapy rehabilitation, including supportive devices

DISPOSITION

- Mortality is approximately 5%-10%. A recent study showed 62% complete recovery, 14% mild weakness, 9% moderate weakness, 4% bed-bound or ventilated, and 8% dead at 1 yr.
- Predictors for poor recovery (inability to walk independently at 1 yr): older age, preceding diarrheal illness, recent CMV infection, fulminant or rapidly progressing course, ventilatory dependence, reduced motor amplitudes (<20% normal), or inexcitable nerves on NCS.

REFERRAL

Tracheostomy may be necessary in patients with prolonged ventilatory support. Percutaneous endoscopic gastrostomy may also be required.

PEARLS & CONSIDERATIONS

COMMENTS

Patient education information may be obtained from the Guillain-Barré Foundation International, Box 262, Wynnewood, PA 19096; phone: (610) 667-0131.

SUGGESTED READINGS

Gorson KC, Ropper AH: Guillain-Barré syndrome (acute inflammatory demyelinating neuropathy) and related disorders. In: Katirji B et al. (eds): *Neuromuscular disorders in clinical practice*. Boston, 2002, Butterworth-Heinemann.

Kuwabara S: Guillain-Barré syndrome: epidemiology, pathophysiology and management, *Drugs* 64:597, 2004.

AUTHOR: **EROBOGHENE E. UBOGU, M.D.**

BASIC INFORMATION

DEFINITION

Congestive heart failure (CHF) is a pathophysiologic state characterized by congestion in the pulmonary or systemic circulation. It is caused by the heart's inability to pump sufficient oxygenated blood to meet the metabolic needs of the tissues. The various classifications for heart failure are described as follows.
The American College of Cardiology and the American Heart Association describe the following four stages of heart failure:

A. At high risk for heart failure, but without structural heart disease or symptoms of heart failure (e.g., CAD, hypertension)
B. Structural heart disease but without symptoms of heart failure
C. Structural heart disease with prior or current symptoms of heart failure
D. Refractory heart failure requiring specialized interventions

The New York Heart Association (NYHA) defines the following functional classes:

I. Asymptomatic
II. Symptomatic with minimal exertion
III. Symptomatic with moderate exertion
IV. Symptomatic at rest

SYNONYMS

CHF
Cardiac failure
Heart failure

ICD-9CM CODES
428.0 Congestive heart failure

EPIDEMIOLOGY & DEMOGRAPHICS

- CHF is the most common admission diagnosis (20%) in elderly patients.
- Heart failure occurs in 4.7 million persons in the U.S. and is the discharge diagnosis in 3.5 million hospitalizations annually.

PHYSICAL FINDINGS & CLINICAL PRESENTATION

The findings on physical examination in patients with CHF vary depending on the severity and whether the failure is right-sided or left-sided.

- Common clinical manifestations are:
  1. Dyspnea on exertion initially, then with progressively less strenuous activity, and eventually manifesting when patient is at rest; caused by increasing pulmonary congestion
  2. Orthopnea caused by increased venous return in the recumbent position

3. Paroxysmal nocturnal dyspnea (PND) resulting from multiple factors (increased venous return in the recumbent position, decreased Pao$_2$, decreased adrenergic stimulation of myocardial function)
4. Fatigue, reduced exercise tolerance, lethargy resulting from low cardiac output, deterioration in ADLs
5. Cognitive impairment, new, or worsening of underlying dementia (i.e., delirium)

- Patients with failure of the left side of the heart may have the following abnormalities on physical examination: pulmonary rales, tachypnea, S$_3$ gallop, cardiac murmurs (AS, AR, MR), paradoxic splitting of S$_2$.
- Patients with failure of right side of the heart manifest with jugular venous distention, peripheral edema, perioral and peripheral cyanosis, congestive hepatomegaly, ascites, hepatojugular reflux.
- In patients with heart failure, elevated jugular venous pressure and a third heart sound each are independently associated with adverse outcomes.
- Acute precipitants of CHF exacerbations are: noncompliance with salt restriction, pulmonary infections, arrhythmias, medications (e.g., calcium channel blockers/antiarrhythmic agents), and failed attempts at reductions in CHF therapy.

ETIOLOGY

LEFT VENTRICULAR FAILURE
- Systemic hypertension
- Valvular heart disease (AS, AR, MR)
- Cardiomyopathy, myocarditis
- Bacterial endocarditis
- Myocardial infarction
- IHSS

Left ventricular failure is further differentiated according to systolic dysfunction (low ejection fraction) and diastolic dysfunction (normal or high ejection fraction), or "stiff ventricle." It is important to make this distinction because treatment is different (see Treatment). Patients with heart failure and a normal ejection fraction have abnormalities in active relaxation and passive stiffness (see Heart Failure, Diastolic in Section I).

- Common causes of systolic dysfunction are post-MI, cardiomyopathy, myocarditis.
- Causes of diastolic dysfunction are hypertensive cardiovascular disease, restrictive cardiomyopathy, ischemic heart disease (see Heart Failure, Diastolic in Section I).

RIGHT VENTRICULAR FAILURE
- Valvular heart disease (mitral stenosis)
- Pulmonary hypertension
- Bacterial endocarditis (right-sided)
- Right ventricular infarction

BIVENTRICULAR FAILURE
- Left ventricular failure
- Cardiomyopathy
- Myocarditis
- Arrhythmias
- Anemia
- Thyrotoxicosis
- AV fistula
- Paget's disease
- Beriberi

DIAGNOSIS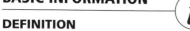

DIFFERENTIAL DIAGNOSIS

- Cirrhosis
- Nephrotic syndrome
- Venous occlusive disease
- COPD, asthma
- Pulmonary embolism
- ARDS
- Heroin overdose
- Pneumonia

WORKUP

- Standard 12-lead ECG is useful to diagnose ischemic heart disease and obtain information about rhythm abnormalities.

LABORATORY TESTS

- CBC (to rule out anemia, infections), BUN, creatinine, liver enzymes, TSH
- B-type natriuretic peptide is a cardiac neurohormone specifically secreted from the ventricles in response to volume expansion and pressure overload. Elevated levels are indicative of CHF. Bedside measurement of B-type natriuretic peptide is useful in establishing or excluding the diagnosis of CHF in patients with acute dyspnea.

IMAGING STUDIES

- Chest x-ray examination:
  1. Pulmonary venous congestion
  2. Cardiomegaly with dilation of the involved heart chamber
  3. Pleural effusions
- Two-dimensional echocardiography is critical to assess global and regional left ventricular function and estimate ejection fraction. The current standard of care requires echocardiography as part of the management of CHF.
- Exercise stress testing may be useful for evaluating concomitant coronary disease and assessing degree of disability in selected patients.
- Cardiac catheterization is an excellent method to evaluate ventricular diastolic properties, significant coronary artery disease, or valvular heart disease; however, it is invasive. The decision to perform cardiac catheterization should be individualized.

TREATMENT

NONPHARMACOLOGIC THERAPY

- Identify and correct precipitating factors (i.e., anemia, thyrotoxicosis, infections, increased sodium load, β-blockers, medical noncompliance).
- Decrease cardiac workload (restrict patients' activity) only during periods of acute decompensation. The risk of thromboembolism during this period can be minimized by using heparin 5000 U SC q12h in hospitalized patients. In patients with mild to moderate symptoms, aerobic training may improve symptoms and exercise capacity.
- Restrict sodium intake to ≤3 g/day.
- Restricting fluid intake to 2 L or less may be useful in patients with hyponatremia.

PHARMACOLOGIC THERAPY

TREATMENT OF CHF SECONDARY TO SYSTOLIC DYSFUNCTION

1. Diuretics: indicated in patients with systolic dysfunction and volume overload. The most useful approach to selecting the dose of, and monitoring the response to, diuretic therapy is by measuring body weight, preferably on a daily basis.
   a. Furosemide: 20 to 80 mg/day produces prompt venodilation and diuresis. IV therapy may produce diuresis when oral therapy has failed; when changing from IV to oral furosemide, doubling the dose is usually necessary to achieve an equal effect. Monitor serum potassium every 6 months (every 3 months if digitalis is also used).
   b. Thiazides are not as powerful as furosemide but are useful in mild to moderate CHF. Monitor serum potassium every 12 months (every 6 months if digitalis is also used). Thiazides are not effective when creatinine clearance is <20 ml/min.
   c. The addition of metolazone to furosemide enhances diuresis. Monitor potassium frequently.
   d. Blockade of aldosterone receptors by spironolactone (12.5 to 25 mg qd) used in conjunction with ACE inhibitors reduces both mortality and morbidity in patients with severe CHF. It is generally not associated with hyperkalemia when used in low doses; however, serum electrolytes and renal function should be closely monitored after initiation of therapy and when changing doses. Spironolactone use should be considered in patients with recent or recurrent class IV (NYHA) symptoms.
   e. Elderly patients have a blunted thirst sensation. They also may have restricted access to water because of mobility impairment or cognitive deficits. As a result, intravascular volume depletion and prerenal failure is a common complication of diuretic therapy. Patients with mild baseline renal failure (e.g., diabetic nephropathy) and patients dependent on others for fluid intake (e.g., nursing home patients) are particularly at risk and need a close monitoring (for clinical signs of dehydration and laboratory evidence of prerenal failure: high BUN/creatinine ratio).
   f. Monitoring fluid intake and output (I&O) is important and appropriate in the hospital. (If a urinary catheter is used for this purpose, its duration should be minimized.) In the nursing home setting, I&O is often unreliable and in outpatients it is impractical. Daily to weekly weight should be monitored in such situations instead of I&O. For reliable patients, a weight-based diuretic sliding scale can be recommended.

2. ACE inhibitors:
   a. Cause dilation of the arteriolar resistance vessels and venous capacity vessels, thereby reducing both preload and afterload.
   b. Are associated with decreased mortality and improved clinical status.
   c. Can be used as first line therapy or can be added to diuretics.
   d. Therapy with ACE inhibitors should be initiated at low dose (e.g., captopril 6.25 mg tid or enalapril 2.5 mg bid) to prevent hypotension and titrated up to high doses if tolerated.
   e. Contraindications to use of ACE inhibitors are renal insufficiency (creatinine >3.0 or creatinine clearance <30 ml/min), renal artery stenosis, persistent hyperkalemia (K+ >5.5 mEQ/L), symptomatic hypotension, and history of adverse reactions (e.g., angioedema).
   f. ACE inhibitors and β-blockers can be used together.

3. Angiotensin II receptor blockers (ARBS) block the A-II type 1 (AT) receptor, which is responsible for many of the deleterious effects of angiotensin II. These receptors are potent vasoconstrictors that may contribute to the impairment of LV function. They are useful in patients unable to tolerate ACE inhibitors because of angioedema or intractable cough. They can also be used in combination with a β-blocker.

4. β-blockers: All patients with stable NYHA class II or III heart failure caused by left ventricular systolic dysfunction should receive a β-blocker unless they have a contraindication to its use or are intolerant to it. β-blockers are especially useful in patients who remain symptomatic despite therapy with ACE inhibitors and diuretics. Effective agents are carvedilol (Coreg) 3.125 mg bid, bisoprolol 1.25 mg qd, or metoprolol 12.5 mg bid initially, titrated upward as tolerated.

5. Digitalis is useful because of its positive inotropic and vagotonic effects in patients with CHF secondary to systolic dysfunction; it is of limited value in patients with mild CHF and normal sinus rhythm. It is more beneficial in patients with rapid atrial fibrillation, severe CHF, or ejection fraction of <30%; it can be added to diuretics and ACE inhibitors in patients with severe CHF. In patients with chronic heart failure and normal sinus rhythm, digoxin does not reduce mortality, but it does reduce the rate of hospitalization both overall and for worsening heart failure. Its beneficial effects are found with a low dose that results in a serum concentration of approximately 0.7 ng/ml. Higher doses may be detrimental.

6. Direct vasodilating drugs (nesiritide, hydralazine, isosorbide) are useful in the therapy of systolic dysfunction with CHF because they can reduce the systemic vascular resistance and pulmonary venous pressure, especially when used in combination.

7. Anticoagulants:
   a. Anticoagulation is not recommended for patients in sinus rhythm and no prior history of stroke, left ventricular thrombi, or arteriolar emboli.
   b. Anticoagulation therapy is appropriate for patients with heart failure and atrial fibrillation or a history of embolism.
   c. Aspirin is appropriate for all patients with ischemic heart disease.

8. Surgical revascularization should be considered in patients with both heart failure and severe limiting angina.

9. Atriobiventricular pacing significantly improves exercise tolerance and quality of life in patients with chronic heart failure and intraventricular conduction delay.

10. Obstructive sleep apnea has an adverse effect on heart failure. Recognition and treatment of coexisting obstructive sleep apnea by continuous positive airway pressure reduces systolic blood pressure and improves left ventricular systolic function.

TREATMENT OF CHF SECONDARY TO STRUCTURAL CARDIAC ABNORMALITIES
1. Aortic stenosis
   a. Diuretics.
   b. Contraindicated medications: ACE inhibitors, ARBs, nitrates, digitalis (except to control rate of atrial fibrillation).
   c. Aortic valve replacement in patients with critical stenosis.
2. Aortic insufficiency and mitral regurgitation
   a. ACE inhibitors increase cardiac output and decrease pulmonary wedge pressure. They are agents of choice along with diuretics.
   b. Hydralazine combined with nitrates can be used if ACE inhibitors are not tolerated.
   c. Surgery.
3. IHSS
   a. β-blockers or verapamil.
   b. Contraindicated medications (they increase outlet obstruction by decreasing the size of the left ventricle in end systole): diuretics, digitalis, ACE inhibitors, ARBs, hydralazine.
   c. Restoration of intravascular volume with IV saline solution if necessary in acute pulmonary edema.
   d. Septal myotomy, DDD pacing are useful in selected patients.
4. Mitral stenosis
   a. Diuretics.
   b. Control of the heart rate and atrial fibrillation with digitalis, verapamil, and/or β-blockers is critical to allow emptying of left atrium and relief of pulmonary congestion.
   c. Repairing or replacing the mitral valve is indicated if CHF is not readily controlled by the previously discussed measures.
   d. Balloon valvuloplasty is useful in selected patients.

TREATMENT OF DIASTOLIC HEART FAILURE
See Heart Failure, Diastolic in Section I.

DISPOSITION

- Annual mortality ranges from 10% in stable patients with mild symptoms to >50% in symptomatic patients with advanced disease.
- Sudden death secondary to ventricular arrhythmias occurs in >40% of patients with heart failure.
- Implantable cardiac defibrillator device in selected patients.
- In patients with advanced heart failure and a prolonged QRS interval, cardiac-resynchronization therapy decreases the combined risk of death from any cause or first hospitalization and, when combined with an implantable defibrillator, significantly reduces mortality.
- Intensive home care by nurses with expertise in the management of heart failure can improve symptom control and reduce hospitalization.
- Cardiac transplantation has a 5-yr survival rate of >70% in many centers and represents a viable option in selected patients.
- The use of a left ventricular assist device in patients with advanced heart failure can result in a clinically meaningful survival benefit and improve quality of life.

SUGGESTED READINGS

Aurigemma GP, Gaasch WH: Diastolic heart failure, *N Engl J Med* 351:1097-1105, 2004.

Bristow MR et al: Cardiac-resynchronization therapy with or without an implantable defibrillator in advanced chronic heart failure, *N Engl J Med* 350:2140-2150, 2004.

Goldstein S: Benefits of β-blocker therapy in heart failure, *Arch Intern Med* 162:641, 2002.

Gutierrez C, Blanchard DG: Diastolic heart failure: challenges of diagnosis and treatment, *Am Fam Physician* 69:2609-2616, 2004.

Jessup M, Brozena S: Heart failure, *N Engl J Med* 348:2007, 2003.

King DE et al: Acute management of heart failure, *Am Fam Physician* 66:249, 2002.

Kukin ML: β-blockers in chronic heart failure, *Mayo Clin Proc* 77:1199, 2002.

Maisel AS et al: Rapid measurement of B-type natriuretic peptide in the emergency diagnosis of heart failure, *N Engl J Med* 347:161, 2002.

Mueller C et al: Use of B-type natriuretic peptide in the evaluation and management of acute dyspnea, *N Engl J Med* 350:647-654, 2004.

Nohria A et al: Medical management of advanced heart failure, *JAMA* 287:628, 2002.

Pfeffer MA et al: Valsartan, captopril, or both in myocardial infarction complicated by heart failure, left ventricular dysfunction, or both, *N Engl J Med* 349(20):1893-1906, 2003.

Zile MR et al: Diastolic heart failure—abnormalities in active relaxation and passive stiffness of the left ventricle, *N Engl J Med* 350:1953-1959, 2004.

AUTHORS: **FRED F. FERRI, M.D.,** and **TOM J. WACHTEL, M.D.**

BASIC INFORMATION

DEFINITION

DIASTOLIC DYSFUNCTION
Abnormality of diastolic distensibility, filling, or relaxation of the left ventricle (LV)

DIASTOLIC HEART FAILURE
Patient with previous pathophysiology and a normal LV ejection fraction who develops congestive heart failure (CHF) symptoms

SYNONYMS

Congestive heart failure with preserved LV function

ICD-9CM CODES
428.0 Congestive heart failure (includes all causes of heart failure)

EPIDEMIOLOGY & DEMOGRAPHICS

- 10% to 15% progression over 5 yr from diastolic dysfunction to diastolic heart failure
- One third patients with CHF
- Ratio increases with age; highest in >75 years of age
- Mortality rate about half that of systolic heart failure
- Morbidity (e.g., hospitalization) same for diastolic and systolic heart failure
- Incidence/prevalence are unknown

PRECIPITANTS OF DIASTOLIC HEART FAILURE

- Uncontrolled hypertension
- Atrial fibrillation
- Other causes of tachycardia
- Myocardial ischemia
- Medication noncompliance
- Dietary noncompliance (salt)
- Anemia
- Renal failure
- Nonsteroidal antiinflammatory drugs (NSAIDs) including COX 2s
- Thioglitazones (TZDs)

PHYSICAL FINDINGS

The symptoms and signs of systolic and diastolic heart failure are indistinguishable (see Heart Failure, Congestive in Section I).
Symptoms include:
- Dyspnea on exertion
- Orthopnea
- Paroxysmal nocturnal dyspnea
- Reduced exercise capacity, fatigue
Physical findings:
- Tachycardia
- Hypertension
- Hypotension
- Pulmonary crackles in the lower parts of the lungs
- Signs of pleural effusion, more likely right-sided: dullness to percussion, reduced breath sounds
- Heart murmurs, S3 gallop
- Peripheral edema
- Hepatomegaly
- Hepatojugular reflux
- Acrocyanosis

PATHOPHYSIOLOGY

- Patients with diastolic heart failure have low stroke volume despite normal ejection fraction.
- Passive stiffness caused by:
  - Increased myocardial mass (hypertensive patient)
  - Alteration in collagen (CAD patient)
- Impaired active relaxation:
  - When chamber compliance is reduced, a small increase in blood volume causes a large increase in left atrial pressure.
- In addition, tachycardia, which may be somewhat helpful to patients with systolic dysfunction, is deleterious when the cause of heart failure is diastolic dysfunction. Indeed, a "stiff" ventricle needs more time to fill during diastole. Thus tachycardia is similar in effect to a pump that loses its prime.

DIAGNOSIS

DIFFERENTIAL DIAGNOSIS

- Pulmonary pathology
  - COPD
  - Asthma
  - Pneumonia
  - ARDS
  - Pulmonary embolism
- Volume overload
  - Cirrhosis
  - Portal hypertension
  - Nephrotic syndrome
  - Lower extremity venous insufficiency
- Pericardial effusion with tamponade
- Constrictive pericarditis
- Other causes of CHF (see Heart Failure, Congestive in Section I)

WORKUP

- Laboratory
  - CBC
  - BUN and creatinine
  - ALT
  - Alkaline, phosphatase
  - TSH
  - Cardiac enzymes
  - B-type natriuretic peptide (BNP)
- ECG
- Chest x-ray
- Two-dimensional echocardiography
- It is probably inappropriate in the 21st century to manage CHF without having the results of a reasonably recent echo.
- Definite diastolic heart failure: LVEF >50%; "probable" diastolic heart failure: LVEF 40%-50%.
- Diagnosis of diastolic heart failure assumes that other diagnoses (e.g., mitral regurgitation, aortic regurgitation, constrictive pericarditis) have been excluded.
- Doppler echo and cardiac cath can also help.

TREATMENT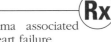

- Pulmonary edema associated with diastolic heart failure
  - Diuretics
  - Oxygen
  - Morphine
  - Nitrates
    1. Treat ischemia if present.
    2. Treat severe hypertension ("hypertensive crisis") if present.
    3. Treat tachycardia (may require urgent cardioversion of atrial fibrillation).
- Chronic management for patients with diastolic heart failure
  - Reduce the congestive state.
    1. Salt restriction
    2. Diuretics
    3. ACE inhibitors
    4. Angiotensin II—receptor blockers
  - Maintain atrial contraction and prevent tachycardia.
    1. β-blockers
    2. Calcium channel blockers
    3. Cardioversion of atrial fibrillation
    4. Sequential atrioventricular pacing
    5. Radiofrequency ablation modification of atrioventricular node and pacing
  - Treat and prevent myocardial ischemia.
    1. Nitrates
    2. β-blockers
    3. Calcium channel blockers
    4. Coronary-artery bypass surgery, percutaneous coronary intervention
  - Control hypertension.
    1. Antihypertensive agents

SUGGESTED READINGS

Aurigemma GP, Gaasch WH: Diastolic heart failure, *N Engl J Med* 351:1097-1105, 2004.
Redfield MM: Understanding "diastolic" heart failure, *N Engl J Med* 350:1930-1931, 2004.
Vasan RS: Diastolic heart failure, *BMJ USA* 4:80-84, 2004.
Zile MR, Baicu CF, Gaasch WH: Diastolic heart failure: abnormalities in active relaxation and passive stiffness of the left ventricle, *N Engl J Med* 350:1953-1959, 2004.

AUTHOR: **TOM J. WACHTEL, M.D.**

BASIC INFORMATION

DEFINITION

HEAT EXHAUSTION: An illness resulting from prolonged heavy activity in a hot environment with subsequent dehydration, electrolyte depletion, and rectal temperature >37.8° C but <40° C.

HEAT STROKE: A life-threatening heat illness characterized by extreme hyperthermia, dehydration, and neurologic manifestations (core temperature >40° C).

SYNONYMS

Heat illness
Hyperthermia

ICD-9CM CODES
992.0 Heat stroke
992.5 Heat exhaustion

EPIDEMIOLOGY & DEMOGRAPHICS

- Heat exhaustion and stroke occur more frequently in elderly patients, especially those taking diuretics or medications that impair heat dissipation (e.g., phenothiazines, anticholinergics, antihistamines, β-blockers).

PHYSICAL FINDINGS & CLINICAL PRESENTATION

HEAT EXHAUSTION:
- Generalized malaise, weakness, headache, muscle and abdominal cramps, nausea, vomiting, hypotension, and tachycardia
- Rectal temperature is usually normal
- Sweating is usually present

HEAT STROKE:
- Neurologic manifestations (seizures, tremor, hemiplegia, coma, psychosis, and other bizarre behavior)
- Evidence of dehydration (poor skin turgor, sunken eyeballs)
- Tachycardia, hyperventilation
- Skin is hot, red, and flushed
- Sweating is often (not always) absent, particularly in elderly patients

ETIOLOGY

- Exogenous heat gain (increased ambient temperature)
- Increased heat production (exercise, infection, hyperthyroidism, drugs)
- Impaired heat dissipation (high humidity, heavy clothing, elderly patients, drugs [phenothiazines, anticholinergics, antihistamines, butyrophenones, amphetamines, cocaine, alcohol, β-blockers])

DIAGNOSIS

DIFFERENTIAL DIAGNOSIS

- Infections (meningitis, encephalitis, sepsis)
- Head trauma
- Epilepsy
- Thyroid storm
- Acute cocaine intoxication
- Malignant hyperthermia
- Heat exhaustion can be differentiated from heat stroke by the following:
  1. Essentially intact mental function and lack of significant fever in heat exhaustion
  2. Mild or absent increases in CPK, AST, LDH, ALT in heat exhaustion

WORKUP

- Heat stroke: comprehensive history, physical examination, and laboratory evaluation
- Heat exhaustion: in most cases, laboratory tests are not necessary for diagnosis

LABORATORY TESTS

Laboratory abnormalities may include the following:
- Elevated BUN, creatinine, Hct
- Hyponatremia or hypernatremia, hyperkalemia or hypokalemia
- Elevated LDH, AST, ALT, CPK, bilirubin
- Lactic acidosis, respiratory alkalosis (secondary to hyperventilation)
- Myoglobinuria, hypofibrinogenemia, fibrinolysis, hypocalcemia

TREATMENT

- Treatment of **heat exhaustion** consists primarily of placing the patient in a cool, shaded area and providing rapid hydration and salt replacement.
  1. Fluid intake should be at least 2 L q4h in patients without history of CHF.
  2. Salt replacement can be accomplished by using one-quarter teaspoon of salt or two 10-grain salt tablets dissolved in 1 L of water.
  3. If IV fluid replacement is necessary in elderly patients, consider using $D_5\frac{1}{2}NS$ IV with rate titrated to cardiovascular status.
- Patients with **heat stroke** should undergo rapid cooling.
  1. Remove the patient's clothes and place the patient in a cool and well-ventilated room.
  2. If unconscious, position patient on his or her side and clear the airway. Protect airway and augment oxygenation (e.g., nasal O_2 at 4 L/min to keep oxygen saturation >90%).
  3. Monitor body temperature every 5 min. Measurement of the patient's core temperature with a rectal probe is recommended. The goal is to reduce the body temperature to 39° C (102.2° F) in 30 to 60 min.
  4. Spray the patient with a cool mist and use fans to enhance airflow over the body (rapid evaporation method).
  5. Immersion of the patient in ice water, stomach lavage with iced saline solution, intravenous administration of cooled fluids, and inhalation of cold air are advisable only when the means for rapid evaporation are not available. Immersion in tepid water (15° C [59° F]) is preferred over ice water immersion to minimize risk of shivering.
  6. Use of ice packs on axillae, neck, and groin is controversial because they increase peripheral vasoconstriction and may induce shivering.
  7. Antipyretics are ineffective because the hypothalamic set point during heat stroke is normal despite the increased body temperature.
  8. Intubate a comatose patient, insert a Foley catheter, and start nasal O_2. Continuous ECG monitoring is recommended.
  9. Insert at least two large-bore IV lines and begin IV hydration with NS or Ringer's lactate.
  10. Draw initial lab studies: electrolytes, CBC, BUN, creatinine, AST, ALT, CPK, LDH, glucose, INR, PTT, platelet count, Ca^{2+}, lactic acid, ABGs.
  11. Treat complications as follows:
      a. Hypotension: vigorous hydration with normal saline or Ringer's lactate.
      b. Convulsions: diazepam 5 to 10 mg IV (slowly).
      c. Shivering: chlorpromazine 10 to 50 mg IV.
      d. Acidosis: use bicarbonate judiciously (only in severe acidosis).
  12. Observe for evidence of rhabdomyolysis, hepatic, renal, or cardiac failure and treat accordingly.

DISPOSITION

Most patients recover completely within 48 hr. Mortality can exceed 30% in patients with prolonged and severe hyperthermia.

SUGGESTED READINGS

Bouchama A, Knochel JP: Heat stroke, *N Engl J Med* 346:1978, 2002.

Wexler RK: Evaluation and treatment of heat-related illness, *Am Fam Physician* 65:230, 2002.

AUTHOR: **FRED F. FERRI, M.D.**

BASIC INFORMATION

DEFINITION

Hematuria is classified as either microscopic or gross in nature. In microscopic hematuria, two or more red blood cells per high power field are identified in a centrifuged urine specimen. In gross hematuria, the blood is visualized by the naked eye. If the RBC per high power field is greater than 20, a tint to the urine will be visible on urinalysis.

ICD-9CM CODES
599.7

EPIDEMIOLOGY & DEMOGRAPHICS

PREVALENCE (IN U.S.): Studies report a range from 0.18% to 16.1%. The prevalence is directly associated with age. In patients over 50 years of age, the prevalence is estimated at 13%.
PREDOMINANT SEX: Several studies have reported a slightly higher prevalence in women.
GENETICS: A family history of renal failure exists in patients with hereditary nephritis and thin basement membrane disease.

ETIOLOGY

To identify the cause of hematuria, the physician should differentiate between a glomerular (medical) or nonglomerular (urologic) source of bleeding. The three most common causes of glomerular hematuria include IgA nephropathy (hematuria, hypertension, rising creatinine), thin basement membrane disease (hematuria, no extrarenal manifestations, rarely renal failure), and hereditary nephritis (hematuria, rising creatinine, <2 gm proteinuria, sensorineural deafness). Nonglomerular causes of hematuria can include lesions in either the kidney or upper urinary tract: neoplasm, nephrolithiasis, cystic disease, and papillary necrosis. Metabolic defects (hypercalciuria or hyperuricosuria) are associated with hematuria. Lower urinary tract lesions, chiefly infectious or neoplastic diseases of the bladder, urethra, and prostate can result in hematuria. Gross hematuria suggests a urologic cause of bleeding and is associated with a much higher risk for a urologic cancer. The suspicion of neoplasm increases with age, with no specific age threshold.

DIAGNOSIS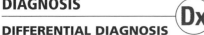

DIFFERENTIAL DIAGNOSIS

False-positive tests can result from substances other than hemoglobin such as myoglobin, vitamin C, beets, and rhubarb. A urinalysis dipstick, which is positive for "blood" but not associated with RBC on microscopic urinalysis, is not hematuria.

WORKUP

Risk factors for bladder cancer: >65 years of age, cigarette smoking, occupational exposure to chemicals (leather, dye, rubber or tire manufacturing), heavy phenacetin use, previous cyclophosphamide treatment, aristolochic acid (found in some weight loss medications). Many clinicians recommend that patients who develop hematuria during anticoagulation therapy should not only have the anticoagulation indices monitored but also undergo an evaluation of the cause of hematuria.

LABORATORY TESTS

Initially a repeat urinalysis should be obtained in a few days. If microscopic hematuria is absent on a repeat test, no further evaluation is warranted if the cause of hematuria is infectious unless the patient has risk factors for bladder cancer. If hematuria is present on repeat testing, a basic chemistry and microscopy are obtained from the patient. Combination of dysmorphic red cells and red cell casts suggests glomerular disease. An elevated creatinine suggests a renal source of the bleeding. A urine dipstick that is positive for protein should then be followed by the spot protein-to-creatinine ratio (P/Cr) or a 24-hour urine protein. A P/Cr greater than 0.3 or >300 mg in a 24-hour period suggests a glomerular source to the bleeding. Anatomic evaluation is indicated in all high-risk patients (age greater than 40 or risk factors for bladder cancer) with hematuria.

IMAGING STUDIES

- Glomerular: no imaging studies will differentiate between the glomerular disease. Biopsy is indicated with worsening renal failure and progressive proteinuria.
- Upper urinary tract: in patients suspected of stone disease, a computer tomography scan without contrast is appropriate. If there is no suspicion for stone disease, CT urography is obtained first without contrast followed by imaging with contrast dye. Ultrasound and excretory urography are most often followed by additional imaging and therefore are not considered cost-saving tests. If a CT scan cannot be performed (unavailable, contrast hypersensitivity, renal failure), ultrasound is the most reasonable alternative test.
- Lower urinary tract: cystoscopy is indicated in all the following patients: over the age of 40 or under the age of 40 in a whom a source of hematuria is not identified with upper urinary tract imaging, with risk factors for bladder cancer, gross hematuria, a urine cytology showing neoplastic cells.

TREATMENT

ACUTE GENERAL Rx

Treat any infection with appropriate antibiotic therapy, nephrolithiasis with hydration and narcotic analgesia, hematuria resulting from metabolic defects will resolve with correction of offending electrolyte imbalance. A risk/benefit analysis including goals of care and quality-of-life expectations should be discussed with the patient before any surgical intervention for neoplastic disease.

CHRONIC Rx

Management of hypertension and proteinuria should include ACE-inhibitor or angiotension receptor blocker therapy. Patients with neoplastic lesions in whom surgery is not performed and the hematuria results in a progressive anemia may require intermittent RBC transfusion therapy.

REFERRAL

When microscopic hematuria accompanies proteinuria or renal insufficiency a nephrology consult is warranted. A nephrology referral should also be obtained if polycystic kidney disease is suspected.

PEARLS & CONSIDERATIONS

COMMENTS

Isolated glomerular hematuria requires repeat testing for proteinuria and renal insufficiency at 6 months and then annually if stable. Urology referral is required whenever cystoscopy will aid in evaluation of hematuria. Isolated urologic hematuria can be monitored every 3 months for 1 yr, yearly for 3 yr, and episodically thereafter.

- The U.S. Preventative Task Force does not recommend routine screening for hematuria due to lack of evidence for effectiveness.
- A diagnosis of nephrolithiasis does not rule out the possibility of an associated urologic malignancy.
- A finding of hematuria in a patient with a recent urinary catheterization should be discarded and have a repeat urinalysis done in 2 to 3 weeks.

SUGGESTED READINGS
Brehmer, M: Imaging for microscopic hematuria, *Curr Opin Urol* 12:155-159, 2002.
Cohen RA, Brown RS: Microscopic hematuria, *N Engl J Med* 348:2330-2338, 2003.
Jaffe JS et al: A new diagnostic algorithm for the evaluation of microscopic hematuria, *Urology* 57:889-894, 2001.
Khadra M, Pickard R, Charlton M: A prospective analysis of 1930 patients with hematuria to evaluate current diagnostic practice., *J Urol* 163:524-527, 2000.

AUTHOR: **MICHAEL P. GERARDO, D.O., M.P.H.**

BASIC INFORMATION

DEFINITION

A hemorrhoid is a varicose dilation of a vein of the superior or inferior hemorrhoidal plexus, resulting from a persistent increase in venous pressure. External hemorrhoids are below the pectinate line (inferior plexus). Internal hemorrhoids are above the pectinate line (superior plexus) (Fig. 1-21).

SYNONYMS

Piles

ICD-9CM CODES
455.6 Hemorrhoids

EPIDEMIOLOGY & DEMOGRAPHICS

Potential for development of symptomatic hemorrhoids in all adults
PREVALENCE: Estimated 50% of the adult population in the U.S.
PREDOMINANT SEX: Males = females

PHYSICAL FINDINGS & CLINICAL PRESENTATION

- Painless bleeding with defecation; bleeding is bright red and staining on toilet paper
- Perianal irritation
- Mucofecal staining of underclothes
- Acute external hemorrhoids: painful, swollen, and often thrombosed
- Pain on sitting, standing, or defecating (thrombosed hemorrhoid)
- Prolapse
- Constipation

ETIOLOGY

- Low-fiber, high-fat diet
- Chronic constipation and straining with defecation
- High resting anal sphincter pressures
- Obesity
- Rectal surgery (i.e., episiotomy)
- Prolonged sitting
- Anal intercourse

DIAGNOSIS

DIFFERENTIAL DIAGNOSIS

- Fissure
- Abscess
- Anal fistula
- Condylomata acuminata
- Hypertrophied anal papillae
- Rectal prolapse
- Rectal polyp
- Neoplasm

WORKUP

- Inspection
- Digital rectal examination
- Anoscopy
- Sigmoidoscopy

TREATMENT

NONPHARMACOLOGIC THERAPY

- Avoidance of constipation and straining with defecation
- Avoidance of prolonged sitting on toilet
- High-fiber diet (20 to 30 g/day)
- Increased fluid intake (six to eight glasses of water per day)

- Cleaning with mild soap and water after defecation
- Warm soaks or ice to soothe
- Sitz baths

ACUTE GENERAL Rx

- Fiber supplements to provide bulk (psyllium extracts or mucilloids)
- Medicated compresses with witch hazel
- Topical hydrocortisone (1% to 3% cream or ointment)
- Topical anesthetic spray
- Glycerin suppositories
- Stool softeners
- Surgically remove during first 72 hr after onset

CHRONIC Rx

- Rubber-band ligation
- Injection sclerotherapy
- Photocoagulation
- Cryodestruction
- Hemorrhoidectomy
- Anal dilation
- Laser or cautery hemorrhoidectomy
- Observance for complications: thrombosis, bleeding, infection, anal stenosis or weakness

DISPOSITION

Should resolve, but there is a high rate of recurrence

REFERRAL

To colorectal or general surgeon for any hemorrhoid that does not respond to conservative therapy

PEARLS & CONSIDERATIONS

COMMENTS

- Patients need to understand the importance of a healthy diet, regular exercise, and rectal hygiene.
- Stress the importance of avoiding prolonged sitting and straining on the toilet.
- Stress the need not to defer the urge to defecate.

SUGGESTED READING

Zuber TJ: Hemorrhoidectomy for thrombosed external hemorrhoids, *Am Fam Physician* 65:1629, 2002.

AUTHOR: **MARIA A. CORIGLIANO, M.D.**

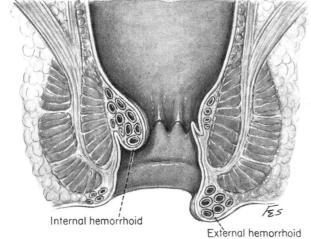

Internal hemorrhoid

External hemorrhoid

FIGURE 1-21 Anatomy of internal and external hemorrhoids. (From Noble J [ed]: *Textbook of primary care medicine,* ed 2, St Louis, 1996, Mosby.)

BASIC INFORMATION

DEFINITION

Herpes zoster is a disease caused by reactivation of the varicella-zoster virus. Following the primary infection (chickenpox) the virus becomes latent in the dorsal root ganglia and reemerges when there is a weakening of the immune system (secondary to disease or advanced age).

SYNONYMS

Shingles

ICD-9CM CODES
053.9 Herpes zoster

EPIDEMIOLOGY & DEMOGRAPHICS

- Herpes zoster occurs during lifetime in 10% to 20% of the population.
- There is an increased incidence in immunocompromised patients (AIDS, malignancy) and the elderly.

PHYSICAL FINDINGS & CLINICAL PRESENTATION

- Pain generally precedes skin manifestation by 3 to 5 days and is generally localized to the dermatome that will be affected by the skin lesions.
- Constitutional symptoms are often present (malaise, fever, headache).
- The initial rash consists of erythematous maculopapules generally affecting one dermatome (thoracic region in majority of cases); some patients (<50%) may have scattered vesicles outside of the affected dermatome.
- The initial maculopapules evolve into vesicles and pustules by the third or the fourth day.
- The vesicles have an erythematous base, are cloudy, and have various sizes (a distinguishing characteristic from herpes simplex in which the vesicles are of uniform size).
- The vesicles subsequently become umbilicated and then form crusts that generally fall off within 3 wk; scarring may occur.
- Pain during and after the rash is generally significant.
- Secondary bacterial infection with *Staphylococcus aureus* or *Streptococcus pyogenes* may occur.
- Regional lymphadenopathy may occur.
- Herpes zoster may involve the trigeminal nerve (most frequent cranial nerve involved); involvement of the geniculate ganglion can cause facial palsy and a painful ear, with the presence of vesicles on the pinna and external auditory canal (*Ramsay Hunt syndrome*).

ETIOLOGY

Reactivation of varicella virus (human herpesvirus III)

DIAGNOSIS

DIFFERENTIAL DIAGNOSIS

- Rash: herpes simplex and other viral infections
- Pain from herpes zoster: may be confused with acute myocardial infarction, pulmonary embolism, pleuritis, pericarditis, renal colic, etc.

LABORATORY TESTS

Laboratory tests are generally not necessary (viral cultures and Tzanck smear will confirm diagnosis in patients with atypical presentation).

TREATMENT

NONPHARMACOLOGIC THERAPY

- Wet compresses (using Burow's solution or cool tap water) applied for 15 to 30 min 5 to 10 times a day are useful to break vesicles and remove serum and crust.
- Care must be taken to prevent any secondary bacterial infection.

ACUTE GENERAL Rx

- Gabapentin 300 to 1800 mg qd is effective in the treatment of pain and sleep interference associated with postherpetic neuralgia.
- Lidocaine patch 5% (Lidoderm) is also effective in relieving postherpetic neuralgia. Patches are applied to intact skin to cover the most painful area for up to 12 hr within a 24-hr period.
- Oral antiviral agents can decrease acute pain, inflammation, and vesicle formation when treatment is begun within 48 hr of onset of rash. Treatment options are:
  1. Acyclovir (Zovirax) 800 mg 5 times daily for 7 to 10 days
  2. Valacyclovir (Valtrex) 1000 mg tid for 7 days
  3. Famciclovir (Famvir) 500 mg tid for 7 days
- Immunocompromised patients should be treated with IV acyclovir 500 mg/m² or 10 mg/kg q8h in 1-hr infusions for 7 days, with close monitoring of renal function and adequate hydration; vidarabine (continuous 12-hr infusion of 10 mg/kg/day for 7 days) is also effective for treatment of disseminated herpes zoster in immunocompromised hosts.

- Patients with AIDS and transplant patients may develop acyclovir-resistant varicella-zoster; these patients can be treated with foscarnet (40 mg/kg IV q8h) continued for at least 10 days or until lesions are completely healed.
- Capsaicin cream (Zostrix) can be useful for treatment of postherpetic neuralgia. It is generally applied three times daily for several weeks after the crusts have fallen off.
- Sympathetic blocks (stellate ganglion or epidural) with 0.25% bupivacaine and rhizotomy are reserved for severe cases unresponsive to conservative treatment.
- Corticosteroids should be considered in older patients if there are no contraindications. Initial dose is prednisone 60 mg/day tapered over a period of 21 days. When used there is a decrease in the use of analgesics and time to resumption of usual activities, but there is no effect on the incidence and duration of postherpetic neuralgia.

DISPOSITION

- The incidence of postherpetic neuralgia (defined as pain that persists more than 30 days after onset of rash) increases with age (>70% by age 70 yr); antivirals reduce the risk of postherpetic neuralgia.
- Incidence of disseminated herpes zoster is increased in immunocompromised hosts (e.g., 15% to 50% of patients with active Hodgkin's disease).
- Immunocompromised hosts are also more prone to neurologic complications (encephalitis, myelitis, cranial and peripheral nerve palsies, acute retinal necrosis). The mortality rate is 10% to 20% in immunocompromised hosts with disseminated zoster.
- Motor neuropathies occur in 5% of all cases of zoster; complete recovery occurs in >70% of patients.

REFERRAL

- Hospitalization for IV acyclovir in patients with disseminated herpes zoster
- Patients with herpes zoster ophthalmicus should be referred to an ophthalmologist
- Surgical referral for rhizotomy in patients with severe pain unresponsive to conventional treatment
- Sympathetic blocks in selected patients

SUGGESTED READING

Gnann JW, Whitley RJ: Herpes zoster, *N Engl J Med* 347:340, 2002.

AUTHOR: **FRED F. FERRI, M.D.**

BASIC INFORMATION

DEFINITION

Hypercholesterolemia refers to a blood cholesterol measurement >200 mg/dl. A cholesterol level of 200 to 239 mg/dl is considered borderline high, and a level of ≥240 mg/dl is considered to be a high cholesterol measurement.

SYNONYMS

Hypercholesteremia

ICD-9CM CODES
272.0 Hypercholesterolemia

EPIDEMIOLOGY & DEMOGRAPHICS

INCIDENCE/PREVALENCE:
- There are well over 100 million Americans with a total serum cholesterol >200 mg/dl.
- Elevated cholesterol requires drug therapy in about 60 million Americans.
- Incidence of heterozygous familial hypercholesterolemia: about 1:500.
- Incidence of homozygous familial hypercholesterolemia: about 1:1 million.
- Prevalence of hypercholesterolemia increases with increasing age.

GENETICS:
- Familial hypercholesterolemia: autosomal dominant disorder
- Familial combined hyperlipidemia: possibly an autosomal dominant disorder
- Multifactorial predilection: apparent in majority of affected individuals

RISK FACTORS:
- Dietary intake
- Genetic predisposition
- Sedentary lifestyle
- Associated secondary causes
- Obesity

PHYSICAL FINDINGS & CLINICAL PRESENTATION
- Most patients: no physical findings
- Possible findings particularly in the familial forms
  1. Tendon xanthomas
  2. Xanthelasma
  3. Arcus corneae
  4. Coronary artery disease
  5. Cerebrovascular disease
  6. Peripheral arterial disease

ETIOLOGY

Primary
1. Genetics
2. Obesity
3. Dietary intake

Secondary
1. Diabetes mellitus
2. Alcohol
3. Hypothyroidism
4. Glucocorticoid use
5. Most diuretics
6. Nephrotic syndrome
7. Hepatoma
8. Extrahepatic biliary obstruction
9. Primary biliary cirrhosis

DIAGNOSIS Dx

DIFFERENTIAL DIAGNOSIS

No real differential diagnosis; however, consider underlying secondary causes/etiologies for the elevated cholesterol.

LABORATORY TESTS

PRIMARY PREVENTION WITHOUT ATHEROSCLEROSIS OR DIABETES MELLITUS:
1. Total cholesterol <200 mg/dl, and the HDL >40: repeat in 5 yr.
2. Cholesterol 200 to 239 mg/dl and the HDL >40: discuss dietary modification, repeat in 1 to 2 yr.
3. Total cholesterol >240 mg/dl or the HDL <40 mg/dl: need a fasting lipid profile (cholesterol, HDL, triglycerides, from which an LDL can be calculated).
4. Fasting lipid profile with LDL <130 mg/dl and 1 or no risk factors: dietary guidance and repeat in 5 yr.
5. Fasting lipid profile with LDL 130 to 159 mg/dl (borderline high risk), and less than two risk factors for CAD: diet and exercise modification, with repeat profile in 12 wk.
6. Fasting lipid profile with LDL >160 mg/dl or borderline LDL and two or more risk factors for CAD: need drug therapy.

SECONDARY PREVENTION WITH ATHEROSCLEROSIS OR DIABETES MELLITUS:
1. All patients: fasting lipid profile
2. If LDL <100 mg/dl: instruction on diet and exercise, and repeat after 3 to 4 months
3. Now classified as very high risk
4. If LDL >70, drug therapy advised

TREATMENT Rx

NONPHARMACOLOGIC THERAPY
- Dietary modifications
  1. Low-cholesterol, low-fat diet (fat intake to 30% or less of the total caloric intake)
  2. Saturated fats <7% of total calories
  3. No more than 200 mg/day of cholesterol
- Increased activity with aerobic exercise: encourage 20 to 30 min of aerobic exercise three to four times a week
- Smoking cessation encouraged
- Counseling on CAD risk factors

ACUTE GENERAL Rx

No acute treatment needed

CHRONIC Rx
- In secondary prevention: needed for patients with known CAD, vascular disease or diabetes mellitus, and LDL >70 mg/dl
- In primary prevention: considered in patients on dietary therapy with LDL >190 mg/dl with no risk factors, LDL >160 mg/dl with two or more risk factors, HDL <30 mg/dl, or LDL 130 to 159 mg/dl with two or more risk factors for CAD
- Medications that can be used (see Table 1-7):
  1. Bile acid sequestrants (poorly tolerated)
  2. Niacin (poorly tolerated)
  3. HMG-CoA reductase inhibitors ("statins")
  4. Fibric acids
  5. Medication tailored to the patient's lipid profile, lifestyle, and the medication's side-effect profile
- Cholesterol absorption inhibitors (ezetimibe)
- Bile acid sequestrants to lower LDL
- Niacin to lower LDL and triglycerides and raise HDL
- HMG-CoA reductase inhibitors to lower LDL
- Fibric acids work to lower triglycerides more than LDL

DISPOSITION
- After initiation of therapy, repeat laboratory tests in 4 to 6 wk, with modifications as necessary.
- Once goal is achieved, lifelong medication and monitoring are needed at least three to four times a year.
- Dietary modification is needed to continue with drug therapy.
- Repeat review for additional CAD risk factors.

PEARLS & CONSIDERATIONS !

COMMENTS

Because the rate of endpoints (coronary and cardiovascular) is higher in older patients, the absolute risk reduction is greater and the number needed to treat is lower in the geriatric patient compared with the middle-aged adult.

SUGGESTED READINGS

Cleeman JI: Detection and evaluation of dyslipoproteinemia, *Endocrinol Metab Clin North Am* 27(3):597, 1998.

Illingworth DR: Management of hypercholesterolemia, *Med Clin North Am* 84(1):23, 2000.

National Cholesterol Education Program: Second Report on the Expert Panel on Detection, Evaluation, and Treatment of High Cholesterol in Adults (adult treatment panel IV), *JAMA* 285:2486, 2001.

Safeer R, Ugalat P: Cholesterol treatment guidelines update, *Am Fam Physician* 65:871, 2002.

AUTHORS: **BETH J. WUTZ, M.D.,** with revisions by **TOM J. WACHTEL, M.D.**

TABLE 1-7 Drugs Affecting Lipoprotein Metabolism

Drug class	Agents and daily doses	Lipid/lipoprotein effects		Side effects	Contraindications
HMG-CoA reductase inhibitors (statins)	Lovastatin (20-80 mg) Pravastatin (20-80 mg) Simvastatin (20-80 mg) Fluvastatin (20-80 mg) Atorvastatin (10-80 mg) Rosuvastain (5-40 mg)	LDL HDL TG	↓18%-55% ↑5%-15% ↓7%-30%	Myopathy Increased liver enzymes	Absolute: • Active or chronic liver disease Relative: • Concomitant use of certain drugs*
Bile acid sequestrants	Cholestyramine (4-16 g) Colestipol (5-20 g) Colesevelam (2.6-3.8 g)	LDL HDL TG	↓1.5%-30% ↑3%-5% No change or increase	Gastrointestinal distress Constipation Decreased absorption of other drugs	Absolute: • Dysbetalipoproteinemia • TG >400 mg/dl Relative: • TG >200 mg/dl
Nicotinic acid	Immediate-release (crystalline) nicotinic acid (1.5-3 g), extended-release nicotinic acid (Niaspan) 1-2 g, sustained-release nicotinic acid (1-2 g)	LDL HDL TG	↓5%-25% ↑15%-35% ↓20%-50%	Flushing Hyperglycemia Hyperuricemia (or gout) Upper GI distress Hepatotoxicity	Absolute: • Chronic liver disease • Severe gout Relative: • Diabetes • Hyperuricemia • Peptic ulcer disease
Fibric acids	Gemfibrozil (600 mg bid) Fenofibrate (160 mg qd) Clofibrate (1000 mg bid)	LDL *(may be increased in patients with high TG)* HDL TG	↓5%-20% ↑10%-20% ↓20%-50%	Dyspepsia Gallstones Myopathy	Absolute: • Severe renal disease • Severe hepatic disease
Cholesterol absorption inhibitors	Ezetimibe (10 mg QD)	LDL HDL TG	↓18% ↑1% ↓7%-8%	Abdominal pain myalgias	• Severe renal disease • Severe hepatic disease

Modified from The National Cholesterol Education Program, *JAMA* 285:2486, 2001.
CoA, Coenzyme A; *GI,* gastrointestinal; *HDL,* high-density lipoprotein; *HMG,* 3-hydroxy-3 methylglutaryl; *LDL,* low-density lipoprotein; *TG,* triglyceride.
*Cyclosporine, macrolide antibiotics, various antifungal agents, and cytochrome P-450 inhibitors (fibrates and niacin should be used with appropriate caution).

BASIC INFORMATION

DEFINITION

Hyperosmolar coma (nonketotic hyperosmolar syndrome) is a state of extreme hyperglycemia, marked dehydration, serum hyperosmolarity, altered mental status, and absence of ketoacidosis.

SYNONYMS

Nonketotic hyperosmolar syndrome
Hyperosmolar nonketotic state

ICD-9CM CODES
250.2 Hyperosmolar coma

PHYSICAL FINDINGS & CLINICAL PRESENTATION

- Evidence of severe dehydration (poor skin turgor, sunken eyeballs, dry mucous membranes)
- Neurologic defects (reversible hemiplegia, focal seizures)
- Orthostatic hypotension, tachycardia
- Evidence of precipitating factors (pneumonia, infected skin ulcer)
- Coma (25% of patients), delirium

ETIOLOGY

- Infections, 20% to 25% (e.g., pneumonia, UTI, sepsis)
- New or previously unrecognized diabetes (30% to 50%)
- Reduction or omission of diabetic medication
- Stress (MI, CVA)
- Drugs: diuretics (dehydration), phenytoin, diazoxide (impaired insulin secretion)

DIAGNOSIS Dx

DIFFERENTIAL DIAGNOSIS

- Diabetic ketoacidosis

LABORATORY TESTS

- Hyperglycemia: serum glucose usually >600 mg/dl.
- Hyperosmolarity: serum osmolarity usually >340 mOsm/L.
- Serum sodium: may be low, normal, or high; if normal or high, the patient is severely dehydrated, because an elevated glucose draws fluid from intracellular space decreasing the serum sodium; the corrected sodium can be obtained by increasing the serum sodium concentration by 1.6 mEq/dl for every 100 mg/dl increase in the serum glucose level over normal.

- Serum potassium: may be low, normal, or high; regardless of the initial serum level, the total body deficit is approximately 5 to 15 mEq/kg.
- Serum bicarbonate: usually >12 mEq/L (average is 17 mEq/L).
- Arterial pH: usually >7.2 (average is 7.26); both serum bicarbonate and arterial pH may be lower if lactic acidosis is present.
- BUN: azotemia (prerenal) is usually present (BUN generally ranges from 60 to 90 mg/dl).
- Phosphorus: hypophosphatemia (average deficit is 70 to 140 mEq).
- Calcium: hypocalcemia (average deficit is 50 to 100 mEq).
- Magnesium: hypomagnesemia (average deficit is 50 to 100 mEq).
- CBC with differential, urinalysis, blood and urine cultures should be performed to rule out infectious etiology.

IMAGING STUDIES

- Chest x-ray examination is useful to rule out infectious process. The initial chest x-ray may be negative if the patient has significant dehydration. Repeat chest x-ray examination after 24 hr of hydration if pulmonary infection is suspected.
- CT scan of head should be performed in patients with suspected CVA.

TREATMENT Rx

NONPHARMACOLOGIC THERAPY

- Monitor mental status, vital signs, urine output qh until improved, then monitor q2-4h.
- Monitor electrolytes, renal function, and glucose level (see Acute General Rx).

ACUTE GENERAL Rx

- Vigorous fluid replacement: the volume and rate of fluid replacement are determined by renal and cardiac function. Typically, infuse 1000 to 1500 ml/hr for the initial 1 to 2 L; then decrease the rate of infusion to 500 ml/hr and monitor urinary output, blood chemistries, and blood pressure; use 0.9% NS (isotonic solution) if the patient is hypotensive; otherwise use 0.45% NS solution. Slower infusion rate may be used initially in patients with compromised cardiovascular or renal status.
- Replace electrolytes and monitor serum levels frequently (e.g., serum sodium and potassium q2h for the first

12 hr). Serum KCl replacement in patients with normal renal function and adequate urinary output is started when the serum potassium level is <5.2 mEq/L (e.g., 10 mEq KCl/hr if potassium level is 4 to 5.2 mEq/L). Continuous ECG monitoring and hourly measurement of urinary output are recommended.
- Correct hyperglycemia. The goal is for plasma glucose to decline by at least 75 to 100 mg/dl/hr.
  1. Vigorous IV hydration will decrease the serum glucose level in most patients by 80 mg/dl/hr; a regular insulin IV bolus (10 U) is often not necessary.
  2. Low-dose insulin infusion at 1 to 2 U/hr (e.g., 25 U of regular insulin in 250 ml of 0.9% saline solution at 20 ml/hr) until the serum glucose level approaches 300 mg/dl; then the patient is started on regular SC insulin with sliding scale coverage. If the plasma glucose does not decrease over 2 to 4 hr despite adequate fluid administration and urine output, consider doubling the hourly insulin dose.
  3. Glucose should be monitored q1-2h in the initial 12 hr.
- In the absence of renal failure, phosphate can be administered at a rate of 0.1 mmol/kg/hr (5 to 10 mmol/hr) to a maximum of 80 to 120 mmol in 24 hr. Magnesium replacement, in absence of renal failure, can be administered IM (0.05 to 0.10 ml/kg of 20% magnesium sulfate) or as IV infusion (4 to 8 ml of 20% magnesium sulfate [0.08 to 0.16 mEq/kg]). Repeat magnesium, phosphate, and calcium levels should be obtained after 12 to 24 hr.

DISPOSITION

Mortality in nonketotic hyperosmolar coma ranges from 20% to 50%.

PEARLS & CONSIDERATIONS

COMMENTS

The typical patient presenting with hyperosmolar coma is an elderly or bedconfined diabetic with impaired ability to communicate thirst who is evaluated after an interval of 1 to 2 wk of prolonged osmotic diuresis.

AUTHOR: **FRED F. FERRI, M.D.**

BASIC INFORMATION

DEFINITION

Primary hyperparathyroidism is an endocrine disorder caused by the excessive secretion of parathyroid hormone (PTH) from the parathyroid glands.

ICD-9CM CODES
252.0 Primary hyperparathyroidism
588.8 Secondary hyperparathyroidism in chronic renal disease

EPIDEMIOLOGY & DEMOGRAPHICS

PREDOMINANT AGE AND SEX:
- Primary hyperparathyroidism occurs most frequently in postmenopausal women; prevalence in this group may be as high as 3%. The condition is asymptomatic in >50% of patients
- Prevalence: 1 case/1000 men and 2 to 3 cases/1000 women
- Primary hyperparathyroidism is the most frequent cause of hypercalcemia in ambulatory patients whereas malignancy is the most frequent cause of hypercalcemia in hospitalized patients.

GENETICS: Hyperparathyroidism can occur in conjunction with MEN I or II.

PHYSICAL FINDINGS & CLINICAL PRESENTATION

Primary hyperparathyroidism can be classified as asymptomatic (75% to 80%) and symptomatic. Physical examination may be entirely normal. The presence of signs and symptoms varies with the rapidity of development and degree of hypercalcemia. The following abnormalities may be present:
- GI: constipation, anorexia, nausea, vomiting, pancreatitis, ulcers
- CNS: confusion, obtundation, psychosis, lassitude, depression, coma
- GU: nephrolithiasis, renal insufficiency, polyuria, decreased urine-concentrating ability, nocturia, nephrocalcinosis
- Musculoskeletal: myopathy, weakness, osteoporosis, pseudogout, bone pain
- Other: hypertension, metastatic calcifications, band keratopathy (found in medial and lateral margin of the cornea), pruritus

ETIOLOGY
- A single adenoma is found in 80% of patients; 90% of the adenomas are found within one of the parathyroid glands, the other 10% are in ectopic sites (lateral neck, thyroid, mediastinum, retroesophagus).
- Parathyroid gland hyperplasia occurs in 20% of patients.
- Primary hyperthyroidism is associated with multiple endocrine neoplasia (MEN) I and II.

DIAGNOSIS

DIFFERENTIAL DIAGNOSIS
Other causes of hypercalcemia:
- Malignancy: neoplasms of breast, lung, kidney, ovary, pancreas; myeloma, lymphoma
- Granulomatous disorders (e.g., sarcoidosis)
- Paget's disease
- Vitamin D intoxication, milk-alkali syndrome
- Thiazide diuretics
- Other: familial hypocalciuric hypercalcemia, thyrotoxicosis, adrenal insufficiency, prolonged immobilization, vitamin A intoxication, recovery from acute renal failure, lithium administration, pheochromocytoma, SLE

WORKUP
- Persistent hypercalcemia, hypophosphatemia, and an elevated serum PTH confirm the diagnosis of primary hyperparathyroidism. Repeated measurements of serum calcium may be necessary because patients may not have persistently elevated serum calcium level. In malnourished patients, the serum calcium level needs to be corrected for low albumin levels by adding 0.8 mg/dl to the total serum calcium level for every 1.0 g/dl by which the serum albumin concentration is lower than 4 g/dl.
- The serum PTH level is the single best test for initial evaluation of confirmed hypercalcemia. The "intact" PTH (iPTH) is the best assay. The iPTH distinguishes primary hyperparathyroidism from hypercalcemia caused by malignancy when the serum calcium level is >12 mg/dl.
- A high level of urinary cyclic AMP is also suggestive of primary hyperparathyroidism.
- Parathyroid hormone–like protein (PLP) is increased in hypercalcemia associated with solid malignancies.
- ECG may reveal shortening of the QT interval secondary to hypercalcemia.

LABORATORY TESTS
- Elevated serum ionized calcium level, low serum phosphorus, and normal or elevated alkaline phosphatase
- Elevated urine calcium level (in contrast with very low urinary calcium levels seen in patients with familial hypocalciuric hypercalcemia)
- Possibly elevated serum chloride levels, decreased serum CO_2, hyperchloremic metabolic acidosis
- A serum albumin level should be obtained when measuring serum calcium and the calcium level should be adjusted (see above) in hypoalbuminemic patients

- The differential diagnosis of hypercalcemia is described in Section II

IMAGING STUDIES
- A bone survey may show evidence of subperiosteal bone resorption (suggesting PTH excess). The classic bone disease of primary hyperparathyroidism is osteitis fibrosa cystica.
- Parathyroid localization with technetium-99m sestamibi has been shown to have a high sensitivity and specificity for single adenomas.
- Screen for osteopenia with measurement of bone mineral density in all postmenopausal women.

TREATMENT

NONPHARMACOLOGIC THERAPY
- Unless contraindicated, patients should maintain a high intake of fluids (3 to 5 L/day) and sodium chloride (>400 mEq/day) to increase renal calcium excretion. Calcium intake should be 1000 mg/day.
- Potential hypercalcemic agents (e.g., thiazide diuretics) should be discontinued.
- Surgery is the only effective treatment for primary hyperparathyroidism. It is generally indicated in all female patients and male patients with complications from hyperthyroidism, such as nephrolithiasis and osteopenia. The conventional surgical approach is bilateral neck exploration under general anesthesia. Minimally invasive adenomectomy guided by preoperative technetium-99-m sestamibi scanning or ultrasound plus spiral CT is an alternative to conventional neck exploration. With the minimally invasive approach, the solitary adenoma is excised through a small unilateral incision with the patient under local cervical block anesthesia.
- Percutaneous ethanol injection into the parathyroid gland should be considered in selected patients who have undergone a subtotal parathyroidectomy for multigland disease and have recurrent hyperparathyroidism as a result of remnant gland.
- Asymptomatic elderly male patients can be followed conservatively with periodic monitoring of serum calcium level and review of symptoms. Serum creatinine and PTH levels should also be obtained at 6- to 12-mo intervals, bone density (cortical and trabecular) yearly. Criteria for medical monitoring of patients with asymptomatic primary hyperparathyroidism are as follows:
  1. Serum calcium level only mildly elevated
  2. Asymptomatic patient

3. Normal bone status (no osteoporosis)
4. Normal kidney function and no urolithiasis or nephrocalcinosis
5. No previous episode of life-threatening hypercalcemia

- Nearly 25% of asymptomatic patients develop indications for surgery during observation.

ACUTE GENERAL Rx

Acute severe hypercalcemia (serum calcium >13 mg/dl) or symptomatic patients can be treated with the following:

- Vigorous IV hydration with NS followed by IV furosemide. Use NS with caution in patients with cardiac or renal insufficiency to avoid fluid overload.
- Calcitonin 4 IU/kg q12h is indicated when saline hydration and furosemide are ineffective or contraindicated.
- Bisphosphonates (pamidronate, etidronate), mithramycin, and gallium nitrate are also effective for severe hypercalcemia.
- Cinacalcet (Sensipar) is an oral calcimimetic agent that directly lowers PTH levels by increasing the calcium-sensing receptor to extracellular calcium. The reduction in PTH is associated with a concomitant decrease in serum calcium levels. It is indicated in treatment of secondary hyperparathyroidism in patients with chronic kidney disease on dialysis and hypercalcemia in parathyroid carcinoma. Initial dose is 30 mg po qd.

PEARLS & CONSIDERATIONS

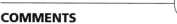

COMMENTS

- Patients with hyperparathyroidism should undergo further evaluation for the presence of MEN I or II.

- Decreased bone mineral density and nephrolithiasis are the major sequelae of untreated hyperparathyroidism.
- An experienced endocrine surgeon cures more than 95% of patients undergoing bilateral neck exploration and incurs <1% perioperative mortality.

SUGGESTED READINGS

Monchik JM et al: Minimally invasive parathyroid surgery in 103 patients with local/regional anesthesia, without exclusion criteria, *Surgery* 131:502, 2002.

Taniegra ED: Hyperparathyroidism, *Am Fam Physician* 69:333, 2004.

Udelsman R: Six hundred fifty-six consecutive explorations for primary hyperparathyroidism, *Ann Surg* 235:665, 2002.

AUTHOR: **FRED F. FERRI, M.D.**

BASIC INFORMATION

DEFINITION

The Joint National Committee on Prevention, Detection, Evaluation, and Treatment of High Blood Pressure (JNC 7) classifies normal blood pressure in adults as <120 mm Hg systolic and <80 mm Hg diastolic. Prehypertension is defined as systolic pressure 120 to 139 mm Hg or diastolic pressure 80 to 89 mm Hg. Stage 1 hypertension is systolic BP 140 to 159 mm Hg or diastolic BP 90 to 99 mm Hg. Stage 2 hypertension is systolic BP ≥160 mm Hg or diastolic BP ≥100 mm Hg.

SYNONYMS

Essential hypertension
Idiopathic hypertension
High blood pressure

ICD-9CM CODES
401.1 Essential hypertension
401.0 Malignant hypertension caused by renal artery stenosis
405.01 Malignant hypertension secondary to renal artery stenosis
437.2 Hypertensive encephalopathy

EPIDEMIOLOGY & DEMOGRAPHICS

- Incidence of hypertension in adult population older than age 60: 65%.
- Two thirds have isolated systolic hypertension, which is no longer considered a separate clinical entity.
- 90% of persons age 55 will develop hypertension in their lifetime.
- 50 million individuals in the U.S. and approximately 1 billion individuals worldwide meet the criteria for diagnosis of hypertension.

PHYSICAL FINDINGS & CLINICAL PRESENTATION

Physical examination may be entirely within normal limits except for the presence of hypertension. A proper initial physical examination on a hypertensive patient should include the following:
- Measure height and weight.
- Evaluate skin for the presence of striae (Cushing's syndrome).
- Perform funduscopic examination: check for papilledema, retinal exudates, hemorrhages, arterial narrowing, AV compression.
- Examine the neck for carotid bruits, distended neck veins, or enlarged thyroid gland.
- Perform cardiopulmonary examination: check for loud aortic component of S_2, S_4, ventricular lift, murmurs, arrhythmias.

- Check abdomen for masses (pheochromocytoma, polycystic kidneys), presence of bruits over the renal artery (renal artery stenosis), dilation of the aorta.
- Obtain two or more BP measurements separated by 2 min with the patient either supine or seated and after standing for at least 2 min (the latter to check for orthostatic hypotension). Measure BP in both upper extremities (if values are discrepant, use the higher value). Blood should be measured at least twice (on separate visits) in the sitting position before making a diagnosis of hypertension.
- Examine arterial pulses (dilated or absent femoral pulses and BP greater in upper extremities than lower extremities suggest aortic coarctation).
- Note the presence of truncal obesity (Cushing's syndrome) and pedal edema (CHF, nephrosis).
- Perform neurologic assessment.
- The clinical evaluation should help determine if the patient has primary or secondary (possibly reversible) hypertension, if there is target organ disease present, and if there are cardiovascular risk factors in addition to hypertension.

ETIOLOGY

- Essential (primary) hypertension (90%)
- Drug induced or drug related (5%)
- Renal parenchymal disease (3%)
- Renovascular hypertension (<2%)
- Endocrine (4% to 5%)
- Primary aldosteronism (0.5%)
- Pheochromocytoma (0.2%)
- Cushing's syndrome and chronic steroid therapy (0.2%)
- Hyperparathyroidism or thyroid disease (0.2%)
- Coarctation of the aorta (0.2%)

DIAGNOSIS

WORKUP

Pertinent history:
- Age of onset of hypertension, previous antihypertensive therapy
- Family history of hypertension, stroke, cardiovascular disease
- Diet, salt intake, alcohol, drugs (e.g., NSAIDs, decongestants, steroids)
- Occupation, lifestyle, socioeconomic status, psychologic factors
- Other cardiovascular risk factors: hyperlipidemia, obesity, diabetes mellitus, carbohydrate intolerance
- Symptoms of secondary hypertension:
  1. Headache, palpitations, excessive perspiration (possible pheochromocytoma)
  2. Weakness, polyuria (consider hyperaldosteronism)
  3. Claudication of lower extremities (seen with coarctation of aorta)

LABORATORY TESTS

- Urinalysis: for evidence of renal disease.
- BUN, creatinine: to rule out renal disease. High-serum creatinine is a predictor of cardiovascular risk in essential hypertension.
- Serum electrolyte levels: low potassium is suggestive of primary aldosteronism, diuretic use, or Cushing's syndrome.
- Fasting serum glucose to screen for Cushing's syndrome.
- Screening for coexisting diseases that may adversely affect prognosis:
  1. Serum lipid panel, uric acid, calcium
  2. If pheochromocytoma is suspected: 24-hr urine for VMA and metanephrines

IMAGING STUDIES

- ECG: check for presence of left ventricular hypertrophy (LVH) with strain pattern.
- Echocardiogram in selected cases.
- MRA of the renal arteries: in suspected renovascular hypertension (renal artery stenosis).

TREATMENT

NONPHARMACOLOGIC THERAPY

Lifestyle modifications:
- Lose weight if overweight.
- Limit alcohol intake to ≤1 oz of ethanol per day in men or ≤0.5 oz in women.
- Exercise (aerobic) regularly (30 min/day, most days).
- Reduce sodium intake.
- Maintain adequate dietary potassium (>3500 mg/day) intake.
- Stop smoking and reduce dietary saturated fat and cholesterol intake for overall cardiovascular health.
- Consume diet rich in fruits and vegetables.

ACUTE GENERAL Rx

According to the Seventh Report of the Joint National Committee on Detection, Evaluation, and Treatment of High Blood Pressure:
- Antihypertensive drug therapy should be initiated in patients with stage 1 hypertension. Diuretics or β-blockers are preferred for initial therapy because a reduction in morbidity and mortality has been demonstrated and because of their lower cost.
- ACE inhibitors, ARBs, calcium channel blockers, and α-β-blockers are also effective.
- Two-drug combination is necessary for most patients with stage 2 hypertension. Fixed dose combinations may improve compliance and cut cost.

- The major advantages and limitations of each class of drugs are described as follows:
  1. Diuretics
     a. Advantages: inexpensive, once per day dosing. Useful in edema states, CHF, chronic renal disease (decreased incidence of hip fractures in patients taking thiazide diuretics; opposite effect for loop diuretics).
     b. Disadvantages: significant adverse metabolic effects, increased risk of cardiac arrhythmias, sexual dysfunction, possible adverse effects on lipids and glucose levels. Avoid in patients with urinary incontinence. Thiazides not effective when creatinine clearance is less than 20 ml/min. (Note: low creatinine clearance can coexist with normal creatinine levels in patients over the age of 85 [see Section IV].)
  2. β-blockers
     a. Advantages: ideal in hypertensive patients with ischemic heart disease or post-MI. Favored in hyperkinetic, younger patients (resting tachycardia, wide pulse pressure, hyperdynamic heart) and stable (Class II-III) CHF patients.
     b. Disadvantages: adverse effect on quality of life (increased incidence of fatigue, depression, impotence, bronchospasm, hypoglycemia, peripheral vascular disease, adverse effects on lipids, masking of signs and symptoms of hypoglycemia in diabetics).
  3. Calcium channel blockers
     a. Advantages: helpful in hypertensive patients with ischemic heart disease. Generally favorable effect on quality of life; can be used in patients with bronchospastic disorders, renal disease, peripheral avascular disease, metabolic disorders, and salt sensitivity. Nondihydropyridine calcium channel blockers (verapamil, diltiazem) are useful in reducing proteinuria.
     b. Disadvantages: diltiazem and verapamil should be avoided in patients with CHF because of their negative chronotropic and inotropic effects; pedal edema may occur with nifedipine and amlodipine; constipation can be a problem in patients receiving verapamil.
  4. ACE inhibitors
     a. Advantages: well tolerated, favorable impact on quality of life; useful in hypertension complicated by CHF; helpful in prevention of diabetic renal disease; effective in decreasing LVH.
     b. Disadvantages: cough is a frequent side effect (5% to 20% of patients); hyperkalemia may occur in patients with diabetes or renal insufficiency; hypotension may occur in volume-depleted patients.
  5. Angiotensin II receptor blockers (ARB)
     a. Advantages: well tolerated, favorable impact on quality of life; useful in patients unable to tolerate ACE inhibitors because of persistent cough and in CHF and diabetic patients; single daily dose.
     b. Disadvantages: cost; hypotension may occur in volume-depleted patients.
  6. α-1 adrenergic blockers
     a. Advantages: no adverse effect on blood lipids or insulin sensitivity; helpful in BPH. May be less effective than other agents.
     b. Disadvantages: postural hypotension; syncope can be avoided by giving an initial low dose at bedtime.
  7. Other agents (e.g., hydralazine, reserpine, guanfacine, methyldopa, minoxidil, clonidine) are infrequently used.
  8. Start with a low dose and titrate upward slowly, monitoring for orthostatic hypotension. Consider titrating down if BP is consistently below 130/80.

TREATMENT OF RENOVASCULAR HYPERTENSION (RVH): Therapeutic approach varies with the cause of the RVH.
1. Medical therapy is advisable in elderly patients with atheromatous renal vascular hypertension; useful agents are:
   a. β-blockers: very effective in patients with elevated plasma renin.
   b. ACE inhibitors: very effective; however, should be avoided in patients with bilateral renal artery stenosis or in patients with solitary kidney and renal stenosis.
   c. Diuretics: often used in combination with ACE inhibitors.
2. Surgical revascularization is generally reserved for atheromatous RVH in patients responding poorly to medical therapy (uncontrolled hypertension, deteriorating renal function).

MALIGNANT HYPERTENSION, HYPERTENSIVE EMERGENCIES, AND HYPERTENSIVE URGENCIES
- Definitions:
  1. Malignant hypertension is a potentially life-threatening situation.
     a. The rate of BP rise is a critical factor.
     b. The clinical manifestations are grade IV hypertensive retinopathy (exudates, hemorrhages, and papilledema), cardiovascular or renal compromise, and encephalopathy.
     c. It requires rapid BP reduction (not necessarily into normal ranges) to prevent or limit target organ disease.
  2. Hypertensive emergencies are situations that require immediate (within 1 hr) lowering of BP to prevent end-organ damage.

The choice of therapeutic agents in malignant hypertension varies with the cause.
1. Nitroprusside is the drug of choice in hypertensive encephalopathy, hypertension and intracranial bleeding, malignant hypertension, hypertension and heart failure, dissecting aortic aneurysm (used in combination with the propranolol); its onset of action is immediate.
2. Fenoldopam is a newer vasodilator agent useful for the short-term (up to 48 hr) management of severe hypertension when rapid but quickly reversible reduction of blood pressure is required.
3. The following are important points to remember when treating hypertensive emergencies:
   a. Introduce a plan for long-term therapy at the time of the initial emergency treatment.
   b. Agents that reduce arterial pressure can cause the kidney to retain sodium and water; therefore, the judicious administration of diuretics should accompany their use.
   c. The initial goal of antihypertensive therapy is not to achieve a normal BP, but rather to gradually reduce the BP; cerebral hyperperfusion may occur if the mean BP is lowered >40% in the initial 24 hr.
   d. Hypertensive emergencies can be treated with oral clonidine 0.1 mg q20 min (to a maximum of 0.8 mg) or intravenous medication.

PEARLS & CONSIDERATIONS

COMMENTS

- In patients with hypertension and chronic renal insufficiency, it is not uncommon to see a small rise in serum creatinine as the blood pressure is lowered. Most physicians will respond by decreasing the dose of the antihypertensive medication. This approach should be discouraged because it is not optimal for the long-term preservation of renal function because a small, nonprogressive increase in serum creatinine in the context of improved blood pressure control is indicative of successful reduction of the intraglomerular pressure.

- The choice of antihypertensive treatment should take comorbidities into account particularly in older patients who are at risk of polypharmacy.
- Home blood pressure monitoring (e.g., once weekly) with a digital measuring device is gaining in popularity. The device should be checked against the physician's equipment from time to time. A blood pressure log should be maintained by the patient. This strategy eliminates "white coat" hypertension and provides a better sampling of BP measurements. However, no one knows what are optimal home blood pressures.

SUGGESTED READINGS

ALLHAT Officers and Coordinators for the ALLHAT Collaborative Research Group: Major outcomes in high-risk hypertensive patients randomized to angiotensin-converting enzyme inhibitor of calcium channel blocker vs diuretic: the Antihypertensive and Lipid-Lowering Treatment to Prevent Heart Attack Trial (ALLHAT) (published erratum appears in *JAMA* 289:178, 2003), *JAMA* 288:2981-2997, 2002.

Aronow WS: Treatment of older persons with hypertension, *Clin Geriatrics* 13:12-16, 2005.

Dickerson LM, Gibson MV: Management of hypertension in older persons, *Am Fam Physician* 71:469-476, 2005.

Francos GC, Schairer HL Jr.: Hypertension. Contemporary challenges in geriatric care, *Geriatrics* 58:44-49, 2003.

Franklin SS et al: Predominance of isolated systolic hypertension among middle-aged and elderly U.S. hypertensives: analysis based on National Health and Nutrition Examination Survey (NHANES) III, *Hypertension* 37:869-874, 2001.

Gueyffier F et al: Antihypertensive drugs in very old people: a subgroup meta-analysis of randomized controlled trials, *Lancet* 353:793-796, 1999.

Magill MK et al: New developments in the management of hypertension, *Am Fam Physician* 68:853, 2003.

Malacco E et al: Treatment of isolated systolic hypertension: the SHELL study results, *Blood Press* 12:160-167, 2003.

Oparil S et al: Pathogenesis of hypertension, *Ann Intern Med* 139:761, 2003.

Seventh Report of the Joint National Committee on Prevention, Detection, Evaluation, and Treatment of High Blood Pressure, *JAMA* 289:2560, 2003.

Staessen JA et al: Risks of untreated and treated isolated systolic hypertension in the elderly: meta-analysis of outcome trials (published erratum appears in *Lancet* 357:724, 2001), *Lancet* 355:865-872, 2000.

Wing LM et al: A comparison of outcomes with angiotensin-converting-enzyme inhibitors and diuretics for hypertension in the elderly, *N Engl J Med* 348:583-592, 2003.

Wright JT et al: Outcomes in hypertensive black and non-black patients, *JAMA* 293:1595-1608, 2005.

AUTHORS: **FRED F. FERRI, M.D.,** and **TOM J. WACHTEL, M.D.**

BASIC INFORMATION

DEFINITION

Hyperthyroidism is a hypermetabolic state resulting from excess thyroid hormone.

SYNONYMS

Thyrotoxicosis

ICD-9CM CODES
242.9 Hyperthyroidism
242.0 Hyperthyroidism with goiter
242.2 Hyperthyroidism, multinodular
242.3 Hyperthyroidism, uninodular

EPIDEMIOLOGY & DEMOGRAPHICS

INCIDENCE/PREVALENCE:
- Hyperthyroidism affects 2% of women and 0.2% of men in their lifetime.
- Toxic multinodular goiter usually occurs in women >55 yr old and is more common than Graves' disease in the elderly.

PHYSICAL FINDINGS & CLINICAL PRESENTATION

- Patients with hyperthyroidism generally present with the following clinical manifestations: tachycardia, tremor, hyperreflexia, anxiety, irritability, emotional lability, panic attacks, heat intolerance, sweating, increased appetite, diarrhea, weight loss; the presentation may be different in elderly patients (see third bullet).
- Patients with Graves' disease may present with exophthalmos, lid retraction (Fig. 1-22, *A*), lid lag (Graves' ophthalmopathy). The following signs and symptoms of ophthalmopathy may be present: blurring of vision, photophobia, increased lacrimation, double vision, deep orbital pressure. Clubbing of fingers associated with periosteal new bone formation in other skeletal areas (Graves' acropachy) and pretibial myxedema (Fig. 1-22, *B*) may also be noted.
- In the elderly the clinical signs of hyperthyroidism may be masked by manifestations of coexisting disease (e.g., new-onset atrial fibrillation, exacerbation of CHF) or may present with failure to thrive (apathetic hyperthyroidism) or dementia.

ETIOLOGY

- Graves' disease (diffuse toxic goiter)
- Toxic multinodular goiter (Plummer's disease)
- Toxic adenoma
- Iatrogenic and factitious
- Transient hyperthyroidism (subacute thyroiditis, Hashimoto's thyroiditis)
- Rare causes: hypersecretion of TSH (e.g., pituitary neoplasms), struma ovarii, ingestion of large amount of iodine in a patient with preexisting thyroid hyperplasia or adenoma (Jod-Basedow phenomenon), carcinoma of thyroid, amiodarone therapy

DIAGNOSIS

DIFFERENTIAL DIAGNOSIS

- Anxiety disorder
- Pheochromocytoma
- Metastatic neoplasm
- Diabetes mellitus

WORKUP

Suspected hyperthyroidism requires laboratory confirmation and identification of its etiology, because treatment varies with its cause. A detailed medical history will often provide clues to the diagnosis and etiology of the hyperthyroidism.

LABORATORY TESTS

- Elevated free thyroxine (T_4)
- Elevated free triiodothyronine (T_3): generally not necessary for diagnosis
- Low TSH (unless hyperthyroidism is a result of the rare hypersecretion of TSH from a pituitary adenoma)
- Thyroid autoantibodies useful in selected cases to differentiate Graves' disease from toxic multinodular goiter (absent thyroid antibodies)

IMAGING STUDIES

- 24-hr radioactive iodine uptake (RAIU) is useful to distinguish hyperthyroidism from iatrogenic thyroid hormone synthesis (thyrotoxicosis factitia) and from thyroiditis.
- An overactive thyroid shows increased uptake, whereas a normal underactive

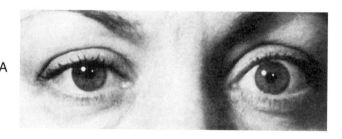

A

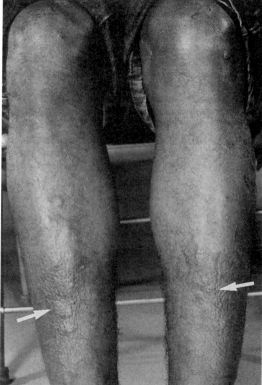

B

FIGURE 1-22 A, Unilateral (*left*) lid retraction in a patient with hyperthyroidism. **B,** Pretibial myxedema (*arrows*) in a patient with Graves' disease. (From Noble J [ed]: *Textbook of primary care medicine,* ed 2, St Louis, 1996, Mosby.)

thyroid (iatrogenic thyroid ingestion, painless or subacute thyroiditis) shows normal or decreased uptake.
- The RAIU results also vary with the etiology of the hyperthyroidism: Graves' disease: increased homogeneous uptake.

Multinodular goiter: increased heterogeneous uptake.

Hot nodule: single focus of increased uptake.
- RAIU is also generally performed before the therapeutic administration of radioactive iodine to determine the appropriate dose.

TREATMENT

NONPHARMACOLOGIC THERAPY

Patient education regarding thyroid disease and discussion of the therapeutic options (medications, radioactive iodine, and thyroid surgery)

ACUTE GENERAL Rx

ANTITHYROID DRUGS (THIONAMIDES): Propylthiouracil (PTU) and methimazole (Tapazole) inhibit thyroid hormone synthesis by blocking production of thyroid peroxidase (PTU and methimazole) or inhibit peripheral conversion of T_4 to T_3 (PTU).
1. Dosage: PTU 50 to 100 mg PO q8h; methimazole 10 to 20 mg PO q8h or 30 to 60 mg/day given as a single dose.
2. Antithyroid drugs can be used as the primary form of treatment or as adjunctive therapy before radioactive therapy or surgery or afterward if the hyperthyroidism recurs.
3. Side effects: skin rash (3% to 5% of patients), arthralgias, myalgias, granulocytopenia (0.5%). Rare side effects are aplastic anemia, hepatic necrosis from PTU, cholestatic jaundice from methimazole.
4. When antithyroid drugs are used as primary therapy, they are usually given for 6 to 24 mo; prolonged therapy may cause hypothyroidism.
5. The use of antithyroid drugs before radioactive iodine therapy is best reserved for patients in whom exacerbation of hyperthyroidism after radioactive iodine therapy is hazardous (e.g., elderly patients with coronary

artery disease or significant coexisting morbidity). In these patients the antithyroid drug can be stopped 2 days before radioactive iodine therapy, resumed 2 days later, and continued for 4 to 6 wk.

RADIOACTIVE IODINE (RAI; ^{131}I):
1. RAI is the treatment of choice for patients with Graves' disease. Radioiodine is also used in hyperthyroidism caused by toxic adenoma or toxic multinodular goiter.
2. A single dose of radioactive iodine is effective in inducing euthyroid state in nearly 80% of patients.
3. There is a high incidence of postradioactive iodine hypothyroidism (>50% within first year and 2%/yr thereafter); therefore these patients should be frequently evaluated for the onset of hypothyroidism (see Chronic Rx).

SURGICAL THERAPY (SUBTOTAL THYROIDECTOMY):
1. Indicated in obstructing goiters and in any patient who refuses radioactive iodine and cannot be adequately managed with antithyroid medications (e.g., patients with toxic adenoma or toxic multinodular goiter).
2. Patients should be rendered euthyroid with antithyroid drugs before surgery.
3. Complications of surgery include hypothyroidism (28% to 43% after 10 yr), hypoparathyroidism, and vocal cord paralysis (1%).
4. Hyperthyroidism recurs after surgery in 10% to 15% of patients.

ADJUNCTIVE THERAPY: Propranolol alleviates the β-adrenergic symptoms of hyperthyroidism; initial dose is 20 to 40 mg PO q6h; dosage is gradually increased until symptoms are controlled; major contraindications to use of propranolol are CHF and bronchospasm.

CHRONIC Rx

Patients undergoing treatment with antithyroid drugs should be seen every 1 to 3 mo until euthyroidism is achieved and every 3 to 4 mo while they remain on antithyroid therapy. After treatment is stopped, periodic monitoring of thyroid function tests with TSH every 3 mo for 1 yr, then every 6 mo for 1 yr, then annually is recommended.

DISPOSITION

Successful treatment of hyperthyroidism requires lifelong monitoring for the onset of hypothyroidism or the recurrence of thyrotoxicosis.

REFERRAL
- Endocrinology referral is recommended at the time of initial diagnosis and during treatment
- Surgical referral in selected patients (see Surgical Therapy)
- Hospitalization of all patients with thyroid storm

PEARLS & CONSIDERATIONS

COMMENTS
- Elderly hyperthyroid patients may have only subtle signs (weight loss, tachycardia, fine skin, brittle nails). This form is known as **apathetic hyperthyroidism** and manifests with lethargy rather than hyperkinetic activity. An enlarged thyroid gland may be absent. Coexisting medical disorders (most commonly cardiac disease) may also mask the symptoms. These patients often have unexplained CHF, worsening of angina, or new-onset atrial fibrillation resistant to treatment.
- **Subclinical hyperthyroidism** is defined as a normal serum free thyroxine and free triiodothyronine levels with a thyroid-stimulating hormone level suppressed below the normal range and usually undetectable. These patients usually do not present with signs or symptoms of overt hyperthyroidism. Treatment options include observation or a therapeutic trial of low-dose antithyroid agents for 6 mo to attempt to induce remission.

SUGGESTED READINGS

Kearns AE, Thompson GB: Medical and surgical management of hyperthyroidism, *Mayo Clin Proc* 77:87, 2002.

Shrier DK et al: Subclinical hyperthyroidism: controversies in management, *Am Fam Physician* 65:431, 2002.

Toft AD: Subclinical hyperthyroidism, *N Engl J Med* 345:512, 2001.

AUTHOR: **FRED F. FERRI, M.D.**

BASIC INFORMATION

DEFINITION

Hypothyroidism is a disorder caused by the inadequate secretion of thyroid hormone.

SYNONYMS

Myxedema

ICD-9CM CODES
244 Acquired hypothyroidism
244.1 Surgical hypothyroidism
244.3 Iatrogenic hypothyroidism
244.8 Pituitary hypothyroidism
246.1 Sporadic goitrous hypothyroidism

EPIDEMIOLOGY & DEMOGRAPHICS

INCIDENCE/PREVALENCE: 1.5% to 2% of women and 0.2% of men
PREDOMINANT AGE: Incidence of hypothyroidism increases with age; among persons older than 60 yr, 6% of women and 2.5% of men have laboratory evidence of hypothyroidism (TSH > twice normal).

PHYSICAL FINDINGS & CLINICAL PRESENTATION

- Hypothyroid patients generally present with the following signs and symptoms: fatigue, lethargy, weakness, constipation, weight gain, cold intolerance, muscle weakness, slow speech, slow cerebration with poor memory.
- Skin: dry, coarse, thick, cool, sallow (yellow color caused by carotenemia); nonpitting edema in skin of eyelids and hands (myxedema) secondary to infiltration of subcutaneous tissues by a hydrophilic mucopolysaccharide substance.
- Hair: brittle and coarse; loss of outer one third of eyebrows.
- Facies: dulled expression, thickened tongue, thick slow-moving lips.
- Thyroid gland: may or may not be palpable (depending on the cause of the hypothyroidism).
- Heart sounds: distant, possible pericardial effusion.
- Pulse: bradycardia.
- Neurologic: delayed relaxation phase of the DTRs, cerebellar ataxia, hearing impairment, poor memory or dementia, peripheral neuropathies with paresthesia.
- Musculoskeletal: carpal tunnel syndrome, muscular stiffness, weakness.

ETIOLOGY

PRIMARY HYPOTHYROIDISM (THYROID GLAND DYSFUNCTION): The cause of >90% of the cases of hypothyroidism
- Hashimoto's thyroiditis is the most common cause of hypothyroidism
- Idiopathic myxedema (nongoitrous form of Hashimoto's thyroiditis)
- Previous treatment of hyperthyroidism (radioiodine therapy, subtotal thyroidectomy)
- Subacute thyroiditis
- Radiation therapy to the neck (usually for malignant disease)
- Iodine deficiency or excess
- Drugs (lithium, PAS, sulfonamides, phenylbutazone, amiodarone, thiourea)
- Prolonged treatment with iodides

SECONDARY HYPOTHYROIDISM: Pituitary dysfunction, postpartum necrosis, neoplasm, infiltrative disease causing deficiency of TSH
TERTIARY HYPOTHYROIDISM: Hypothalamic disease (granuloma, neoplasm, or irradiation causing deficiency of TRH)
TISSUE RESISTANCE TO THYROID HORMONE: Rare

DIAGNOSIS **Dx**

DIFFERENTIAL DIAGNOSIS

- Depression
- Dementia from other causes
- Systemic disorders (e.g., nephrotic syndrome, CHF, amyloidosis)

LABORATORY TESTS

- Increased TSH: TSH may be normal if patient has secondary or tertiary hypothyroidism, is receiving dopamine or corticosteroids, or the level is obtained following severe illness
- Decreased free T_4
- Other common laboratory abnormalities: hyperlipidemia, hyponatremia, and anemia
- Increased antimicrosomal and antithyroglobulin antibody titers: useful when autoimmune thyroiditis is suspected as the cause of the hypothyroidism

TREATMENT **Rx**

NONPHARMACOLOGIC THERAPY

Patients should be educated regarding hypothyroidism and its possible complications. Patients should also be instructed about the need for lifelong treatment and monitoring of their thyroid abnormality.

ACUTE GENERAL Rx

Start replacement therapy with levothyroxine (Synthroid, Levothroid) 25 μg/day. The dose may be increased by 25 μg/day every 6 to 8 wk, depending on the clinical response and serum TSH level. Elderly patients with coronary artery disease should be started with 12.5 μg/day (higher doses may precipitate angina). The average maintenance dose of levothyroxine is 1.7 μg/kg/day (100 to 150 μg/day in adults). The elderly may require <1 μg/kg/day.

CHRONIC Rx

- Periodic monitoring of TSH level is an essential part of treatment. Patients should be evaluated initially with office visit and TSH levels every 6 to 8 wk until the patient is clinically euthyroid and the TSH level is normalized. The frequency of subsequent visits and TSH measurement can then be decreased to every 6 to 12 mo.
- For monitoring therapy in patients with central hypothyroidism, measurement of serum free thyroxine (free T_4 level) is appropriate and should be maintained in the upper half of the normal range.

REFERRAL

Admission to the hospital ICU is recommended in all patients with myxedema coma.

PEARLS & CONSIDERATIONS

COMMENTS

Subclinical hypothyroidism occurs in as many as 15% of elderly patients and is characterized by an elevated serum TSH and a normal free T_4 level. Treatment is individualized. Generally, replacement therapy is recommended for all patients with serum TSH >10 mU/L, patients with presence of goiter, patients with cognitive deficits, or obese patients. Some patients who report no symptoms prior to thyroid replacement feel more energetic when euthyroidism is restored.

AUTHOR: **FRED F. FERRI, M.D.**

BASIC INFORMATION

DEFINITION

Fecal incontinence is the involuntary loss of stool through the anal canal.

SYNONYMS

Uncontrollable loss of stool

ICD-9CM CODES
787.6 Fecal incontinence

EPIDEMIOLOGY & DEMOGRAPHICS

PREVALENCE:
- Extremely variable dependent on definition, site, and mode of collection of data
- Average range: 0.004% to 18%
- U.S. nursing homes report 47%

DEMOGRAPHICS:
- Over age 65: 30%
- Females: 63%
- Notable with advanced age, severe debility, and multiple comorbidities

FREQUENCY (IN U.S. STUDY):
- Daily: 2.7% of patients
- Weekly: 4.5%
- Monthly or less: 7.1%

RISK FACTORS:
- Constipation
- Age >80
- Urinary incontinence
- Impaired mobility
- Dementia
- Neurologic disease

PHYSICAL FINDINGS & CLINICAL PRESENTATION

- Uncontrolled loss of fecal matter or staining of underclothing
- Often unreported to physicians, or reported as pruritus, diarrhea, or urgency
- May cause complications, such as pressure sores and urinary infections, and may lead to isolation, avoidance of normal activities, and depression

- Inspection of anal area for deformed perineal body, scar formation, skin breakdown, gaping of anus
- Digital rectal exam to evaluate anal tone and to identify fecal impaction
- Evaluation of perineal sensation and anal wink reflex

ETIOLOGY

- Anatomic:
  - Sphincteric disruption, from vaginal deliveries, anorectal surgery, and trauma
  - Pelvic floor neuropathy with rectal prolapse, chronic straining at stool, and pelvic floor descent
  - Isolated degeneration of internal anal sphincter
- Neurologic:
  - CNS damage or malfunction, including dementia
  - Diabetes mellitus, multiple sclerosis, and other specific entities
- Functional:
  - Fecal impaction
  - Abnormal GI function with excessive stool volume and rapid gut transport
  - Laxative abuse
  - Transient fecal incontinence associated with diarrhea

DIAGNOSIS

DIFFERENTIAL DIAGNOSIS

- Mainly requires establishing applicable etiology by history and physical exam
- Uncontrolled diarrhea from diseases of the gut
- Medication abuse, primarily laxatives

WORKUP

- Colonoscopy for masses and inflammatory conditions when pathology suspected
- Anorectal physiology testing: imaging, manometry, and EMG

LABORATORY TESTS

- TSH
- Electrolytes

IMAGING STUDIES

- Abdominal x-ray

TREATMENT

NONPHARMACOLOGIC THERAPY

- Dietary changes: avoid food stimulants (e.g., lactose), add fiber
- Habit training
- Barrier creams to protect skin
- Biofeedback by trained personnel

ACUTE GENERAL Rx

- Antidiarrheal meds: loperamide, diphenoxylate, and bile-acid binders
- If diarrhea is present, identify its etiology and treat it

REFERRAL

- Gastroenterologist
- Colorectal surgeon
  - Sphincteroplasty
  - Diversion of fecal stream (ostomy)

PEARLS & CONSIDERATIONS

COMMENTS

- Severely annoying problem requiring proper protection and skin care.
- Most cases are reversible, controllable, and manageable by generalist.
- Complex and anatomic distortions will require specialist intervention.
- Dementia and other neurologic problems may prevent cure.

SUGGESTED READINGS

Madoff RD et al: Faecal incontinence in adults, *Lancet* 364:621, 2004.

AUTHOR: **E. GORDON MARGOLIN, M.D.**

BASIC INFORMATION

DEFINITION

Urinary incontinence is defined as the uncontrolled loss of urine, generally in an undesirable place, creating social and hygienic problems. Recently, the definition has been broadened to encompass the related problem of the overactive bladder even when there is no accompanying loss of urine.

SYNONYMS

Uncontrolled loss of urine
Bladder accidents
Overactive bladder

ICD-9CM CODES

788.30 Urinary incontinence, including urge and functional
788.33 Mixed
625.6 Stress (females)
788.32 Stress (males)
788.39 Other
596.51 Overactive bladder

EPIDEMIOLOGY & DEMOGRAPHICS

- Can present at any age.
- Prevalence increases with advancing age.
- More common in women than in men.
- Estimated prevalence in elders: 30% in community dwellers, 50% in hospitalized individuals, and 70% or more in nursing home residents.
- Annual costs in U.S. are estimated at $30 billion reflecting labor, laundry, institutional costs, products, and complicating events.

PHYSICAL FINDINGS & CLINICAL PRESENTATION

- Types of incontinence—defined by duration:
  - Acute or transient (less than 2 months' duration): may be due to, or associated with, delirium, infection, atrophic urethritis and vaginitis, pharmaceuticals, psychologic issues, excessive urine production, restricted mobility, and stool impaction (DIAPPERS).
  - Chronic or established (more than 2 months' duration): described as follows.
- Types of established incontinence—defined by manifestations:
  - Stress: incompetence of sphincteric mechanism, allowing spurts of urine when there are increases in intraabdominal pressure (such as coughing, lifting, etc.). Constant leakage can occur with totally incompetent sphincter (continuous incontinence).
  - Urge: overactivity of detrusor muscle, creating sudden losses of variable amounts of urine both with and without warning. *Overactive bladder syndrome* is the same mechanism with severe urgency but with capability to toilet quickly enough to prevent urinary losses.
  - Overflow: sudden and uncontrolled emptying of an overdistended bladder, due to either obstruction to outflow or paralysis of the musculature of the detrusor. Symptoms may mimic those of Urge.
  - Functional: despite normal lower urinary system, there is failure to toilet appropriately because of cognitive, physical, or environmental constraints.
  - Mixed: combinations of any of the previous four types—especially Stress, Urge, and Functional—are common in the elderly.

PHYSICAL FINDINGS & CLINICAL PRESENTATION

- Incontinence is frequently not reported to, or identified by, the physician.
- Careful history taking can often determine the clinical type(s) of incontinence, but not necessarily the cause. It is essential to evaluate all medications being taken.
- Abdominal, pelvic, and rectal examinations help identify enlarged bladder, anatomic distortions of pelvic organs, enlargement of prostate, impaction of stool.
- Neurologic exam describes cerebral or spinal cord disease, peripheral neuropathy, gait limitations, and dexterity.
- Levels of cognition, awareness, and motivation determine functional issues.

ETIOLOGY

- Partly related to aging changes in physiology and anatomy of the lower urinary tract
  - Shrinkage of bladder
  - Increased number of uncontrolled detrusor contractions
  - Increase in postvoid volume and a decrease in bladder contractility
  - Loss of hormonal support of genitourinary tissues
  - Impaired responses to sensory stimuli
  - Frailty
  - Alteration of diurnal rhythms resulting in larger urinary flows at night
- Changes of supporting tissues, often related to damage from childbirth
- Enlargement of prostate in men

- Neurologic diseases, involving either the spinal cord or the brain
- Infections and stones of the bladder and kidneys
- Trauma to the bladder and its outlet, mechanical or radiation induced
- Hormonal changes
- Selected medications, such as α-agonists, anticholinergics, sedatives
- Diabetes mellitus and its consequences

DIAGNOSIS

DIFFERENTIAL DIAGNOSIS

- Urinary tract infection
- Rectal mass or impaction
- Volume overload
- Atrophic vaginitis
- Benign prostatic hypertrophy
- Spinal cord injury
- Diabetes mellitus

WORKUP

- Careful history and focused physical exam are the mainstay of evaluation.
- Fluid intake and presence of edema are important considerations.
- Voiding diary.
- Urodynamic testing is not routinely indicated as first line.

LABORATORY TESTS

- Urinalysis and urine culture and sensitivity
- Renal function tests

IMAGING STUDIES

- Bladder ultrasound.
- Measurement of postvoid residual may be essential to identify Overflow and to distinguish it from Urge.

TREATMENT

ACUTE GENERAL Rx

STRESS:
- Pharmaceutical
  - α-agonists (pseudoephedrine)
  - Local estrogen creams
- Behavioral—see treatment for Urge
- Products
  - Pessaries may benefit women with vaginal or uterine prolapse
  - Small pads for small losses
  - Briefs
- Surgical
  - Needs as defined by surgical specialists include prostatectomy, pelvic repair, etc.

URGE:

- Pharmaceutical—anticholinergic drugs
  - Tolterodine
  - Oxybutynin
  - Darifenacin
  - Caution: systemic complications of these drugs and urination retention in BPH
  - Overactive bladder syndrome is also managed with these drugs
- Behavioral
  - Bladder training (i.e., timed voiding and control)
  - Pelvic muscle exercises (Kegel)
- Products
  - Large variety available to accommodate particular needs
- Surgical
  - Experimental use of excisional techniques
  - Placement of "pacemaker-type" devices

OVERFLOW:

- Neurogenic causes may be helped with parasympathetic agonists (bethanechol).
- Repeated catheterizations to empty the bladder may be necessary.
- Obstructive causes are mechanical, requiring surgical intervention.
  - Especially after trials with α_1-blockers used to relax the sphincter or finasteride to shrink the size of the prostate

  - See Benign Prostatic Hyperplasia (BPH) in Section I

FUNCTIONAL:

- Dependent on cause
  - May require redirection
  - Frequent toileting
  - Assistive devices for mobility enhancement
  - Proximal placement of commode

MIXED:

- Best to treat each type separately, starting with the type causing the greatest nuisance.

DISPOSITION

PROGNOSIS

- In the more frail and dependent elderly individual, success rates are limited by virtue of noncompliance, complications and side effects of medicationss.
- Use of products to contain urine when other measures fail can be most useful in management, in reduction of embarrassment, and to provide comfort and sense of security for the troubled patient.

REFERRAL

Gynecologic, urologic, and urodynamic studies are required only with refractory or uncertain cases, when associated with hematuria or uncontrolled infections, where anatomic distortions need interventions, or when symptoms are atypical.

PEARLS & CONSIDERATIONS

COMMENTS

- A careful history should precede any further workup, including a diary maintained by the patient or caregiver.
- Usual workup includes focused physical examination and limited laboratory measurement.
- Behavioral therapy is preferred, if effective.
- Current medications are fraught with side effects and must be used cautiously. New medications are in study.
- Advising regarding products and activities, as well as supporting the patient, is an ongoing process.

SUGGESTED READINGS

Holroyd-Leduc JM, Straus SE: Management of urinary incontinence in women, *JAMA* 291:996, 2004.

Ouslander JG: Management of overactive bladder, *N Engl J Med* 350:786, 2004.

Scientific Committee of the First International Consultation on Incontinence: Assessment and treatment of urinary incontinence, *Lancet* 355(9221):2153, 2000.

Weiss BD: Diagnostic evaluation of urinary incontinence in geriatric patients, *Am Fam Physician* 57:2675, 1998.

AUTHOR: **E. GORDON MARGOLIN, M.D.**

BASIC INFORMATION

DEFINITION

Influenza is an acute febrile illness caused by infection with influenza type A or B virus.

SYNONYMS

Flu

ICD-9CM CODES
487.1 Influenza

EPIDEMIOLOGY & DEMOGRAPHICS

INCIDENCE (IN U.S.): Annual incidence of influenza-related deaths is approximately 20,000 deaths/yr
PREDOMINANT SEX: Male = female
PEAK INCIDENCE: Winter outbreaks lasting 5 to 6 wk

PHYSICAL FINDINGS & CLINICAL PRESENTATION

- "Classic flu" is characterized by abrupt onset of fever, headache, myalgias, anorexia, and malaise after a 1- to 2-day incubation period.
- Clinical syndromes are similar to those produced by other respiratory viruses, including pharyngitis, common colds, tracheobronchitis, bronchiolitis, croup.
- Respiratory symptoms such as cough, sore throat, and nasal discharge are usually present at the onset of illness, but systemic symptoms predominate.
- Elderly patients may experience fever, weakness, and confusion without any respiratory complaints.
- Acute deterioration to status asthmaticus may occur in patients with asthma.
- Influenza pneumonia: rapidly progressive cough, dyspnea, and cyanosis may occur after typical flu onset.

ETIOLOGY

- Variation in the surface antigens of the influenza virus, hemagglutinin (HA) and neuraminidase (NA), leading to infection with variants to which resistance is inadequate in the population at risk
- Transmitted by small-particle aerosols and deposited on the respiratory tract epithelium

DIAGNOSIS

DIFFERENTIAL DIAGNOSIS

- Adenovirus, parainfluenza virus infection
- Secondary bacterial pneumonia or mixed bacterial-viral pneumonia

WORKUP

- Virus isolation from nasal or throat swab or sputum specimens is the most rapid diagnostic method in the setting of acute illness.
- Specimens are placed into virus transport medium and processed by a reference laboratory.
- For serologic diagnosis:
  1. Paired serum specimens, acute and convalescent, the latter obtained 10 to 20 days later
  2. Fourfold rises or falls in the titer of antibodies (various techniques) considered diagnostic of recent infection

LABORATORY TESTS

Septic syndrome presentation: CBC, ABG analysis, blood cultures

IMAGING STUDIES

- Chest x-ray examination to demonstrate findings of viral pneumonia: peribronchial and patchy interstitial infiltrates in multiple lobes with atelectasis
- Possible progression to diffuse interstitial pneumonitis

TREATMENT

NONPHARMACOLOGIC THERAPY

- Bed rest
- Hydration

ACUTE GENERAL Rx

- Supportive care: antipyretics
- Antibiotics if bacterial pneumonia is proven or suspected
- Amantadine (100 mg PO once daily in patients >65 yr) and rimantadine (same dose schedule as amantadine)
  1. Further dose adjustments needed with renal insufficiency
  2. Fewer CNS side effects with rimantadine
- Neuraminidase inhibitors block release of virions from infected cells, resulting in shortened duration of symptoms and decrease in complications; effective against both influenza A and B
  1. Zanamivir, administered via inhaler, 10 mg bid
  2. Oseltamivir, administered orally
- Placebo-controlled studies have suggested that antiviral therapy with any of the above mentioned agents must be initiated within 1 to 2 days of the onset of symptoms and reduces the duration of illness by approximately 1 day

DISPOSITION

Patients are hospitalized if signs of pneumonia are present.

REFERRAL

Infectious disease and/or pulmonary consultation when influenza pneumonia is suspected

PEARLS & CONSIDERATIONS

COMMENTS

- Prevention of influenza in patients at high risk is an important goal of primary care.
- Vaccines reduce the risk of infection and the severity of illness.
  1. Antigenic composition of the vaccine is updated annually.
  2. Vaccination should be given at the start of the flu season (October) for the following groups:
     a. Adults ≥65 yr
     b. Adults with chronic cardiac or pulmonary disease, including asthma
     c. Adults with illness requiring frequent follow-up (e.g., hemoglobinopathies, diabetes mellitus)
     d. Immunocompromised patients
     e. Household contacts of persons in the previous groups
     f. Health-care workers
  3. Only contraindication to vaccination is hypersensitivity to hen's eggs.
  4. Special efforts should be made to vaccinate high-risk patients <65 yr, only 10% to 15% of whom are vaccinated each year.
- Chemoprophylaxis:
  1. Amantadine and rimantadine approved for prophylaxis against influenza A; they are ineffective against influenza B
  2. Consider:
     a. For high-risk patients in whom vaccination is contraindicated
     b. When the available vaccine is known not to include the circulating strain
     c. To provide added protection to immunosuppressed patients likely to have a diminished response to vaccination
     d. In the setting of an outbreak, when immediate protection of unvaccinated or recently vaccinated patients is desired (e.g., in a nursing home)
  3. Give for 2 wk in the case of late vaccination and for the duration of the flu season in all other patients

SUGGESTED READINGS

Colgan R et al: Antiviral drugs in the immunocompetent host: part II. Treatment of influenza and respiratory syncytial virus infections, *Am Fam Physician* 67(4):763, 2003.

Montalto NJ: An office-based approach to influenza: clinical diagnosis and laboratory testing, *Am Fam Physician* 67(1):111, 2003.

AUTHOR: **CLAUDIA L. DADE, M.D.**

BASIC INFORMATION

DEFINITION

Insomnia is a disturbance of initiating or maintaining sleep. Restless, nonrestorative sleep may also be described as insomnia. The disturbance may be subjective without daytime sequelae but still a cause of distress, or may be objectively measurable with poor sleep efficiency and daytime consequences of sleepiness and functional impairment.

SYNONYMS

Sleeplessness, sleep disorder, sleep disturbance, dyssomnia. The terms sleep disorder, sleep disturbance, and dyssomnia are generic and can refer to disorders of wakefulness (hypersomnia) or sleep-related behavior disorders (parasomnias).

ICD-9CM CODES
780.52 Insomnia
780.51 Insomnia with sleep apnea
307.41 Insomnia nonorganic origin
307.42 Insomnia persistent (primary)
307.41 Insomnia transient
307.49 Subjective complaint
DSM IV-TR Codes:
307.42 Primary insomnia
307.45 Circadian rhythm disorders
780.52 Insomnia due to a general
         medical condition
291.89 Substance-induced insomnia
         due to alcohol
292.89 Substance-induced insomnia
         due to other (i.e., caffeine,
         drug)

EPIDEMIOLOGY & DEMOGRAPHICS

INCIDENCE (IN U.S.): 30%-45% of adults experience insomnia per year.
PREVALENCE (IN U.S.): 1%-15% of all adults develop persistent insomnia, 25% of older adults.
PREDOMINANT SEX: More common in women.
PREDOMINANT AGE: Transient insomnia is common at any age, persistent insomnia is more common in those >60 yrs. Older adults usually have more sleep maintenance difficulty.
GENETICS: Both idiopathic primary insomnia and chronobiologic forms of insomnia run in families and may be genetically determined.

CLINICAL PRESENTATION

• Complain of difficulty falling asleep, difficulty staying asleep, early morning awakening, restless or nonrestorative sleep, or difficulty sleeping at desired times.
• May or may not complain of daytime sleepiness or fatigue.

• Symptoms may be acute and self-limited, chronic but intermittent, or chronic and frequent.

ETIOLOGY

• Transient insomnia:
  1. Stress
  2. Illness
  3. Travel
  4. Environmental disruptions (noise, heat, cold, poor bedding, unfamiliar surroundings, etc.)
• Persistent insomnia:
  1. Mood disorders (depression, hypomania/mania)
  2. Primary or psychophysiologic (with or without poor sleep hygiene)
  3. Sleep-related breathing disorders (e.g., obstructive apnea)
  4. Chronobiologic (a.k.a. circadian rhythm) disorder (delayed sleep phase, advanced sleep phase, shift work, free-running rhythm secondary to blindness)
  5. Drug and alcohol abuse
  6. Restless legs and periodic leg movements
  7. Neurodegenerative (Alzheimer's disease, Parkinson's disease, etc.)
  8. Medical (pain, GERD, nocturia, orthopnea, medications, etc.)

DIAGNOSIS **Dx**

DIFFERENTIAL DIAGNOSIS

• Primary or psychophysiologic insomnia is diagnosed when other etiologies (see above) are ruled out.

WORKUP

• History (with bed partner interview, if possible)
• Sleep diary for 2 weeks to document severity, frequency, daytime function, and distress (sample sleep diary can be downloaded from the National Sleep Foundation website: http://www.sleepfoundation.org)

• Validated sleep-quality rating scale (optional)
  1. Pittsburgh Sleep Quality Index or similar questionnaire
  2. Epworth Sleepiness Scale (see Daytime Sleepiness Test at http://www.sleepfoundation.org)

LABORATORY TESTS

• Evaluate for anemia, uremia (for restless legs), thyroid function (if other signs present)
• Polysomnography (in home or in sleep lab) for symptoms suggesting something other than primary insomnia: daytime sleepiness (obstructive sleep apnea, narcolepsy), nonrestorative sleep (periodic leg movements), or sleep behavior suggesting parasomnia (somnambulism, REM sleep behavior)

IMAGING STUDIES

• Not generally helpful for insomnia
• Brain CT or MRI for severe daytime sleepiness of acute onset

TREATMENT

NONPHARMACOLOGIC THERAPY

• Sleep hygiene measures (see Box 1-3).
• Cognitive-behavioral therapy (CBT) to address anxiety and insomnia-perpetuating behaviors.
• Bright light exposure timed to correct a circadian phase disturbance can be helpful for insomnia secondary to delayed or advanced sleep phase, jet lag, or shift work.

ACUTE GENERAL Rx

• Benzodiazepine sedative-hypnotics (e.g., temazepam 7.5-30 mg, triazolam 0.125-0.25 mg) should generally be avoided in the geriatric population.
  1. In critical care: lorazepam 0.25-0.5 mg PO, SL, or IV as needed for sleep.

BOX 1-3   Sleep Habits (Sleep Hygiene Measures) That May Improve Insomnia

1. Reduce caffeine, alcohol, or tobacco late in the day or evening.
2. Avoid heavy meals at night.
3. Increase daytime activity.
4. Increase daytime exposure to natural light.
5. Take warm bath as part of bedtime ritual.
6. Restrict bed to sleep and sex.
7. Get out of bed if not asleep after 30 minutes and return when drowsy.
8. Repeat above if awakened during the night.
9. Maintain regular sleep and wake times.
10. Go to bed with calm mind; resolve arguments or deal with problems earlier in day.

- Benzodiazepine receptor agonists (e.g., zolpidem 5-10 mg for sleep-onset and maintenance insomnia, zaleplon 5-10 mg for sleep-onset insomnia) eszopiclone 1 mg qhs for sleep initiation or 2 mg qhs for sleep maintenance.
- Avoid antihistamines.
- Optimize treatment of medical symptoms, especially pain.

CHRONIC Rx

- Ramelteon 8 mg qhs is a melatonin agonist and can be used on a long-term basis.
- Eszopiclone and zolpidem CR (6.25 or 12.5 mg tablets) can also be used long-term.
- Some evidence that benzodiazepines and benzodiazepine receptor agonists can be used for chronic insomnia on either intermittent or nightly use with moderate risk of tolerance and dependence but low risk of addiction.
- Sedating antidepressants (e.g., trazodone 25-150 mg, mirtazapine 7.5-30 mg) in widespread use but limited data on safety and efficacy for insomnia. Treatments of choice for comorbid depression or anxiety. Amitriptyline should be avoided if possible in older adults.
- Sedating antipsychotics (e.g., quetiapine 25-200 mg, olanzapine 2.5-10 mg) for severe mood or psychotic disorders associated with insomnia.

COMPLEMENTARY & ALTERNATIVE MEDICINE

Melatonin is the only substance that has been studied in larger controlled trials. It may shorten sleep-onset latency in some individuals. Melatonin can be very effective for insomnia due to circadian rhythm disturbances if scheduled to correct the underlying circadian phase disturbance.

DISPOSITION

- Transient insomnia: usually self-limited, but may require follow-up if stress- or illness-related because of risk of depression or persistent insomnia.
- Persistent insomnia: patients have a chronic and recurrent disorder and will need periodic follow-up to reinforce good sleep hygiene measures and to reassess need for pharmacologic and nonpharmacologic therapies.

REFERRAL

- Excessive daytime sleepiness not obviously due to insomnia (e.g., narcolepsy, sleep-related breathing disorder, etc.)
- Nighttime behavior suggestive of a parasomnia (e.g., somnambulism, REM behavior disorder, etc.)
- Severe insomnia not responsive to basic interventions

PEARLS & CONSIDERATIONS

COMMENTS

Treatment of insomnia should focus on reducing daytime sleepiness and improving daytime function, rather than trying to achieve the elusive goal of uninterrupted nighttime sleep.

PREVENTION

Not much is known about prevention of insomnia. Effective treatment of transient insomnia may reduce the risk of developing persistent insomnia.

PATIENT/FAMILY EDUCATION

The National Sleep Foundation (http://www.sleepfoundation.org) is a comprehensive resource for health care providers and patients.

SUGGESTED READINGS

Jacobs GD et al: Cognitive behavior therapy and pharmacotherapy for insomnia: a randomized controlled trial and direct comparison, *Arch Int Med* 164(17):1888, 2004.

Krystal AD: The changing perspective on chronic insomnia management, *J Clin Psychiatry* 65(Suppl 8):20, 2004.

Ringdahl EN, Pereira SL, Delzell JE: Treatment of primary insomnia, *J Am Board Fam Pract Behavioural Medicine in Primary Care: A Practical Guide,* ed 2, New York, 2003, Lange Medical Books/McGraw Hill.

Smith MT et al: Comparative meta-analysis of pharmacotherapy and behaviour therapy for persistent insomnia, *Am J Psychiatry* 159:5, 2002.

AUTHOR: **CLIFFORD MILO SINGER, M.D.**

BASIC INFORMATION

DEFINITION

Irritable bowel syndrome (IBS) is a chronic functional disorder manifested by alteration in bowel habits and recurrent abdominal pain and bloating.

SYNONYMS

Irritable colon
Spastic colon
IBS

ICD-9CM CODES
564.1 Irritable bowel syndrome

EPIDEMIOLOGY & DEMOGRAPHICS

- IBS occurs in 20% of population of industrialized countries and is responsible for >50% of GI referrals. Worldwide adult prevalence is 12%.
- Female:male ratio is 2:1.
- Nearly 50% of patients have psychiatric abnormalities, with anxiety disorders being most common.

PHYSICAL FINDINGS & CLINICAL PRESENTATION

- The clinical presentation of IBS consists of abdominal pain and abnormalities of defecation, which may include loose stools usually after meals and in the morning, alternating with episodes of constipation.
- Physical examination is generally normal.
- Nonspecific abdominal tenderness and distention may be present.

ETIOLOGY

- Unknown
- Associated pathophysiology includes altered GI motility and increased gut sensitivity
- Risk factors: anxiety, depression, personality disorders, history of childhood sexual abuse, and domestic abuse in women

DIAGNOSIS

DIFFERENTIAL DIAGNOSIS

- IBD
- Diverticulitis
- Colon malignancy
- PUD
- Biliary liver disease
- Chronic pancreatitis

WORKUP

Diagnostic workup is aimed primarily at excluding the conditions listed in the differential diagnoses. It is important to identify "red flags" of other diseases, such as weight loss, rectal bleeding, onset in patients 50 years of age, fever, nocturnal pain, family history of malignancy.

The criteria for diagnosis of IBS are: more than 3 months of symptoms *including* abdominal pain that is relieved by a bowel movement, *or* pain accompanied by a change in bowel pattern, *and* abnormality in bowel movement 25% of the time, characterized by two of the following features:
- Abdominal distention
- Abnormal consistency
- Abnormal defecation (e.g., straining, sense of incomplete evacuation)
- Abnormal frequency
- Mucus with bowel movement

LABORATORY TESTS

- Blood work is generally normal. The presence of anemia should alert to the possibility of a colonic malignancy or IBD.
- Testing of stool for ova and parasites and for celiac disease should be considered in patients with chronic diarrhea.

IMAGING STUDIES

- Small bowel series and barium enema are normal and not necessary for diagnosis.
- Lower endoscopy is generally normal except for the presence of some spasms.

TREATMENT

NONPHARMACOLOGIC THERAPY

- The patient should be encouraged to maintain a high-fiber diet and to eliminate foods that aggravate symptoms. Avoidance of dietary caffeine and dietary excesses is also helpful.
- Behavioral therapy is also recommended because psychosocial stressors are important triggers of IBS.
- Importance of regular exercise and adequate fluid intake should be stressed.

GENERAL Rx

- The mainstay of treatment of IBS is high-fiber diet. Because symptoms are chronic, the use of laxatives should be avoided.
- Fiber supplementation with psyllium 1 to 2 tablespoons bid or calcium polycarbophil (FiberCon) 2 tablets one to four times daily followed by 8 oz of water may be necessary in some patients.
- Patients should be instructed that there might be some increased bloating on initiation of fiber supplementation, which should resolve within 2 to 3 wk. It is important that patients take these fiber products on a regular basis and not only prn. Slow titration may help.
- Antispasmodics-anticholinergics may be useful in refractory cases (e.g., di-

cyclomine [Bentyl] 10 to 20 mg up to three times daily).
- Patients who appear anxious can benefit from use of sedatives and anticholinergics such as chlordiazepoxide-clidinium (Librax) or SSRIs.
- Loperamide is effective for diarrhea.
- Tegaserod (Zelnorm), a 5-HT$_4$ receptor partial agonist, increases GI motility and can be used to relieve symptoms in patients whose predominant symptom is constipation. Usual dose is 2 to 6 mg PO bid before meals. Tegaserod is contraindicated in patients with severe renal insufficiency, moderate to severe hepatic impairment, intestinal adhesions, or a history of bowel obstruction.

DISPOSITION

Greater than 60% of patients respond successfully to treatment over the initial 12 mo; however, IBS is a chronic relapsing condition and requires prolonged therapy.

REFERRAL

GI referral is recommended in patients with rectal bleeding, fever, nocturnal diarrhea, anemia, weight loss, or onset of symptoms after age 40 yr.

PEARLS & CONSIDERATIONS

COMMENTS

- Patients should be educated regarding maintenance of high-fiber diet and elimination of stressors, which can precipitate attacks of IBS. They should be reassured that their condition cannot lead to cancer.
- The modified Rome criteria define IBS as:
  A. The presence of ≥12 wk of continuous or recurrent abdominal pain or discomfort that cannot be explained by structural or biochemical abnormalities and
  B. The presence of at least two of the following three features:
    1. Pain is relieved with defecation
    2. Its onset is associated with a change in the frequency of bowel movement
    3. Its onset is associated with a change in the form of the stool.

SUGGESTED READINGS

Mertz HR: Irritable bowel syndrome, *N Engl J Med* 349:22, 2003.
Viera AJ et al: Management of irritable bowel syndrome, *Am Fam Physician* 66:1867, 2002.

AUTHOR: **FRED F. FERRI, M.D.**

BASIC INFORMATION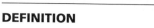

DEFINITION

Cancer of the larynx, including the vocal cords (glottis), supraglottis, and subglottis.

SYNONYMS

Laryngeal cancer
Head and neck cancer (subsite); other sites include oral cavity, pharynx, perinasal sinus, and salivary glands

ICD-9CM CODES

231.0 Carcinoma of larynx

EPIDEMIOLOGY & DEMOGRAPHICS

- 12,000 new cases per year in the U.S.
- 80% male predominance (current, with past and projected increase in female rates as a result of changing smoking habits)
- Peak incidence in sixth decade

PHYSICAL FINDINGS & CLINICAL PRESENTATION

- Glottis

Early diagnosis possible because of voice change (hoarseness). Any voice change of more than 2 wk duration should prompt a laryngeal examination.

- Supraglottis
  1. No early symptom
  2. Cervical lymphadenopathy
  3. Neck pain or ear pain
  4. Discomfort during swallowing
  5. Odynophagia
  6. Later: hoarseness, dysphagia, airway obstruction
- Subglottis

Even more subtle than supraglottic lesion; the same signs occur, only later in the course

ETIOLOGY

- Smoking (cigarette, cigar, or pipe)
- Alcohol intake/abuse
- Diet and nutritional deficiencies
- Gastroesophageal reflux
- Voice abuse
- Chronic laryngitis
- Exposure to wood dust
- Asbestosis
- Exposure to radiation
- Possible role of human papilloma virus

DIAGNOSIS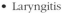

DIFFERENTIAL DIAGNOSIS

- Laryngitis
- Allergic and nonallergic rhinosinusitis
- Gastroesophageal reflux
- Voice abuse leading to hoarseness
- Laryngeal papilloma

- Vocal cord paralysis secondary to a neurologic condition or secondary to entrapment of the recurrent laryngeal nerve caused by mediastinal compression
- Tracheomalacia

STAGING:

Supraglottic

T1 Tumor limited to one subsite with normal cord mobility

T2 Tumor invades mucosa of more than one subsite (e.g., base of tongue, vallecula, pyriform sinus) without fixation of larynx

T3 Tumor limited to larynx with vocal cord fixation or invasion of postcricoid area or preepiglottis

T4 Tumor invades thyroid cartilage or extends into soft tissue of the neck, thyroid, or esophagus

Glottic

T1 Tumor limited to vocal cord with normal mobility

T1a Tumor limited to one vocal cord

T1b Tumor involves both vocal cords

T2 Tumor extends to supra- or subglottis or impairs cord mobility

T3 Tumor limited to larynx with cord fixation

T4 Tumor invades through cartilage or other tissues beyond larynx

Stage grouping

Stage I: T1, N0, M0
Stage II: T2, N0, M0
Stage III: T3, N0, M0
T1, T2, T3, N1, M0
Stage IV: T4, N0, N1, M0
Any T, N2, N3, M0
Any T, any N or M >0

WORKUP

- Laboratory: none
- Endoscopic laryngeal inspection
- After (and only after) diagnosis of the malignancy, imaging with CT or MRI should be undertaken to stage the disease

HISTOLOGIC CLASSIFICATION:

Epithelial cancers
- Squamous cell carcinoma in situ
- Superficially invasive cancer
- Verrucous carcinoma
- Pseudosarcoma
- Anaplastic cancer
- Transitional cell carcinoma
- Lymphoepithelial cancer
- Adenocarcinoma
- Neuroendocrine tumors, including small cell and carcinoid
Sarcomas
Metastatic malignancies

TREATMENT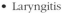

ACUTE GENERAL Rx

- Early Stage (T or T₂): two options
  1. Conservative surgery (partial laryngectomy) with neck dissection
  2. Primary radiation

- Intermediate Stage: four options
  1. Primary radiation alone
  2. Supraglottic laryngectomy with neck dissection
  3. Supraglottic laryngectomy with postoperative radiation
  4. Chemotherapy with radiation
- Advanced Stage

Chemotherapy and radiation with total laryngectomy reserved for treatment failure

Glottis
- Carcinoma in situ
  1. Microexcision
  2. Laser vaporization
  3. Radiation
- Early Stage (T or T₂): two options
  1. Voice conservation surgery
  2. Radiation
- Intermediate Stage (T₃)
  1. Combined radiation and chemotherapy (cisplatin and 5FU)
  2. Total laryngectomy for treatment failure
- Advanced Stage (T₄)
  1. Combined radiation and chemotherapy
  2. Total laryngectomy and neck dissection followed by postoperative radiation in unfavorable lesion or treatment failure

Subglottis

Total laryngectomy and approximate neck surgery to excise the tumor, followed by radiation

Unresected Cancers
- Induction chemotherapy and radiation followed by neck dissection in chemosensitive tumors, or by laryngectomy and neck dissection in chemoresistant tumors
- If hypopharyngeal involvement exists: laryngopharyngectomy, neck dissection, and postoperative radiation

DISPOSITION

Supraglottis 5-yr control
- T₁ 95% to 100%
- T₂ 80% to 90%
- T₃ 65% to 85%
- T₄ 40% to 55%

Glottis 5-yr control
- T₁ 95% to 100%
- T₂ 50% to 85%
- T₃ 35% to 85%
- T₄ 20% to 65%

SUGGESTED READING

Sessions RB, Harrison LB, Forastiere AA: Tumors of the larynx and hypopharynx. In *Cancer: Principles and Practice of Oncology*, ed 6, Philadelphia, 2001, Lippincott Williams & Wilkins.

AUTHOR: **TOM J. WACHTEL, M.D.**

BASIC INFORMATION

DEFINITION

Chronic lymphocytic leukemia (CLL) is a lymphoproliferative disorder characterized by proliferation and accumulation of mature-appearing neoplastic lymphocytes.

SYNONYMS

CLL

ICD-9CM CODES
204.1 Leukemia, chronic lymphocytic

EPIDEMIOLOGY & DEMOGRAPHICS

- Most frequent form of leukemia in Western countries (10,000 new cases/yr in the U.S.)
- Generally occurs in middle-aged and elderly patients (median age of 65 yr)
- Male:female ratio of 2:1

PHYSICAL FINDINGS & CLINICAL PRESENTATION

- Lymphadenopathy, splenomegaly, and hepatomegaly in the majority of patients
- Variable clinical presentation according to stage of the disease
- Abnormal CBC: many cases are diagnosed on the basis of laboratory results obtained after routine physical examination
- Some patients come to medical attention because of weakness and fatigue (secondary to anemia) or lymphadenopathy

ETIOLOGY

Unknown

DIAGNOSIS

DIFFERENTIAL DIAGNOSIS

- Hairy cell leukemia
- Adult T cell lymphoma
- Prolymphocytic leukemia
- Viral infections
- Waldenström's macroglobulinemia

WORKUP

- Laboratory evaluation
- Bone marrow aspirate
- Chromosome analysis

LABORATORY TESTS

- Proliferative lymphocytosis ($\geq$15,000/dl) of well-differentiated lymphocytes is the hallmark of CLL.
- There is monotonous replacement of the bone marrow by small lymphocytes (marrow contains $\geq$30% of well-differentiated lymphocytes).

- Hypogammaglobulinemia and elevated LDH may be present at the time of diagnosis.
- Anemia or thrombocytopenia, if present, indicates poor prognosis.
- Trisomy-12 is the most common chromosomal abnormality, followed by 14 q+, 13 q, and 11 q; these all indicate a poor prognosis.
- New laboratory techniques (CD 38, fluorescence in situ hybridization [FISH]) can identify patients with early-stage CLL at higher risk of rapid disease progression.

STAGING

- Rai et al divided CLL into five clinical stages:

Stage 0—Characterized by lymphocytosis only ($\geq$15,000/mm^3 on peripheral smear, bone marrow aspirate $\geq$40% lymphocytes). The coexistence of lymphocytosis and other factors increases the clinical stage.

Stage 1—Lymphadenopathy

Stage 2—Lymphadenopathy/hepatomegaly

Stage 3—Anemia (Hgb <11 g/mm^3)

Stage 4—Thrombocytopenia (platelets <100,000/mm^3)

- Another well-known staging system developed by Binet divides chronic lymphocytic leukemia into three stages:

Stage A—Hgb $\geq$10 g/dl, platelets $\geq$100,000/mm^3, and fewer than three areas involved (the cervical, axillary, and inguinal lymph nodes [whether unilaterally or bilaterally]; the spleen; and the liver)

Stage B—Hgb $\geq$10 g/dl, platelets $\geq$100,000/mm^3, and three or more areas involved

Stage C—Hgb <10 g/dl, low platelets (<100,000/mm^3), or both (independent of the areas involved)

IMAGING STUDIES

CT scan of abdomen to evaluate for hepatomegaly and splenomegaly

TREATMENT

NONPHARMACOLOGIC THERAPY

- Treatment goals are relief of symptoms and prolongation of life.
- Observation is appropriate for patients in Rai Stage 0 or Binet Stage A.

ACUTE GENERAL Rx

- Symptomatic patients in Rai Stage I and II or Binet Stage B: chlorambucil; local irradiation for isolated symptomatic lymphadenopathy and lymph nodes that interfere with vital organs

- Fludarabine is an effective treatment for CLL that does not respond to initial treatment with chlorambucil. Recent reports indicate that when used as the initial treatment for CLL, fludarabine yields higher response rates and a longer duration of remission and progression-free survival than chlorambucil; overall survival, however, is not enhanced.
- Rai Stages III and IV, Binet Stage C: chlorambucil chemotherapy with or without prednisone
  1. Fludarabine, CAP (cyclophosphamide, Adriamycin, prednisone), or cyclophosphamide, doxorubicin, vincristine, and prednisone (mini-CHOP) can be used in patients who respond poorly to chlorambucil.
  2. Splenic irradiation can be used in selected patients with advanced disease.

CHRONIC Rx

Treatment of systemic complications:

- Hypogammaglobulinemia is frequent in CLL and is the chief cause of infections. Immune globulin (250 mg/kg IV every 4 wk) may prevent infections but has no effect on survival. Infections should be treated with broad-spectrum antibiotics. Patients should be monitored for opportunistic infections.
- Recombinant hematopoietic cofactors (e.g., granulocyte-macrophage colony–stimulating factor and granulocyte colony–stimulating factor) may be useful to overcome neutropenia related to treatment.
- Erythropoietin may be useful to treat anemia that is unresponsive to other measures.

DISPOSITION

The patient's prognosis is directly related to the clinical stage (e.g., the average survival in patients in Rai Stage 0 or Binet Stage A is >120 mo, whereas for RAI Stage 4 or Binet Stage C it is approximately 30 mo). Overall 5-yr survival is 60%.

PEARLS & CONSIDERATIONS

COMMENTS

Long-term follow-up and frequency of follow-up are generally determined by the pace of the disease.

SUGGESTED READING

Shanafelt TD, Call TG: Current approach to diagnosis and management of chronic lymphocytic leukemia, *Mayo Clin Proc* 79:388, 2004.

AUTHOR: **FRED F. FERRI, M.D.**

BASIC INFORMATION

DEFINITION

Chronic inflammatory condition of the skin usually affecting the vulva, perianal area, and groin

ICD-9CM CODES
701.0 Lichen sclerosus

EPIDEMIOLOGY & DEMOGRAPHICS

- Most common in postmenopausal women and men between ages 40 and 60 yr
- More common in females

PHYSICAL FINDINGS & CLINICAL PRESENTATION

- Erythema may be the only initial sign. A characteristic finding is the presence of ivory-white atrophic lesions on the involved area.
- Close inspection of the affected area will reveal the presence of white-to-brown follicular plugs on the surface (dells).
- When the genitals are involved, the white parchmentlike skin assumes an hourglass configuration around the introital and perianal area ("keyhole" distribution, see Fig. 1-23). Inflammation, subepithelial hemorrhages, and chronic ulceration may develop.
- Dyspareunia, genital bleeding, and anal bleeding are common.

ETIOLOGY

Unknown. There may be an autoimmune association and a genetic familial component.

DIAGNOSIS **Dx**

DIFFERENTIAL DIAGNOSIS

- Localized scleroderma (morphea)
- Cutaneous discoid lupus erythematosus
- Atrophic lichen planus
- Psoriasis

WORKUP

Diagnosis is based on close examination of the lesions for the presence of ivory-white atrophic lesions and typical location.

LABORATORY TESTS

Punch or deep shave biopsy can be used to confirm the diagnosis when in doubt.

IMAGING STUDIES

Not indicated

TREATMENT **Rx**

NONPHARMACOLOGIC THERAPY

Attention to hygiene and elimination of irritants or excessive bathing with harsh soaps

GENERAL Rx

- Application of clobetasol propionate 0.05% topically bid for up to 4 wk is usually effective. Repeat courses of corticosteroids may be necessary because of the chronic nature of this disorder. Continual application of topical steroids may lead to atrophy of the vulva.
- Use of topical testosterone (2%) has been found to be less effective than topical corticosteroids.
- Lubricants (e.g., Nutraplus cream) are useful to soothe dry tissues.
- Hydroxyzine 25 mg at hs is effective in decreasing nocturnal itching.
- Use of intralesional steroids, etretinate, and surgical management are usually reserved for refractory cases.

DISPOSITION

- The disease persists in approximately one third of patients.
- Squamous cell carcinoma can develop within the lesions in 3% to 10% of older patients; therefore, periodic examination and biopsy of suspicious areas are indicated.

PEARLS & CONSIDERATIONS **!**

COMMENTS

- Lichen sclerosus of the vulva (kraurosis vulvae) usually occurs after menopause and is generally chronic. It can be painful and interfere with sexual activity.
- Lichen sclerosus of the penis (balanitis xerotica obliterans) is seen more commonly in uncircumcised males. It affects the glans and prepuce and may lead to stricture if it encroaches into the urinary meatus.

AUTHOR: **FRED F. FERRI, M.D.**

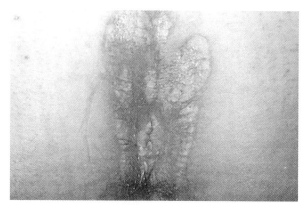

FIGURE 1-23   Lichen sclerosus. Perianal area is thinned and chalk white (keyhole distribution). (Courtesy Department of Dermatology, University of North Carolina at Chapel Hill. From Goldstein BG, Goldstein AO: *Practical dermatology*, ed 2, St Louis, 1997, Mosby.)

BASIC INFORMATION

DEFINITION

Lumbar disk syndromes are diseases resulting from disk disorder, either herniation or degenerative change (spondylosis). Massive disk protrusion may rarely lead to paralysis in the lower extremity, a condition termed *cauda equina syndrome*. Gradual narrowing of the spinal canal (lumbar stenosis), usually from spondylosis, may also cause lower extremity symptoms.

ICD-9CM CODES

722.10 Lumbar disk displacement
724.02 Lumbar stenosis
344.60 Cauda equina syndrome
721.3 Lumbar spondylosis

EPIDEMIOLOGY & DEMOGRAPHICS

PREVALENCE:
- Variable
- At least one episode in 80% of adults

PREVALENT SEX: Approximately equal

PHYSICAL FINDINGS & CLINICAL PRESENTATION (TABLE 1-8)

- Overlapping clinical syndromes that may result:
  1. Mild herniation without nerve root compression
  2. Herniation with nerve root compression
  3. Cauda equina syndrome
  4. Chronic degenerative disease with or without leg symptoms
  5. Spinal stenosis
- Low back pain, often worsened by activity or coughing and sneezing
- Local lumbar or lumbosacral tenderness
- Paresthesias, usually unilateral
- Restricted low back motion
- Increased pain on bending toward affected side
- Weakness and reflex changes
- Sensory examination usually not helpful
- Lumbar stenosis that possibly produces symptoms (pseudoclaudication), which are often misinterpreted as being vascular

- Positive straight leg raising test if nerve root compression is present
- Also see Spinal Stenosis in Section I

ETIOLOGY

Unknown

DIAGNOSIS (Dx)

DIFFERENTIAL DIAGNOSIS

- Soft-tissue strain/sprain
- Tumor
- Degenerative arthritis of hip
- Insufficiency fracture of hip or pelvis

Section II describes the differential diagnosis of common low back pain syndromes.

WORKUP

In most cases, the diagnosis can be established on a clinical basis alone.

IMAGING STUDIES

- Plain roentgenograms may be indicated within the first few weeks; they are usually normal in soft disk herniation, but with chronic degenerative disk disease, loss of height of the disk space and osteophyte formation can occur.
- CT scanning and MRI may be indicated in patients whose symptoms do not resolve or when other spinal pathology may be suspected.
- Electrodiagnostic studies may confirm the diagnosis or rule out peripheral nerve disorders.

TREATMENT (Rx)

NONPHARMACOLOGIC THERAPY

- Short course (3 to 5 days) of bed rest for severe pain; prolonged rest for acute disk herniation with leg pain
- Physical therapy for modalities plus a careful gradual exercise program
- Lumbosacral corset brace during rehabilitation process in conjunction with exercise program

- Percutaneous electrical nerve stimulation (PENS) may be beneficial in selected patients with chronic back pain

PHARMACOLOGIC THERAPY

- NSAIDs
- Muscle relaxants for sedative effect
- Analgesics
- Epidural steroid injection for leg symptoms in selected patients

DISPOSITION

- Almost all lumbar disk syndromes improve with time.
- Recurrent episodes usually respond to medical management.
- Recovery from the rare paralytic event is often incomplete.

REFERRAL

- For orthopedic or neurosurgical consultation for intractable pain or significant neurologic deficit
- Emergency referral for cauda equina syndrome

PEARLS & CONSIDERATIONS

COMMENTS

- Surgery is more consistently helpful when leg pain (not back pain) predominates.
- A clinical algorithm for evaluation of back pain is described in Section III.

SUGGESTED READINGS

Biyani A, Andersson GB: Low back pain: Pathophysiology and management, *J Am Acad Orthop Surg* 12:106, 2004.

Brodke DS, Ritter SM: Nonoperative management of low back pain and lumbar disc degeneration, *J Bone Joint Surg* 86A:1810, 2004.

Buchner M, Schiltenwolf M: Cauda equina syndrome caused by intervertebral lumbar disc prolapse: mid-term results of 22 patients and literature review, *Orthopedics* 25:727, 2002.

Butterman GR: Treatment of lumbar disc herniation: epidural steroid infection compared with discectomy: a prospective, randomized study, *J Bone Joint Surg* 86A:670, 2004.

TABLE 1-8   Diagnosis of Lower Lumbar and Sacral Radiculopathy

	Pain	Weakness (Selected Muscles)	Sensory Loss	Reflex Loss
L4	Across thigh and medial leg to medial malleolus	Quadriceps, thigh adductors, tibialis anterior	Medial leg	Knee
L5	Posterior thigh and lateral calf, dorsum of foot	Extensor digitorum brevis and longus, peronei	Dorsum of foot	
S1	Buttock and posterior thigh, calf, and lateral foot	Extensor digitorum brevis, peronei, gastrocnemius, soleus	Sole or lateral border of foot	Ankle
S2-4	Posterior thigh, buttock, and genitalia	Gastrocnemius, soleus, abductor hallucis, abductor digiti quinti pedis, sphincter muscles	Buttocks, anal region, and genitalia	Bulbocavernosus, anal

From Goldman L, Bennett JC (eds): *Cecil textbook of medicine*, ed 21, Philadelphia, 2000, WB Saunders.

Dreyfuss P et al: Sacroiliac joint pain, *J Am Acad Orthop Surg* 12:255, 2004.

Kawaguchi Y et al: The association of lumbar disc disease with vitamin-D receptor gene polymorphism, *J Bone Joint Surg* 84(a):2022, 2002.

Paassilta P et al: Identification of a novel common genetic risk factor for lumbar disc disease, *JAMA* 285:1843, 2001.

Robinson LR: Role of neurophysiologic evaluation in diagnosis, *J Am Acad Orthop Surg* 8:190, 2000.

Silber JS et al: Advances in surgical management of lumbar degenerative disc disease, *Orthopedics* 25:767, 2002.

Simotas AC: Non-operative treatment for lumbar spinal stenosis, *Clin Orthop* 384:153, 2001.

Swenson R, Haldeman S: Spinal manipulation for low back pain, *J Am Acad Orthop Surg* 11:228, 2003.

Tribus CB: Degenerative lumbar scoliosis: evaluation and management, *J Am Acad Orthop Surg* 11:174, 2003.

Wetzel FT, McNally TA: Treatment of chronic discogenic low back pain with intradiskal electrothermal therapy, *J Am Acad Orthop Surg* 11:6, 2003.

Yoshihara K et al: Atrophy of the multifidus muscle in patients with lumbar disc herniation: histochemical and electromyographic study, *Orthopedics* 26:493, 2003.

AUTHOR: **LONNIE R. MERCIER, M.D.**

BASIC INFORMATION

DEFINITION

A primary lung neoplasm is a malignancy arising from lung tissue. The World Health Organization distinguishes 12 types of pulmonary neoplasms. Among them, the major types are *squamous cell carcinoma, adenocarcinoma, small cell carcinoma,* and *large cell carcinoma.* However, the crucial difference in the diagnosis of lung cancer is between small cell and non–small cell types, because the therapeutic approach is different. Selective characteristics of lung carcinomas:

ADENOCARCINOMA: Represents 35% of lung carcinomas; frequently located in mid lung and periphery; initial metastases are to lymphatics, frequently associated with peripheral scars

SQUAMOUS CELL (EPIDERMOID): 20% to 30% of lung cancers; central location; metastasis by local invasion; frequent cavitation and obstructive phenomena

SMALL CELL (OAT CELL): 20% of lung carcinomas; central location; metastasis through lymphatics; associated with lesion of the short arm of chromosome 3; high cavitation rate

LARGE CELL: 15% to 20% of lung carcinomas; frequently located in the periphery; metastasis to CNS and mediastinum; rapid growth rate with early metastasis

BRONCHOALVEOLAR: 5% of lung carcinomas; frequently located in the periphery; may be bilateral; initial metastasis through lymphatic, hematogenous, and local invasion; no correlation with cigarette smoking; cavitation rare

SYNONYMS

Lung cancer

ICD-9CM CODES
162.9 Malignant neoplasm of bronchus and lung, unspecified

EPIDEMIOLOGY & DEMOGRAPHICS

- Lung cancer is responsible for >30% of cancer deaths in males and >25% of cancer deaths in females.
- Tobacco smoking is implicated in 85% of cases; second-hand smoke is responsible for approximately 20% of cases.
- There are >180,000 new cases of lung cancer yearly in the U.S., most occurring >age 50 yr.

PHYSICAL FINDINGS & CLINICAL PRESENTATION

- Weight loss, fatigue, fever, anorexia, dysphagia
- Cough, hemoptysis, dyspnea, wheezing
- Chest, shoulder, and bone pain

- Paraneoplastic syndromes:
  1. *Eaton-Lambert syndrome:* myopathy involving proximal muscle groups
  2. Endocrine manifestations: hypercalcemia, ectopic ACTH, SIADH
  3. Neurologic: subacute cerebellar degeneration, peripheral neuropathy, cortical degeneration
  4. Musculoskeletal: polymyositis, clubbing, hypertrophic pulmonary osteoarthropathy
  5. Hematologic or vascular: migratory thrombophlebitis, marantic thrombosis, anemia, thrombocytosis, or thrombocytopenia
  6. Cutaneous: acanthosis nigricans, dermatomyositis
- Pleural effusion (10% of patients), recurrent pneumonias (secondary to obstruction), localized wheezing
- *Superior vena cava syndrome:*
  1. Obstruction of venous return of the superior vena cava is most commonly caused by bronchogenic carcinoma or metastasis to paratracheal nodes.
  2. The patient usually complains of headache, nausea, dizziness, visual changes, syncope, and respiratory distress.
  3. Physical examination reveals distention of thoracic and neck veins, edema of face and upper extremities, facial plethora, and cyanosis.
- *Horner's syndrome:* constricted pupil, ptosis, facial anhidrosis caused by spinal cord damage between C8 and T1 secondary to a superior sulcus tumor (bronchogenic carcinoma of the extreme lung apex); a superior sulcus tumor associated with ipsilateral Horner's syndrome and shoulder pain is known as *"Pancoast" tumor.*

ETIOLOGY

- Tobacco abuse
- Environmental agents (e.g., radon) and industrial agents (e.g., ionizing radiation, asbestos, nickel, uranium, vinyl chloride, chromium, arsenic, coal dust)

DIAGNOSIS

DIFFERENTIAL DIAGNOSIS

- Pneumonia
- TB
- Metastatic carcinoma to the lung
- Lung abscess
- Granulomatous disease
- Carcinoid tumor
- Mycobacterial and fungal diseases
- Sarcoidosis
- Viral pneumonitis
- Benign lesions that simulate thoracic malignancy:
  1. Lobar atelectasis: pneumonia, TB, chronic inflammatory disease, allergic bronchopulmonary aspergillosis

  2. Multiple pulmonary nodules: septic emboli, Wegener's granulomatosis, sarcoidosis, rheumatoid nodules, fungal disease, multiple pulmonary AV fistulas
  3. Mediastinal adenopathy: sarcoidosis, lymphoma, primary TB, fungal disease, silicosis, pneumoconiosis, drug-induced (e.g., phenytoin, trimethadione)
  4. Pleural effusion: CHF, pneumonia with parapneumonic effusion, TB, viral pneumonitis, ascites, pancreatitis, collagen-vascular disease

WORKUP

Workup generally includes chest x-ray, CT scan of chest, PET scan, and tissue biopsy.

LABORATORY TESTS

Obtain tissue diagnosis. Various modalities are available:

- Biopsy of any suspicious lymph nodes (e.g., supraclavicular node)
- Flexible fiberoptic bronchoscopy: brush and biopsy specimens are obtained from any visualized endobronchial lesions
- Transbronchial needle aspiration: done via a special needle passed through the bronchoscope; this technique is useful to sample mediastinal masses or paratracheal lymph nodes
- Transthoracic fine-needle aspiration biopsy with fluoroscopic or CT scan guidance to evaluate peripheral pulmonary nodules
- Mediastinoscopy and anteromedial sternotomy in suspected tumor involvement of the mediastinum
- Pleural biopsy in patients with pleural effusion
- Thoracentesis of pleural effusion and cytologic evaluation of the obtained fluid: may confirm diagnosis

IMAGING STUDIES

- Chest x-ray: The radiographic presentation often varies with the cell type. Pleural effusion, lobar atelectasis, and mediastinal adenopathy can accompany any cell types.
- CT scan of chest: to evaluate mediastinal and pleural extension of suspected lung neoplasms.
- Positron emission tomography (PET) with 18F-fluorodeoxyglucose (18 FDG-PET), a metabolic marker of malignant tissue, is superior to CT scan in detecting mediastinal and distant metastases in non–small cell lung cancer. It is useful for preoperative staging of non–small cell lung cancer.

STAGING

- Following confirmation of diagnosis, patients should undergo staging:
  1. The international staging system is the most widely accepted staging

system for non–small cell lung cancer. In this system, stage 1 (N0 [no lymph node involvement]), stage 2 (N1 [spread to ipsilateral bronchopulmonary or hilar lymph nodes]) include localized tumors for which surgical resection is the preferred treatment. Stage 3 is subdivided into 3A (potentially resectable) and 3B. The surgical management of stage 3A disease (N2 [involvement of ipsilateral mediastinal nodes]) is controversial. Only 20% of N2 disease is considered minimal disease (involvement of only one node) and technically resectable. Stage 4 indicates metastatic disease. The pathologic staging system uses a tumor/nodal involvement/metastasis system.

2. In patients with small cell lung cancer, a more practical accepted staging system is the one developed by the Veterans Administration Lung Cancer Study Group (VALG). This system contains two stages:
    a. Limited stage: disease confined to the regional lymph nodes and to one hemithorax (excluding pleural surfaces)
    b. Extensive stage: disease spread beyond the confines of limited stage disease

3. Pretreatment staging procedures for lung cancer patients, in addition to complete history and physical examination, generally include the following tests:
    a. Chest x-ray (PA and lateral), ECG
    b. Laboratory evaluation: CBC, electrolytes, platelets, calcium, phosphorus, glucose, renal and liver function studies, ABGs, and skin tests for TB
    c. Pulmonary function studies
    d. CT scan of chest and PET scan: A recent Dutch trial revealed a 51% relative reduction in futile thoracotomies for patients with suspected non–small cell lung cancer who underwent preoperative assessment with PET with the tracer 18FDG-PET in addition to conventional workup
    e. Mediastinoscopy or anterior mediastinotomy in patients being considered for possible curative lung resection
    f. Biopsy of any accessible suspect lesions
    g. CT scan of liver and brain; radionuclide scans of bone in all patients with small cell carcinoma of the lung and patients with non–small cell lung neoplasms suspected of involving these organs
    h. Bone marrow aspiration and biopsy only in selected patients with small cell carcinoma of the lung. In the absence of an increased LDH or cytopenia, routine bone marrow examination is not recommended

TREATMENT

NONPHARMACOLOGIC THERAPY

- Nutritional support
- Avoidance of tobacco or other substances toxic to the lungs
- Supplemental O_2 prn

ACUTE GENERAL Rx

NON–SMALL CELL CARCINOMA:

- Surgery
    1. Surgical resection is indicated in patients with limited disease (not involving mediastinal nodes, ribs, pleura, or distant sites). This represents approximately 15% to 30% of diagnosed cases.
    2. Preoperative evaluation includes review of cardiac status (e.g., recent MI, major arrhythmias) and evaluation of pulmonary function (to determine if the patient can tolerate any loss of lung tissue). Pneumonectomy is possible if the patient has a preoperative $FEV_1 \geq 2$ L or if the MVV is >50% of predicted capacity.
    3. Preoperative chemotherapy should be considered in patients with more advanced disease (stage 3A) who are being considered for surgery, because it increases the median survival time in patients with non–small cell lung cancer compared with the use of surgery alone.
- Treatment of unresectable non–small cell carcinoma of the lung:
    1. Radiotherapy can be used alone or in combination with chemotherapy; it is used primarily for treatment of CNS and skeletal metastases, superior vena cava syndrome, and obstructive atelectasis; although thoracic radiotherapy is generally considered standard therapy for stage 3 disease, it has limited effect on survival. Palliative radiotherapy should be delayed until symptoms occur since immediate therapy offers no advantage over delayed therapy and results in more adverse events from the radiotherapy.
    2. Chemotherapy: various combination regimens are available. Current

drugs of choice are paclitaxel plus either carboplatin or cisplatin; cisplatin plus vinorelbine; gemcitabine plus cisplatin; carboplatin or cisplatin plus docetaxel. The overall results are disappointing, and none of the standard regimens for non–small cell lung cancer is clearly superior to the others. Gefitinib (Iressa), an inhibitor of epidermal growth factor receptor (EGFR) tyrosine kinase, is an oral preparation currently undergoing clinical trials for advanced non–small cell lung cancer.
    3. The addition of chemotherapy to radiotherapy improves survival in patients with locally advanced, unresectable non–small cell lung cancer. The absolute benefit is relatively small, however, and should be balanced against the increased toxicity associated with the addition of chemotherapy.

TREATMENT OF SMALL CELL LUNG CANCER:

- Limited stage disease: standard treatments include thoracic radiotherapy and chemotherapy (cisplatin and etoposide)
- Extensive stage disease: standard treatments include combination chemotherapy (cisplatin or carboplatin plus etoposide or combination of irinotecan and cisplatin)
- Prophylactic cranial irradiation for patients in complete remission to decrease the risk of CNS metastasis

DISPOSITION

- The 5-yr survival of patients with non–small cell carcinoma when the disease is resectable is approximately 30%.
- Median survival time in patients with limited stage disease and small cell lung cancer is 15 mo; in patients with extensive stage disease, it is 9 mo.

SUGGESTED READINGS

Kris MG et al: Efficacy of gefitinib, an inhibitor of the epidermal growth factor receptor tyrosine kinase, in symptomatic patients with non-small cell lung cancer, *JAMA* 290:2149, 2003.

Lardinois D et al: Staging of non-small cell lung cancer with integrated positron-emission tomography and computed tomography, *N Engl J Med* 348:2500, 2003.

Schiller JH et al: Comparison of four chemotherapy regimens for advanced non-small-cell lung cancer, *N Engl J Med* 346:92, 2002.

Spira A, Ettinger DS: Multidisciplinary management of lung cancer, *N Engl J Med* 350:379, 2004.

AUTHOR: **FRED F. FERRI, M.D.**

BASIC INFORMATION

DEFINITION

Non-Hodgkin lymphoma is a heterogeneous group of malignancies of the lymphoreticular system.

SYNONYMS

NHL

ICD-9CM CODES
201.9 Lymphoma, non-Hodgkin

EPIDEMIOLOGY & DEMOGRAPHICS

- Sixth most common neoplasm in the U.S. (56,000 new cases/yr)
- Increasing incidence with age

PHYSICAL FINDINGS & CLINICAL PRESENTATION

- Patients often present with asymptomatic lymphadenopathy.
- Approximately one third of NHL originates extranodally. Involvement of extranodal sites can result in unusual presentations (e.g., GI tract involvement can simulate PUD).
- NHL cases associated with HIV occur predominantly in the brain.
- Pruritus, fever, night sweats, weight loss are less common than in Hodgkin's disease.
- Hepatomegaly and splenomegaly may be present.

DIAGNOSIS

DIFFERENTIAL DIAGNOSIS

- Hodgkin's disease
- Viral infections
- Metastatic carcinoma
- A clinical algorithm for evaluation of lymphadenopathy is described in Section III
- The differential diagnosis of lymphadenopathy is described in Section II

WORKUP

Initial laboratory evaluation may reveal only mild anemia and elevated LDH and ESR. Proper staging of non-Hodgkin's lymphoma requires the following:

- A thorough history, physical examination, and adequate biopsy
- Routine laboratory evaluation (CBC, ESR, urinalysis, LDH, BUN, creatinine, serum calcium, uric acid, LFTs, serum protein electrophoresis)
- Chest x-ray examination (PA and lateral)
- Bone marrow evaluation (aspirate and full bone core biopsy)
- CT scan of abdomen and pelvis; CT scan of chest if chest x-ray films abnormal
- Bone scan (particularly in patients with histiocytic lymphoma)

- Depending on the histopathology, the results of the above studies and the planned therapy, some other tests may be performed: gallium scan (e.g., in patients with high-grade lymphomas), liver/spleen scan, PET scan, lymphangiography, lumbar puncture
- β-2 Microglobulin levels should be obtained initially (prognostic value) and serially in patients with low-grade lymphomas (useful to monitor therapeutic response of the tumor)
- Serum interleukin levels have prognostic value in diffuse large cell lymphoma

CLASSIFICATION: The Working Formulation of non-Hodgkin lymphoma for clinical usage subdivides lymphomas into low grade, intermediate grade, high grade, and miscellaneous (Table 1-9).

STAGING: The Ann Arbor classification is used to stage non-Hodgkin lymphomas, and histopathology has greater therapeutic implications in NHL than in Hodgkin's disease.

IMAGING STUDIES

See "Workup."

TREATMENT

ACUTE GENERAL Rx

The therapeutic regimen varies with the histologic type and pathologic stage. Following are the commonly used therapeutic modalities:

LOW-GRADE NHL (E.G., NODULAR, POORLY DIFFERENTIATED):

1. Local radiotherapy for symptomatic obstructive adenopathy
2. Deferment of therapy and careful observation in asymptomatic patients
3. Single-agent chemotherapy with cyclophosphamide or chlorambucil and glucocorticoids
4. Combination chemotherapy alone or with radiotherapy: generally indicated only when the lymphoma becomes more invasive, with poor response to less aggressive treatment; commonly used regimens: CVP, CHOP, CHOP-BLEO, COPP, BACOP; addition of recombinant alpha interferon at low doses to chemotherapy prolongs remission duration in patients with low-grade NHL
5. Monoclonal antibodies directed against B-cell surface antigens can also be used to treat follicular lymphomas that are resistant to conventional therapy. The anti-CD20 monoclonal antibody rituximab is a targeted, minimally toxic treatment effective against low-grade NHL in patients who have not received previous treatment
6. The addition of rituximab to CHOP is generally well tolerated; however, ad-

ditional studies may be necessary to clarify the role of CHOP plus rituximab in patients with indolent NHL

7. Ibritumomab tiuxetan (Zevalin), an immunoconjugate that combines the linker-chelator tiuxetan with the monoclonal antibody ibritumomab, can be used as part of a two-step regimen for treatment of patients with relapsed or refractory low-grade, follicular, or transformed B-cell NHL refractory to rituximab
8. New purine analogs (FLAMP, 2CDA) can be used in salvage treatment of refractory lymphomas. They all have activity in follicular lymphomas

INTERMEDIATE- AND HIGH-GRADE LYMPHOMAS (E.G., DIFFUSE HISTIOCYTIC LYMPHOMA):

Combination chemotherapy regimens (e.g., CHOP, PRO-MACE-CYTABOM, MACOP-B, M-BACOD). An anthracycline-containing regimen (such as CHOP) given in standard doses and schedule is generally best for treatment of older patients with advanced stage, aggressive-histology lymphoma who do not have significant comorbid illness.

1. High-dose sequential therapy is superior to standard-dose MACOP-B for patients with diffuse large-cell lymphoma of the B-cell type.
2. Dose-modified chemotherapy should be considered for most HIV-infected patients with lymphoma. As compared with treatment with standard doses of cytotoxic chemotherapy (M-BACOD), reduced doses cause significantly fewer hematologic toxic effects yet have similar efficacy in patients with HIV-related lymphoma.

- Three cycles of CHOP followed by involved-field radiotherapy may be superior to eight cycles of CHOP alone in patients with localized intermediate- and high-grade NHL.
- The addition of rituximab against CD20 B-cell lymphoma to the CHOP regimen increases the complete response rate and prolongs event-free and overall survival in elderly patients with diffuse large B-cell lymphoma without a clinically significant increase in toxicity. Bexxar, a combination of the mononuclear antibody tositumomab and radiolabeled iodine-131 tositumomab can be used for a single treatment of relapsed follicular NHL in patients who are refractory to rituximab. It results in complete remission in 25% of patients and clinical response in 60% of patients.
- Granulocyte colony-stimulating factor (G-CSF): may be effective in reducing the risk of infection in patients with aggressive lymphoma undergoing chemotherapy

- Radioimmunotherapy with (^{131}I) anti-B1 antibody therapy for NHL either by itself or in combination with other treatments
- Treatment with high-dose chemotherapy and autologous bone marrow transplant: as compared with conventional chemotherapy, increases event-free and overall survival in patients with chemotherapy-sensitive non-Hodgkin lymphoma in relapse

DISPOSITION

- Patients with low-grade lymphoma, despite their long-term survival (6 to 10 yr average), are rarely cured, and the great majority (if not all) eventually die of the lymphoma, whereas patients with a high-grade lymphoma may achieve a cure with aggressive chemotherapy.
- Complete remission occurs in 35% to 50% of patients with intermediate- and high-grade lymphoma. Prognostic factors include the histologic subtype, age of patient, and bulk of disease.

AUTHOR: **FRED F. FERRI, M.D.**

TABLE 1-9   Classification Systems for Grading Lymphomas

Kiel Classification	Working Formulation	Revised European-American Classification
Low-grade malignancy	Low grade	B-cell lymphomas
Lymphocytic, CLL	A. Malignant lymphoma, small lymphocytic	
Lymphocytic, other	Consistent with chronic lymphocytic leukemia	B-CLL/SLL
Lymphoplasmacytoid		Lymphoplasmacytoid lymphoma
Centrocytic	B. Malignant lymphoma, follicular, predominantly small cleaved cell	Follicle center lymphomas
Centroblastic/Centrocytic		Marginal zone lymphomas (MALT)
Follicular without sclerosis	Diffuse areas	Mantle cell lymphoma
Follicular with sclerosis	Sclerosis	
Follicular and diffuse, without sclerosis	C. Malignant lymphoma, follicular mixed, small cleaved and large cell	
Follicular and diffuse, with sclerosis	Diffuse areas	Diffuse large B-cell lymphoma
Diffuse	Sclerosis	Primary mediastinal large B-cell lymphoma
Low-grade malignant lymphoma, unclassified	Intermediate grade	Burkitt's lymphoma
High-grade malignancy	D. Malignant lymphoma, follicular	T-cell lymphomas
Centroblastic	Diffuse areas	
Lymphoblastic, Burkitt's type	E. Malignant lymphoma, diffuse small cleaved cell	
Lymphoblastic, convoluted cell type		T-CLL
Lymphoblastic, other (unclassified) immunoblastic		Mycosis fungoides/Sézary syndrome
High-grade malignant lymphoma, unclassified	F. Malignant lymphoma, diffuse mixed, small and large cell sclerosis	
Malignant lymphoma unclassified (unable to specify high grade or low grade)	G. Malignant lymphoma diffuse	Peripheral T-cell lymphoma, unspecified
Composite lymphoma	Large cell	Angioimmunoblastic T-cell lymphoma
	Cleaved cell	Angiocentric lymphoma
	Noncleaved cell	Intestinal T-cell lymphoma
	Sclerosis	Adult T-cell lymphoma/leukemia
	High grade	Anaplastic large cell lymphoma
	H. Malignant lymphoma large cell, immunoblastic	Precursor T-lymphoid lymphoma/leukemia
	Plasmacytoid	
	Clear cell	
	Polymorphous	
	Epithelioid cell component	
	I. Malignant lymphoma lymphoblastic	
	Convoluted cell	
	Nonconvoluted cell	
	J. Malignant lymphoma small noncleaved cell	
	Burkitt's	
	Follicular areas	

From Abeloff MD: *Clinical oncology,* ed 2, New York, 2000, Churchill Livingstone.
B-CLL, B-cell chronic lymphoid leukemia; *MALT,* mucosa-associated lymphoid tumor; *SLL,* lymphoid leukemia; *T-CLL,* T-cell CLL.

BASIC INFORMATION

DEFINITION

Macular degeneration refers to a group of diseases associated with loss of central vision and damage to the macula. Degenerative changes occur in the pigment, neural, and vascular layers of the macula. The dry macular degeneration is usually ischemic in etiology, and a wet macular degeneration is associated with leakage of fluid from blood vessels, usually referred to as age-related macular degeneration (ARMD).

ICD-9CM CODES
362.5 Degeneration of macula
and posterior pole

EPIDEMIOLOGY & DEMOGRAPHICS

INCIDENCE (IN U.S.):
- Main cause of blindness in the U.S. in 40 yr and older
- Increases with age
- 1.75 million individuals in the U.S. currently affected; 3 million by year 2020

PREDOMINANT SEX: Male = female (15% of white women >80 have severe ARMD)

PREDOMINANT AGE: >50 yr

PEAK INCIDENCE:
- 75 to 80 yr old
- Dramatic increases in incidence and prevalence with age until approximately 80% of people 75 yr or older have senile macular degeneration.

GENETICS:
- Different syndrome: senile macular degeneration is age related.
- Several rare neurologic syndromes are associated with macular degeneration.
- Vascular disease closely related to macular degeneration.

PHYSICAL FINDINGS
- Decreased central vision
- Macular hemorrhage, pigmentation, edema, atrophy
- The most common abnormality seen in age-related macular degeneration (AMD) is the presence of drusen, or yellowish deposits deep to the retina; this may be early in course of disease

ETIOLOGY
- Subretinal neovascular membrane early
- Pigmentary and vascular changes with exudate, edema, and scar tissue development
- Early in course, possible subretinal neovascularization
- Dry type atrophy of macular pigment epithelium

DIAGNOSIS

DIFFERENTIAL DIAGNOSIS
- Diabetic retinopathy
- Hypertension
- Histoplasmosis
- Trauma with scar

WORKUP
- Complete eye examination, including visual field and fluorescein angiography
- Optical coherence tomography (OCT)

LABORATORY TESTS
Evaluate for diabetes and other metabolic problems, as well as vascular diseases.

IMAGING STUDIES
- Optical coherence tomography (OCT)
- Fluorescein angiography

TREATMENT

NONPHARMACOLOGIC THERAPY
- Laser treatment to stop progression of disease—photo dynamic treatment with verteporfin IV
- Laser (Argon)
- Diet, exercise
- Vitamins with zinc and antioxidants

ACUTE GENERAL Rx
Intravitral steroids, photodynamic treatment (PDT) with laser

CHRONIC Rx
- Repeated laser treatments
- Antioxidants and zinc may slow down progression of ARMD

DISPOSITION
- Follow closely by ophthalmologist.
- If vision deteriorates, refer urgently to an ophthalmologist.

REFERRAL
- To ophthalmologist early in the course of the disease if the sight is to be saved
- Immediate referral if any change in vision

PEARLS & CONSIDERATIONS

COMMENTS
- Sildenafil has no significant effect on macular degeneration.
- The vision of only 1 out of 10 people can be saved, but the disease is so devastating that vigorous therapy should be attempted.
- Statins plus aspirin may slow down progression.
- Vitamins with zinc and antioxidants may slow down progression of ARMD.

SUGGESTED READINGS
Friedman DS et al: Prevalence of age-related macular degeneration in the US, *Arch Ophthalmol* 122(4):564, 2004.

Gottlieb JL: Age-related macular degeneration, *JAMA* 288:2233, 2002.

Jonas JB: Verteporfin theory of subfoveal choroidal neovascularization in age-related macular degeneration, *Am J Ophthalmol* 133(6):F57, 2002.

Liu M, Regillo CD: A review of treatments for macular degeneration: a synopsis of currently approved treatments and ongoing clinical trials, *Curr Opin Ophthalmol* 15(3):221, 2004.

Makenzie PJ, Chang TS: ETN assessment of vision-related emotion in patients with age related macular degeneration, *Ophthalmology* 109(4):720, 2002.

Ting TD et al: Decreased visual acuity associated with cystoid macular edema in neovascular or age-related macular degeneration, *Arch Ophthamol* 120(6):731, 2002.

AUTHOR: **MELVYN KOBY, M.D.**

BASIC INFORMATION

DEFINITION

Meniere's disease is a syndrome characterized by recurrent vertigo with fluctuating hearing loss, tinnitus, and fullness in the ear.

SYNONYMS

Endolymphatic hydrops
Meniere's syndrome

ICD-9CM CODES
386.01 Meniere's disease, cochleovestibular (active)

EPIDEMIOLOGY & DEMOGRAPHICS

INCIDENCE (IN U.S.): 15 cases/100,000 persons
PREVALENCE (IN U.S.): 100-200 cases/ 100,000 persons
PREDOMINANT SEX: Male = female
PREDOMINANT AGE: Adults
GENETICS: Not known to be genetic

PHYSICAL FINDINGS & CLINICAL PRESENTATION

- Hearing may be unilaterally decreased
- Pallor, sweating, and nausea may occur during a severe attack
- Usually the patient develops a sensation of fullness and pressure along with decreased hearing and tinnitus in a single ear
- The patient typically experiences severe vertigo, which peaks within minutes, then slowly subsides over hours
- Persistent sense of disequilibrium for days is typical after an acute episode

ETIOLOGY

- Unknown; viral and autoimmune etiologies have been suggested
- Associated with endolymphatic hydrops

DIAGNOSIS

DIFFERENTIAL DIAGNOSIS

- Acoustic neuroma
- Migrainous vertigo
- Multiple sclerosis
- Autoimmune inner ear syndrome
- Otitis media
- Vertebrobasilar disease
- Viral labyrinthitis

WORKUP

- Electronystagmography may show peripheral vestibular deficit.
- Electrocochleography and glycerol test used by some otoneurologists and ENT specialists.

LABORATORY TESTS

Audiogram may show sensorineural hearing loss, with lower frequencies primarily affected.

IMAGING STUDIES

MRI to rule out acoustic neuroma, especially if cerebellar or CNS dysfunction is present

TREATMENT

NONPHARMACOLOGIC THERAPY

Limit activity during attacks.

ACUTE GENERAL Rx

- Prochlorperazine 5 to 10 mg PO q6h or 25 mg PO bid
- Promethazine 12.5 to 25 mg PO q4-6h
- Diazepam 5 to 10 mg IV/PO for acute attack
- Meclizine 12.5 to 25 mg tid
- Scopolamine patch

CHRONIC Rx

Diuretics such as hydrochlorothiazide or acetazolamide, salt restriction, and avoidance of caffeine are traditional.

DISPOSITION

- Usual course of disease consists of alternating attacks and remissions
- Majority of patients can be managed medically; fewer than 10% of patients will undergo surgical intervention for persistent incapacitating vertigo

REFERRAL

To an otolaryngologist for surgical intervention if attacks persist despite medical therapy

PEARLS & CONSIDERATIONS

COMMENTS

- Many variations of the classical clinical picture. The essential features for diagnosis are episodic vertigo and sensorineural hearing loss audiometrically documented on at least one occasion.
- In one-third of patients both ears are eventually involved.
- Some evidence that Meniere's disease and migraine may be pathophysiologically linked.

SUGGESTED READINGS

Baloh RW, Fife TD, Furman JM, Zee DS: Recurrent spontaneous attacks of vertigo, *Continuum Lifelong Learning in Neurology* 2(2):56, 1996.

Radtke A et al: Migraine and Meniere's disease: is there a link? *Neurology* 59(11):1700, 2002.

Thai-Von H, Bounaix MJ, Fraysse B: Meniere's disease: pathophysiology and treatment, *Drugs* 61(8):1089, 2001.

Weber PC, Adkins WY Jr: The differential diagnosis of Meniere's disease, *Otolaryngol Clin North Am* 30(6):977, 1997.

AUTHOR: **SHARON S. HARTMAN, M.D., PH.D.**

BASIC INFORMATION

DEFINITION

Menopause is the occurrence of no menstrual periods for 1 yr after age 40 yr or permanent cessation of ovulation following lost ovarian activity. It is a climacteric reproductive stage of life marked by waxing and waning estrogen levels followed by decreasing ovarian function. Premature ovarian failure and no menstrual periods may also occur because of depletion of ovarian follicles before the age of 40 yr.

SYNONYMS

Change of life
Climacteric ovarian failure

ICD-9CM CODES
627.2 Menopausal or female climacteric states
627.4 States associated with artificial menopause
716.3 Climacteric arthritis

EPIDEMIOLOGY & DEMOGRAPHICS

- Average age of menopause in the U.S. is 51 yr.
- Age at which menopause occurs is genetically determined.
- Smokers experience menopause an average of 1.5 yr earlier than nonsmokers.
- More than one third of a woman's life will be spent after menopause.
- Onset of perimenopause is usually in a woman's mid- to late 40s.
- Approximately 4000 women each day begin menopause.

PHYSICAL FINDINGS & CLINICAL PRESENTATION

- Atrophic vaginitis, which can cause burning, itching, bleeding, dyspareunia
- Either complete cessation of menses or a period of irregular cycles and diminished or heavier bleeding
- Osteoporosis
- Psychologic dysfunction:
  1. Anxiety
  2. Depression
  3. Insomnia
  4. Nervousness
  5. Irritability
  6. Inability to concentrate
- Sexual changes, decreased libido, dyspareunia
- Urinary incontinence
- Vasomotor symptoms (hot flashes, flushes), night sweats, cardiovascular disease, coronary artery disease, atherosclerosis, headaches, tiredness, and lethargy

ETIOLOGY

- The most common etiology: physiologic, caused by degenerating theca cells that fail to react to endogenous gonadotropins, producing less estrogen; decreased negative feedback in the hypothalamic pituitary access, increased follicle-stimulating hormone (FSH), and increased luteinizing hormone (LH), which leads to stromal cells that continue to produce androgens as a result of the LH stimulation
- Surgical castration
- Family history of early menopause, cigarette smoking, blindness, abnormal chromosomal karyotype (Turner's syndrome, gonadal dysgenesis), precocious puberty, and left-handedness

DIAGNOSIS

DIFFERENTIAL DIAGNOSIS

- Asherman's syndrome
- Hypothalamic dysfunction
- Hypothyroidism
- Pituitary tumors
- Adrenal abnormalities
- Ovarian abnormalities
- Polycystic ovarian syndrome
- Ovarian neoplasm
- TB

WORKUP

- If the clinical picture is highly suggestive of menopause, estrogen can be prescribed. If all symptoms resolve, then diagnosis has essentially been made. Before estrogen is prescribed, a complete history and physical examination are needed. If a patient has estrogen-dependent malignancy, unexplained abnormal uterine bleeding, history of thrombophlebitis, or acute liver disease, estrogen therapy is contraindicated.
- Progesterone challenge test: progesterone 100 mg is given IM to induce withdrawal bleeding. If no withdrawal bleeding is obtained, it would be safe to assume that a hypoestrogenic state is present.
- Physical examination, height, weight, blood pressure, breast examination, and pelvic examination are needed.
- Assess risk for coronary artery disease, osteoporosis, cigarette smoking, personal history, history of breast cancer, liver disease, active coagulation disorder, or any unexplained vaginal bleeding.

LABORATORY TESTS

- FSH, LH, and estrogen levels: if the FSH is markedly elevated and the estrogen level is markedly depressed, constitutes laboratory diagnosis of ovarian failure

- TSH to rule out thyroid dysfunction and prolactin level if patient has symptoms of galactorrhea and if suspicion of pituitary adenoma exists
- A general chemistry profile to check for any systemic diseases
- Pap smear, endometrial biopsy, or D&C in patients who have had irregular periods or intermenstrual or postmenopausal bleeding
- Mammogram

IMAGING STUDIES

- CT scan or MRI of head if pituitary tumor is suspected
- Bone density studies
- Pelvic ultrasound to check endometrial stripe

TREATMENT

NONPHARMACOLOGIC THERAPY

- A balanced diet: low in fat, with total fat intake being <30% of calories; total calories sufficient to maintain body weight or to produce weight loss if that is needed
- Avoidance of smoking, excessive alcohol or caffeine intake
- Exercise: weight-bearing exercise for osteoporosis prevention
- Kegel exercises for strengthening the pelvic floor
- Adequate calcium intake: 1500 mg qd and vitamin D 600 units qd are necessary to maintain calcium balance in postmenopausal women and prevent osteoporosis
- Change in the ambient temperature (may ameliorate hot flashes and reduce night sweats)
- Vitamin E
- Avoidance of caffeine, alcohol, and spicy foods if they trigger hot flashes
- Vaginal lubricants to help with the dyspareunia secondary to vaginal dryness (e.g., Replens, K-Y Jelly, or Gyne-Moistrin cream)

ACUTE GENERAL Rx

Estrogen replacement in symptomatic patients can be done in a variety of forms, including oral estrogen and transdermal estrogen patch.

- Examples of oral estrogen would include conjugated estrogens:
  1. Premarin: start with 0.625 mg qd and increase up to 1.25 mg qd, depending on symptoms. Cenestin (synthetic conjugated estrogens, A) available in 0.625-, 0.9-, and 1.25-mg doses.
  2. Estradiol (Estrace): start with 1 mg qd and increase to 2 mg qd; also

available in 0.5 mg tablet for patients who experience side effects from the estrogen.

3. Esterified estrogens (Estratab): start with 0.3 to 1.25 mg qd.
4. Estropipate (Ogen, Ortho-Est): start with 0.625 to 1.25 mg qd.
5. Esterified estrogen/testosterone combination: give 1.25 mg and methyltestosterone 2.5 mg (Estratest) and esterified estrogen 0.625 mg and methyltestosterone 1.25 mg (Estratest HS). May improve sexual enjoyment and libido.

- If the patient has had a hysterectomy for benign disease, estrogen alone is sufficient. However, if she still has her uterus, progestin should be added for its protective effect against endometrial cancer. Medroxyprogesterone acetate (Provera) is the most commonly prescribed progestin. It can be prescribed in a continual daily dose of 2.5 mg or of 5 mg if continual breakthrough bleeding is encountered. This can also be prescribed in a 5-mg cyclic fashion for the first 14 days of the month or as 10-mg tablets for the first 10 days of the month. Patients need to be advised that this generally will cause withdrawal bleeding but in a fairly regular fashion. Continuous hormone replacement therapy is preferred, because after a period of time the patient should be amenorrheic. Patients should be counseled that they may experience some irregular spotting for the first 6 to 9 mo after starting the hormone replacement therapy.
- Combination oral preparations Femhrt ⅕ (1 mg norethindrone acetate/5 μg ethinyl estradiol) one pill daily. Ortho—Prefest 1 mg 17β-estradiol (white pill) alternating with 1 mg 17β-estradiol and 0.9 mg norgestimate (pink pill) q3d Prempro 0.625 mg conjugated estrogen/2.5 mg medroxyprogesterone one pill daily Prempro 0.625 mg conjugated estrogen/5.0 mg medroxyprogesterone one pill daily Activella 1 mg estradiol and 0.5 mg norethindrone acetate Premphase 0.625 mg conjugated estrogen with 5 mg medroxyprogesterone last 14 days.
- Transdermal patches can be either estradiol (Estraderm, Vivelle, Fempatch) 0.025 to 0.1 mg applied twice weekly or Climara 0.025 to 0.1 mg used once a week. With these preparations, progesterone should be used in a similar fashion. Combipatch—apply twice weekly (combination estrogen and progesterone).
- Vaginal creams can be used, and these should be reserved for local therapy of atrophic vaginitis. Systemic absorption does occur; however, blood levels are unpredictable. Start with a loading dose of 2 to 4 g of estrogen-containing cream nightly for 1 to 2 wk. When symptoms improve, once to twice weekly is adequate maintenance.
- Vagifem estradiol vaginal tablets. Initial dosage: one Vagifem tablet, inserted vaginally, once daily for 2 wk. Maintenance dose: one Vagifem tablet, inserted vaginally, twice weekly.
- Femring vaginal ring delivering the equivalent of 50 micrograms per day inserted every 3 months.
- EstroGel 0.06% (estrodiol gel) One Pump (1.25 g/day) applied to one arm from wrist to shoulder.
- For women in whom estrogen is contraindicated or for those who do not wish to take estrogen, the following regimens can be used:
  1. Depo-Provera 150 mg IM every month (may be helpful in alleviating hot flashes)
  2. Clonidine 0.05 to 0.15 mg qd
  3. Bellergal-S
  4. Fosamax (alendronate sodium) or Actonel (risedronate) 5 mg qd or 35 mg weekly are approved for prophylactic prevention of osteoporosis. They should be taken on an empty stomach; wait at least 30 min before ingesting any substance, including liquids, because this decreases absorption into the body. They should be swallowed on arising for the day with a full glass of water, 6 to 8 oz, and patients should not lie down for at least 30 min and until after their first food of the day.
  5. Evista (Raloxifene) 60 mg daily PO has positive bone effect, a total cholesterol–lowering effect, and LDL cholesterol–lowering effect; it is a selective estrogen receptor agonist; it does not affect estrogen receptors in the breast or uterus. It does not ameliorate vasomotor symptoms or vaginal atrophy.
- Tibolone significantly improves vasomotor symptoms, libido, and vaginal lubrication.

CHRONIC Rx

Hormone replacement therapy should be used only for the short term unless benefits outweigh the risks of long-term use.

DISPOSITION

If treated, the patient should have resolution of her symptoms and reduced incidence of osteoporosis. Lifelong medical supervision is necessary to monitor adequacy of treatment and prevention of complications. This should include annual Pap smears, pelvic examinations, breast examinations, mammography, and endometrial sampling of any type of abnormal bleeding. If untreated, the vasomotor symptoms will eventually disappear; however, this takes many years, and some women who are in their 80s have experienced hot flashes. Urogenital atrophy will continue to worsen. Osteoporosis and coronary artery disease risks will increase with every passing year.

REFERRAL

This condition can be managed adequately by the patient's primary care physician who has an interest in treating menopausal women.

PEARLS & CONSIDERATIONS

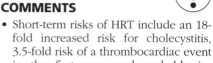

COMMENTS

- Short-term risks of HRT include an 18-fold increased risk for cholecystitis, 3.5-fold risk of a thrombocardiac event in the first year, and probably increased risk of stroke and MI.
- Results of the WHI study found that for every 10,000 women taking HRT for 1 yr (10,000 person-yr), 7 more would have coronary events, 8 more strokes, 8 more pulmonary emboli, and 8 more with early breast cancer than would 10,000 women taking placebo. Benefits of HRT were 6 fewer cases of colorectal cancer and 5 fewer hip fractures per 10,000 women.
- HRT should not be initiated or continued for the primary or secondary prevention of CHD or osteoporosis.
- Patient education materials can be obtained through the American College of Obstetricians and Gynecologists, 409 12th Street SW, Washington, DC 20024, and *Menopause News,* 2074 Union Street, San Francisco, CA 94123; phone: 1-800-241-MENO. Multiple patient educational brochures are produced by pharmacologic companies.

SUGGESTED READINGS

Gambrell RD: The Women's Health Initiative Reports: critical review of the findings, the female patient, *Menopause* 29:(11):23, 2004.

Han KK et al: Benefits of soy isoflavone therapeutic regimen on menopausal symptoms, *Obstet Gynecol* 99:389, 2002.

Lacey JV et al: Menopausal hormone replacement therapy and risk of ovarian cancer, *JAMA* 288:334, 2002.

Nelson H et al: Postmenopausal hormone replacement therapy, *JAMA* 288:872, 2002.

Santoro N: The menopause transition: an update, *Human Reproduction Update* 8(2):155, 2002.

Speroff L: Efficacy and tolerability of a novel estradiol vaginal ring for relief of menopausal symptoms, *Obstet Gynecol* 102(4):823, 2003.

Writing Group for the Women's Health Initiative Investigators: Risks and benefits of estrogen plus progestin in healthy postmenopausal women, *JAMA* 288:321, 2002.

AUTHOR: **GEORGE T. DANAKAS, M.D.**

BASIC INFORMATION

DEFINITION

Mitral regurgitation (MR) is retrograde blood flow through the left atrium secondary to an incompetent mitral valve. Eventually there is an increase in left atrial and pulmonary pressures, which may result in right ventricular failure.

SYNONYMS

Mitral insufficiency
MR

ICD-9CM CODES
424.0 Mitral regurgitation

EPIDEMIOLOGY & DEMOGRAPHICS

The incidence of MR has increased over the past 30 yr; however, this may be because of increasing availability of echocardiography rather than any real increases in this condition.

PHYSICAL FINDINGS & CLINICAL PRESENTATION

- Patients with MR generally present with the following symptoms:
  1. Fatigue, dyspnea, orthopnea, frank CHF
  2. Hemoptysis (caused by pulmonary hypertension)
  3. Possible systemic emboli in patients with left atrial mural thrombi associated with atrial fibrillation
- Hyperdynamic apex, often with palpable left ventricular lift and apical thrill
- Holosystolic murmur at apex with radiation to base or to left axilla; poor correlation between the intensity of the systolic murmur and the degree of regurgitation
- Apical early- to mid-diastolic rumble (rare)

ETIOLOGY

- Papillary muscle dysfunction (as a result of ischemic heart disease)
- Ruptured chordae tendineae
- Infective endocarditis
- Calcified mitral valve annulus
- Left ventricular dilation
- Rheumatic valvulitis
- Primary or secondary mitral valve prolapse
- Hypertrophic cardiomyopathy
- Idiopathic myxomatous degeneration of the mitral valve
- Myxoma
- SLE

DIAGNOSIS

DIFFERENTIAL DIAGNOSIS

- Hypertrophic cardiomyopathy
- Pulmonary regurgitation
- Tricuspid regurgitation
- VSD

WORKUP

Diagnostic workup consists of echocardiography, ECG, and chest x-ray.

IMAGING STUDIES

- Echocardiography: enlarged left atrium, hyperdynamic left ventricle (erratic motion of the leaflet is seen in patients with ruptured chordae tendineae); Doppler electrocardiography will show evidence of MR. The most important aspect of the echocardiographic examination is the quantification of left ventricular systolic performance.
- Chest x-ray study:
  1. Left atrial enlargement (usually more pronounced in mitral stenosis)
  2. Left ventricular enlargement
  3. Possible pulmonary congestion
- ECG:
  1. Left atrial enlargement
  2. Left ventricular hypertrophy
  3. Atrial fibrillation

TREATMENT

NONPHARMACOLOGIC THERAPY

Salt restriction

ACUTE GENERAL Rx

- Medical: Medical therapy is primarily directed toward treatment of complications (e.g., atrial fibrillation) and prevention of bacterial endocarditis.
  1. Consider digitalis for inotropic effect and to control ventricular response if atrial fibrillation with fast ventricular response is present
  2. Afterload reduction (to decrease the regurgitant fraction and to increase cardiac output): may be accomplished with nifedipine, hydralazine plus nitrates, ACE inhibitors, or RRBs
  3. Anticoagulants if atrial fibrillation occurs
  4. Antibiotic prophylaxis before dental and surgical procedures

- Surgery: Surgery is the only definitive treatment for MR. Transesophageal echocardiography allows accurate assessment of the feasibility of valve repair and is indicated before surgical intervention. The timing of surgical repair is controversial; generally surgery should be considered early in symptomatic patients despite optimal medical therapy and in patients with moderate to severe MR and minimal symptoms if there is echocardiographic evidence of rapidly progressive increase in left ventricular end-diastolic and end-systolic dimension (echocardiographic evidence of systolic failure includes end-systolic dimension >55 mm and fractional shortening <31%). Surgery is also indicated in asymptomatic patients with preserved ventricular function if there is a high likelihood of valve repair or if there is evidence of pulmonary hypertension or recent atrial fibrillation.

DISPOSITION

Prognosis is generally good unless there is significant impairment of left ventricle or significantly elevated pulmonary artery pressures. Most patients remain asymptomatic for many years (average interval from diagnosis to onset of symptoms is 16 yr).

REFERRAL

Surgical referral in selected patients (see "Acute General Rx"); emergency surgery may be necessary in patients with MR caused by ruptured chordae tendineae following MI.

PEARLS & CONSIDERATIONS

COMMENTS

Patients should be counseled regarding weight reduction (if obese), avoidance of tobacco, and maintenance of normal (nonstrenuous) activities.

SUGGESTED READING

Otto CM: Evaluation and management of chronic mitral regurgitation, *N Engl J Med* 345:740, 2001.

AUTHOR: **FRED F. FERRI, M.D.**

BASIC INFORMATION

DEFINITION

Mitral stenosis is a narrowing of the mitral valve orifice. The cross section of a normal orifice measures 4 to 6 cm². A murmur becomes audible when the valve orifice becomes smaller than 2 cm². When the orifice approaches 1 cm², the condition becomes critical, and symptoms become more evident.

SYNONYMS

MS

ICD-9CM CODES

394.0 Mitral stenosis

EPIDEMIOLOGY & DEMOGRAPHICS

- The occurrence of mitral valve stenosis has decreased worldwide over the past 30 yr (particularly in developed countries) as a result of declining incidence of rheumatic fever.
- The incidence of mitral stenosis is higher in women.

PHYSICAL FINDINGS & CLINICAL PRESENTATION

- Exertional dyspnea initially, followed by orthopnea and PND
- Acute pulmonary edema (may develop after exertion)
- Systemic emboli (caused by stagnation of blood in the left atrium; may occur in patients with associated atrial fibrillation)
- Hemoptysis (may be present as a result of persistent pulmonary hypertension)
- Prominent jugular A waves are present in patients with normal sinus rhythm.
- Opening snap occurs in early diastole; a short (<0.07-second) A_2 to opening snap interval indicates severe mitral stenosis.
- Apical middiastolic or presystolic rumble that does not radiate is present.
- Accentuated S_1 (because of delayed and forceful closure of the valve) is present.
- If pulmonary hypertension is present, there may be an accentuated P_2 and/or a soft, early diastolic decrescendo murmur (Graham Steell murmur) caused by pulmonary regurgitation (it is best heard along the left sternal border and may be confused with aortic regurgitation).
- A palpable right ventricular heave may be present at the left sternal border.
- Patients with mitral stenosis usually have symptoms of left-sided heart failure: dyspnea on exertion, PND, orthopnea.

- Right ventricular dysfunction (in late stages) may be manifested by peripheral edema, enlarged and pulsatile liver, and ascites.

ETIOLOGY

- Progressive fibrosis, scarring, and calcification of the valve
- Rheumatic fever (still a common cause in underdeveloped countries); heart valves most frequently affected in rheumatic heart disease (in descending order of occurrence): mitral, aortic, tricuspid, and pulmonary
- Rare causes: endomyocardial fibroelastosis, malignant carcinoid syndrome, SLE

DIAGNOSIS

DIFFERENTIAL DIAGNOSIS

- Left atrial myxoma
- Other valvular abnormalities (e.g., tricuspid stenosis, mitral regurgitation)
- Atrial septal defect

WORKUP

Physical examination and echocardiography

IMAGING STUDIES

- Echocardiography:
  1. The characteristic finding on echocardiogram is a markedly diminished E to F slope of the anterior mitral valve leaflet during diastole; there is also fusion of the commissures, resulting in anterior movement of the posterior mitral valve leaflet during diastole (calcification in the valve may also be noted).
  Two-dimensional echocardiogram can accurately establish valve area.
- Chest x-ray:
  1. Straightening of the left cardiac border caused by dilated left atrial appendage
  2. Left atrial enlargement on lateral chest x-ray (appearing as double density of PA chest x-ray)
  3. Prominence of pulmonary arteries
  4. Possible pulmonary congestion and edema (Kerley B lines)
- ECG:
  1. Right ventricular hypertrophy; right axis deviation caused by pulmonary hypertension
  2. Left atrial enlargement (broad notched P waves)
  3. Atrial fibrillation
- Cardiac catheterization to help establish the severity of mitral stenosis and

diagnose associated valvular and coronary lesions. Findings on cardiac catheterization include:
1. Normal left ventricular function
2. Elevated left atrial and pulmonary pressures

TREATMENT

NONPHARMACOLOGIC THERAPY

Decrease level of activity in symptomatic patients.

ACUTE GENERAL Rx

- Medical:
  1. If the patient is in atrial fibrillation, control the rate response with diltiazem, digitalis, or esmolol. Although digitalis is the drug of choice for chronic heart rate control, IV diltiazem or esmolol may be acutely preferable when a rapid decrease in heart rate is required.
  2. If the patient has persistent atrial fibrillation (because of large left atrium), permanent anticoagulation is indicated to decrease the risk of serious thromboembolism.
  3. Treat CHF with diuretics and sodium restriction.
  4. Give antibiotic prophylaxis with dental and surgical procedures (see Section V).
- Surgical: valve replacement is indicated when the valve orifice is <0.7 to 0.8 cm² or if symptoms persist despite optimal medical therapy; commissurotomy may be possible if the mitral valve is noncalcified and if there is pure mitral stenosis without significant subvalvular disease.
- Percutaneous transvenous mitral valvotomy (PTMV) is becoming the therapy of choice for many patients with mitral stenosis responding poorly to medical therapy, particularly those who are poor surgical candidates and whose valve is not heavily calcified; balloon valvotomy gives excellent mechanical relief, usually resulting in prolonged benefit.

DISPOSITION

- Prognosis is generally good except in patients with chronic pulmonary hypertension.
- Operative mortality rates for mitral valve replacement are 1% to 5% in most institutions.

AUTHOR: **FRED F. FERRI, M.D.**

BASIC INFORMATION

DEFINITION

Mitral valve prolapse (MVP) is the posterior bulging of interior and posterior leaflets in systole. Mitral valve prolapse syndrome refers to a constellation of MVP and associated symptoms (e.g., autonomic dysfunction, palpitations) or other physical abnormalities (e.g., pectus excavatum).

SYNONYMS

MVP
Mitral click murmur syndrome

ICD-9CM CODES
424.0 Mitral valve disorders
394.9 Other and unspecified mitral valve diseases

EPIDEMIOLOGY & DEMOGRAPHICS

- MVP can be found by 2-D echocardiogram in 4% of the general population (females > males).
- Increased incidence is seen with autoimmune thyroid disorders, Ehlers-Danlos syndrome, Marfan's syndrome, pseudoxanthoma elasticum, pectus excavatum, anorexia nervosa, and bulimia.

PHYSICAL FINDINGS & CLINICAL PRESENTATION

- Usually, female patient with narrow AP chest diameter, low body weight, low blood pressure
- Mid to late click, heard best at the apex
- Crescendo mid to late diastolic murmur
- Findings accentuated in the standing position
- Most patients with MVP are asymptomatic; symptoms (if present) consist primarily of chest pain and palpitations
- Neurologic abnormalities (e.g., TIA or stroke) are rare
- Patients may also complain of anxiety, fatigue, and dyspnea

ETIOLOGY

- Myxomatous degeneration of connective tissue of mitral valve
- Congenital deformity of mitral valve and supportive structures
- Secondary to other disorders (e.g., Ehlers-Danlos, pseudoxanthoma elasticum)

DIAGNOSIS

DIFFERENTIAL DIAGNOSIS

- Other valvular abnormalities
- Constrictive pericarditis
- Ventricular aneurysm

WORKUP

- Medical history and physical examination
- Workup consists primarily of echocardiography in patients with a systolic click or murmur on careful auscultation

IMAGING STUDIES

Echocardiography shows the anterior and posterior leaflets bulging posteriorly in systole.

TREATMENT

NONPHARMACOLOGIC THERAPY

Avoidance of stimulants (e.g., caffeine, nicotine) in patients with palpitations

ACUTE GENERAL Rx

- The empiric use of antiarrhythmic drugs to prevent sudden death in patients with uncomplicated MVP is not advisable; β-blockers may be tried in symptomatic patients (e.g., palpitations, chest pain); they decrease the heart rate, thus decreasing the stretch on the prolapsing valve leaflets.
- Antibiotic prophylaxis for infective endocarditis when undergoing dental, GI, or GU procedures is indicated only in patients with MVP who have a systolic murmur and echocardiographic evidence of mitral regurgitation.

CHRONIC Rx

Monitoring for complications:

- Bacterial endocarditis (risk is three to eight times that of the general population)
- TIA or stroke secondary to embolic phenomena (from fibrin and platelet thrombi)
- Cardiac arrhythmias (usually supraventricular)
- Sudden death (rare occurrence, most often caused by ventricular arrhythmias)
- Mitral regurgitation (most common complication of MVP)

DISPOSITION

The incidence of complications of MVP is very low (<1%/yr) and generally associated with an increase in mitral leaflet thickness to ≥5 mm.

REFERRAL

Surgical referral may be necessary in patients who develop symptomatic progressive mitral regurgitation.

PEARLS & CONSIDERATIONS

COMMENTS

- Recent studies suggest that the prevalence of MVP and its propensity to cause symptoms and serious complications have been overestimated in the past.
- Asymptomatic patients with MVP and mild or no mitral regurgitation can be evaluated clinically every 3 to 5 yr. High-risk patients should undergo a follow-up examination once a year.

SUGGESTED READINGS

Bouknight DP, O'Rourke RA: Current management of mitral valve prolapse, *Am Fam Physician* 61:3343, 2000.
Freed LA: Prevalence and clinical outcome of mitral valve prolapse, *N Engl J Med* 341:1, 1999.

AUTHOR: **FRED F. FERRI, M.D.**

BASIC INFORMATION

DEFINITION

Multiple myeloma is a malignancy of plasma cells characterized by overproduction of intact monoclonal immunoglobulin or free monoclonal kappa or lambda chains.

ICD-9CM CODES
203.0 Multiple myeloma

EPIDEMIOLOGY & DEMOGRAPHICS

ANNUAL INCIDENCE: 4 cases/100,000 persons (blacks affected twice as frequently as whites); multiple myeloma accounts for 10% of all hematologic cancers

PREDOMINANT AGE: Peak incidence in the seventh decade at a median age of 69 yr

PHYSICAL FINDINGS & CLINICAL PRESENTATION

The patient usually comes to medical attention because of one or more of the following:

- Bone pain (back, thorax) or pathologic fractures caused by osteolytic lesions
- Fatigue or weakness because of anemia secondary to bone marrow infiltration with plasma cells
- Recurrent infections as a result of impaired neutrophil function and deficiency of normal immunoglobulins
- Nausea and vomiting caused by constipation and uremia
- Delirium secondary to hypercalcemia
- Neurologic complications, such as spinal cord or nerve root compression, blurred vision from hyperviscosity
- Pallor and generalized weakness from anemia
- Purpura, epistaxis from thrombocytopenia
- Evidence of infections from impaired immune system
- Bone pain, weight loss
- Swelling on ribs, vertebrae, and other bones

DIAGNOSIS **Dx**

DIFFERENTIAL DIAGNOSIS

- Metastatic carcinoma
- Lymphoma
- Bone neoplasms (e.g., sarcoma)
- Monoclonal gammopathy of undetermined significance (MGUS)

LABORATORY TESTS

- Normochromic, normocytic anemia; rouleaux formation on peripheral smear
- Hypercalcemia is present in 15% of patients at diagnosis
- Elevated BUN, creatinine, uric acid, and total protein
- Proteinuria secondary to overproduction and secretion of free monoclonal kappa or lambda chains (Bence Jones protein)
- Tall homogeneous monoclonal spike (M spike) on protein immunoelectrophoresis (IEP) in approximately 75% of patients; decreased levels of normal immunoglobulins
  1. The increased immunoglobulins are generally IgG (75%) or IgA (15%).
  2. Approximately 17% of patients have flat level of immunoglobulins but increased light chains in the urine by electrophoresis.
  3. A very small percentage (<2%) of patients have nonsecreting myeloma (no increase in immunoglobulins and no light chains in the urine) but have other evidence of the disease (e.g., positive bone marrow examination).
- Reduced ion gap resulting from the positive charge of the M proteins and the frequent presence of hyponatremia in myeloma patients
- Hyponatremia, serum hyperviscosity (more common with production of IgA)
- Bone marrow examination: usually demonstrates nests or sheets of plasma cells, which comprise >30% of the bone marrow, and ≥10% are immature
- Serum β-2 microglobulin has little diagnostic value; it is useful for prognosis because levels >8 mg/L indicate high tumor mass and aggressive disease
- Elevated serum levels of LDH at the time of diagnosis define a subgroup of myeloma patients with very poor prognosis
- Increased interleukin-6 in serum during active stage of myeloma
- The production of DKK1, an inhibitor of osteoblast differentiation, by myeloma cells is associated with the presence of lytic bone lesions in patients with multiple myeloma.

IMAGING STUDIES

X-ray films of painful areas may demonstrate punched-out lytic lesions or osteoporosis. Bone scans are not useful, because lesions are not blastic.

TREATMENT **Rx**

NONPHARMACOLOGIC THERAPY

Prevention of renal failure with adequate hydration and avoidance of nephrotoxic agents and dye contrast studies

ACUTE GENERAL Rx

- Newly diagnosed patients with good performance status are best treated with autologous stem cell transplantation, resulting in improved survival. Useful guidelines (from the Hematology Disease Site Group of the Cancer Care Ontario Practice Guidelines Initiative) regarding the role of high-dose chemotherapy and stem-cell transplantation are as follows:
  1. Autologous transplantation is recommended for patients with stage II or III myeloma and good performance status.
  2. Allogenic transplantation is not recommended as routine therapy.
  3. Patients potentially eligible for transplantation should be referred for assessment early after diagnosis and should not be extensively exposed to alkylating agents before collection of stem cells.
  4. Autologous peripheral stem cells should be harvested early in the patient's treatment course (best when performed as part of initial therapy).
  5. A single transplant with high-dose melphalan, with or without total body irradiation, is suggested for patients undergoing transplantation outside a clinical trial.
  6. At this time no conclusion can be reached about the role of interferon therapy after transplantation.
- Chemotherapeutic agents effective in multiple myeloma are:
  1. Melphalan and prednisone: the rates of response to this treatment range from 40% to 60%. Adding continuous low-dose interferon to standard melphalan-prednisone therapy does not improve response rate or survival; however, response duration and plateau phase duration are prolonged by maintenance therapy with interferon.
  2. Vincristine, doxorubicin (Adriamycin), and dexamethasone (VAD) can be used in patients not responding or relapsing after treatment with melphalan and prednisone; methylprednisolone is substituted for dexamethasone (VAMP) in some centers.
  3. High-dose chemotherapy (HDCT) with vincristine, melphalan, cyclophosphamide, and prednisone (VMCP) alternating with vincristine, carmustine, doxorubicin, and prednisone (BVAP) combined with bone marrow transplantation improves the response rate, event-free survival, and overall survival in patients with myeloma.

4. Current HDCT regimen with autologous stem-cell support achieve complete response in approximately 20% to 30% of patients, with best results seen in good-risk patients, defined as young patients (<50 yr of age) with good performance status and a low tumor burden (β_2 microglobulin ≤2.5 mg/L).

5. Thalidomide, an agent with antiangiogenic properties, is useful to induce responses in patients with multiple myeloma refractory to chemotherapy.

6. Bortezomib (Velcade) is a newer protease inhibitor that is cytotoxic for multiple myeloma. It is indicated for treatment of refractory multiple myeloma. It is expensive, with an average course of treatment (5 cycles) costing >$20,000.

CHRONIC Rx

- Promptly diagnose and treat infections. Common bacterial agents are *Streptococcus pneumoniae* and *Haemophilus influenzae*. Prophylactic therapy against *Pneumocystis carinii* with trimethoprim sulfamethoxazole must be considered in patients receiving chemotherapy and high-dose corticosteroid regimens.
- Control hypercalcemia and hyperuricemia.
- Control pain with analgesics; radiation therapy and surgical stabilization may also be indicated.
- Treat anemia with epoetin alfa.
- Monthly infusions of the bisphosphonate pamidronate provide significant protection against skeletal complications and improve the quality of life of patients with advanced multiple myeloma. Zoledronic acid (Zometa) can be infused over 15 min and is more effective than pamidronate for treatment of hypercalcemia of malignancy. Bisphosphonates (pamidronate, zoledranate, and ibandronate) also appear to have an antitumor effect.

DISPOSITION

- Prognosis is better in asymptomatic patients with indolent or smoldering myeloma: median survival time is approximately 10 yr in persons with no lytic bone lesions and a serum myeloma protein concentration <3 g/dl.
- As compared with a single autologous stem-cell transplantation, double transplantation (two successive autologus stem-cell transplantations) improves survival among patients with myeloma, especially those who do not have a very good partial response after undergoing one transplantation.

SUGGESTED READINGS

Attal M et al: Single versus double autologous stem-cell transplantation for multiple myeloma, *N Engl J Med* 349:2495, 2003.

Imrie K et al: The role of high dose chemotherapy and stem-cell transplantation in patients with multiple myeloma: a practice guideline of the Cancer Care Ontario Practice Guidelines Initiative, *Ann Intern Med* 136:619, 2002.

Rajkumar SV et al: Current therapy for multiple myeloma, *Mayo Clin Proc* 77:813, 2002.

Tian E et al: The role of WNT-signaling antagonist DKK1 in the development of osteolytic lesions in multiple myeloma, *N Engl J Med* 349:2483, 2003.

AUTHOR: **FRED F. FERRI, M.D.**

BASIC INFORMATION

DEFINITION

Myelodysplastic syndromes (MDS) are a group of acquired clonal disorders affecting the hemopoietic stem cells and characterized by cytopenias with hypercellular bone marrow and various morphologic abnormalities in the hemopoietic cell lines. MDSs show abnormal (dysplastic) hemopoietic maturation. Marrow cellularity is increased, reflecting an effective hematopoiesis, but inadequate maturation results in peripheral cytopenias. Myelodysplasia encompasses several heterogenous syndromes. The French-American-British classification of myelodysplastic syndromes includes the following: refractory anemia, refractory anemia with ringed sideroblasts, refractory anemia with excess blasts, chronic myelomonocytic leukemia, and refractory anemia with excess blasts in transformation.

SYNONYMS

MDS
Preleukemia
Dysmyelopoietic syndrome

ICD-9CM CODES
238.7 Myelodysplastic syndrome

EPIDEMIOLOGY & DEMOGRAPHICS

INCIDENCE (IN U.S.): Approximately 82 cases/100,000 persons/yr
PREDOMINANT AGE: More common in elderly patients, with a median age of >65 yr

PHYSICAL FINDINGS & CLINICAL PRESENTATION

- Splenomegaly, skin pallor, mucosal bleeding, ecchymosis may be present.
- Patients often present with fatigue.
- Fever, infection, and dyspnea are common.

ETIOLOGY

Unknown. However, exposure to radiation, chemotherapeutic agents, benzene, or other organic compounds is associated with myelodysplasia.

DIAGNOSIS

DIFFERENTIAL DIAGNOSIS

- Vitamin B_{12}/folate deficiency
- Exposure to toxins (drugs, alcohol, chemotherapy)
- Renal failure
- Irradiation
- Autoimmune disease
- Infections (TB, viral infections)
- Paroxysmal nocturnal hemoglobinuria

WORKUP

- Diagnostic workup includes laboratory evaluation and bone marrow examination.
- An algorithmic approach to patients with suspected myelodysplastic syndromes is described in Section III.

LABORATORY TESTS

- Anemia with variable MCV (normal or increased)
- Reduced reticulocyte count (in relation to the degree of anemia)
- Hypogranular or agranular neutrophils
- Thrombocytopenia or normal platelet count
- Hypogranular platelets may be present
- Hypercellular bone marrow, with frequent clonal chromosomal abnormalities

IMAGING STUDIES

Abdominal CT scan may reveal hepatosplenomegaly.

TREATMENT

NONPHARMACOLOGIC THERAPY

RBC transfusions in patients with severe symptomatic anemia

ACUTE GENERAL Rx

- Results of chemotherapy are generally disappointing.
- The role of myeloid growth factors (granulocyte colony–stimulating factor, granulocyte-macrophage colony–stimulating factor) and immunotherapy is undefined. In a recent trial, 34% of patients treated with antithymocyte globulin (40 mg/kg for 4 days) became transfusion independent. Response was also associated with a statistically significantly longer survival.
- Allogeneic stem-cell transplantation should be considered in patients <60 yr old because this is the established procedure with cure potential.

CHRONIC Rx

Monitor for infections, bleeding, and complications of anemia.

DISPOSITION

- Cure rates in patients with allogeneic bone marrow transplantations approach 30% to 50%.
- The risk of transformation to acute myelogenous leukemia varies with the percentage of blasts in the bone marrow.
- Advanced age, male sex, and deletion of chromosomes 5 and 7 are associated with a poor prognosis.
- According to the International Myelodysplastic Syndrome Risk Analysis Workshop, the most important variables in disease outcome are the specific cytogenetic abnormalities, the percentage of blasts in the bone marrow, and the number of hematopoietic lineages involved in the cytopenias.

REFERRAL

Hematology referral in all patients with MDS

PEARLS & CONSIDERATIONS

COMMENTS

- Erythropoietin (epoetin alfa) SC three times weekly may be effective in increasing the Hgb and reducing the RBC transfusion requirement in some patients.
- Lenalidomide, a novel analogue of thalidomide, has demonstrated hematologic activity in patients with low-rise myelodysplastic syndrome who have no response to erythropoietin or who are unlikely to benefit from conventional therapy.
- Patients with cytogenetic abnormalities associated with poor prognosis should be considered for aggressive treatment with high-dose chemotherapy and stem-cell transplantation.
- Nearly 50% of the deaths that result from myelodysplastic syndromes are the result of cytopenia associated with bone marrow failure.

SUGGESTED READINGS

List A et al: Efficacy of lenalidomide in myelodysplastic syndromes, *N Engl J Med* 352:549, 2005.

Molldrem JJ et al: Antithymocyte globulin for treatment of the bone marrow failure associated with myelodysplastic syndromes, *Ann Intern Med* 137:156, 2002.

AUTHOR: **FRED F. FERRI, M.D.**

BASIC INFORMATION

DEFINITION

Acute coronary syndromes are manifestations of ischemic heart disease and represent a broad clinical spectrum that includes unstable angina/non-ST elevation MI and ST-elevation MI.

1. **Myocardial infarction** is characterized by necrosis resulting from an insufficient supply of oxygenated blood to an area of the heart. According to the joint European Society of Cardiology/ American College of Cardiology, either one of the following criteria for acute evolving or recent MI satisfies the diagnosis:
   a. Typical rise and gradual fall (troponin) or more rapid rise and fall (CK-MB) of biochemical markers of myocardial necrosis with at least one of the following:
      i. Ischemic symptoms
      ii. Development of pathologic Q waves on ECG
      iii. ECG changes indicative of ischemia (ST-segment elevation or depression)
      iv. Coronary artery intervention (e.g., coronary angioplasty)
   b. Pathologic findings of acute MI
2. **ST elevation MI:** area of ischemic necrosis that penetrates the entire thickness of the ventricular wall and results in ST-segment elevation.
3. **Unstable angina:** coronary arterial plaque rupture with fragmentation and distal arterial embolization resulting in myocardial necrosis. Usually occurs without ST elevation and is thus termed **non-ST elevation MI.**

SYNONYMS

MI
Non-ST elevation MI
ST-elevation MI
Heart attack
Coronary thrombosis
Coronary occlusion

ICD-9CM CODES
410.9 Acute myocardial infarction, unspecified site

EPIDEMIOLOGY & DEMOGRAPHICS

INCIDENCE/PREVALENCE (IN U.S.):
- >500 cases/100,000 persons.
- >500,000 MIs in the U.S. yearly.
- More prominent in males between the ages of 40 and 65 yr; no predominant sex after age 65 yr.
- Women experience more lethal and severe first acute MIs than men, regardless of comorbidity, previous angina, or age.
- At least one fourth of all myocardial infections are clinically unrecognized.

PHYSICAL FINDINGS & CLINICAL PRESENTATION

Clinical presentation:
- Crushing substernal chest pain usually lasts longer than 30 min.
- Pain is unrelieved by rest or sublingual nitroglycerin or is rapidly recurring.
- Pain radiates to the left or right arm, neck, jaw, back, shoulders, or abdomen and is not pleuritic in character.
- Pain may be associated with dyspnea, diaphoresis, nausea, or vomiting.
- There is no pain in approximately 20% of infarctions (usually in diabetic or elderly patients).

Physical findings:
- Skin may be diaphoretic, with pallor (because of decreased oxygen).
- Rales may be present at the bases of lungs (indicative of CHF).
- Cardiac auscultation may reveal an apical systolic murmur caused by mitral regurgitation secondary to papillary muscle dysfunction; S_3 or S_4 may also be present.
- Physical examination may be completely normal

ETIOLOGY

- Coronary atherosclerosis
- Coronary artery spasm
- Coronary embolism (caused by infective endocarditis, rheumatic heart disease, intracavitary thrombus)
- Periarteritis and other coronary artery inflammatory diseases
- Dissection into coronary arteries (aneurysmal or iatrogenic)
- Congenital abnormalities of coronary circulation
- Hypercoagulable states, increased blood viscosity (polycythemia vera)

DIAGNOSIS

DIFFERENTIAL DIAGNOSIS

The various causes of myocardial ischemia are described in Section II along with the differential diagnosis of chest pain.

LABORATORY TESTS

- Cardiac troponin levels: cardiac-specific troponin T (cTnT) and cardiac-specific troponin I (cTnI) are highly specific for myocardial injury. Increases in serum levels of cTnT and cTnI may occur relatively early after muscle damage (3-12 hr), peak within 24 hr, and may be present for several days after MI (up to 7 days for cTnI and up to 10-14 days for cTnT). Troponin T tests can be falsely positive in patients with renal failure. The threshold level of troponin T considered positive for MI is 0.1 ng/ml in patients with normal renal function or 0.5 ng/ml in patients with renal impairment.

- Creatine kinase MB isoenzyme is a useful marker for MI. It is released in the circulation in amounts that correlate with the size of the infarct.
- Neither CK-MB nor troponin consistently appears in the blood within 6 hr after an ischemic event; therefore serial testing (e.g., on presentation and after 8 hr) is necessary to definitely rule out MI.
- ECG:
1. In ST-elevation MI, there is development of:
   a. Inverted T waves, indicating an area of ischemia
   b. Elevated ST segment, indicating an area of injury
   c. Q waves, indicating an area of infarction (usually develop over 12 to 36 hr)
2. In unstable angina/non-ST elevation MI, Q waves are absent, but the following indications are present:
   a. History and myocardial enzyme elevations are compatible with MI.
   b. ECG shows ST segment elevation, depression, or no change followed by T wave inversion.

IMAGING STUDIES

- Chest radiography is useful to evaluate for pulmonary congestion and exclude other causes of chest pain.
- Echocardiography can evaluate wall motion abnormalities and identify mural thrombus or mitral regurgitation, which can occur acutely after MI.

TREATMENT **Rx**

NONPHARMACOLOGIC THERAPY

- Limit patient's activity: bed rest for the initial 24 hr; if the patient remains stable, gradually increase activity.
- Diet: NPO until stable, then no added salt and a low-cholesterol diet.
- Patient education to decrease the risk of subsequent cardiac events (proper diet, cessation of smoking, regular exercise) should be initiated when the patient is medically stable.

ACUTE GENERAL Rx

- Any patient with suspected acute MI should immediately receive the following:
1. Aspirin: give 160 to 325 mg PO unless true aspirin allergy is suspected. If the first dose is chewed, a blood level is achieved more rapidly than if it is swallowed. Clopidogrel may be substituted if true allergy is present.
2. Nitrates: they increase the supply of oxygen by reducing coronary vasospasm and decrease consumption of oxygen by reducing

ventricular preload. Sublingual nitroglycerin can be administered immediately on suspicion of MI (unless systolic blood pressure is <90 mm Hg or heart rate is <50 bpm or >100 bpm); IV nitroglycerin can be subsequently used. Nitroglycerin should be used with great caution in patients with inferior wall MI; nitrate usage can result in hypotension because these patients are sensitive to change in preload. It should also be avoided in patients suspected of having right ventricular infarction (increased risk of preload reduction) and if a patient has used sildenafil (Viagra), or vardenafil (Levitra) within the previous 24 hr or tadalafil (Cialis) in the previous 36 to 48 hr.

3. Adequate analgesia: morphine sulfate 2 mg IV q5min PRN can be given for severe pain unrelieved by nitroglycerin. Hypotension secondary to morphine can be treated with careful IV hydration with saline solution. If sinus bradycardia accompanies hypotension, use atropine (0.5 to 1.0 mg IV q 5 min PRN to a total dose of 2.5 mg). Respiratory depression caused by morphine can be reversed with naloxone (Narcan) 0.8 mg.

4. Nasal oxygen: administer at 2 to 4 L/min.

- If readily available without delay, percutaneous coronary intervention (PCI) with adjunctive glycoprotein IIb/IIIa is preferred over thrombolytic therapy. It is effective and generally results in more favorable outcomes than thrombolytic therapy. When PCI is performed, use of IV heparin is recommended. Coronary stents are useful to decrease ischemia, improve long-term patency, and lower the rate of restenosis of the infarct-related artery.

- Thrombolytic therapy: if the duration of pain has been <6 hr and primary angioplasty is not readily available, recanalization of the occluded arteries should be attempted with thrombolytic agents, possibly in combination with glycoprotein IIb/IIIa inhibition. Because the effectiveness of thrombolytics is time-dependent, ideally these agents should be administered either in the field or within 30 min of the patient's arrival in the emergency department. When tPA or rPA is used, IV heparin is given to increase the likelihood of patency in the infarct-related artery. In patients receiving streptokinase or APSAC, IV heparin is not indicated, because it does not offer any additional benefit and can result in increased bleeding complications. Tenecteplase and reteplase are comparable with accelerated infusion recombinant TPA in terms of efficacy and safety, but are more convenient because they are administered by bolus injection. Lanoplase and heparin bolus plus infusion is as effective as TPA with regard to mortality, but the rate of intracranial hemorrhage is significantly higher. Absolute contraindications to thrombolytic therapy include active internal bleeding, intracranial neoplasm or arteriovenous malformation, intracranial surgery in past 6 mo, stroke in past year, head trauma with loss of consciousness in past 6 mo, surgery in noncompressible location in past 6 wk, alteration in mental status, and infectious endocarditis.

- β-adrenergic blocking agents should be given to all patients with evolving acute MI, provided that there are no contraindications (see below). β-Blockers are useful to reduce myocardial oxygen consumption and prevent tachyarrhythmias. Early IV β-blockage (in the initial 24 hr) followed by institution of an oral maintenance regimen is also effective in reducing recurrent infarction and ischemia. Frequently used agents are:

1. Metoprolol (Lopressor): IV 5 mg q2min × 3 doses, then PO 25 to 50 mg q6h, given 15 min after last IV dose, continued for 48 hr; maintenance dosage is 50 to 100 mg bid.

2. Atenolol (Tenormin): IV 5 mg over 5 min, repeat in 10 min if initial dose is well tolerated, then start PO dose 10 min after the last IV dose; PO 50 mg qd, increasing to 100 mg as tolerated.

Before using β-blockers, some of the contraindications and side effects (i.e., exacerbation of asthma, CNS effects, hypertension, bradycardia) must be carefully assessed.

- ACE inhibitors reduce left ventricular dysfunction and dilation and slow the progression of CHF during and after acute MI. They should be initiated within hours of hospitalization, provided that the patient does not have hypotension or a contraindication (bilateral renal stenosis, renal failure, or history of angioedema caused by previous treatment with ACE inhibitors).

1. Commonly used agents are captopril 12.5 mg PO bid, enalapril 2.5 mg bid, or lisinopril 2.5 to 5 mg qd initially, with subsequent titration as needed.

2. ACE inhibitors may be stopped in patients without complications and no evidence of left ventricular dysfunction after 6 to 8 wk.

3. ACE inhibitors should be continued indefinitely in patients with impaired left ventricular function (ejection fraction <40%) or clinical CHF.

- Glycoprotein IIb receptor inhibitors (tirofiban, eptifibatide), when administered with heparin and aspirin, further reduce the incidence of ischemic events in patients with non-Q wave MI. The use of IV glycoprotein IIb/IIIa inhibitors (e.g., abciximab) before and during PTCA also reduces the risk of closure postangioplasty.

- Initiation of statin therapy before hospital discharge.

CHRONIC Rx

Discharge medications in all patients with MI/NSTEMI (unless contraindicated) should include antiischemic medications (e.g., nitroglycerin, β-blocker), lipid-lowering agents, and aspirin (81-325 mg/day). Clopidogrel (Plavix) 75 mg/day can be given in addition to aspirin for up to nine months or in place of aspirin in those who cannot tolerate aspirin. The addition of ACE inhibitors is also recommended in all patients with diabetes, CHF, and in those with EF <40%.

Evaluation of post-MI patients

- Submaximal (low level) treadmill test (can be done 1 to 3 wk after MI) in stable patients without any clinical evidence of significant left ventricular dysfunction or post-MI angina

1. Useful to assess the patient's functional capacity and formulate an at-home exercise program

2. Helpful to determine the patient's prognosis

- Radionuclide angiography or two-dimensional echocardiography

1. To evaluate patient's left ventricular ejection fraction

2. To evaluate ventricular size and segmental wall motion

3. Echocardiography to rule out presence of mural thrombi in patients with anterior wall infarction; transesophageal echo is preferred if mural thrombosis is suspected

- A 24-hr Holter monitor study to evaluate patients who have demonstrated significant arrhythmias during their hospital stay; selected patients with complex ventricular ectopy may be candidates for programmed electrical stimulation studies and antiarrhythmic therapy and/or implanted defibrillator, depending on the results of these studies

DISPOSITION

The prognosis after MI depends on multiple factors:

- Use of β-blockers: the mortality of patients on a regular regimen of β-blockers is significantly decreased when compared with that of control groups. Discharge medication in patients with MI/NSTEMI should include a β-blocker in all patients without contraindications.

- Presence of arrhythmias, frequent ventricular ectopy (≥10/hr), or repetitive forms of ventricular ectopic beats (couplets, triplets) indicates an increased risk (two to three times greater) of sudden cardiac death. New bundle branch block, Mobitz II second-degree block, and third-degree heart block also adversely affect outcome.

- Size of infarct: the larger it is, the higher the post-MI mortality rate. Significant myocardial stunning with subsequent improvement of ventricular function occurs in most patients after anterior MI. A lower level of creatine kinase, an estimate of the extent of necrosis, is independently predictive of recovery of function.
- Site of infarct: inferior wall MI carries a better prognosis than anterior wall MI; however, patients with inferior wall MI and right ventricular involvement have a high risk for arrhythmic complications and cardiac shock.
- Ejection fraction after MI: the lower the left ventricular ejection fraction, the higher the mortality after MI.
- Presence of post-MI angina indicates a high mortality rate.
- Performance on low-level exercise test: the presence of ST segment changes during the test is a predictor of high mortality during the first year.
- Presence of pericarditis during the acute phase of MI increases mortality at 1 yr.
- Type A behavior (competitive drive, ambitiousness, hostility) is associated with a lower mortality rate after symptomatic MI.
- The Killip classification is an independent predictor of all-cause mortality in patients with non-ST elevation acute coronary syndromes.

- Self-reported moderate alcohol consumption in the year before acute MI is associated with reduced 1-yr mortality.
- Discharge medication in patients with MI/NSTEMI should include lipid-lowering agents in patients with hyperlipidemia unresponsive to exercise and dietary restrictions. Statins may also lower vascular inflammation and damage by mechanisms other than reduction of LDL cholesterol. Early initiation of statin treatment in patients with acute MI is associated with reduced 1-yr mortality.
- Additional poor prognostic factors include the following: cigarette smoking, history of hypertension or prior MI, presence of ST segment depression in acute MI, increasing age, diabetes mellitus, and female sex.

SUGGESTED READINGS

Andersen HR et al: A comparison of coronary angioplasty with fibrinolytic therapy in acute myocardial infarction, *N Engl J Med* 349:733, 2003.

Becker RC: Antithrombotic therapy after myocardial infarction, *N Engl J Med* 347:1019, 2002.

Birnbaum Y et al: Ventricular septal rupture after acute myocardial infarction, *N Engl J Med* 347:1426, 2002.

Brennan ML et al: Prognostic value of myeloperoxidase in patients with chest pain. N Engl J Med 349:1595, 2003.

Cannon CP, Baim DS: Expanding the reach of primary percutaneous coronary intervention for the treatment of acute myocardial infarction, *J Am Coll Cardiol* 39:1720, 2002.

Cannon CP et al: Intensive versus moderate lipid lowering with statins after acute coronary syndromes, *N Engl J Med* 350:1495, 2004.

Dickstein K et al: Effects of losartan and captopril on mortality and morbidity in high-risk patients after acute myocardial infarction: the OPTIMAAL randomized trial, *Lancet* 360:752, 2002.

Hurlen et al: Warfarin, aspirin, or both after myocardial infarction, *N Engl J Med* 347:969, 2002.

Khot UN et al: Prognostic importance of physical examination for heart failure in Non-ST elevation acute coronary syndromes, *JAMA* 290:2174, 2003.

Meier MA et al: The new definition of myocardial infarction, *Arch Intern Med* 162:1585, 2002.

Moss AJ et al: Prophylactic implantation of a defibrillator in patients with myocardial infarction and reduced ejection fraction, *N Engl J Med* 346:877, 2002.

Newby LK et al: Early statin initiation and outcomes in patients with acute coronary syndromes, *JAMA* 287:3087, 2002.

Stenestrand U, Wallentin L: Early revascularisation and 1-year survival in 14-day survivors of acute myocardial infarction: a prospective cohort study, *Lancet* 359:1805, 2002.

Stone GW et al: Comparison of angioplasty with stenting, with or without abciximab, in acute myocardial infarction, *N Engl J Med* 346:957, 2002.

Wiviott SD, Braunwauld E: Unstable Angina and Non-ST-Segment Elevation Myocardial Infarction, *Am Fam Physician* 70:525, 2004.

Zimetbaum PJ, Josephson ME: Use of electrocardiogram in acute myocardial infarction, *N Engl J Med* 348:933, 2003.

AUTHOR: **FRED F. FERRI, M.D.**

BASIC INFORMATION

DEFINITION

Liver disease occurring in patients who do not abuse alcohol and manifested histologically by mononuclear cells and/or polymorphonuclear cells, hepatocyte ballooning, and spotty necrosis.

SYNONYMS

- Nonalcoholic steatohepatitis (NASH)
- Fatty liver hepatitis
- Diabetes hepatitis

ICD-9CM CODES
571.8 Fatty liver

EPIDEMIOLOGY & DEMOGRAPHICS

- Nonalcoholic fatty liver disease affects 10% to 24% of general population
- Increased prevalence in obese persons (57% to 74%), type 2 diabetes mellitus, and hyperlipidemia (primarily hypertriglyceridemia)
- Most common cause of abnormal liver test results in adults in the U.S. (accounts for up to 90% of cases of asymptomatic ALT elevations)
- 30 million obese adults have steatosis, 8.6 million may have steatohepatitis

PHYSICAL FINDINGS & CLINICAL PRESENTATION

- Most patients are asymptomatic
- Patients may report a sensation of fullness or discomfort on the right side of the upper abdomen
- Nonspecific complaints of fatigue or malaise may be reported
- Hepatomegaly is generally the only positive finding on physical examination

ETIOLOGY

- Insulin resistance is the most reproducible factor in the development of nonalcoholic fatty liver disease
- Risk factors are obesity (especially truncal obesity), diabetes mellitus, hyperlipidemia

DIAGNOSIS

DIFFERENTIAL DIAGNOSIS

- Alcohol-induced liver disease (a daily alcohol intake of 20 g in females and 30 g in males [three 12-oz beers or 12 oz of wine] may be enough to cause alcohol-induced liver disease)
- Viral hepatitis
- Autoimmune hepatitis
- Toxin or drug-induced liver disease

WORKUP

Diagnosis is usually suspected on the basis of hepatomegaly, asymptomatic elevations of transaminases, or "fatty liver" on sonogram of abdomen in obese patients with little or no alcohol use. Liver biopsy will confirm diagnosis and provide prognostic information. It should be considered in patients with suspected advanced liver fibrosis (presence of obesity or type 2 diabetes, AST/ALT ratio 1).

LABORATORY TESTS

- Elevated ALT, AST: AST/ALT ratio is usually <1, but can increase as fibrosis advances
- Negative serology for infectious hepatitis; generally normal GGTP, and serum alkaline phosphatase
- Hyperlipidemia (primarily hypertriglyceridemia) may be present
- Elevated glucose levels may be present
- Prolonged prothrombin time, hypoalbuminuria, and elevated bilirubin may be present in advanced stages
- Elevated serum ferritin and increased transferrin saturation may be found in up to 10% of patients; however, hepatic iron index and hepatic iron level are normal
- Liver biopsy may show a wide spectrum of liver damage, ranging from simple steatosis to advanced fibrosis and cirrhosis

IMAGING STUDIES

- Ultrasound generally reveals diffuse increase in echogenicity as compared with that of the kidneys; CT scan reveals diffuse low-density hepatic parenchyma.

- Occasionally patients may have focal rather than diffuse steatosis, which may be misinterpreted as a liver mass on ultrasound or CT; use of MRI in these cases will identify focal fatty infiltration.

TREATMENT

NONPHARMACOLOGIC THERAPY

Weight reduction in all obese patients. Exercise is also effective.

GENERAL THERAPY

- No medications have been proved to directly improve liver damage from nonalcoholic fatty liver disease.
- Medications to control hyperlipidemia (e.g., fenofibrates for elevated triglycerides) and hyperglycemia (e.g., metformin) can lead to improvement in abnormal liver test results. Metformin, pioglitazone, and rosiglitazone may be effective but are not yet FDA-aproved for this purpose.

DISPOSITION

- Patients with pure steatosis on liver biopsy generally have a relatively benign course.
- The presence of steatohepatitis or advanced fibrosis on liver biopsy is associated with a worse prognosis.

REFERRAL

Liver transplantation should be considered in patients with decompensated, end-stage disease; however, in these patients there may be a recurrence of nonalcoholic fatty liver disease posttransplantation.

SUGGESTED READINGS

Angulo P: Nonalcoholic fatty liver disease, *N Engl J Med* 346:1221, 2002.

Clark JM: Nonalcoholic fatty liver disease, *JAMA* 289:3000, 2003.

Dixon JB et al: Nonalcoholic fatty liver disease: predictors of nonalcoholic steatohepatitis and liver fibrosis in the severely obese, *Gastroenterology* 121:91, 2001.

AUTHOR: FRED F. FERRI, M.D.

BASIC INFORMATION

DEFINITION

Obesity refers to excess body fat defined as a body mass index (BMI) $\geq$30 kg/m^2. Overweight is defined as BMI of 25 to 29.9 kg/m^2. These conditions result from a problem of imbalance between energy intake and expenditure.

SYNONYMS

Overweight

ICD-9CM CODES
278.0 Obesity

EPIDEMIOLOGY & DEMOGRAPHICS

- Approximately 97 million adults in the U.S. and 310 million people worldwide are overweight or obese.
- The present costs of obesity in the U.S. population are estimated to run at 5%-8% of total healthcare spending, which equates to $92.6-$99.2 billion annually (1998 data normalized to 2002 dollars).
- From 1960 to 1999, the prevalence of excess weight (BMI $\geq$25 kg/m^2) increased from 44% to 61% of the adult population, and the prevalence of obesity (BMI $\geq$30 kg/m^2) doubled, from 13% to 27%. Estimates in 2003 suggest that 31% of the U.S. population is now obese.
- In the U.S., the progression of obesity is 3-4 yr ahead of the problem in Europe.
- Overweight and obesity are defined as stated previously on the basis of epidemiologic data showing increased mortality with BMIs above 25 kg/m^2.
- For persons with a BMI of $\geq$30 kg/m^2, all-cause mortality is increased by 50% to 100% above that of persons with BMIs in the range of 20 to 25 kg/m^2.
- Obese individuals are at increased risk of morbidity/mortality from type 2 diabetes, hypertension, CVD, cancer (particularly breast cancer), sleep apnea, osteoarthritis, and skin disorders.
- The effects of obesity on health outcome appear to be reversible with weight loss.
- Obesity is more prevalent in black and Hispanic women compared with non-Hispanic white women and men. Approximately 50% of the black female population is estimated to be obese.
- People in the U.S. with low incomes or low education are 5% more likely to be obese than those of higher socioeconomic status.
- In 1993 the Deputy Assistant Secretary for Health (J. Michael McGinnis) and the former Director of the Centers for Disease Control and Prevention (CDC) (William Foege) coauthored a journal article, "Actual Causes of Death in the U.S." It concluded that a combination of dietary factors and sedentary activity patterns accounts for at least 300,000 deaths each year, and obesity is the second leading cause of preventable death in the United States.

PHYSICAL FINDINGS & CLINICAL PRESENTATION

- Obesity is self-evident on examination.
- Measuring the height in meters and weight in kilograms determines your BMI.
- Increased waist circumference (>40 inches in men and >35 inches in women) is apparent.
- Hypertension is related to obesity.
- Symptoms of diabetes (e.g., polyuria, polydipsia, retinopathy, and neuropathy) may be present.
- Joint pain and swelling are associated with osteoarthritis and obesity.
- Dyspnea may be present.

ETIOLOGY

- The cause of obesity is multifactorial, involving social, cultural, behavioral, physiologic, metabolic, and genetic factors.
- Supporting genetic factors come from identical twins reared apart and "obesity genes" encoding for the appetite-suppressant hormone leptin.
- Environmental factors are a major determinant of obesity with the underlying theme of excess calorie intake and lack of physical activity.
- Genetics and environmental factors exert their effects on energy balance and obesity via effects on behavior and physiology. There is no direct link between genetics and body weight or obesity. Obesity develops as a result of excessive energy intake, inadequate energy expenditure, or both.
- Over the last 2 decades, fat consumption has declined in parallel with the increased prevalence of obesity in both the U.S. and Europe, and the decline is matched by a parallel increase in carbohydrate consumption, suggesting a role for excessive dietary carbohydrate in the development of obesity.

DIAGNOSIS

- Determination of the BMI establishes the diagnosis of obesity according to the previous definition and assesses the individual's risk for disease.
- BMI is defined as the weight in kilograms divided by the square of the height in meters (W$\div$H^2).
- Strict BMI measurements should be used with caution in making a diagnosis of obesity.

DIFFERENTIAL DIAGNOSIS

It is important to rule out specific causative medical disorders in obese patients. Hypothalamic disorders, hypothyroidism, Cushing's syndrome, insulinoma, and chronic corticosteroid use can cause obesity.

WORKUP

The workup of an obese patient typically requires laboratory work to assess for risks and complications as well as to rule out underlying causative medical conditions.

LABORATORY TESTS

- Laboratory tests are not specific in diagnosing obesity; however, they are used to identify diabetes and hyperlipidemia commonly related to excess weight.
- In the proper clinical setting, thyroid function studies (TSH, free T$_4$), AM cortisol level, and insulin level with C-peptide measurements will exclude hypothyroidism, Cushing's syndrome, and insulinoma as underlying causes of obesity.

IMAGING STUDIES

- X-ray imaging studies are not specific in the diagnosis of obesity.
- Several methods are available for determining or calculating total body fat but offer no significant advantage over the BMI.
  1. Total body water
  2. Total body potassium
  3. Bioelectrical impedance
  4. Dual-energy x-ray absorptiometry
- Buoyancy testing is the most accurate method for determining total body fat composition.

TREATMENT

- Treatment is aimed at weight reduction and risk factor modification (e.g., diabetes, lipids, hypertension).
- Once a joint decision between patient and clinician has been made to lose weight, the expert panel recommends as an initial goal the loss of 10% of baseline weight, to be lost at a rate of 1 to 2 lb/wk over a 6- to 12-mo period followed by long-term maintenance of reduced weight.

NONPHARMACOLOGIC THERAPY

- The three major components of weight loss therapy are:
  1. Many studies demonstrate that obese adults can lose about 0.5 kg per wk by decreasing their daily intake to 500 to 1000 kcal below the caloric intake required for the maintenance of their current weight.

2. Increased physical activity initially by walking 30 min 3 times/wk and gradually build up to intense walking 45 min 5 days/wk. The eventual goal is at least 30 min of moderate intense walking.

3. Behavioral therapy is also necessary.

ACUTE GENERAL Rx

- Medications for the treatment of obesity are currently approved as an adjunct to diet and physical activity for patients with a BMI of ≥30 with no concomitant obesity-related risk factors or diseases, and for patients with a BMI ≥27 with concomitant obesity-related risk factors or diseases.
- Medications approved for the treatment of obesity include
  1. Sibutramine 5-15 mg/day
  2. Orlistat 120 mg 3 times/day with or within 1 hour after fat-containing meals, plus a daily vitamin.
- Only sibutramine and orlistat are approved for long-term use. The safety and efficacy of weight loss medications beyond 2 yr of use have not been established, nor have they been established for the geriatric population.
- Medications are divided into appetite suppressants (e.g., sibutramine) and those that decrease nutrient absorption (e.g., orlistat).
- Side effects of sibutramine include increases in blood pressure and pulse, dry mouth, headache, insomnia, and constipation. Side effects of orlistat include oily spotting, flatus with discharge, and fecal urgency.
- Other medications in clinical trials include bupropion (Wellbutrin), topiramate (Topamax), and metformin (Glucophage).

CHRONIC Rx

- Bariatric surgery is a consideration in clinically severe obesity (e.g., BMI ≥ 40 or ≥ 35 with comorbid conditions).
- Gastroplasty, gastric banding, gastric partitioning, and gastric bypass are the surgical procedures performed.

DISPOSITION

- Obesity increases the risk of developing hypertension, hyperlipidemia, type 2 diabetes, coronary artery disease, cerebrovascular disease, osteoarthritis, sleep apnea, and endometrial, breast, prostate, and colon cancers.
- All-cause mortality is increased in obese patients.

REFERRAL

Obesity is commonly seen in the primary care setting. If pharmacologic therapy is considered, consultation with physicians specializing in obesity and experienced with the use of the drug is recommended. In addition, consultation with nutritionists and behavioral therapists is helpful. A consultation with general surgery is indicated in patients being considered for surgical intervention.

PEARLS & CONSIDERATIONS

COMMENTS

- The National Heart, Lung, and Blood Institute's (NHLBI) Obesity Education Initiative in cooperation with the National Institute of Diabetes convened the Expert Panel on the Identification, Evaluation, and Treatment of Overweight and Obesity in Adults in May 1995 and have since published evidence-based clinical guidelines for treatment of obesity.

- Only about 20% of adult men and women actually restrict caloric intake and increase physical activity to consciously control body weight.
- As knowledge of the physiologic process governing maintenance of body weight increases, newer drug therapies are emerging, which will target lipid metabolic enzymes involved in digestion, absorption, synthesis, storage, and mobilization of fat within the human body

SUGGESTED READINGS

Blanck HM et al: Use of non-prescription weight loss products: results from a multistate survey, *JAMA* 286:930, 2001.

Clinical Guidelines on the Identification, Evaluation, and Treatment of Overweight and Obesity in Adults. The Evidence Report. National Institute of Health, National Heart, Lung, and Blood Institute. *www.nhlbi.nih.gov/guidelines/obesity/ob_gdlns.pdf*

Executive Summary of the Clinical Guidelines on the Identification, Evaluation, and Treatment of Overweight and Obesity in Adults, *Arch Intern Med* 158(17):1855, 1867, 1998.

Korner J, Aronne LJ: Pharmacological approaches to weight reduction: Therapeutic targets, *J Clin End Metab* 89(6)2616, 2004.

Lyznicki JM et al: Obesity: assessment and management in primary care, *Am Fam Physician* 63:2185, 2001.

McTigue KM et al: Screening and interventions for obesity in adults: summary of the evidence for the U.S. Preventive Services Task Force, *Ann Intern Med* 139:933, 2003.

Speakman JR: Obesity: the integrated roles of environment and genetics, *J Nutr* 134:2090S, 2004.

Weil E et al: Obesity among adults with disabling conditions, *JAMA* 288:1265, 2002.

Wilson PW et al: Overweight and obesity as determinants of cardiovascular risk, *Arch Intern Med* 162:1867, 2002.

Yanovski SZ, Yanovski JA: Obesity: drug therapy, *N Engl J Med* 346(8):591, 2002.

AUTHORS: **JASON IANNUCCILLI, M.D.,** and **PETER PETROPOULOS, M.D.**

BASIC INFORMATION

DEFINITION

Onychomycosis is defined as a persistent fungal infection affecting the toenails and fingernails.

SYNONYMS

Tinea unguium
Ringworm of the nails

ICD-9CM CODES
110.1 Onychomycosis

EPIDEMIOLOGY & DEMOGRAPHICS

- Onychomycosis is most commonly found in people above age 40.
- Onychomycosis rarely occurs before puberty.
- Incidence: 20 to 100 cases/1000 population.
- Toenail infection is four to six times more common than fingernail infections.
- Onychomycosis affects men more often than women.
- Occurs more frequently in patients with diabetes, peripheral vascular disease, and any conditions resulting in the suppression of the immune system.
- Occlusive footwear, physical exercise followed by communal showering, and incompletely drying the feet predisposes the individual to developing onychomycosis.

PHYSICAL FINDINGS & CLINICAL PRESENTATION

- Onychomycosis causes nails to become thick, brittle, hard, distorted, and discolored (yellow to brown color). Eventually, the nail may loosen, separate from the nail bed, and fall off (Fig. 1-24).

- Onychomycosis is frequently associated with tinea pedis (athlete's foot).

ETIOLOGY

- The most common causes of onychomycosis are dermatophyte, yeast, and nondermatophyte molds.
- The dermatophyte *Trichophyton rubrum* accounts for 80% of all nail infections caused by fungus.
- *Trichophyton interdigitale* and *Trichophyton mentagrophytes* are other fungi causing onychomycosis.
- The yeast *Candida albicans* is responsible for 5% of the cases of onychomycosis.
- Nondermatophyte molds *Scopulariopsis brevicaulis* and *Aspergillus niger,* although rare, can also cause onychomycosis.
- Onychomycosis is classified according to the clinical pattern of nail bed involvement. The main types are:
  1. Distal and lateral subungual onychomycosis (DLSO)
  2. Superficial onychomycosis
  3. Proximal subungual onychomycosis
  4. Endonyx onychomycosis
  5. Total dystrophic onychomycosis

DIAGNOSIS

The diagnosis of onychomycosis is based on the clinical nail findings and confirmed by direct microscopy and culture.

DIFFERENTIAL DIAGNOSIS

- Psoriasis
- Contact dermatitis
- Lichen planus
- Subungual keratosis
- Paronychia
- Infection (e.g., *Pseudomonas*)
- Trauma
- Peripheral vascular disease
- Yellow nail syndrome

WORKUP

The workup of suspected onychomycosis is directed at confirming the diagnosis of onychomycosis by visualizing hyphae under the microscope or by growing the organism in culture.

LABORATORY TESTS

- Blood tests are not specific in the diagnosis of onychomycosis
- KOH prep
- Fungal cultures on Sabouraud medium

IMAGING STUDIES

- Imaging studies are not very specific in making the diagnosis of onychomycosis.
- If an infection is present and osteomyelitis is a consideration, an x-ray of the specific area and a bone scan may help establish the diagnosis.

TREATMENT Rx

NONPHARMACOLOGIC THERAPY

- Surgical removal of the nail plate is a treatment option; however, the relapse rate is high.
- Prevention of reinfection by wearing properly fitted shoes, avoiding public showers, and keeping feet and nails clean and dry.

ACUTE GENERAL Rx

- Topical antifungal creams are used for early superficial nail infections.
  1. Miconazole 2% cream applied over the nail plate bid
  2. Clotrimazole 1% cream bid
- Oral agents
  1. *Itraconazole*
     a. For toenails: 200 mg qd × 3 mo
     b. For fingernails: 200 mg PO bid × 7 days, followed by 3 wk of no medicine, for two pulses

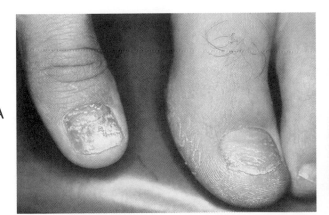
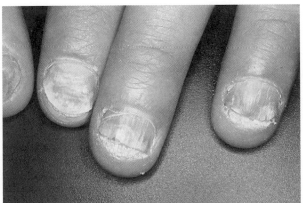

FIGURE 1-24 **A,** Superficial white onychomycosis. **B,** Distal subungual onychomycosis. (From Noble J [ed]: *Textbook of primary care medicine,* ed 3, St Louis, 2002, Mosby.)

2. *Terbinafine*
   a. For toenails: 250 mg/day for 3 mo
   b. For fingernails: 250 mg/day for 6 wk
3. *Fluconazole*
   a. For toenails: 150 to 300 mg once weekly, until infection clears
   b. For fingernails: 150 to 300 mg once weekly until infection clears

- All oral agents used for onychomycosis require periodic monitoring of liver function blood tests.
- Itraconazole is contraindicated in patients taking cisapride, astemizole, triazolam, midazolam, and terfenadine. Statins should be discontinued during itraconazole therapy.
- Fluconazole is contraindicated in patients taking cisapride and terfenadine.
- Ciclopirox, a topical nail lacquer antifungal agent, is FDA approved for treatment of mild to moderate disease not involving the lunula.

CHRONIC Rx

See under "Acute General Rx."

DISPOSITION

- Spontaneous remission of onychomycosis is rare.
- A disease-free toenail is reported to occur in approximately 25% to 50% of patients treated with the oral antifungal agents mentioned previously.

REFERRAL

- Podiatry consultation is indicated in diabetic patients for proper instruction in foot care, footwear, and nail debridement or surgical removal of the toenail.
- Dermatology consultation is indicated in patients refractory to treatment or if another diagnosis is considered (e.g., psoriasis).

PEARLS & CONSIDERATIONS

COMMENTS

- The growth of fungus on an infected nail typically begins at the end of the nail and spreads under the nail plate to infect the nail bed as well.

- Please review informational insert regarding drug-drug interactions and contraindications before initiating oral antifungal agents.

SUGGESTED READINGS

Elewski BE, Hay RJ: Update on the management of onychomycosis: highlights of the Third International Summit on Cutaneous Antifungal Therapy, *Clin Infect Dis* 23:305, 1996.

Epstein E: How often does oral treatment of toenail onychomycosis produce a disease-free nail? an analysis of published data, *Arch Dermatol* 134(12):1551, 1998.

Gupta AK: The new oral antifungal agents for onychomycosis of the toenails, *J Eur Acad Dermatol Venereol* 13(1):1, 1999.

Rodgers P, Bassler M: Treating onychomycosis, *Am Fam Physician* 63:663, 2001.

Scher RK, Coppa LM: Advances in the diagnosis and treatment of onychomycosis, *Hosp Med* 34(4):11, 1998.

AUTHOR: **DENNIS MIKOLICH, M.D.**

BASIC INFORMATION

DEFINITION

Osteoarthritis is a joint condition in which degeneration and loss of articular cartilage occur, leading to pain and deformity. Two forms are usually recognized: primary (idiopathic) and secondary. The primary form may be localized or generalized.

SYNONYMS

Degenerative joint disease
Osteoarthrosis
Arthrosis

ICD-9CM CODES
715.0 Osteoarthrosis and allied disorders

EPIDEMIOLOGY & DEMOGRAPHICS

PREVALENCE: 2% to 6% of general population
PREDOMINANT SEX: Female = male
PREDOMINANT AGE: >50 yr

PHYSICAL FINDINGS & CLINICAL PRESENTATION

- Similar symptoms in most forms: stiffness, pain, and crepitus
- Joint tenderness, swelling
- Decreased range of motion
- Crepitus with motion
- Bony hypertrophy
- Pain with range of motion
- DIP joint involvement possibly leading to development of nodular swellings called Heberden's nodes (Fig. 1-25)
- PIP joint involvement possibly leading to development of nodular swellings called Bouchard's nodes

ETIOLOGY

Primary osteoarthritis is of unknown cause. Secondary osteoarthritis may result from a number of disorders including trauma, metabolic conditions, and other forms of arthritis.

DIAGNOSIS

DIFFERENTIAL DIAGNOSIS

- Bursitis, tendinitis
- Radicular spine pain
- Inflammatory arthritides
- Infectious arthritis

WORKUP

- No diagnostic test exists for degenerative joint disease.
- Laboratory evaluation is normal.
- Rheumatoid factor, ESR, CBC, and ANA tests may be required if inflammatory component is present.
- Synovial fluid examination is generally normal.

IMAGING STUDIES

- Roentgenographic evaluation reveals:
  1. Joint space narrowing
  2. Subchondral sclerosis
  3. New bone formation in the form of osteophytes
- When knee is involved, standing AP x-ray

TREATMENT

ACUTE GENERAL Rx

- Rest, restricted use or weight bearing, and heat
- Walking aids such as a cane (often helpful for weight-bearing joints)
- Suitable footwear
- Gentle range of motion and strengthening exercise
- Local creams and liniments to provide a counterirritant effect
- Education, reassurance

PHARMACOLOGIC THERAPY

- Mild analgesics for joint pain
- NSAIDs if inflammation is present
- Occasional local corticosteroid injections
- Viscosupplementation (injection of hyaluronic acid products into the degenerative joint) is of uncertain benefit
- Nutritional supplements (glucosamine and chondroitin) are unproven

DISPOSITION

Progression is not always inevitable, and the prognosis is variable depending on the site and extent of the disease.

REFERRAL

Surgical consultation for patients not responding to medical management

PEARLS & CONSIDERATIONS

COMMENTS

Surgical intervention is generally helpful in degenerative joint disease. Arthroplasty, arthrodesis, and realignment osteotomy are the most common procedures performed. Arthroscopic debridement (of the knee) appears to be of only limited value.

SUGGESTED READINGS

Callahan JJ et al: Results of Charnley total hip arthroplasty at a minimum of thirty years, *J Bone Joint Surg* 86A:690, 2004.
Felson DT: Hyaluronate sodium injections for osteoarthritis: hope, hype and hard truths, *Arch Intern Med* 162:245, 2002.
Hartofilakidis G, Karachalios T: Idiopathic osteoarthritis of the hip: incidence, classification and natural history of 272 cases, *Orthopedics* 26:161, 2003.
Hinton R et al: Osteoarthritis: diagnosis and therapeutic considerations, *Am Fam Physician* 65:841, 2002.
Hunt SA, Jazrawi LM, Sherman OH: Arthroscopic management of osteoarthritis of the knee, *J Am Orthop Surg* 10:356, 2002.
Kelly MA et al: Osteoarthritis and beyond: a consensus on the past, present and future of hyaluronans in orthopedics, *Orthopedics* 26:1064, 2003.
Leopold S et al: Corticosteroid compared with hyaluronic acid injections for the treatment of osteoarthritis of the knee, *J Bone Joint Surg* 85:1197, 2003.
Lo HG: Intra-articular hyaluronic acid in treatment of knee osteoarthritis, *JAMA* 290:3115, 2003.
Moseley JB et al: A controlled trial of arthroscopic surgery for osteoarthritis of the knee, *N Engl J Med* 347:81, 2002.
Scott WN, Clarke HD: Early knee arthritis: the role of arthroscopy, *Orthopedics* 26:943, 2003.
Wai EK, Kreder HJ, Williams JI: Arthroscopic debridement of the knee for osteoarthritis in patients fifty years of age or older, *J Bone Joint Surg* 84(A):17, 2002.
Wang C et al: Therapeutic effects of hyaluronic acid in osteoarthritis of the knee, *J Bone Joint Surg* 86A:538, 2004.
Wegman A et al: Nonsteroidal antiinflammatory drugs or acetaminophen for osteoarthritis of the hip or knee? A systematic review of evidence and guidelines, *J Rheumatol* 31:344, 2004.

AUTHOR: **LONNIE R. MERCIER, M.D.**

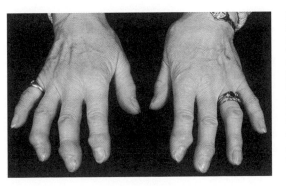

FIGURE 1-25 Osteoarthritis of the distal interphalangeal (DIP) joints. This patient has the typical clinical findings of advanced osteoarthritis of the DIP joints, including large, firm swellings (Heberden's nodes), some of which are tender and red because of associated inflammation of the periarticular tissues as well as of the joint. (From Klippel J, Dieppe P, Ferri F [eds]: *Primary care rheumatology,* London, 1999, Mosby.)

BASIC INFORMATION

DEFINITION

Osteomyelitis is an acute or chronic infection of the bone secondary to the hematogenous or contiguous source of infection or direct traumatic inoculation, which is usually bacterial.

SYNONYMS

Bone infection

ICD-9CM CODES
730.1 Chronic osteomyelitis
730.2 Acute or subacute osteomyelitis

EPIDEMIOLOGY & DEMOGRAPHICS

PREDOMINANT SEX: Male > female
PREDOMINANT AGE: All ages

PHYSICAL FINDINGS

HEMATOGENOUS OSTEOMYELITIS:
- Localized inflammation: often secondary to trauma with accompanying hematoma or cellulitis
- Fever
- Lethargy
- Irritability
- Pain in involved bone

VERTEBRAL OSTEOMYELITIS: Usually hematogenous.
- Fever: 50%
- Localized pain/tenderness
- Neurologic defects: motor/sensory

CONTIGUOUS OSTEOMYELITIS: DIRECT INOCULATION.
- Associated with trauma, fractures, surgical fixation, pressure ulcer
- Chronic infection of skin/soft tissue
- Fever, drainage from surgical site

CHRONIC OSTEOMYELITIS:
- Bone pain
- Sinus tract drainage, nonhealing ulcer
- Chronic low-grade fever
- Chronic localized pain

ETIOLOGY

- *Staphylococcus aureus*
- *S. aureus* (methicillin-resistant)
- *Pseudomonas aeruginosa*
- Enterobacteriaceae
- *Streptococcus pyogenes*
- *Enterococcus*
- Mycobacteria
- Fungi
- Coagulase-negative staphylococci
- *Salmonella* (in sickle cell disease)

DIAGNOSIS **Dx**

DIFFERENTIAL DIAGNOSIS

- Bone infarction
- Charcot's joint
- Gout
- Fracture

WORKUP

- ESR, C-reactive protein
- Blood culturing
- Bone culture
- Pathologic evaluation of bone biopsy for acute/chronic changes consistent with necrosis or acute inflammation

IMAGING STUDIES

- Bone x-ray examination
- Bone scan (Fig. 1-26)
- Gallium scan
- Indium scan
- MRI (most accurate imaging study)
- Doppler studies: useful in patients with suspected peripheral vascular disease to determine vascular adequacy

TREATMENT **Rx**

Surgical debridement in biopsy-positive cases will guide direction for antibiotic therapy. This will vary with type of osteomyelitis. Duration of therapy is usually 6 wk for acute osteomyelitis; chronic osteomyelitis may need a longer course of medication.

- *S. aureus:* cefazolin IV, nafcillin IV, vancomycin IV (in patient allergic to penicillin)
- *S. aureus* (methicillin resistant): vancomycin IV
- *Streptococcus* spp.: cefazolin or ceftriaxone
- *P. aeruginosa:* piperacillin plus aminoglycoside or ceftazidime plus aminoglycoside
- Enterobacteriaceae: ceftriaxone or fluoroquinolone
- Hyperbaric oxygen therapy: may be useful in treatment of chronic osteomyelitis, especially with associated wound healing
- Surgical debridement of all devitalized bone and tissue
- Immobilization of affected bone (plaster, traction) if bone is unstable
- Bone grafts using a vascularized or open graft may be necessary if the remaining bone is inadequate

SUGGESTED READINGS

Boutin RD et al: Update on imaging of orthopedic infections, *Orthop Clin North Am* 29:41, 1998.
Carek PJ et al: Diagnosis and management of osteomyelitis, *Am Fam Physician* 63:2413, 2001.

AUTHORS: **GLENN G. FORT, M.D.,** and **DENNIS J. MIKOLICH, M.D.**

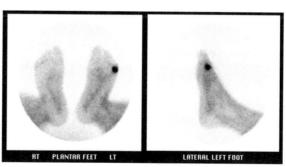

FIGURE 1-26 Osteomyelitis. Intense accumulation of Tc-99m WBC in proximal phalanx of fifth digit of left foot at 4 hours after injection. (From Specht N [ed]: *Practical guide to diagnostic imaging,* St Louis, 1998, Mosby.)

BASIC INFORMATION

DEFINITION

Osteoporosis is a systemic skeletal disease characterized by low bone mass and microarchitectural deterioration of bone tissue resulting in reduced bone strength and increased risk of fracture. Other definitions:

- Bone strength: bone density plus bone quality (bone mineral density accounts for 70% of bone strength)
- Bone density: grams of mineral per volume
- Bone mineral density: grams of mineral per area
- Bone quality: factors that influence bone strength, including microarchitecture, turnover, damage accumulation, and mineralization
- Microarchitecture: describes number of trabeculae, trabecular thickness, trabecular spacing, etc.
  Note: macroarchitecture also affects bone strength but is not related to osteoporosis.

SYNONYMS

None, but osteopenia describes a milder phase of this disease

ICD-9CM CODES
733.0 Osteoporosis

EPIDEMIOLOGY & DEMOGRAPHICS

- 44 million adults in the U.S. have abnormally low bone mass (osteopenia or osteoporosis).
- 40% of all women and 25% of all men will experience a fragility (or low-impact) fracture in their lifetime.
- 80% of all osteoporotic persons are women.
- Osteoporosis (and osteopenia) account for 800,000 vertebral compression fractures, 300,000 hip fractures, and 250,000 wrist fractures, annually.
- The consequences of those fractures are significant for the patients:
  - The mortality for hip fracture is 24% in the first 12 months; of those who survive, 50% fail to regain full ambulatory capability and 25% need long-term institutional care.
  - Vertebral fractures can be asymptomatic but they can also be associated with back pain (twofold increased risk of back pain associated with vertebral fractures), reduced activity or bed rest, 70,000 annual U.S. hospital admissions, and increased mortality.
- Osteoporotic fractures are responsible for 4.1 million hospital days, 44.6 million nursing home days, and 3.4 million outpatient visits and an economic impact of $20 billion annually.

RISK FACTORS FOR PRIMARY OSTEOPOROSIS AND FRAGILITY FRACTURES

- Personal history of a prior fragility fracture is the strongest predictor of a subsequent fracture regardless of bone density
- Family history of fracture
- Cigarette smoking
- Low body mass index/poor nutrition
- Female gender
- Early menopause (natural or surgical)
- Age
- Alcoholism
- Low calcium intake
- Sedentary life style
- General fragility
- Race/ethnicity (Whites and Asians at higher risk than African Americans and Hispanics.)
- "Excessive" caffeine intake
- History of falls
- Unsteady gait
- Risk factors for falls and unsteady gait such as impaired vision, vertigo, orthostatic hypotension, arthritis, neurologic disorders, dementia medications

PHYSICAL FINDINGS & CLINICAL PRESENTATION

- Often silent with no signs or symptoms. The prevalence of osteoporosis is 22% in white women ages 60 to 69, 38% in those ages 70 to 79, and 70% in those older than 80. This means that osteoporosis should be presumed to exist in all elderly women until proven otherwise.
- The most common sign of osteoporosis is height loss. All elderly women (and probably men also) should be measured yearly. Most people know their adult height (or what it used to be).
- Other signs include thoracic kyphosis (dowager's hump), back pain associated with vertebral compression fractures (osteoporosis without resulting fractures does not cause back pain), symptoms/signs associated with the causes of secondary osteoporosis.

ETIOLOGY

PRIMARY OSTEOPOROSIS

Multifactorial resulting from a combination of factors including nutrition, peak bone mass, genetics, level of physical activity, age of menopause (spontaneous vs. surgical), and estrogen status. Postmenopausal osteoporosis is by far the most common form of primary osteoporosis. Increased bone resorption results in net bone loss, most rapidly during the first 5 years following menopause. In men, primary osteoporosis is also related to decreasing levels of sex hormones.

SECONDARY OSTEOPOROSIS

- Endocrine/metabolic
  - Vitamin D deficiency
  - Primary hyperparathyroidism
  - Thyrotoxicosis
  - Hypercortisolism (Cushing's syndrome)
  - (Male) hypogonadism
  - Type I diabetes mellitus
  - Anorexia nervosa
  - Hyperprolactinemia
  - Porphyria
  - Hypophosphatasia
- Gastrointestinal
  - Malabsorption syndromes
  - Chronic liver disease
  - Inflammatory bowel disease
- Malignancies
  - Multiple myeloma
  - Lymphoma
  - Paraneoplastic syndromes
  - Other malignancies
- Rheumatoid arthritis and variants
- COPD
- Osteogenesis imperfecta
- Marfan's syndrome
- Homocystinuria
- Mastocytosis
- Drugs
  - Glucocorticoids
  - Thyroid hormones
  - Antiepileptic drug (e.g., phenytoin and phenobarbital)
  - Loop diuretics
  - GNRH antagonists

DIAGNOSIS

DIFFERENTIAL DIAGNOSIS

Differential diagnosis of low bone density: none
Differential diagnosis of fractures:

- Traumatic fracture resulting from a force that exceeds the strength of normal bone
- Pathologic fractures involving a bone whose strength is weakened by a disease other than osteoporosis including:
  - Primary bone cancer
  - Metastatic bone cancer
  - Benign bone tumor
  - Paget's disease
  - Osteomalacia
  - Osteopetrosis and other acquired causes of brittle bone
- Osteoporotic (or fragility or low impact) fractures

WORKUP

Diagnosis of osteoporosis is made by densitometry. It is indicated in:

- All women 65 and over
- Postmenopausal women under age 65 with osteoporosis risk factors
- All adults with fragility fractures
- Anyone expected to be treated with glucocorticoids drugs for longer than 3 months (cumulative)

- Selectively in adults with known diseases associated with secondary osteoporosis
- Men 70 and older (controversial)

TECHNOLOGIES FOR MEASURING BONE MINERAL DENSITY (BMD)

- Quantitative ultrasound (QUS)
  - Advantages:
    1. Low cost
    2. Safe (no radiation)
  - Disadvantages
    1. Only peripheral sites (finger, wrist, heel)
    2. Imprecise
- Dual-energy x-ray absorptiometry (DXA)
  - Advantages
    1. The "gold standard"
    2. Epidemiologic studies have correlated and standardized BMD data obtained by DXA with fracture risk
    3. Precise
    4. Can measure peripheral and central sites (hip and spine)
  - Disadvantages
    1. More costly than QUS
    2. Radiation exposure
    3. Variable results among different machines
    4. Any dense structure between radiation source and film (e.g., osteophytes, vascular calcifications) will give a false high reading, because density is measured from a two-dimensional image
- Quantitative computed tomography (QCT)
  - Advantages
    1. Central or peripheral site
    2. Precise
    3. Measures the intended targeted bone only as a three-dimensional structure
  - Disadvantages
    1. Most expensive technology
    2 Radiation exposure
    3. Not yet fully standardized

INTERPRETATION

- All BMD measurement results are expressed in T scores and Z scores regardless of what technology is used.
- World Health Organization Criteria for the Diagnosis of Osteoporosis
  - Normal: T-score >-1
  - Osteopenia: T-score -1 to -2.5
  - Osteoporosis: T-score ≤ -2.5
  - Severe osteoporosis: T-score <-2.5 plus fragility fracture(s)

T SCORES AND Z SCORES

See Fig. 1-27.
DXA values are reported by comparison to age and gender reference groups with T scores (standard deviations or percentage above or below values for young normals) and Z scores (standard deviations or percentage above or below age-matched values). A T score more than 2 standard deviations below young normals indicates an increased risk of frac-

ture and should lead to consideration of active therapy to prevent further bone loss. A Z score of more than 1 to 2 standard deviations below the age-matched mean value should prompt a thorough evaluation for secondary causes of bone loss.

The workup for secondary causes of osteoporosis is presented in Table 1-10.

TREATMENT   **Rx**

See Table 1-11.
The goal of treatment is fracture prevention. The strongest predictors of fracture are previous fracture, falls, low BMD, and advancing age (see Fig. 1-28).

NONPHARMACOLOGIC THERAPY
RESISTIVE EXERCISES

- Walking
- Rowing machine
- Weight lifting
- Evidence suggests that the strongest predictor of compliance is enjoyability, which therefore should always be considered in providing recommendations.

FALL PREVENTION

- Assess gait and fall risk
- Consider referral for gait training, lower extremity muscle strengthening, and balance training
- Home safety evaluation
- Assistive devices as appropriate
- Hip protectors

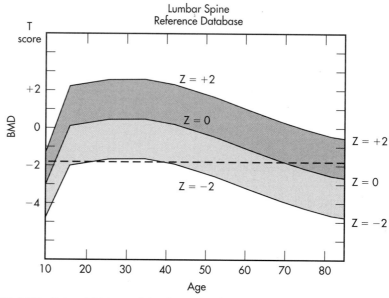

FIGURE 1-27 Natural history of lumbar spine bone mineral density, lumbar spine in women age 10 to 85. The band is a mean ± 2 standard deviation representation of bone density. The X-axis represents age; the Y-axis represents bone density in T scores. The middle of the ribbon represents a Z score of 0 (i.e., the statistical average woman's bone density as she ages).

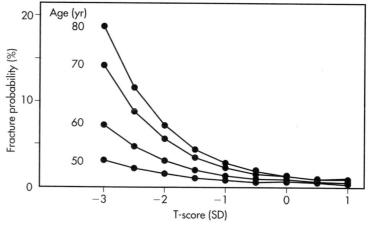

FIGURE 1-28 Ten-year probability (%) of hip fracture in women according to age and T score for bone mineral density at the femoral neck. (Reproduced from *Osteoporosis International*, 13: 527-536, 2002 with permission. All rights reserved.)

SUPPLEMENTS

- Calcium: provide 1500 mg per day from diet or supplements.
  - Examples of dietary sources include:
    1. Milk = 300 mg per cup
    2. Yogurt = 350 mg per cup
    3. Cheese = 200 mg per oz
    4. Broccoli = 100 mg per cup
  - Calcium preparations
    1. Calcium carbonate
    2. Calcium citrate
    3. Calcium gluconate
- Vitamin D: 800 IU per day from diet, sun exposure, or supplements. Many calcium supplements also contain vitamin D

PHARMACOLOGIC THERAPY

- Indication for treatment (according to the National Osteoporosis Foundation)
  - T score <-2.0 (by central DXA)
  - T score <-1.5 (by central DXA) plus at least one additional fracture risk factor

---

TABLE 1-10 **Workup for the Secondary Cause of Osteoporosis (Low Z Score)**

Differential Diagnosis	Screening	Positive Screen	Confirmatory Test
Endocrine/Metabolism			
• Hyperparathyroidism	Ca++, Phos	↑ Ca++ and/or ↓ Phos	Parathormone (PTH) level
• Low vitamin D state*	Ca++, Phos	Lowish Ca++ and ↓ Phos	25-OH-vit D level
• Hypercortisolism	FBS, K+	↑ FBS, ↓ K+	overnight dexamethasone suppression test
• Hyperthyroidism	TSH	↓ TSH	TT$_4$, TT$_3$, T$_3$ RU
• Hypogonadism	Testosterone, FSH, LH in men	↓ testo, ↑ FSH, ↑ LH ↑ FSH, ↑ LH	
Neoplasia			
• Multiple myeloma	CBC, ESR, Ca++, creat	Anemia, ↑ ESR, ↑ Ca++ or ↑ crest	SPEP, UEP
• Lymphoma	CBC ? Imaging	Anemia, lymphadenopathy	More imaging
• Leukemia	CBC	↑ WBC	Bone marrow aspirate
• Metastatic cancer	N/A		
Chronic Illness			
• Hepatic failure	SGPT, Alk Phos, PT	Abn LFTs	Variable
• Renal failure	Creat	↑ Creat	Variable
• Rheumatoid arthritis	Steroid use (for longer than 3 months)		
Gastrointestinal			
• Malabsorption	CBC, PT, Carotene	Anemia, ↑ PT, ↓ carotene	D-xylose absorption anemia evaluation
Drugs			
• Glucocorticoids	Medication history		
• Thyroid hormone			
• Loop diuretics			
• Dilantin			

*In high-risk populations (e.g., nursing home, northern latitude residence) a screening 25-OH-vit D level is recommended.

TABLE 1-11 **Interventions for the Prevention and Treatment of Postmenopausal Osteoporosis**

	Therapy	Dosage
Nonpharmacologic Measures		
	Calcium	1500 mg/d
	Vitamin D	800 IU/d
	Exercise (weight bearing)	30 min, 3 days/wk
Pharmacologic Therapies		
	Risedronate	5 mg/d or 35 mg/wk (prevention and treatment)
	Alendronate	5 mg/d or 35 mg/wk (prevention) 10 mg/d or 70 mg/wk (treatment)
	Raloxifene	60 mg/d (prevention and treatment)
	Salmon calcitonin	200 IU/d intranasally 50-100 IU/d SC or IM (treatment)
	HRT/ERT	0.625 mg/d conjugated estrogens in women with bothersome menopausal symptoms
	Teriparatide	20 mcg/d SC (treatment)

- Any prior history of fragility vertebral or hip fracture: such patients should be treated even if a DXA is not available.
- Preventive treatment for osteoporosis and treatment of osteopenia are controversial.
- Antiresorptive (i.e., antiosteoclastic) treatments
  - Estrogen: effective at the dose of conjugated estrogens 0.625 mg daily in preventing hip and vertebral fractures; however, the overall risk outweighs the benefit. This treatment is no longer recommended for osteoporosis either as single therapy or combined with progesterone.
  - Selective estrogen receptor modulators (SERM): two drugs, raloxifen 60 mg daily and tamoxifen 20 mg daily, are available in the U.S.; however, only raloxifen is approved for the treatment (and prevention) of osteoporosis. Evidence exists that raloxifen is effective in reducing the risk of vertebral fractures. It is not known if it can reduce the risk of hip fracture. Both SERMs reduce the risk of breast cancer. Side effects are hot flashes, leg cramps, and increased risk of deep vein thrombosis and of endometrial cancer.
  - Calcitonin nasal spray 200 IU per day reduces the risk of vertebral fractures. It is not known if it can reduce the risk of hip fracture. The drug is well tolerated, but probably less effective than other agents.
  - Bisphosphonates: several bisphosphonates are available, but only three are widely used from the treatment or prevention of osteoporosis. They are alendronate (70 mg po weekly or 10 mg po daily), risedronate (35 mg po weekly or 5 mg po daily), and ibandronate (150 mg PO monthly). All three drugs are efficacious in reducing the risk of vertebral and hip fracture. The principal side effect for these drugs is potential esophageal ulceration and diarrhea. Alendronate may be marginally more potent at increasing bone density and risedronate may have better gastrointestinal tolerability, but both drugs are probably interchangeable. They are considered the first line of pharmacologic treatment for osteoporosis.
- Bone-building treatments (i.e., osteoblastic stimulant): recombinant human parathyroid hormone (rh-PTH or teriparatide) is a potent stimulant of osteoblastic cells when administered as pulse therapy. (Continuous exposure to parathormone stimulates osteoclasts more than osteoblasts and results in a net bone loss.) Teriparatide is administered at the dose of 20 mcg injected SC daily and results in a reduction of both vertebral and nonvertebral fractures (not specifically hip as is the case for alendronate and risedronate). The main concern of teriparatide is its potential to cause osteosarcoma at high doses in rats. It is also very expensive.

MONITORING TREATMENT

- No evidence exists currently to demonstrate effectiveness of a monitoring strategy. Most clinicians recommend a central DXA at baseline, at 2 years, and at 4 years into treatment (the technology is not precise enough to recommend shorter intervals). Treatment success can be defined by an improvement or no change in BMD over time and no fracture. However, a decline in BMD over time does not necessarily indicate failure: treatment trials show efficacy in fracture reduction compared with placebo even in subjects with declining BMD. Nonetheless, many clinicians consider declining BMD or fracture to be indicative of treatment failure and need to change treatment. Evidence to support combined treatment is not convincing.
- Markers of bone turnover are used by some clinicians to monitor response to treatment. The most common markers of bone resorption include acid phosphatase, hydroxyproline, and N-telopeptide (a metabolite of collagen cross-links). The most common markers of bone formation are alkaline phosphatase and osteocalcin. Change in those markers only takes 3 months to observe, but such changes correlate only poorly with fracture risk.

OSTEOPOROSIS IN MEN

Twenty percent of all osteoporotic persons in the U.S. are men. Secondary causes (e.g., hypogonadism or vitamin D deficiency) are more likely than in women who typically have primary osteoporosis. Bisphosphonates, calcitonin, and teriparatide are used to treat osteoporotic men; however, only alendronate and teriparatide are approved.

DURATION OF TREATMENT

Most treatment trials were not conducted for periods longer than 5 years (alendronate has 10-yr data from trial extension open label studies). Some clinicians hesitate to treat for longer than 5 years (for lack of any evidence base), whereas others treat indefinitely because BMD declines after treatment withdrawal.

SUGGESTED READINGS

Bone HG et al: Ten years' experience with alendronate for osteoporosis in postmenopausal women, *N Engl J Med* 350:1189-1199, 2004.

Cauley JA et al: Effects of estrogen plus progestin on risk of fracture and bone mineral density: the Women's Health Initiative randomized trial, *JAMA* 290:1729-1738, 2003.

Elliott ME et al: Fracture risks of women in long-term care: high prevalence of calcaneal osteoporosis and hypovitaminosis D, *Pharmacotherapy* 23:702-710, 2003.

Greenspan SL et al: Alendronate improves bone mineral density in elderly women with osteoporosis residing in long-term care facilities: a randomized, double-blind, placebo-controlled trial, *Ann Intern Med* 136:742-746, 2002.

Jolly EE et al: Prevention of osteoporosis and uterine effects in postmenopausal women taking raloxifene for 5 years, *Menopause* 10:337-344, 2003.

Keller MI: Treating osteoporosis in postmenopausal women: a case approach, *Cleve J Med* 71:829, 2004.

Kiebzak GM, Miller PD: Determinants of bone strength, *J Bone Miner Res* 18:383-384, 2003.

Lindsay R et al: Risk of new vertebral fracture in the year following a fracture, *JAMA* 285:320-323, 2001.

Marshall D, Johnell O, Wedel H: Meta-analysis of how well measures of bone mineral density predict occurrence of osteoporotic fractures, *BMJ* 312:1254-1259, 1996.

National Osteoporosis Foundation: *Physician's Guide to Prevention and Treatment of Osteoporosis*, Washington, DC, 2003, National Osteoporosis Foundation.

Neer RM et al: Effect of parathyroid hormone (1-34) on fractures and bone mineral density in postmenopausal women with osteoporosis, *N Engl J Med* 344:1434-1441, 2001.

Roux C et al: Efficacy of risedronate on clinical vertebral fractures within six months, *Curr Med Res Opin* 20:433-439, 2004.

Siris ES et al: Identification and fracture outcomes of undiagnosed low bone mineral density in postmenopausal women: results from the National Osteoporosis Risk Assessment, *JAMA* 286:2815-2822, 2001.

Sorensen OH et al: Long-term efficacy of risedronate: a 5-year placebo-controlled clinical experience, *Bone* 32:120-126, 2003.

Zimmerman SI et al: The prevalence of osteoporosis in nursing home residents, *Osteoporos Int* 9:151-157, 1999.

AUTHOR: **TOM J. WACHTEL, M.D.**

BASIC INFORMATION

DEFINITION

Ovarian tumors can be benign, requiring operative intervention but not recurring or metastasizing; malignant, recurring, metastasizing, and having decreased survival; or borderline, having a small risk of recurrence or metastases but generally having a good prognosis.

SYNONYMS

Epithelial ovarian cancer
Germ cell tumor
Sex cord stromal tumor
Ovarian tumor of low malignant potential

ICD-9CM CODES
183.0 Malignant neoplasm of ovary

EPIDEMIOLOGY & DEMOGRAPHICS

INCIDENCE: 12.9 to 15.1 cases/100,000 persons; approximately 25,000 new cases annually
PREDOMINANCE: Median age of 61 yr, peaks at age 75 to 79 yr (54/100,000)
GENETICS: Familial susceptibility has been shown with the BRCA1 gene located on 17q12 to 21. This correlates with breast-ovarian cancer syndrome.
RISK FACTORS: Low parity, delayed childbearing, use of talc on the perineum, high-fat diet, fertility drugs (possibly), Lynch II syndrome (nonpolyposis colon cancer, endometrial cancer, breast cancer, and ovarian cancer clusters in first- and second-degree relatives), breast-ovarian familial cancer syndrome, site-specific familial ovarian cancer (NOTE: Use of oral contraceptives appears to have a protective effect.)

PHYSICAL FINDINGS & CLINICAL PRESENTATION

- 60% present with advanced disease
- Abdominal fullness, early satiety, dyspepsia
- Pelvic pain, back pain, constipation
- Pelvic or abdominal mass
- Lymphadenopathy (inguinal)
- Sister Mary Joseph nodule (umbilical mass)

ETIOLOGY

- Can be inherited as site-specific familial ovarian cancer (two or more first-degree relatives have ovarian cancer)

- Breast-ovarian cancer syndrome (clusters of breast and ovarian cancer among first- and second-degree relatives)
- Lynch syndrome
- No family history and unknown etiology in the majority of ovarian cancer cases

DIAGNOSIS

DIFFERENTIAL DIAGNOSIS

- Primary peritoneal cancer
- Benign ovarian tumor
- Functional ovarian cyst
- Ovarian torsion
- Pelvic kidney
- Pedunculated uterine fibroid
- Primary cancer from breast, GI tract, or other pelvic organ metastasized to the ovary

WORKUP

- Definitive diagnosis made at laparotomy
- Careful physical and history including family history
- Exclusion of nongynecologic etiologies

LABORATORY TESTS

- CBC
- Chemistry profile
- CA-125 or lysophosphatidic acid level
- Consider: hCG, Inhibin, AFP, neuron-specific enolase (NSE), and LDH in patients at risk for germ cell tumors
- Osteopontin-Potential new biomarker for ovarian cancer

IMAGING STUDIES

- Ultrasound (has not been shown to be effective as a screening mechanism but is useful in the evaluation of a pelvic mass)
- Chest x-ray examination
- Mammogram
- CT scan to help evaluate extent of disease
- Other studies (BE, MRI, IVP, etc.) as clinically indicated

TREATMENT

NONPHARMACOLOGIC THERAPY

Virtually all cases of ovarian cancer involve surgical exploration. This includes:
- Abdominal cytology
- Total abdominal hysterectomy and bilateral salpingo-oophorectomy

- Omentectomy
- Diaphragm sampling
- Selective lymphadenectomy (pelvis and paraaortic)
- Primary cytoreduction with a goal of residual tumor diameter <2 cm
- Bowel surgery, splenectomy if needed to obtain optimal (<2 cm) cytoreduction

ACUTE GENERAL Rx

- Optimal cytoreduction is generally followed by chemotherapy (except in some early-stage disease).
- Cisplatin-based combination chemotherapy is used for stage II or greater, 6 mo treatment.
- Chemotherapy regimens continue to change as research continues.
- Consider second-look surgery when chemotherapy is complete.

CHRONIC Rx

- If CA-125 have recurrent disease
- Physical and pelvic examinations every 3 mo for 2 yr, every 4 mo during third year, then every 6 mo
- CA-125 every visit
- Yearly Pap smear

DISPOSITION

- Overall 5-yr survival rates remain low because of the preponderance of late-stage disease:
Stage I and II 80% to 100%
Stage III 15% to 20%
Stage IV 5%

REFERRAL

- Studies have shown that optimal cytoreduction is most likely to occur in the hands of a gynecologic oncologist.
- Have gynecologic/oncology backup available if suspicious of malignancy.

SUGGESTED READINGS

Haber D: Prophylactic oophorectomy to reduce the risk of ovarian and breast cancer in carriers of BRCA mutations, *N Engl J Med* 346:1660, 2002.

Kim JH et al: Osteopontin as a potential diagnostic biomarker for ovarian cancer, *JAMA* 287:1671, 2002.

Modan B et al: Parity, oral contraceptives and the risk of ovarian cancer among carriers and noncarriers of a brca1 or brca2 mutation, *N Engl J Med* 345:235, 2001.

Olson SH et al: Symptoms of ovarian cancer, *Obstet Gynecol* 98:212, 2001.

AUTHOR: **GIL FARKASH, M.D.**

BASIC INFORMATION

DEFINITION

Paget's disease of the bone is a non-metabolic disease of bone characterized by repeated episodes of osteolysis and excessive attempts at repair that results in a weakened bone of increased mass. Monostotic (solitary lesion) and polyostotic (numerous lesions) disease are both described.

SYNONYMS

Osteitis deformans

ICD-9CM CODES

731.0 Paget's disease (osteitis deformans)

EPIDEMIOLOGY & DEMOGRAPHICS

PREVALENCE: Localized lesions in 3% of patients >50 yr
PREVALENT SEX: Male:female ratio of 2:1

PHYSICAL FINDINGS & CLINICAL PRESENTATION

- Many lesions are asymptomatic.
- Onset is variable.
- Symptoms result mainly from the effects of complications:
  1. Skeletal pain, especially hip and pelvis
  2. Bowing of long bones, sometimes leading to pathologic fracture
  3. Increased heat of extremity (resulting from increased vascularity)
  4. Skull enlargement and spinal involvement caused by characteristic bone enlargement, which can produce neurologic complications (vision, hearing loss, radicular pain, and cord compression)
  5. Thoracic kyphoscoliosis
  6. Secondary osteoarthritis, especially of hip
  7. Heart failure as a result of chest and spine deformity and blood shunting

ETIOLOGY

Unknown

DIAGNOSIS

DIFFERENTIAL DIAGNOSIS

- Fibrous dysplasia
- Skeletal neoplasm (primary or metastatic)
- Osteomyelitis
- Hyperparathyroidism
- Vertebral hemangioma

LABORATORY TESTS

- Increased serum alkaline phosphatase (SAP)

- Normal serum calcium and phosphorus levels
- Increased urinary excretion of pyridinoline cross-links, although test is expensive and not usually required in routine cases
- Other: bone biopsy only in uncertain cases or if sarcomatous degeneration is suspected

IMAGING STUDIES

- Appropriate radiographs reflect the characteristic radiolucency and opacity (Fig. 1-29).
- Bone scanning usually reflects the activity and extent of the disease.

TREATMENT

ACUTE GENERAL Rx

- Counseling regarding home environment to prevent falls
- Cane for balance and weight-bearing pain

PHARMACOLOGIC THERAPY

- Calcitonin
- Bisphosphonates
- NSAIDs for pain relief
- General indications for treatment
  1. All symptomatic patients
  2. Asymptomatic patients with high level of metabolic activity or those at risk for deformity
  3. Preoperative, if surgery involves pagetic site

DISPOSITION

- Many monostotic lesions probably remain asymptomatic.
- Progression of the disease is common.
- Malignant degeneration occurs in <1% of patients and should be considered when there is a sudden increase in pain.

- Sarcomatous change carries a grave prognosis.

REFERRAL

- For dental evaluation if there is involvement of the mandible or maxilla
- For ENT evaluation if there is hearing loss
- For ophthalmologic evaluation if there is impaired vision
- For orthopedic consultation for assessment of pain in bone or joint

PEARLS & CONSIDERATIONS

COMMENTS

Surgical intervention is often required for neurologic complications or joint symptoms

- Often associated with profuse blood loss
- Elective cases: benefit from preoperative treatment to suppress bone activity and vascularity

SUGGESTED READINGS

Crandall C: Risedronate: a clinical review, *Arch Intern Med* 161:353, 2001.
Kotocvicz MA: Paget's disease of bone: Diagnosis and indications for treatment, *Aust Fam Physician* 33(3):127, 2004.
Langston AL, Ralston SH: Management of Paget's disease of bone, *Rheumatology* 43(8):955, 2004.
Lin JT, Lane JM: Bisphosphonates, *J Am Acad Orthop Surg* 11:1, 2003.
Roodman GD: Studies in Paget's disease and their relevance to oncology, *Semin Oncol* 28:15, 2001.
Schneider D et al: Diagnosis and treatment of Paget's disease of bone, *Am Fam Physician* 65:2069, 2002.

AUTHOR: **LONNIE R. MERCIER, M.D.**

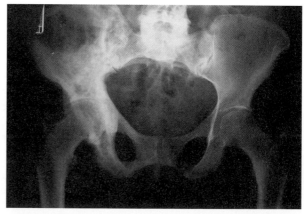

FIGURE 1-29 Frontal radiograph of the pelvis shows marked prominence to the trabeculae in the right ilium, ischium, and pubic bones with small lytic areas identified compatible with the later stages of Paget's disease. (From Specht N [ed]: *Practical guide to diagnostic imaging,* St Louis, 1998, Mosby.)

BASIC INFORMATION

DEFINITION

Pancreatic cancer is an adenocarcinoma derived from the epithelium of the pancreatic duct.

ICD-9CM CODES
157.9 Pancreatic cancer
157.0 (head)
157.1 (body)
157.2 (tail)
157.3 (duct)
230.9 (in situ)

EPIDEMIOLOGY & DEMOGRAPHICS

INCIDENCE: 1 case/10,000 persons/yr
PEAK AGE: Seventh and eighth decades of life
PREDOMINANT SEX: Male:female ratio of 2:1

PHYSICAL FINDINGS & CLINICAL PRESENTATION

Presenting symptoms:
• Jaundice
• Abdominal pain
• Weight loss
• Anorexia/change in taste
• Nausea
• Uncommonly: depression, GI bleeding, acute pancreatitis, back pain
Physical findings:
• Icterus
• Cachexia
• Excoriations from scratching pruritic skin

ETIOLOGY

Unknown, but several conditions have been associated with pancreatic cancer:
• Smoking
• Alcoholism
• Gallstones
• Diabetes mellitus
• Chronic pancreatitis
• Diet rich in animal fat
• Occupational exposures: oil refining, paper manufacturing, chemical industry

DIAGNOSIS

DIFFERENTIAL DIAGNOSIS

• Common duct cholelithiasis
• Cholangiocarcinoma
• Common duct stricture
• Sclerosing cholangitis
• Primary biliary cirrhosis
• Drug-induced cholestasis (e.g., phenothiazines)
• Chronic hepatitis
• Sarcoidosis
• Other pancreatic tumors (islet cell tumor, cystadenocarcinoma, epidermoid carcinoma, sarcomas, lymphomas)

WORKUP

Routine laboratory tests	% abnormal
Alkaline phosphatase	80
Bilirubin	55
Total protein	15
Amylase	15
Hematocrit	60

IMAGING STUDIES

Noninvasive imaging	% abnormal
Abdominal ultrasonography	60
Abdominal CT scan (Fig. 1-30) (without or with contrast [IV or oral])	90
Abdominal MRI scan	90
Invasive imaging	
Endoscopic retrograde cholangiopancreatography (ERCP)	90
CT scan or ultrasonography-guided needle aspiration cytology	90-95

TREATMENT **Rx**

• Surgery
Curative pancreatectomy (Whipple's procedure) appropriate for only 10% to 20% of patients whose lesion is <5 cm, solitary, and without metastases. Surgical mortality is 5%. Adjunct chemotherapy may improve postoperative survival.
Palliative surgery (for biliary decompression/diversion)
Palliative therapeutic endoscopic retrograde cholangiopancreatography (ERCP) using stents
• Chemotherapy
The best combination chemotherapy using streptozotocin, mitomycin C, and 5-FU provides only a 19-wk median survival.
• Radiation
External beam radiation for palliation of pain.
• Combined chemotherapy and radiation provides a median survival of 11 mo.
• Celiac plexus block by an experienced anesthesiologist provides pain relief in 80% to 90% of cases.

DISPOSITION

Adjunct chemotherapy has a significant survival benefit in patients with resected pancreatic cancer, whereas adjuvant chemotherapy has a deleterious effect on survival.

SUGGESTED READINGS

Cello JP: Pancreatic cancer. In Feldman M, Scharschmidt BF, Sleisenger MH (eds): *Gastrointestinal and Liver Disease,* ed 6, Philadelphia, 1998, WB Saunders.
Michaud DS et al: Physical activity, obesity, height, and the risk of pancreatic cancer, *JAMA* 286:821, 2001.
Neoptolemos JP et al: A randomized trial of chemotherapy and radiochemotherapy after resection of pancreatic cancer, *N Engl J Med* 350:1200, 2004.
Wong GY: Effect of neurolytic celiac plexus block on pain relief, quality of life, and survival in patients with unresectable pancreatic cancer, *JAMA* 291:1092, 2004.

AUTHOR: **TOM J. WACHTEL, M.D.**

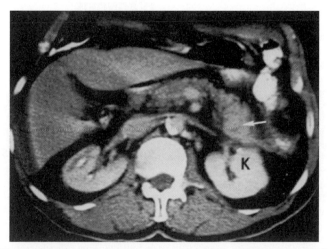

FIGURE 1-30 CT scan of a patient with adenocarcinoma of the body and tail of the pancreas. The tumor *(arrow)* is seen anterior and adjacent to the left kidney *(K)*. At operation, the tumor was invading Gerota's fascia. (From Sabiston D: *Textbook of surgery,* ed 15, Philadelphia, 1997, WB Saunders.)

BASIC INFORMATION

DEFINITION

Idiopathic Parkinson's disease (PD) is a progressive neurodegenerative disorder characterized clinically by rigidity, tremor, and bradykinesia. The major manifestations of the disease are due to loss of dopamine in the substantia nigra pars compacta. Its pathologic hallmark is the Lewy body, which is a cytoplasmic eosinophilic inclusion body.

SYNONYMS

Paralysis agitans

ICD-9CM CODES
332.0 Idiopathic Parkinson's disease, primary
332.1 Parkinson's disease, secondary

EPIDEMIOLOGY & DEMOGRAPHICS

PREVALENCE

- Affects over 1 million people in North America
- In age group >70 yr, 700/100,000 are affected
- Highest incidence in whites, lowest incidence in Asians and black Africans

PHYSICAL FINDINGS & CLINICAL PRESENTATION

- Tremor—typically a resting tremor with a frequency of 4-6 Hz that is often first noted in the hand as a pill-rolling tremor (thumb and forefinger). Can also involve the leg and lip. Tremor improves with purposeful movement. Usually starts asymmetrically but can eventually involve the other hemibody.
- Rigidity—increased muscle tone. This, too, is usually asymmetric in onset, involving the arm, leg, or both. It is resistance that persists throughout the range of passive movement of a joint.
- Akinesia/Bradykinesia—slowness in initiating movement.
- Mask facies—face seems expressionless, giving the appearance of depression. Decreased blink, often there is excess drooling.
- Gait disturbance. In the elderly, falls (particularly backwards) may be the first sign of PD.
- Stooped posture, decreased arm swing.
- Difficulty initiating the first step; small shuffling steps that increase in speed (festinating gait) as if the patient is chasing his or her center of gravity (steps become progressively faster and shorter while the trunk inclines further forward).
- Other complaints and findings early on include micrographia—handwriting becomes smaller, and hypophonia—voice becomes softer.
- Postural instability—tested by "pull test." Ask patient to stand in place with back to examiner. Examiner pulls patient back by the shoulders, and proper response would be to take no steps back or very few steps back without falling. Retropulsion is a positive test as is falling straight back. This is not usually severe early on. If falls and postural reflexes are greatly impaired early on, then consider other disorders.

ETIOLOGY

- Primary
  - Unknown
  - Most cases are sporadic, with age being the most common risk factor, although there is probably a combination of both environmental and genetic factors contributing to disease expression. There are rare familial forms.
- Secondary (acquired) parkinsonism
  - Postinfectious parkinsonism—von Economo's encephalitis
  - Parkinson's pugilistica—after repeated head trauma
  - Iatrogenic—any of the neuroleptics and antipsychotics. The high potency D_2-blocker neuroleptics are most likely to cause parkinsonism. Quetiapine is an atypical antipsychotic with a lower risk of causing parkinsonism. Clozaril does not cause parkinsonism.
  - Toxins (e.g., manganese, carbon monoxide)
  - Cerebrovascular disease (basal ganglia infarcts)

DIAGNOSIS

A presumptive clinical diagnosis can be based on history and physical examination. The combination of asymmetric signs, resting tremor, and good response to levodopa best differentiates idiopathic Parkinson's disease from other causes of parkinsonism (see Differential Diagnosis).

DIFFERENTIAL DIAGNOSIS

- Multisystem atrophy—distinguishing features include autonomic dysfunction, including urinary incontinence, orthostatic hypotension, and erectile dysfunction, parkinsonism, cerebellar signs, and normal cognition.
- Diffuse Lewy body disease—parkinsonism with concomitant dementia. Patients often have early hallucinations and fluctuations in level of alertness and mental status.
- Corticobasal degeneration—often begins asymmetrically with apraxia, cortical sensory loss in one limb, and sometimes alien limb phenomenon.
- Progressive supranuclear palsy—tends to have axial rigidity greater than appendicular (limb) rigidity. These patients have early and severe postural instability. Hallmark is supranuclear gaze palsy that involves vertical gaze before horizontal. Progressive dementia is part of this syndrome.
- Essential tremor—bilateral postural and action tremor.

WORKUP

Identification of clinical signs and symptoms associated with Parkinson's disease (see Physical Findings & Clinical Presentation) and elimination of conditions that may mimic it with a comprehensive history and physical examination

IMAGING STUDIES

CT scan has almost no role in investigations. MRI of the head may sometimes distinguish between idiopathic Parkinson's disease and other conditions that present with signs of parkinsonism (see Differential Diagnosis).

TREATMENT

NONPHARMACOLOGIC THERAPY

- Physical therapy, patient education and reassurance, treatment of associated conditions (e.g., depression)
- Avoidance of drugs that can induce or worsen parkinsonism: neuroleptics (especially high potency), certain antiemetics (prochlorperazine, trimethobenzamide), metoclopramide, nonselective MAO inhibitors (may induce hypertensive crisis), reserpine, methyldopa

PHARMACOLOGIC THERAPY

- Whether levodopa should always be the initial treatment is controversial, but is the prevailing practice in the U.S.
- Pharmacotherapy should be initiated when required by symptoms; prior practice of waiting for limitation of ADLs is now outdated.
- Motor complications that develop during the course of the disease may reflect the combination of disease progression and side effects of dopaminergic medications.

CHRONIC Rx

- Levodopa therapy
  1. Cornerstone of symptomatic therapy—should be used with a peripheral dopa decarboxylase inhibitor (carbidopa) to minimize side effects (nausea, mood changes, postural hypotension). The combination of the two drugs is marketed under the trade name Sinemet.
  2. Usual starting dose is 25/100 mg (carbidopa/levodopa) tid 1 hr before meals.
  3. Controlled-release preparations (Sinemet CR [200 mg levodopa/50 mg carbidopa, or 100 mg levodopa/25 mg carbidopa]) are available.
- Entacapone (Comtan) is a reversible inhibitor of catechol-o-methyl transferase and is used as an adjunct to levodopa/carbidopa. Side effects include orthostatic hypotension, diarrhea, hallucinations. Not to be used with any nonselective MAO inhibitor. Initial dose is 200 mg tid given with each dose of Sinemet.
- Dopamine receptor agonists (ropinirole, pramipexole, pergolide, and bromocriptine) are not as potent as levodopa, but they are often used as initial treatment in younger patients to attempt to delay the onset of complications (dyskinesias, motor fluctuations) associated with levodopa therapy. These medications are more expensive than levodopa. In general they cause more side effects than levodopa. These include nausea, vomiting, light-headedness, peripheral edema, confusion, and somnolence.
  1. Ropinirole (Requip): initial dose is 0.25 mg tid
  2. Pramipexole (Mirapex): initial dose of 0.125 mg tid
  3. Pergolide (Permax): initial dose, 0.05 mg for first 2 days increased by 0.1 mg every third day over next 12 days. There have been cases of restrictive valvulopathy, most commonly in tricuspid valve, associated with Permax use. All patients on this medication need a good clinical cardiac examination, and if any concern, an echo
  4. Bromocriptine (Parlodel): initial dose, 1.25 mg qhs
- Selegiline (Eldepryl), an inhibitor of MAO B, can be used early as initial therapy in those with mild disease or as adjunctive therapy. Selegiline was once advocated as early, first line therapy because of proposed neuroprotective effects; however, those benefits are probably less robust than once thought. Usual dose is 5 mg bid with breakfast and lunch. It can be useful in treating the fatigue that is commonly associated with PD. Concurrent use of stimulants and sympathomimetics should be avoided.
- Amantadine (Symmetrel) is an antiviral agent that augments release and decreases reuptake of dopamine. It can be used alone early in the disease or in combination with levodopa; dosage is 100 mg tid (titrate q week from 100 mg qd). Must adjust for age and renal impairment. Most notable side effect, especially in elderly, is confusion.
- Anticholinergic agents are helpful in treating the tremor and drooling in patients with Parkinson's disease and can be used alone or in combination with levodopa; potential side effects include constipation, urinary retention, memory impairment, and hallucinations. They should generally be avoided in the elderly.
  1. Trihexyphenidyl (Artane): initial dose, 1 mg tid po
  2. Benztropine (Cogentin): usual dose, 0.5 to 1 mg qd or bid
- Surgical options:
  1. Pallidal (globus pallidus interna) and subthalamic deep brain stimulation are currently the surgical options of choice; thalamic DBS may be useful for refractory tremor.
  2. Surgery is limited to patients with disabling, medically refractory problems, and patients must still have a good response to L-dopa to undergo surgery. DBS results in decreased dyskinesias, fluctuations, rigidity, and tremor.
- Associated depression should be identified and treated.
- Coexisting dementia may represent either diffuse Lewy body disease or a late complication of PD. An acetylcholinesterase inhibitor trial should be prescribed.

DISPOSITION

Parkinson's disease usually follows a slowly progressive course leading to disability over the course of several years. However, every patient will progress individually and patients should be reassured that this diagnosis does not always result in debilitation.

REFERRAL

- Neurology consultation is recommended on initial diagnosis of Parkinson's disease.
- Participation in outpatient physical therapy, occupational, or speech program is recommended for patients with moderate to advanced disease. Falls are a common problem and require special attention.

PEARLS & CONSIDERATIONS

- Asymmetry of symptoms at onset is very useful in distinguishing PD from other causes of parkinsonism.
- Although resting tremor is a common presenting symptom, up to one fourth of patients with idiopathic PD do not have classic resting tremor.
- Management of delirium and hallucinations is often difficult because most antipsychotic drugs have extrapyramidal side effects that worsen Parkinsonian symptoms. The atypical antipsychotic drugs of choice in PD are Clozaril (watch for agranulocytosis) and quetiapine.
- Walkers, if prescribed, should always be wheeled (to reduce the risk of falling backwards when lifting a nonwheeled walker).

COMMENTS

Additional patient information on Parkinson's disease can be obtained from www.parkinson.org and from the National Parkinson Foundation, Inc., 1501 Ninth Avenue NW, Miami, FL 33136; phone: (800) 327-4545.

SUGGESTED READINGS

Ahlskog, JE: Parkinson's disease: medical and surgical treatment, *Neurol Clin* 19:3, 2001.
Lang AE et al: Parkinson's disease, *N Engl J Med* 339(15):1044, 1998.
Lang AE et al: Parkinson's disease, *N Engl J Med* 339(16):1130, 1998.
Siderowf A: Parkinson's disease: clinical features, epidemiology, and genetics, *Neurol Clin* 19:3, 2001.

AUTHOR: **CINDY ZADIKOFF, M.D.**

BASIC INFORMATION

DEFINITION

Peptic ulcer disease (PUD) is an ulceration in the stomach or duodenum resulting from an imbalance between mucosal protective factors and various mucosal damaging mechanisms (see "Etiology").

SYNONYMS

PUD
Duodenal ulcer (DU)
Gastric ulcer (GU)

ICD-9CM CODES
536.8 Peptic ulcer disease
531.3 Peptic ulcer, stomach, acute
531.7 Peptic ulcer, stomach, chronic
532.3 Peptic ulcer, duodenum, acute
532.7 Peptic ulcer, duodenum, chronic

EPIDEMIOLOGY & DEMOGRAPHICS

- Incidence: 250,000 to 500,000 (200,000 to 400,000 DU; 50,000 to 100,000 GU) annually; duodenal ulcer:gastric ulcer ratio is 4:1.
- Anatomic location: >90% of DUs occur in the first portion of the duodenum; GU occurs most frequently in the lesser curvature near the incisura angularis.

PHYSICAL FINDINGS & CLINICAL PRESENTATION

- Physical examination is often unremarkable.
- Patient may have epigastric tenderness, tachycardia, pallor, hypotension (from acute or chronic blood loss), nausea and vomiting (if pyloric channel is obstructed), boardlike abdomen and rebound tenderness (if perforated), and hematemesis or melena (with a bleeding ulcer).

ETIOLOGY

Often multifactorial; the following are common mucosal damaging factors:
- *Helicobacter pylori* infection
- Medications (NSAIDs, including aspirin, and glucocorticoids)
- Incompetent pylorus or LES
- Bile acids
- Impaired proximal duodenal bicarbonate secretion
- Decreased blood flow to gastric mucosa
- Acid secreted by parietal cells and pepsin secreted as pepsinogen by chief cells
- Cigarette smoking
- Alcohol

DIAGNOSIS

DIFFERENTIAL DIAGNOSIS

- GERD
- Cholelithiasis syndrome
- Pancreatitis
- Gastritis
- Nonulcer dyspepsia
- Neoplasm (gastric carcinoma, lymphoma, pancreatic carcinoma)
- Angina pectoris, MI, pericarditis
- Dissecting aneurysm
- Other: high small bowel obstruction, pneumonia, subphrenic abscess, early appendicitis

WORKUP

- Comprehensive history and physical examination to exclude other diagnoses. Diagnostic modalities include endoscopy or UGI series. Endoscopy is invasive and more expensive; however, it is preferred for the following reasons:
  1. Highest accuracy (approximately 90% to 95%)
  2. Useful to identify superficial or very small ulcerations
  3. Essential to diagnose gastric ulcers (1% to 4% of gastric ulcers diagnosed as benign by UGI series are eventually diagnosed as gastric carcinoma)
  4. Additional advantages over UGI series include:
     - Biopsy of suspicious looking ulcers
     - Electrocautery of bleeding ulcers
     - Measurement of gastric pH in suspected gastrinoma (e.g., patient with multiple ulcers)
     - Diagnosis of esophagitis, gastritis, duodenitis
     - Endoscopic biopsy for *H. pylori*

LABORATORY TESTS

- Routine laboratory evaluation is usually unremarkable.
- Anemia may be present in patients with significant GI bleeding.
- *H. pylori* testing via endoscopic biopsy, urea breath test, stool antigen test (*H. pylori* stool antigen), or specific antibody test is recommended:
  1. Serologic testing for antibodies to *H. pylori* is easy and inexpensive; however, the presence of antibodies demonstrates previous but not necessarily current infection. Antibodies to *H. pylori* can remain elevated for months to years after infection has cleared; therefore antibody levels must be interpreted in light of patient's symptoms and other test results (e.g., PUD seen on UGI series).
  2. The urea breath test documents active infection. The patient ingests a small amount of urea labeled with carbon 13 (^{13}C) or carbon 14. If urease is present (produced by the organism), the urea is hydrolyzed and the patient exhales labeled carbon dioxide that is then collected and measured. This test is more expensive and not as readily available. Use of proton pump inhibitors within 2 wk of the urea breath test may interfere with test results.
  3. Histologic evaluation of endoscopic biopsy samples is currently the gold standard for accurate diagnosis of *H. pylori* infection.
  4. Stool antigen test is as accurate as the urea breath test for follow-up evaluation of patients treated for *H. pylori*. This test detects the presence of infection by measuring the fecal excretion of *H. pylori* antigens. A negative result on the stool antigen test 8 wk after completion of therapy identifies patients in whom eradication of *H. pylori* was successful.
- Additional laboratory evaluation is indicated only in specific cases (e.g., amylase level in suspected pancreatitis, serum gastrin level in suspected Zollinger-Ellison [Z-E] syndrome).

IMAGING STUDIES

Conventional UGI barium studies identify approximately 70% to 80% of PUD; accuracy can be increased to approximately 90% by using double contrast.

TREATMENT

NONPHARMACOLOGIC THERAPY

- Stop cigarette smoking; cigarette smoking increases the risk of PUD, decreases the healing rate, and increases the frequency of recurrence.
- Avoid NSAIDs and alcohol.
- Special diets have been proved *unrelated* to ulcer development and healing; however, avoid foods that cause symptoms.

ACUTE GENERAL Rx

Eradication of *H. pylori*, when present, can be accomplished with various regimens:
1. Proton pump inhibitors (PPI) bid (e.g., omeprazole 20 mg bid or lansoprazole 30 mg bid) *plus* clarithromycin 500 mg bid *and* amoxicillin 1000 mg bid for 7 to 10 days
2. PPI bid *plus* amoxicillin 500 mg bid *plus* metronidazole 500 mg for 7 to 10 days
3. PPI bid *plus* clarithromycin 500 mg bid *and* metronidazole 500 mg bid for 7 days

4. Recent trials indicate that a 1-day quadruple therapy may be as effective as a 7-day triple therapy regimen. The 1-day quadruple therapy regimen consists of two tablets of 262 mg bismuth subsalicylate qid, one 500 mg metronidazole tablet qid, 2 g of amoxicillin suspension qid, and two capsules of 30 mg of lansoprazole.

5. Bismuth compound qid *plus* tetracycline 500 mg qid *and* metronidazole 500 mg qid for 14 days

6. A 5-day treatment with three antibiotics (amoxicillin 1 g bid, clarithromycin 250 mg bid, and metronidazole 400 mg bid) plus either lansoprazole 30 mg bid or ranitidine 300 mg bid is an efficacious cost-saving option for patients older than 55 yr with no prior history of PUD

PUD patients testing negative for *H. pylori* should be treated with antisecretory agents:

- Histamine-2 receptor antagonists (H$_2$RAs): cimetidine, ranitidine, famotidine, and nizatidine are all effective; they are usually given in split dose or at nighttime.
- Proton pump inhibitors (PPIs): can also induce rapid healing; they are usually given 30 min before meals.

Antacids and sucralfate are also effective agents for the treatment and prevention of PUD.

CHRONIC Rx

Maintenance therapy in duodenal ulcer patients is indicated in the following situations:

- Persistent smokers
- Recurrent ulcerations
- Chronic treatment with NSAIDs, glucocorticoids

- Elderly or debilitated patients
- Aggressive or complicated ulcer disease (e.g., perforation, hemorrhage)
- Asymptomatic bleeders

Misoprostol therapy (100 μg qid with food, increased to 200 μg qid if well tolerated) is useful for the prevention of NSAID-induced gastric ulcers in all patients on long-term NSAID therapy. Proton pump inhibitors are also effective at healing ulcers and maintaining remission in patients on long-term NSAIDs.

DISPOSITION

- The recurrence rate for untreated PUD is approximately 60% (>70% in smokers). Treatment decreases the recurrence rate by nearly 30%.
- Patients with recurrent ulcers should be retreated for an additional 8 wk and then placed on maintenance therapy with H$_2$RAs, PPIs, sucralfate, or antacids.
- An ulcer is considered refractory to treatment if healing is not evident after 8 wk for duodenal ulcers and 12 wk for gastric ulcers. In these patients maximum acid inhibition (e.g., esomeprazole 40 mg bid) is preferred over continued therapy with standard antiulcer therapy.
- Eradication of *H. pylori* (when present) is indicated in all patients. A negative stool antigen test for *H. pylori* 6 weeks after treatment accurately confirms cure of *H. pylori* infection with reasonable sensitivity in initially seropositive healthy subjects.
- Screening for Zollinger-Ellison (Z-E) syndrome should also be considered in patients with multiple recurrent ulcers; in patients with Z-E, the serum gastrin level is >1000 pg/ml and the basal acid output is usually >15 mEq/hr.

- Surgery for refractory ulcers is now only rarely performed; it consists of highly selective vagotomy for duodenal ulcers or ulcer removal with antrectomy or hemigastrectomy without vagotomy for gastric ulcers.

REFERRAL

- GI referral for patients requiring endoscopy
- Surgical referral for patients with non-healing ulcers despite appropriate medical therapy

PEARLS & CONSIDERATIONS

COMMENTS

- Patients with gastric ulcers should have repeat endoscopy after 4 to 6 wk of therapy to document healing and test exfoliative cytology for gastric carcinoma.
- After endoscopic treatment of bleeding peptic ulcers, bleeding recurs in up to 20% of patients. PPI administration intravenously by continuous infusion substantially reduces the risk of recurrent bleeding.

SUGGESTED READINGS

Graham DY et al: Ulcer prevention in long-term users of nonsteroidal anti-inflammatory drugs, *Arch Intern Med* 162:169, 2002.

Lai KC et al: Lansoprazole for the prevention of recurrences of ulcer complications from long-term low-dose aspirin use, *N Engl J Med* 346:2033, 2002.

Lara LF et al: One day quadruple therapy compared with 7-day triple therapy for helicobacter pylori infection, *Arch Intern Med* 163:2079, 2003.

AUTHOR: **FRED F. FERRI, M.D.**

BASIC INFORMATION

DEFINITION

Peripheral arterial disease (PAD) usually refers to atherosclerotic obstruction of the arteries to the lower extremity.

ICD-9CM CODES
443.9 Peripheral vascular disease

EPIDEMIOLOGY & DEMOGRAPHICS

- Age-adjusted prevalence of PAD is approximately 12%.
- PAD affects men and women equally.
- An estimated 27 million people in Europe and North America (or 16% of the population 55 yr of age and older) have PAD.
- African Americans and Hispanics with diabetes have a higher prevalence of PAD than whites.
- PAD is a marker for systemic vascular disease.
- Patients with newly diagnosed PAD are 6 times more likely to die within the next 10 yr when compared with patients without PAD.
- Risk factors associated with PAD are similar to coronary artery disease, including tobacco, diabetes, hyperlipidemia, hypertension, and advanced age.
- Smoking is the major determinant of disease progression.
- Other potential risk factors include elevated levels of C-reactive protein, fibrinogen, homocysteine, apolipoprotein (a), and plasma viscocity.
- An inverse relationship has been suggested between PAD and alcohol consumption.

PHYSICAL FINDINGS & CLINICAL PRESENTATION

- Nearly 50% of the patients with PAD experience no symptoms, making PAD an underdiagnosed and undertreated condition
- Approximately one third of patients with PAD present with intermittent claudication described as an aching or cramping leg pain brought on by exertion and relieved with rest that can progress with time; however, relying on the classic history of claudication alone will miss 85%-90% of patients with PAD
- Pain at rest occurring commonly at night when the patient is supine
- Diminished pulses
- Bruits heard over the distal aorta, iliac, or femoral arteries
- Rubor with prolonged capillary refill on dependency
- Cool skin temperature
- Trophic changes of hair loss and muscle atrophy
- Nonhealing ulcers, necrotic tissue, and gangrene possible

ETIOLOGY

The primary cause of peripheral arterial disease is atherosclerosis: atherosclerotic lesions of the arteries to the lower extremities subsequently leading to stenosis of peripheral vessels and inability to supply oxygenated blood to working limb muscles.

DIAGNOSIS

DIFFERENTIAL DIAGNOSIS

- Spinal stenosis
- Degenerative joint disease of the lumbar spine and hips
- Muscle cramps
- Compartment syndrome

WORKUP

- The initial workup in any patient suspected of having PAD includes measuring the ankle-brachial index (ABI). The ABI is calculated by dividing the highest ankle systolic pressure using either the dorsalis pedis or posterior tibial artery by the highest systolic pressure from either arm.
- A diagnosis of PAD is based on the presence of limb symptoms or an ABI
- The severity of PAD is based on the ABI at rest and during treadmill exercise (1 to 2 mph, 5 min, or symptom-limited) and is classified as follows:
  1. Mild: ABI at rest 0.71 to 0.90 or ABI during exercise >0.50
  2. Moderate: ABI at rest 0.41 to 0.70 or ABI during exercise >0.20
  3. Severe: ABI at rest <0.40 or ABI during exercise <0.20

LABORATORY TESTS

- Lipid profile
- Blood glucose
- HgbA1c levels in diabetic patients
- Homocysteine
- Fibrinogen

IMAGING STUDIES

- Duplex ultrasound can be used to locate the occluded areas and assess the patency of the distal arterial system or prior vein grafts.
- Rest or exercise pulse volume recordings. Pulse volume recordings measure volume of limb flow per pulse in different segments of the limb (e.g., thigh, calf, ankle, metatarsal, and toes). It helps to localize the site of the stenosis since the contour of the pulse wave changes distal to the occlusion.
- MRA can be used as a noninvasive approach to visualize the aorta and peripheral lower extremity arteries. A major advantage of MRA is that it does not require contrast agents.
- Angiography remains the gold standard for visualizing the arterial anatomy before revascularization.

TREATMENT

NONPHARMACOLOGIC THERAPY

- PAD patients with no prior history of a cardiac event are to be considered as a cardiovascular "equivalent" with risks of future cardiovascular events similar to patients with prior MIs
- Diet counseling (e.g., salt restriction in hypertension, ADA calorie diets in diabetics)
- Exercise training walking 30 to 60 min/day at about 2 mi/hr every day improves exercise capacity, walking distance, and quality of life
- Aggressive management of risk factors for PAD including:
  1. Tobacco counseling and smoke cessation programs are indispensable in decreasing the progression of disease as well as reducing the mortality rate from cardiovascular events in patients with PAD.
  2. Management of hypertension.
  3. Tight glycemic control (A1C <7%) in diabetic patients with PAD results in prevention of microvascular complications.
  4. Control of dyslipidemia reduces severity of claudication symptoms.

ACUTE GENERAL THERAPY

Most patients with PAD respond to conservative management mentioned previously. If this fails, medicines can be tried (see "Chronic Rx"). Surgical reconstitution has its specific indications reserved for patient with impending limb loss (see "Chronic Rx").

CHRONIC Rx

- Aspirin 81 mg to 325 mg daily is recommended for secondary disease prevention in patients with cardiovascular disease.
- Clopidogrel 75 mg daily also provides protection from cardiovascular and cerebrovascular events associated with PAD.
- Pentoxyphylline (Trental, Pentoxil) 400 mg tid may provide a small benefit in walking distance when compared with placebo.

- Cilostazol (Pletal) 100 mg bid has been shown to significantly increase the distance patients with claudication can walk when compared with placebo, but should not be given to patients with congestive heart failure and an ejection fraction <40.
- Surgical reconstruction is indicated in patients with refractory rest pain, limb ischemia, nonhealing ulcers, or gangrene, and in a select group of patients with functional disability. Common surgical procedures:
  1. Aortoiliofemoral reconstruction
  2. Infrainguinal bypass (e.g., femoropopliteal, femorotibial)
  3. Extraanatomic bypass (e.g., axillofemoral or femorofemoral bypass)
- Angioplasty is used on short, discrete stenotic lesions in the iliac or femoropopliteal artery.

DISPOSITION

Risk factor modification with aggressive pharmacotherapy in the treatment of hyperlipidemia, diabetes, hypertension, and smoking is essential in the prevention of progression, limb ischemia, and cardiovascular events in patients with PAD.

REFERRAL

Consultation with a vascular surgeon is recommended in patients with PAD and rest pain, functional disability from pain, ABI less than 0.50 at rest, any signs of limb ischemia, or gangrene.

PEARLS & CONSIDERATIONS

COMMENTS

- Asymptomatic PAD, similar to symptomatic PAD, is associated with an increased risk of atherothrombotic events (e.g., MI and CVA).
- Although the prevalence of PAD in Europe and North America is estimated at approximately 27 million people, PAD remains underdiagnosed and undertreated.

When PAD limits a patient's ability to walk and exercise, percutaneous revascularization can be considered. Data reveal excellent outcomes with angioplasty and stenting. Outcomes will likely be better as peripheral interventional technology and skills improve.

SUGGESTED READINGS

American Diabetes Association: Peripheral arterial disease in people with diabetes, *Diabetes Care* 26:3333, 2003.

Belch JJ et al: Critical issues in peripheral arterial disease detection and management, *Arch Intern Med* 163;884, 2003.

Burns P, Gaugh S, Bradbury AW: Management of peripheral arterial disease in primary care, *British Medical Journal* 326:584, 2003.

Hiatt WR: Medical treatment of peripheral arterial disease and claudication, *N Engl J Med* 344:21, 2001.

Hirsch AT et al: Peripheral arterial disease detection, awareness, and treatment in primary care, *JAMA* 286:11, 2001.

Lesho E et al: Management of peripheral arterial disease, *Am Fam Physician* 69:525, 2004.

Mukheijee D, Yadav JS: Update on peripheral vascular diseases: from smoking cessation to stenting, *Cleve Clinic J Med* 68:8, 2001.

AUTHORS: **PRANAV M. PATEL, M.D.,** and **WEN-CHIH WU, M.D.**

BASIC INFORMATION

DEFINITION

The term *peripheral neuropathy* refers to any disorder involving the peripheral nerves. It encompasses:

- Polyneuropathy—a symmetric, usually length-dependent disorder of peripheral nerves; a distinction is often made between predominantly small-fiber (often painful) and large-fiber neuropathies.
- Mononeuropathy—disorder of a single peripheral nerve (e.g., median or ulnar neuropathy).
- Mononeuropathy multiplex—a multifocal disorder characterized by dysfunction of many individual peripheral nerves (when extensive, dysfunction may become confluent and resemble a generalized neuropathy).

ICD-9CM CODES
356.9 Unspecified idiopathic peripheral neuropathy

PHYSICAL FINDINGS & CLINICAL PRESENTATION

Polyneuropathy—symptoms usually begin distally in the feet and gradually spread proximally.

- Sensory
  - Numbness, paresthesiae, neuropathic pain
  - Sensory ataxia (result of impairment of position sense)
  - Reduced or absent deep tendon reflexes
- Motor
  - Weakness, muscle atrophy
  - Foot deformities (high arches, hammer toes)—especially with hereditary neuropathy
- Autonomic
  - Postural hypotension

Mononeuropathy—symptoms and signs depend on the peripheral nerve affected

- Median nerve (carpal tunnel syndrome)—numbness, tingling in the thumb and adjacent two fingers; pain in the wrist and forearm; often worse at night and with activities like driving

Mononeuropathy multiplex

- Pain in the distribution of individual peripheral nerves
- Multifocal motor and sensory deficits

ETIOLOGY

HEREDITARY NEUROPATHIES

- Charcot-Marie-Tooth syndrome
  1. Most common familial motor and sensory neuropathy
  2. Type I (most common) is demyelinating; type II is axonal
  3. Foot deformities (high arches, hammer toes) are common

ACQUIRED NEUROPATHIES

- Demyelinating
  1. Guillain-Barré syndrome—acute (progression over <4 wk) ascending flaccid paralysis with areflexia; may be accompanying sensory loss, pain, and autonomic dysfunction (see Guillain-Barré Syndrome in Section I)
  2. Chronic inflammatory demyelinating polyradiculoneuropathy (CIDP)—subacute to chronic (progression over >2 mo) sensorimotor polyneuropathy (may be associated with monoclonal gammopathy)
- Axonal
  1. Diabetes mellitus: frequently painful, usually affects sensory fibers more than motor
  2. Nutritional deficiency—B_{12}, folate
  3. Toxins—alcohol, drugs (e.g., isoniazid, vincristine, cisplatin, colchicines, amiodarone, phenytoin, antiretrovirals, metronidazole, dapsone, nitrofurantoin, disulfiram), chemicals (lead, arsenic, mercury)
  4. Thyroid disease (hypothyroidism)
  5. Paraproteinemia—monoclonal gammopathy of undetermined significance (MGUS), multiple myeloma, Waldenstrom's macroglobulinemia, primary systemic amyloidosis
  6. Collagen vascular disorders—SLE, rheumatoid arthritis, Sjögren's syndrome, polyarteritis nodosa (may cause polyneuropathy and mononeuropathy multiplex)
  7. Sarcoidosis: cranial nerve palsies (most common is facial nerve)
  8. Paraneoplastic
  9. Infections (leprosy, herpes zoster, TB, diphtheria, Lyme disease, HIV); may cause polyneuropathy or mononeuropathy
  10. Uremia
  11. Compression—typically causes mononeuropathy

DIAGNOSIS

WORKUP

- History should be directed toward inquiry about specific etiologies—systemic disease (e.g., diabetes mellitus, collagen disorder), alcohol intake, medication use, toxin exposure, dietary practices (e.g., veganism may cause B_{12} deficiency), risk factors for HIV infection, family history (of neuropathy or foot deformities).
- Neurophysiology (nerve conduction studies and electromyography) to determine the pattern of involvement (e.g., polyneuropathy vs. mononeuropathy multiplex) as well as the physiology (axonal vs. demyelinating).
- Lumbar puncture may be indicated when vasculitis or amyloid suspected.
- Fig. 3-84 in Section III describes an approach to the patient with peripheral neuropathy.

LABORATORY TESTS

Some or all of these tests may be appropriate, depending on clinical suspicion:

- Fasting blood sugar and/or 2-hr glucose tolerance test
- Serum B_{12}, homocysteine, methylmalonic acid as well as folate
- Renal function
- Thyroid function tests
- Serum protein and immunoelectrophoresis; urine protein electrophoresis
- ANA, RF, cryoglobulins
- HIV, RPR, hepatitis serologies, Lyme titers
- Heavy metal screen; urinary porphyrins

IMAGING STUDIES

Usually, imaging studies are not required. Certain clinical conditions may require the following:

- Chest x-ray—when sarcoid or underlying lung cancer suspected
- Skeletal survey (long bone x-rays) to identify plasmacytoma
- MRI of lumbosacral (or cervical spine) if spinal cord pathology or polyradiculopathy suspected

TREATMENT

NONPHARMACOLOGIC THERAPY

- Stop offending agent (drugs or toxins) if any identified.
- Surgical referral for entrapment neuropathy.
- Physical or occupational therapy as well as splinting (e.g., ankle-foot orthosis) as appropriate.

ACUTE GENERAL Rx

- Treatment of underlying systemic disease (e.g., diabetes, uremia, multiple myeloma)
- Nutritional replacement when appropriate (e.g., B_{12} injections)

- Symptomatic treatment of neuropathic pain—many options available:
  - Neurontin—start 100 mg tid (more slowly in the very elderly); gradually increase as needed and as tolerated, aiming initially for 600 mg tid.
  - Topamax—start 25 mg qd, then 25 mg bid, then 50 mg bid, increasing as tolerated and needed.
  - Lamictal—start 50 mg qd for 2 wk, then 50 mg bid for 2 wk; then increase by 50 mg per week as tolerated and needed (Stevens-Johnson rash may occur if dose escalates too quickly).
  - Narcotic analgesics—may be used, but the aforementioned agents should be tried first.

SUGGESTED READINGS

Hughes RAC: Peripheral neuropathy, *BMJ* 324:466, 2002.

Mendell JR, Sahenk Z: Clinical practice—painful sensory neuropathy, *N Engl J Med* 348:1243, 2003.

Stevens JC et al: Symptoms of 100 patients with electromyographically verified carpal tunnel syndrome, *Muscle Nerve* 22:1448, 1999.

AUTHOR: **MICHAEL BENATAR, M.B.CH.B., D.PHIL.**

BASIC INFORMATION

DEFINITION

Plantar fasciitis is a common, painful inflammation or degeneration of the plantar fascia, a tissue that extends from the calcaneus to the proximal phalanges of each toe.

SYNONYMS

Painful heel syndrome
Painful heel spur

ICD-9CM CODES
728.71 Plantar fasciitis
726.73 Calcaneal spur

EPIDEMIOLOGY & DEMOGRAPHICS

PREVALENT SEX: Males = females
Bilateral in 10% to 20% of cases

PHYSICAL FINDINGS & CLINICAL PRESENTATION

- Pain is characteristically worse on arising and after periods of rest; "warming up" often lessens the pain
- Local tenderness at site involvement, usually the medial tubercle of the calcaneus, sometimes in the midfascia
- Pain sometimes elicited by passive dorsiflexion of toes and ankle, which stretches the plantar fascia
- A tight heel cord may be present

ETIOLOGY

- Uncertain
- Inflammation, microscopic tears, and/or degeneration
- The role of the calcaneal traction osteophyte (spur) is unclear
- May be associated with tight heel cord

DIAGNOSIS

DIFFERENTIAL DIAGNOSIS

- Other regional tendonitis
- Stress fracture
- Tarsal tunnel syndrome
- Tumor, infection

IMAGING STUDIES

Traction osteophyte or minor soft tissue calcification may be present on plain radiography. Other studies are usually not required.

TREATMENT

- Sensible activity restriction
- Gentle stretching exercises
- NSAIDS
- Local steroid/lidocaine injections (Fig. 1-31)
- Heel lift
- Night brace, daytime cast brace

DISPOSITION

Disorder is usually self-limited, although full recovery may take 1 to 2 yr.

REFERRAL

- If symptoms fail to respond to medical management
- For surgical consideration (plantar fascia release, excision of osteophyte)

PEARLS & CONSIDERATIONS

COMMENTS

- Various cushions and heel cups are generally ineffective because stretching, not heel strikes, is probably cause of disorder.
- Surgical intervention is rarely necessary.
- Shock wave therapy is of unproven benefit.

SUGGESTED READINGS

Aldridge J: Diagnosing heel pain in adults, *Am Fam Physician* 70:332, 2004.

Bachbinder R et al: Ultrasound-guided extracorporeal shockwave therapy for plantar fasciitis, *JAMA* 288:1364, 2002.

Bachbinder R: Plantar fasciitis, *N Engl J Med* 350:2159, 2004.

DiGiovanni BF et al: Tissue specific plantar fascia stretching exercises enhances outcomes in patients with chronic heel pain, *J Bone Joint Surg* 85:1270, 2003.

Haake M et al: Extra-corporeal shockwave therapy for plantar fasciitis: randomized controlled multicentre trial, *Br Med J* 327:75, 2003.

Riddle DL et al: Risk factors for plantar fasciitis: a matched case-control study, *J Bone Joint Surg* 85:872, 2003.

Rompe JD et al: Evaluation of low-energy extracorporeal shockwave application for chronic plantar fasciitis, *J Bone Joint Surg* 84(A):335, 2002.

Young CC et al: Treatment of plantar fasciitis, *Am Fam Physician* 63:467, 2001.

AUTHOR: **LONNIE R. MERCIER, M.D.**

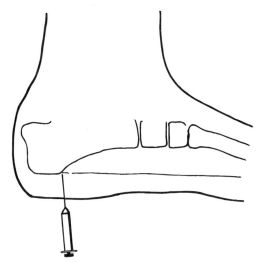

FIGURE 1-31 Injection site for plantar fasciitis. Injection should be through the sole into the area of maximum tenderness. A 25- or 27-gauge needle should be used and the medication injected slowly as some pain may occur. The total volume should be no greater than 1.5 ml. (From Mercier L: *Practical orthopedics*, ed 5, St Louis, 2002, Mosby.)

BASIC INFORMATION

DEFINITION

Aspiration pneumonia is a lung infection caused by bacterial organisms aspirated from nasopharyngeal space.

ICD-9CM CODES
507.0 Aspiration pneumonia

EPIDEMIOLOGY & DEMOGRAPHICS

INCIDENCE (IN U.S.):
- Few reliable data
- 20% to 35% of all pneumonias
- 5% to 15% of all community acquired pneumonias

PREVALENCE (IN U.S.): Unreliable data
PREDOMINANT SEX: Equal
PREDOMINANT AGE: Elderly
PEAK INCIDENCE: Elderly patients in hospitals or nursing homes

PHYSICAL FINDINGS & CLINICAL PRESENTATION

- Shortness of breath, tachypnea, cough, sputum, fever after vomiting, or difficulty swallowing
- Rales, rhonchi, often diffusely throughout lung

ETIOLOGY

Complex interaction of etiologies, ranging from chemical (often acid) pneumonitis following aspiration of sterile gastric contents (generally not requiring antibiotic treatment) to bacterial aspiration

COMMUNITY-ACQUIRED ASPIRATION PNEUMONIA:
- Generally results from predominantly anaerobic mouth bacteria (anaerobic and microaerophilic streptococci, fusobacteria, gram-positive anaerobic non–spore-forming rods), *Bacteroides* species *(melaninogenicus, intermedius, oralis, ureolyticus),* *Haemophilus influenzae,* and *Streptococcus pneumoniae*
- Rarely caused by *Bacteroides fragilis* (of uncertain validity in published studies) or *Eikenella corrodens*
- High-risk groups: elderly, alcoholics, IV drug users, patients who are obtunded, those with esophageal disorders, seizures, poor dentition, stroke victims, or recent dental manipulations

HOSPITAL-ACQUIRED ASPIRATION PNEUMONIA:
- Often occurs among elderly patients and others with diminished gag reflex; those with nasogastric tubes, intestinal obstruction, or ventilator support; and especially those exposed to contaminated nebulizers or unsterile suctioning
- High-risk groups: seriously ill hospitalized patients (especially patients with coma, acidosis, alcoholism, uremia, diabetes mellitus, nasogastric intubation, or recent antimicrobial therapy, who are frequently colonized with aerobic gram-negative rods); patients undergoing anesthesia; those with strokes, dementia, swallowing disorders; the frail elderly; and those receiving antacids or H_2 blockers (but not sucralfate)
- Hypoxic patients receiving concentrated O_2 have diminished ciliary activity, encouraging aspiration
- Causative organisms:
  1. Anaerobes listed previously, although in many studies gram-negative aerobes (60%) and gram-positive aerobes (20%) predominate
  2. *E. coli, P. aeruginosa, S. aureus, Klebsiella, Enterobacter, Serratia,* and *Proteus* spp. *H. influenzae, S. pneumoniae, Legionella,* and *Acinetobacter* spp. (sporadic pneumonias) in two thirds of cases
  3. Fungi, including *Candida albicans,* in fewer than 1%

DIAGNOSIS

DIFFERENTIAL DIAGNOSIS

- Other necrotizing or cavitary pneumonias (especially tuberculosis, gram-negative pneumonias)
- See "Pulmonary Tuberculosis"

WORKUP

- Chest x-ray examination
- CBC, blood cultures
- Sputum Gram stain and culture
- Consideration of tracheal aspirate

LABORATORY TESTS

- CBC: leukocytosis often present
- Sputum Gram stain
  1. Often useful when carefully prepared immediately after obtaining suctioned or expectorated specimen, examined by experienced observer.
  2. Only specimens with multiple WBCs and rare or absent epithelial cells should be examined.
  3. Unlike nonaspiration pneumonias (e.g., pneumococcal), multiple organisms may be present.
  4. Long, slender rods suggest anaerobes.
  5. Sputum from pneumonia caused by acid aspiration may be devoid of organisms.
  6. Cultures should be interpreted in light of morphology of visualized organisms.

IMAGING STUDIES

- Chest x-ray examination often reveals bilateral, diffuse, patchy infiltrates, in posterior segment upper lobes or at the bases.
- Aspiration pneumonias of several days' or longer duration may reveal necrosis (especially community-acquired anaerobic pneumonias) and even cavitation with air-fluid levels, indicating lung abscess.

TREATMENT ℞

NONPHARMACOLOGIC THERAPY

- Airway management to prevent repeated aspiration—swallowing evaluation (may include a modified barium swallow test)
- Ventilatory support if necessary
- NPO and G-tube feeding do not effectively prevent aspiration

ACUTE GENERAL Rx

Acute aspiration of acidic gastric contents without bacteria may not require antibiotic therapy; consult infectious diseases or pulmonary expert.

FOR COMMUNITY-ACQUIRED ANAEROBIC ASPIRATION PNEUMONIA:
- Levofloxacin 500 mg qd or ceftriaxone 1 to 2 g/day

NURSING HOME ASPIRATIONS:
- Levofloxacin 500 mg qd or piperacillin-tazobactam 3.375 g q6h or ceftazidime 2 g q8h

HOSPITAL-ACQUIRED ASPIRATION PNEUMONIA:
- Piperacillin-tazobactam 3.375 g IV q6h, or clindamycin 450-900 mg IV q8h, or cefoxitin 2 g IV q8h
- Knowledge of resident flora in the microenvironment of the aspiration within the hospital is crucial to intelligent antibiotic selection; consult infection control nurses or hospital epidemiologist.
- Confirmed *Pseudomonas* pneumonia should be treated with antipseudomonal β-lactam agent plus an aminoglycoside until antimicrobial sensitivities confirm that less toxic agents may replace aminoglycoside.
- Do not use metronidazole alone for anaerobes.

DISPOSITION

Repeat chest x-ray examination in 6 to 8 wk.

REFERRAL

For consultation with infectious disease and/or pulmonary experts for patients with respiratory distress, hypoxia, ventilatory support, pneumonia in more than one lobe, necrosis or cavitation on x-ray examination, or not responding to antibiotic therapy within 2 to 3 days

SUGGESTED READING

Marik PE: Aspiration pneumonitis and aspiration pneumonia, *N Engl J Med* 344:665, 2001.

AUTHOR: **BETH J. WUTZ, M.D.**

BASIC INFORMATION

DEFINITION

Bacterial pneumonia is an infection involving the lung parenchyma

ICD-9CM CODES
486.0 Pneumonia, acute
507.0 Pneumonia, aspiration
482.9 Pneumonia, bacterial
481 Pneumonia, pneumococcal
482.1 Pneumonia, *Pseudomonas*
482.4 Pneumonia, staphylococcal
428.0 Pneumonia, *Klebsiella*
482.2 Pneumonia, *Haemophilus influenzae*

EPIDEMIOLOGY & DEMOGRAPHICS

- Incidence of community-acquired pneumonia is 1/100 persons.
- Incidence of nosocomial pneumonia is 8 cases/1000 persons/yr.
- Primary care physicians see an average of 10 cases of pneumonia annually.
- Hospitalization rate for pneumonia is 15% to 20%.
- Most cases of pneumonia occur in the winter and in elderly patients.

PHYSICAL FINDINGS & CLINICAL PRESENTATION

- Fever, tachypnea, chills, tachycardia, cough
- Presentation varies with the cause of pneumonia, the patient's age, and the clinical situation:
  1. Patients with streptococcal pneumonia usually present with high fever, shaking chills, pleuritic chest pain, cough, and copious production of purulent sputum.
  2. Elderly or immunocompromised hosts may initially present with only minimal symptoms (e.g., low-grade fever, confusion); respiratory and nonrespiratory symptoms are less commonly reported by older patients with pneumonia.
  3. Generally, auscultation reveals crackles and diminished breath sounds.
  4. Percussion dullness is present if the patient has pleural effusion.

ETIOLOGY

- *Streptococcus pneumoniae*
- *Haemophilus influenzae*
- *Legionella pneumophila* (1% to 5% of adult pneumonias)
- *Klebsiella, Pseudomonas, E. coli*
- *Staphylococcus aureus*
- Pneumococcal infection is responsible for 50% to 75% of community-acquired pneumonias, whereas gram-negative organisms cause >80% of nosocomial pneumonias

- Predisposing factors are:
  1. COPD: *H. influenzae, S. pneumoniae, Legionella*
  2. Seizures: aspiration pneumonia
  3. Compromised hosts: *Legionella,* gram-negative organisms
  4. Alcoholism: *Klebsiella, S. pneumoniae, H. influenzae*
  5. HIV: *S. pneumoniae*
  6. IV drug addicts with right-sided bacterial endocarditis: *S. aureus*

DIAGNOSIS

DIFFERENTIAL DIAGNOSIS

- Exacerbation of chronic bronchitis
- Pulmonary embolism or infarction
- Lung neoplasm
- Bronchiolitis
- Sarcoidosis
- Hypersensitivity pneumonitis
- Pulmonary edema
- Drug-induced lung injury
- Viral pneumonias
- Fungal pneumonias
- Parasitic pneumonias
- Atypical pneumonia
- Tuberculosis

WORKUP

Laboratory evaluation and chest x-ray examination

LABORATORY TESTS

- In hospitalized patients, attempt to obtain an adequate sputum specimen for Gram stain and cultures.
  1. An expectorated sputum sample is often inadequate because of many false positive results (secondary to contamination from oral flora) and many false negative results; a specimen may be considered adequate if the Gram stain shows >25 PMNs and <10 epithelial cells per low-power field.
  2. Aerosol induction with hypertonic saline solution (3% to 10%) may increase the diagnostic yield of sputum.
  3. The use of fiberoptic bronchoscopy to obtain a sputum sample is generally reserved for critically ill patients responding poorly to initial antimicrobial therapy.
  4. Gram stain of sputum may reveal the following:
  Lancet-shaped, gram-positive cocci indicate streptococcal pneumonia.
  Pleomorphic, small coccobacillary, gram-negative organisms indicate *H. influenzae.*
  Encapsulated gram-negative bacilli: *K. pneumoniae*
- WBC count is elevated, usually with left shift

- Blood cultures: positive in approximately 20% of cases of pneumococcal pneumonia
- Pulse oximetry or ABGs: hypoxemia with partial pressure of oxygen <60 mm Hg while the patient is breathing room air is a standard criterion for hospital admission
- Direct immunofluorescent examination of sputum when suspecting *Legionella* (e.g., direct fluorescent antibody [DFA] stain is a highly specific and rapid test for detecting legionellae in clinical specimen)
- Serologic testing for HIV in selected patients

IMAGING STUDIES

Chest x-ray: findings vary with the stage and type of pneumonia and the hydration of the patient (Fig. 1-32).
- Classically, pneumococcal pneumonia presents with a segmental lobe infiltrate.
- Diffuse infiltrates on chest x-ray can be seen with *L. pneumophila, M. pneumoniae,* viral pneumonias, *P. carinii,* miliary TB, aspiration, aspergillosis.
- An initial chest x-ray is also useful to rule out the presence of any complications (pneumothorax, empyema, abscesses).

TREATMENT

NONPHARMACOLOGIC THERAPY

- Avoidance of tobacco use
- Oxygen to maintain partial oxygen pressure in arterial blood >60 mm Hg
- IV hydration, correction of dehydration
- Assisted ventilation in patients with significant respiratory failure

ACUTE GENERAL Rx

- Initial antibiotic therapy should be based on clinical, radiographic, and laboratory evaluation.
- Macrolides (azithromycin or clarithromycin) or levofloxacin is recommended for empirical out-patient treatment of community-acquired pneumonia; cefotaxime or a beta-lactam/beta-lactamase inhibitor can be added in patients with more severe presentation who insist on out-patient therapy. Duration of treatment ranges from 7 to 14 days.
- In the hospital setting, patients admitted to the general ward can be treated empirically with a second- or third-generation cephalosporin (ceftriaxone, ceftizoxime, cefotaxime, or cefuroxime) plus a macrolide (azithromycin or clarithromycin) or doxycycline. An antipseudomonal quinolone (levo-

floxacin, moxifloxacin, or gatifloxacin) may be substituted in place of the macrolide or doxycycline.

- In hospitalized patients at risk for *P. aeruginosa* infection, empirical treatment should consist of an antipseudomonal beta-lactam (cefepime or piperacillin-tazobactam) *plus* an aminoglycoside *plus* an antipseudomonal quinolone or macrolide.

CHRONIC Rx

Parapneumonic effusion-empyema can be managed with chest tube placement for drainage. Instillation of fibrinolytic agents (streptokinase, urokinase) via the chest tube may be necessary in resistant cases.

DISPOSITION

- Most patients respond well to antibiotic therapy.
- Indications for hospital admission are:
  1. Hypoxemia (oxygen saturation <90% while patient is breathing room air)
  2. Hemodynamic instability
  3. Inability to tolerate medications
  4. Active co-existing condition requiring hospitalization
- The decision to treat a nursing home patient at the facility or in the hospital depends on the condition of the patient (e.g., stable vital signs and ability to maintain O_2 sat above 90%), the resources available at the nursing home (e.g., staffing, access to IV therapy), and the overall plan of care for the patient (e.g., advance directives).

PEARLS & CONSIDERATIONS

COMMENTS

Causes of slowly resolving or nonresolving pneumonia:

- Difficult to treat infections: viral pneumonia, *Legionella*, pneumococci, or staphylococci with impaired host response, TB, fungi
- Neoplasm: lung, lymphoma, metastasis
- CHF
- Pulmonary embolism
- Immunologic or idiopathic: Wegener's granulomatosis, pulmonary eosinophilic syndromes, SLE
- Drug toxicity (e.g., amiodarone)

SUGGESTED READINGS

Davidson R et al: Resistance to levofloxacin and failure of treatment of pneumococcal pneumonia, *N Engl J Med* 346:747, 2002.

Halm EA, Teirstein AS: Management of community-acquired pneumonia, *N Engl J Med* 347:2039, 2002.

AUTHOR: **FRED F. FERRI, M.D.**

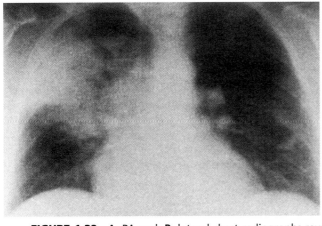 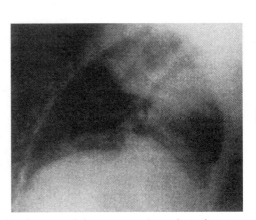

FIGURE 1-32   **A,** PA and, **B,** lateral chest radiographs reveal right upper lobe pneumonia and patchy left lower lobe infiltrate. A variety of organisms can produce this pattern, including *S. pneumoniae* and *H. influenzae.* (From Marx J [ed]: Rosen's *Emergency medicine,* ed 5, St Louis, 2003, Mosby.)

BASIC INFORMATION

DEFINITION

Polymyalgia rheumatica is a disorder of unknown cause affecting older patients. It is characterized by shoulder and hip stiffness and an elevated erythrocyte sedimentation rate (ESR).

SYNONYMS

Anarthritic rheumatoid syndrome

ICD-9CM CODES
725.0 Polymyalgia rheumatica

EPIDEMIOLOGY & DEMOGRAPHICS

PREVALENCE: 1 case/135 persons >50 yr old
PREDOMINANT SEX: Female:male ratio of 2:1
PREDOMINANT AGE: Average age at onset: 70 yr

PHYSICAL FINDINGS & CLINICAL PRESENTATION

- Symptoms are frequently of sudden onset but are often present for months before the diagnosis is made.
- Neck, shoulder, low back, and thigh pain are common complaints.
- Morning stiffness lasting 2 to 3 hr is typical, and patients often have difficulty getting out of bed.
- Malaise, weight loss, depression, and a low-grade fever are common constitutional symptoms and may suggest systemic inflammation.
- Physical findings are usually limited. Synovitis may be present in peripheral joints and may also be responsible for the proximal girdle symptoms in spite of the fact that they appear to be "muscular" in nature.
- Mild soft tissue tenderness may be present.
- Distal extremity manifestations (knee, wrist, metacarpophalangeal joints) may occur in 25% to 45% of patients.
- The temporal arteries should be carefully examined because of the strong relation of polymyalgia rheumatica with temporal or giant cell arteritis.

ETIOLOGY

Unknown

DIAGNOSIS

DIFFERENTIAL DIAGNOSIS
(Table 1-12)

- Rheumatoid arthritis: rheumatoid factor is negative in polymyalgia.
- Polymyositis: enzyme studies are negative in polymyalgia.
- Fibromyalgia

WORKUP

The diagnosis of polymyalgia rheumatica is suggested by the following findings:
- Pain and stiffness of pectoral and pelvic musculature
- Patient >50 yr old
- Morning stiffness >1 hr
- Normal motor strength
- Symptoms for at least 4 to 6 wk
- Elevated ESR (>45)
- Rapid clinical response to low-dose corticosteroid therapy

LABORATORY TESTS

- CBC, ESR, and rheumatoid factor should be performed.
- Mild anemia may be present.

TREATMENT

ACUTE GENERAL Rx

- Prednisone 10 to 20 mg/day is given. The response is often so dramatic that it can be used to confirm the diagnosis. Improvement is usually noted within 24 to 48 hr. Generally, if the initial prednisone dose is 20 mg/day, reduce by 2.5 mg every wk to 10 mg/day, then by 1 mg/day every month if tolerated.
- Steroids are gradually tapered over the next few weeks as soon as symptoms permit, but small doses (5 mg/day) may be needed for 2 yr.
- NSAIDs may be tried in mild cases.
- Physical therapy is usually unnecessary.

PEARLS & CONSIDERATIONS

COMMENTS

The prognosis is generally favorable. Relapse occasionally occurs in several years, but again responds well to prednisone.

TABLE 1-12 Differential Features in Polymyalgia Rheumatica and Similar Disorders

Signs/Symptoms	Polymyalgia Rheumatica	Giant Cell Arteritis	Rheumatoid Arthritis	Dermatomyositis	Fibromyalgia
Morning stiffness >30 min	+	±	+*	±	Variable
Headache and/or scalp tenderness	0	+	0	0	Variable
Pain with active joint movement	+	0	+*	0	Inconstant
Tender joints	±	0	+*	0	Tender spots
Swollen joints	±	±	+	0	0
Muscle weakness	±†	0	+*	+	0
Normochromic anemia	+	+	+	0	0
Elevated erythrocyte sedimentation rate	+	+	+	±	0
Elevated serum creatine kinase	0	0	0	+	0
Serum rheumatoid factor	0	0	70%	0	0
Distinct electromyographic abnormality	0	0	0	+	0
Response to nonsteroidal antiinflammatory drug	±	0	+	0	0

From Goldman L, Ausiello D, (eds): *Cecil textbook of medicine*, ed 22, Philadelphia, 2004, WB Saunders.
0, Absent; +, present; ±, present in minority of cases.
*Associated with affected joints
†Pain inhibits movement. Disuse atrophy may occur.

SUGGESTED READINGS

Cimmino MA, Macchioni P et al: Pulse steroid treatment of polymyalgia rheumatica, *Clin Exp Rheumatol* 22(3):381, 2004.

Clough JD: Polymyalgia rheumatica: not well understood, but important to consider, *Cleve Clin J Med* 71(6):446, 2004.

Cohen MD, Abril A: Polymyalgia rheumatica revisited, *Bull Rheum Dis* 50:1, 2001.

De Jager JP: Polymyalgia rheumatica and giant cell arteritis: avoiding management traps, *Aust Fam Physician* 30:643, 2001.

Mandell BF: Polymyalgia rheumatica: clinical presentation is key to diagnosis and treatment, *Cleve Clin J Med* 71(6):489, 2004.

Marti J, Anton E: Polymyalgia rheumatica complication influenza vaccination, *J Am Geriatr Soc* 52(8):1412, 2004.

Meskimen S, Cook TD, Blake RL: Management of giant cell arteritis and polymyalgia rheumatica, *Am Fam Physician* 61:2061, 2000.

Salvarani C et al: Polymyalgia rheumatica and giant-cell arteritis, *N Engl J Med* 347:261, 2002.

AUTHOR: **LONNIE R. MERCIER, M.D.**

BASIC INFORMATION

DEFINITION

Prostate cancer is a neoplasm involving the prostate; various classifications have been developed to evaluate malignancy potential and prognosis:

- The degree of malignancy varies with the stage:

Stage A: Confined to the prostate, no nodule palpable

Stage B: Palpable nodule confined to the gland

Stage C: Local extension

Stage D: Regional lymph nodes or distant metastases

- In the Gleason classification, histologic patterns are independently assigned numbers 1 to 5 (best to least differentiated). These numbers are added to give a total tumor score:
  1. Prognosis is generally good if score is ≤5.
  2. Score of 6, 7, or 8 carries an intermediate prognosis.
  3. Score ≥9 correlates with anaplastic lesions with poor prognosis.

ICD-9CM CODES
185 Malignant neoplasm of prostate

EPIDEMIOLOGY & DEMOGRAPHICS

- Prostate cancer has surpassed lung cancer as the most common nonskin cancer in men.
- More than 100,000 cases are diagnosed yearly, and nearly 30,000 men die from prostate cancer each year (second leading cause of death from cancer in U.S. men).
- Incidence of prostate cancer increases with age: 80% of new cases are diagnosed in patients ≥65 yr.
- Average age at time of diagnosis is 72 yr.
- Blacks in the U.S. have the highest incidence of prostate cancer in the world (one in every nine males).
- Incidence is low in Asians.
- Approximately 9% of all prostate cancers may be familial.

PHYSICAL FINDINGS & CLINICAL PRESENTATION

- Generally silent disease until it reaches advanced stages.
- Bone pain and pathologic fractures may be initial symptoms of prostate cancer.
- Local growth can cause symptoms of urinary outflow obstruction.
- Digital rectal examination (DRE) may reveal an area of increased firmness. An asymmetric prostate is also suspicious for cancer. 10% of patients will have a negative DRE.

- Prostate may be hard, fixed, with extension of tumor to the seminal vesicles in advanced stages.

DIAGNOSIS

DIFFERENTIAL DIAGNOSIS

- Benign prostatic hypertrophy
- Prostatitis
- Prostate stones

LABORATORY TESTS

- Measurement of PSA is useful in early diagnosis of prostate cancer (screening) and in monitoring response to therapy as well as an early sign of recurrence. Normal PSA is found in >20% of patients with prostate cancer (lack of sensitivity), whereas only 20% of men with PSA levels between 4 ng/ml and 10 ng/ml have prostate cancer (lack of specificity). PSA >10 ng/ml is associated with more advanced prostate cancer. The American Cancer Society recommends offering the PSA test and digital rectal examination yearly to men 50 years or older who have a life expectancy of at least 10 years. Earlier testing, starting at age 40, is recommended for men at high risk (e.g., African Americans and men with a family history of prostate cancer). The most common causes of false-positive PSA are BPH, prostatitis, and ejaculation within 48 hours of testing. Rectal exam causes only a minimal rise in PSA (of 0.2 ng/ml over baseline). Finasteride and dutasteride reduce PSA values by 50%.
- Ideally, prostate cancer should be diagnosed when the PSA is between 4 and 10 mg/ml (between 2.6 and 10 ng/ml for African American men). Unfortunately, in this range of PSA, many men do not have cancer (false-positive test) and prostate biopsies are invasive, uncomfortable, and themselves subject to false-negative results from sampling. To cope with this, many clinicians use the PSA velocity concept. In the absence of cancer, the PSA rises slowly over time in a linear pattern. With cancer, the rate of PSA increase can be exponential. Instead of repeating the PSA annually when the result is between 4 and 10 mg/ml, it is repeated every 3 months until a pattern of increase can be ascertained. Also, PSA should not rise by more than 0.85 mg/ml per year and should take 4 years to double in the absence of cancer.
- The use of serum-free PSA for prostate screening has been proposed by some urologists as a means to decrease unwarranted biopsies without missing a significant number of prostate cancers. This approach is based on the higher

free PSA in men with benign prostatic hyperplasia and the higher protein-bound PSA levels in men with prostate cancer. For example, in men with total PSA levels of 4 to 10 ng/ml, the cancer probability is 0.25, but if the percentage of free PSA is <10%, the probability of cancer increases to 0.45, and if the percentage of free PSA is >25%, the probability of cancer decreases to 8%.

- If the PSA is <2 mg/ml in non–African American men, the frequency of screening can drop from yearly to every 2 years.
- If the DRE reveals a suspicious prostate for cancer, referral to a urologist for prostate biopsy is appropriate regardless of PSA level.
- Prostatic acid phosphatase (PAP) can be used for evaluation of nonlocalized disease.
- Transrectal biopsy and fine-needle aspiration of prostate can confirm the diagnosis.

IMAGING STUDIES

- According to the AUA screening, transrectal ultrasonography adds little to the combination of PSA and digital rectal examination.
- Bone scan is useful to evaluate bone metastasis. However, according to the American Urological Association (AUA), the routine use of bone scanning is not required for staging of prostate cancer in asymptomatic men with clinically localized cancer if the PSA level is ≤20 ng/ml.
- CT scan, MRI, and transrectal ultrasonography may be useful in selected patients to assess extent of prostate cancer. CT and MRI imaging are generally not indicated for cancer staging in men with clinically localized cancer and PSA <25 ng/ml. With regard to pelvic lymph node dissection in staging, the AUA states that it may not be required in patients with PSA levels <10 ng/ml and when PSA level is <20 ng/ml and the Gleason score is <6. High-resolution MRI with magnetic nanoparticles has been used for the detection of small and otherwise undetectable lymph node metastases in patients with prostate cancer.

TREATMENT

NONPHARMACOLOGIC THERAPY

Watchful waiting is reasonable in patients with early stage (T-IA) and projected life expectancy <10 yr, or in patients with focal and moderately differentiated carcinoma.

ACUTE GENERAL Rx

- Therapeutic approach varies with the following:
  1. Stage of the tumor
  2. Patient's life expectancy
  3. General medical condition
  4. Patient's treatment preference (e.g., patient may be opposed to orchiectomy)
- The optimal treatment of clinically localized prostate cancer is unclear.
  1. Radical prostatectomy is generally performed in patients with localized prostate cancer and life expectancy >10 yr.
  2. Radiation therapy (external beam irradiation or implantation of radioactive pellets [seeds]) represents an alternative in patients with localized prostate cancer, especially poor surgical candidates or patients with a high-grade malignancy.
  3. Watchful waiting is reasonable in patients who are too old or too ill to survive longer than 10 yr. If the cancer progresses to the point where it becomes symptomatic, palliation can be attempted with several methods.
- Patients with advanced disease and projected life expectancy <10 yr are candidates for radiation therapy and hormonal therapy (DES, LHRH analogs, antiandrogens, bilateral orchiectomy).
- Recommended treatment of patients with regional metastatic prostate cancer with projected life expectancy ≥10 yr includes radical prostatectomy, radiation therapy, hormonal therapy.
- Androgen-deprivation therapy with a gonadotropin-releasing hormone agonist is the mainstay of treatment for metastatic prostate cancer. Adjuvant treatment with GnRH agonists (goserelin leuprolide, or triptorelin) plus antiandrogens (flutamide, bicalutamide, or nilutamide), when started simultaneously with external irradiation, improves local control and survival in patients with locally advanced prostate cancer. Bisphosphonates inhibit osteoclast-mediated bone resorption and prevent bone loss in the hip and lumbar spine in men receiving treatment for prostate cancer with a GnRH.

CHRONIC Rx

- Patients should be monitored at 3- to 6-mo intervals with clinical examination, and PSA for the first year, then every 6 mo for the second year, then yearly if stable. For patients who have undergone radical prostatectomy, a rising PSA level suggests evidence of residual or recurrent prostate cancer.
- Chest x-ray examination, bone scan should be performed yearly or sooner if patient develops symptoms.

DISPOSITION

- Prognosis varies with the stage of the disease and the Gleason classification (see Definition & Classification).
- The ploidy of the tumor also has prognostic value: prognosis is better with diploid tumor cells, worse with aneuploid tumor cells.
- For Stage A tumors, the extended 10-yr, disease-specific survival is similar for patients with prostatectomy (94%), radiotherapy (90%), and conservative management (93%); survival rate is better with surgery than with radiotherapy or conservative management in patients with Stage B or C localized prostate cancer.
- Expression of the gene EZH2 has been identified as an important factor in the determination of the aggressiveness of prostate cancer. A recent study revealed that expression of the EZH2 gene may be a better predictor of clinical failure than Gleason score, tumor stage, or surgical margin status. Testing for EZH2 protein in prostate cancer tissue may be useful to determine prognosis and direct treatment.

SUGGESTED READINGS

Gann PH et al: Strategies combining total and percent free prostate specific antigen for detecting prostate cancer: a perspective evaluation, *J Urol* 167:2427, 2002.

Harisinghani MG et al: Noninvasive detection of clinically occult lymph-node metastases in prostate cancer, *N Engl J Med* 348:2491, 2003.

Homberg L et al: A randomized trial comparing radical prostatectomy with watchful waiting in early prostate cancer, *N Engl J Med* 347:781, 2002.

Makinen T et al: Family history and prostate cancer screening with prostate specific antigen, *J Clin Oncol* 20:2658, 2002.

Nelson WG: Prostate cancer, *N Engl J Med* 349:366, 2003.

Steineck G et al: Quality of life after radical prostatectomy or watchful waiting, *N Engl J Med* 347:790, 2002.

Varambally S et al: The polycarb group protein EZH2 is involved in progression of prostate cancer, *Nature* 419:624, 2002.

AUTHORS: **FRED F. FERRI, M.D.,** and **TOM J. WACHTEL, M.D.**

BASIC INFORMATION

DEFINITION

Prostatitis refers to inflammation of the prostate gland. There are four major categories:
- Acute bacterial prostatitis
- Chronic bacterial prostatitis
- Nonbacterial prostatitis
- Prostatodynia

ICD-9CM CODES
601.0 Prostatitis (acute)
601.1 Prostatitis (chronic)
099.54 Prostatitis (chlamydial)

EPIDEMIOLOGY & DEMOGRAPHICS

- 50% of men experience symptoms of prostatitis in their lifetime
- Acute bacterial prostatitis is uncommon
- The relative prevalence of the other three entities among men with inflammatory prostatic symptoms is:
  1. 5% to 10% chronic bacterial prostatitis
  2. 10% to 65% nonbacterial prostatitis
  3. 30% to 80% prostatodynia

The figures are imprecise because nonbacterial prostatitis and prostatodynia are very difficult to differentiate.

PHYSICAL FINDINGS & CLINICAL PRESENTATION

ACUTE BACTERIAL PROSTATITIS:
- Sudden or rapidly progressive onset of:
  1. Dysuria
  2. Frequency
  3. Urgency
  4. Nocturia
  5. Perineal pain that may radiate to the back, the rectum, or the penis
- Hematuria or a purulent urethral discharge may occur.
- Occasionally urinary retention complicates the course.
- Fever, chills, and signs of sepsis can also be part of the clinical picture.
- On rectal examination the prostate is typically tender.

CHRONIC BACTERIAL PROSTATITIS:
- May be asymptomatic when the infection is confined to the prostate
- May present as an increase in severity of baseline symptoms of benign prostatic hypertrophy
- When cystitis is also present, urinary frequency, urgency, and burning may be reported
- Hematuria may be a presenting complaint
- In elderly men, new onset of urinary incontinence may be noted

NONBACTERIAL PROSTATITIS AND PROSTATODYNIA:
- Present similarly with symptoms of bladder irritation (urinary frequency, urgency, dysuria, increase in nocturia episodes) and perineal discomfort
- The symptoms can be of variable severity, but tend to be more bothersome in prostatodynia

ETIOLOGY

ACUTE BACTERIAL PROSTATITIS:
- Acute usually gram-negative infection of the prostate gland
  1. Generally associated with cystitis
  2. Resulting from the ascent of bacteria in the urethra
- Occasionally the route of infection is hematogenous or a lymphatogenous spread of rectal bacteria
- The condition is more likely to occur in young or middle-aged men

CHRONIC BACTERIAL PROSTATITIS:
- Often asymptomatic
- Exacerbation of symptoms of benign prostatic hypertrophy caused by the same mechanism as in acute bacterial prostatitis

NONBACTERIAL PROSTATITIS:
- Refers to symptoms of prostatic inflammation associated with the presence of WBCs in prostatic secretions with no identifiable bacterial organism
- Chlamydia infection may be etiologically implicated in some cases

PROSTATODYNIA:
- Refers to symptoms of prostatic inflammation with no or few WBCs in the prostatic secretion
- Spasm in the bladder neck or urethra is felt to be the cause of symptoms

DIAGNOSIS **Dx**

DIFFERENTIAL DIAGNOSIS
- Benign prostatic hypertrophy with lower urinary tract symptoms
- Prostate cancer
- Also see differential diagnosis of hematuria

WORKUP
- Rectal examination
  1. Tender prostate most suggestive of acute bacterial prostatitis
  2. Enlarged prostate common in chronic bacterial prostatitis
  3. Normal prostate is consistent with chronic bacterial and nonbacterial prostatitis and is typical in prostatodynia
- Expression of prostatic secretions (EPS) by prostate massage is contraindicated in acute bacterial prostatitis but is appropriate in the other three situations

LABORATORY TESTS
- Urinalysis
- Urine culture and sensitivity
- Bacterial localization studies can be performed but are cumbersome and impractical in most clinical settings
- Cell count and culture of expressed prostatic secretions
- The yield of a urine culture may be increased if the specimen is obtained after a prostatic massage
- PSA is not used to diagnose prostatitis; however, a rapid rise over baseline should raise the possibility of prostatitis even in the absence of symptoms. In such cases, a follow-up PSA after treatment of prostatitis is appropriate
- CBC and blood cultures if fever, chills, or signs of sepsis exist
- If hematuria is present, a workup to rule out a urologic malignancy should be considered if the hematuria does not clear after treatment of prostatitis

TREATMENT

ACUTE BACTERIAL PROSTATITIS:
Culture guided antibiotic therapy for 4 wk (beginning with a few days of intravenous antibiotics if the infection is serious or if the patient is bacteremic).

CHRONIC BACTERIAL PROSTATITIS:
- Trimethoprim-sulfamethoxazole is first-line choice for 4 wk if the organism is sensitive.
- Second-line choice for treatment failure or organisms resistant to TMP-SMX is with a fluoroquinolone.
- Patient with refractory infection or with multiple relapses may be offered long-term suppressive therapy.

NONBACTERIAL PROSTATITIS AND PROSTATODYNIA:
- No specific treatment
- Antibiotics are not effective
- A trial of treatment with an α-adrenergic blocker (terazosin, doxazosin, or tamsulosin) may be considered
- Any underlying bladder pathology should be ruled out by cystoscopy and treated if identified

SUGGESTED READINGS

Fowler JE: Prostatitis. In Gillenwater JY et al (eds): *Adult and Pediatric Urology*, St Louis, 1996, Mosby.
McNaughton Collins M, MacDonald R, Wilt TJ: Diagnosis and treatment of chronic abacterial prostatitis: a systemic review, *Ann Intern Med* 133:367, 2000.

AUTHOR: **TOM J. WACHTEL, M.D.**

BASIC INFORMATION

DEFINITION

Pseudogout is one of the clinical patterns associated with a crystal-induced synovitis resulting from the deposition of calcium pyrophosphate dehydrate (CPPD) crystals in joint hyaline and fibrocartilage. The cartilage deposition is termed *chondrocalcinosis.*

SYNONYMS

Calcium pyrophosphate dehydrate crystal deposition disease (CPDD)
Chondrocalcinosis
Pyrophosphate arthropathy

ICD-9CM CODES
275.4 Chondrocalcinosis

EPIDEMIOLOGY & DEMOGRAPHICS

PREVALENCE:
- Uncertain
- Probably similar to gout (3/1000 persons)
- Chondrocalcinosis is present in >20% of all people at age 80 yr, but most are asymptomatic

PREDOMINANT SEX: Female:male ratio of approximately 1.5:1
PREVALENT AGE: 60 to 70 yr at onset

PHYSICAL FINDINGS & CLINICAL PRESENTATION

- Symptoms are similar to those of gouty arthritis with acute attacks and chronic arthritis
- Knee joint is most commonly affected
- Swelling, stiffness, and increased heat in affected joint

ETIOLOGY

- Unknown
- Often associated with various medical conditions, including hyperparathyroidism and amyloidosis

DIAGNOSIS

DIFFERENTIAL DIAGNOSIS

- Gouty arthritis
- Rheumatoid arthritis
- Osteoarthritis
- Neuropathic joint

Section II describes the differential diagnosis of acute monoarticular and oligoarticular arthritis and crystal-induced arthritides. An algorithm for evaluation of arthralgia is described in Section III, "Arthralgia Limited to One or Few Joints."

WORKUP

- Variable clinical presentation
- Diagnosis dependent on the identification of CPPD crystals
- The American Rheumatism Association revised diagnostic criteria for CPPD crystal deposition disease (pseudogout) are often used:

1. Criteria
   I. Demonstration of CPPD crystals (obtained by biopsy, necroscopy, or aspirated synovial fluid) by definitive means (e.g., characteristic "fingerprint" by x-ray diffraction powder pattern or by chemical analysis)
   II. (a) Identification of monoclinic and/or triclinic crystals showing either no or only a weakly positive birefringence by compensated polarized light microscopy (b) Presence of typical calcifications in roentgenograms
   III. (a) Acute arthritis, especially of knees or other large joints, with or without concomitant hyperuricemia
   (b) Chronic arthritis, especially of knees, hips, wrists, carpus, elbow, shoulder, and metacarpophalangeal joints, especially if accompanied by acute exacerbations; the following features are helpful in differentiating chronic arthritis from osteoarthritis:
      1. Uncommon site—for example, wrist, MCP, elbow, shoulder
      2. Appearance of lesion radiologically—for example, radiocarpal or patellofemoral joint space narrowing, especially if isolated (patella "wrapped around" the femur)
      3. Subchondral cyst formation
      4. Severity of degeneration—progressive, with subchondral bony collapse (microfractures), and fragmentation, with formation of intraarticular radiodense bodies
      5. Osteophyte formation—variable and inconstant
      6. Tendon calcifications, especially Achilles, triceps, obturators

2. Categories
   Definite—Criteria I or II(a) plus (b) must be fulfilled.
   Probable—Criteria II(a) or II(b) must be fulfilled.
   Possible—Criteria III(a) or (b) should alert the clinician to the possibility of underlying CPPD deposition.

LABORATORY TESTS

Crystal analysis of the synovial fluid aspirate to reveal rhomboid calcium pyrophosphate crystals

IMAGING STUDIES

Plain radiographs to reveal the following:
- Stippled calcification in bands running parallel to the subchondral bone margins
- Crystal deposition in menisci, synovium, and ligament tissue; triangular wrist cartilage and symphysis pubis are often affected

TREATMENT

NONPHARMACOLOGIC THERAPY

General measures such as heat, rest, and elevation as needed

ACUTE GENERAL Rx

- NSAIDs (as for gout)
- Colchicine
- Aspiration/steroid injection

DISPOSITION

Structural joint damage may occasionally occur, requiring arthroplasty in rare cases.

REFERRAL

For orthopedic consultation for destructive joint changes

PEARLS & CONSIDERATIONS

COMMENTS

As with gout, acute attacks may be triggered by various surgical or medical events.

SUGGESTED READINGS

Agudelo CA, Wise CM: Crystal-associated arthritis in the elderly, *Rheum Dis Clin North Am* 26:527, 2000.

Canhao H et al: Cross-sectional study of 50 patients with calcium pyrophosphate dihydrate crystal arthropathy, *Clin Rheumatol* 20:119, 2001.

Halverson PB, Derfus BA: Calcium crystal-induced inflammation, *Curr Opin Rheumatol* 13:221, 2001.

Mader B: Calcium pyrophosphate dihydrate deposition disease of the wrist, *Clin Rheumatol* 23(1):95, 2004.

Rosenthal AK: Crystal arthropathies and other unpopular rheumatic diseases, *Curr Opin Rheumatol* 16(3):262, 2004.

Sagarin MJ: Pseudogout, *Emerg Med* 18:373, 2000.

AUTHOR: **LONNIE R. MERCIER, M.D.**

BASIC INFORMATION

DEFINITION

Pseudomembranous colitis is the occurrence of diarrhea and bowel inflammation associated with antibiotic use.

SYNONYMS

Antibiotic-induced colitis
Clostridium dificile colitis

ICD-9CM CODES
008.45 *Clostridium difficile,*
      pseudomembranous colitis

EPIDEMIOLOGY & DEMOGRAPHICS

- Cephalosporins are the most frequent offending agent in pseudomembranous colitis because of their high rates of use.
- The antibiotic with the highest incidence is clindamycin (10% incidence of pseudomembranous colitis with its use).
- *Clostridium difficile* causes more than 250,000 cases of diarrhea and colitis in the U.S. every year.

PHYSICAL FINDINGS & CLINICAL PRESENTATION

- Abdominal tenderness (generalized or lower abdominal)
- Fever
- In patients with prolonged diarrhea, poor skin turgor, dry mucous membranes, and other signs of dehydration may be present

ETIOLOGY

Risk factors for *C. difficile* (the major identifiable agent of antibiotic-induced diarrhea and colitis):

- Administration of antibiotics: can occur with any antibiotic, but occurs most frequently with clindamycin, ampicillin, and cephalosporins
- Prolonged hospitalization
- Advanced age
- Abdominal surgery
- Hospitalized, tube-fed patients are at risk for *C. difficile*–associated diarrhea. Clinicians should consider testing for *C. difficile* in tube-fed patients with diarrhea unrelated to the feeding solution

DIAGNOSIS **Dx**

The clinical signs of pseudomembranous colitis generally include diarrhea, fever, and abdominal cramps following use of antibiotics.

DIFFERENTIAL DIAGNOSIS

- GI bacterial infections (e.g., *Salmonella, Shigella, Campylobacter, Yersinia*)
- Enteric parasites (e.g., *Cryptosporidium, Entamoeba histolytica*)
- IBD
- Celiac sprue
- Irritable bowel syndrome

WORKUP

- All patients with diarrhea accompanied by current or recent antibiotic use should be tested for *C. difficile* (see "Laboratory Tests").
- Sigmoidoscopy (without cleansing enema) may be necessary when the clinical and laboratory diagnosis is inconclusive and the diarrhea persists.
- In antibiotic-induced pseudomembranous colitis, the sigmoidoscopy often reveals raised white-yellow exudative plaques adherent to the colonic mucosa (Fig. 1-33).

LABORATORY TESTS

- *C. difficile* toxin can be detected by cytotoxin tissue-culture assay (gold standard for identifying *C. difficile* toxin in stool specimen) and by enzyme-linked immunoabsorbent assay (ELISA) for *C. difficile* toxins A and B. The latter is used most widely in the clinical setting. It has a sensitivity of 85% and a specificity of 100%.
- Fecal leukocytes (assessed by microscopy or lactoferrin assay) are generally present in stool samples.
- CBC usually reveals leukocytosis.

IMAGING STUDIES

Abdominal film (flat plate and upright) is useful in patients with abdominal pain or evidence of obstruction on physical examination.

TREATMENT **Rx**

NONPHARMACOLOGIC THERAPY

- Discontinue offending antibiotic
- Fluid hydration and correct electrolyte abnormalities

ACUTE GENERAL Rx

- Metronidazole 500 mg PO tid for 10 to 14 days
- Vancomycin 125 mg PO qid for 10 to 14 days in cases resistant to metronidazole
- Cholestyramine 4 g PO qid for 10 days in addition to metronidazole to control severe diarrhea (avoid use with vancomycin)
- When parenteral therapy is necessary (e.g., patient with paralytic ileus), IV metronidazole 500 mg qid can be used. It can also be supplemented with vancomycin 500 mg via NG tube or enema

CHRONIC Rx

Judicious future use of antibiotics to prevent recurrences (e.g., avoid prolonged antibiotic therapy)

DISPOSITION

Most patients recover completely with appropriate therapy. Fever resolves within 48 hr and diarrhea within 4 to 5 days. Mortality exceeds 10% in untreated patients.

REFERRAL

Hospital admission and IV hydration in severe cases

PEARLS & CONSIDERATIONS **(!)**

COMMENTS

Possible complications of pseudomembranous colitis include dehydration, bowel perforation, toxic megacolon, electrolyte imbalance, and reactive arthritis.

SUGGESTED READINGS

Bartlett JG: Antibiotic-associated diarrhea, *N Engl J Med* 346:334, 2002.
Hurley BW, Nguyen CC: The spectrum of pseudomembranous enterocolitis and antibiotic-associated diarrhea, *Arch Intern Med* 162:2177, 2002.

AUTHOR: **FRED F. FERRI, M.D.**

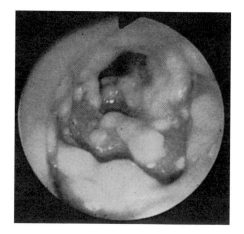

FIGURE 1-33 Pseudomembranous plaques seen with colonoscopy in a patient with *C. difficile*-associated PMC. (From Gorbach SL: *Infectious diseases,* ed 2, Philadelphia, 1998, WB Saunders.)

BASIC INFORMATION

DEFINITION

Pulmonary embolism (PE) refers to the lodging of a thrombus or other embolic material from a distant site in the pulmonary circulation.

SYNONYMS

Pulmonary thromboembolism
PE

ICD-9CM CODES

415.1 Pulmonary embolism and infarction

EPIDEMIOLOGY & DEMOGRAPHICS

- 650,000 cases of PE occur in the U.S. each year; 50,000 result in death (increased incidence in women and with advanced age).
- More than 90% of pulmonary emboli originate in the deep venous system of the lower extremities.
- Pulmonary thromboembolism is associated with >200,000 hospitalizations each year in the U.S.
- 8% to 10% of victims of PE die within the first hour.

PHYSICAL FINDINGS & CLINICAL PRESENTATION

- Most common symptom: dyspnea
- Chest pain: may be nonpleuritic or pleuritic (infarction)
- Syncope (massive PE)
- Fever, diaphoresis, apprehension
- Hemoptysis, cough
- Evidence of DVT may be present (e.g., swelling and tenderness of extremities)
- Cardiac examination: may reveal tachycardia, increased pulmonic component of S_2, murmur of tricuspid insufficiency, right ventricular heave, right-sided S_3
- Pulmonary examination: may demonstrate rales, localized wheezing, friction rub
- Most common physical finding: tachypnea

ETIOLOGY

- Thrombus, fat, or other foreign material
- Risk factors for PE:
  1. Prolonged immobilization
  2. Postoperative state
  3. Trauma to lower extremities
  4. Estrogen-containing birth control pills
  5. Prior history of DVT or PE
  6. CHF
  7. Visceral cancer (lung, pancreas, alimentary and genitourinary tracts)
  8. Trauma, burns
  9. Advanced age
  10. Obesity
  11. Hematologic disease (e.g., antithrombin III deficiency, protein C deficiency, protein S deficiency, lupus anticoagulant, polycythemia vera, dysfibrinogenemia, paroxysmal nocturnal hemoglobinuria, factor V Leiden mutation, G20210A prothrombin mutation)
  12. COPD, diabetes mellitus
  13. Prolonged air travel

DIAGNOSIS

DIFFERENTIAL DIAGNOSIS

- Myocardial infarction
- Pericarditis
- Pneumonia
- Pneumothorax
- Chest wall pain
- GI abnormalities (e.g., peptic ulcer, esophageal rupture, gastritis)
- CHF
- Pleuritis
- Anxiety disorder with hyperventilation
- Pericardial tamponade
- Dissection of aorta
- Asthma

WORKUP

- Clinical assessment alone is insufficient to diagnose or rule out PE. It is also important to remember that no single noninvasive test has both high sensitivity and high specificity for PE. Consequently, in addition to clinical assessment, most patients will require several noninvasive tests or pulmonary angiography to diagnose PE.
- Spiral CT of chest or lung scan may be diagnostic. Pulmonary angiogram (when indicated) will confirm the diagnosis.
- Serial compressive duplex ultrasonography of lower extremities can be used in patients with "low-probability" lung scan and high clinical suspicion (see "Imaging Studies"). It is useful if positive, negative results do not exclude pulmonary embolism.

LABORATORY TESTS

- ABGs generally reveal decreased Pao_2 and $Paco_2$ and increased pH; normal results do not rule out PE.
- Alveolar-arteriolar (A-a) oxygen gradient, a measure of the difference in oxygen concentration between alveoli and arterial blood, is a more sensitive indicator of the alteration in oxygenation than Pao_2; it can easily be calculated using the information from ABGs; a normal A-a gradient among patients without history of PE or DVT makes the diagnosis of PE unlikely.
- Plasma D-dimer measurement: D-dimer assays by ELISA detect the presence of plasmin-mediated degradation products of fibrin that contain cross-linked D fragments in the whole blood or plasma. A normal plasma D-dimer level is useful to exclude pulmonary embolism in patients with a nondiagnostic lung scan and a low pretest probability of PE. However, it cannot be used to "rule in" the diagnosis because it increases with many other disorders (e.g., metastatic cancer, trauma, sepsis, postoperative state). Plasma D-dimer can also be used in conjunction with lower-extremity compression ultrasonography in patients with indeterminate V/Q and spiral CT scans. Absence of DVT and presence of a normal D-dimer level in these settings generally rules out clinically significant pulmonary embolism.
- Elevated cardiac troponin levels also occur in patients with pulmonary embolism because of right ventricular dilation and myocardial injury; therefore, PE should be considered in the differential diagnosis of all patients presenting with chest pain or dyspnea and elevated cardiac troponin levels.
- ECG is abnormal in 85% of patients with acute PE. Frequent abnormalities are sinus tachycardia; nonspecific ST-segment or T wave changes; S-I, Q-III, T-III pattern (10% of patients); S-I, S-II, S-III pattern; T wave inversion in V_1 to V_6; acute RBBB; new-onset atrial fibrillation; ST segment depression in lead II; right ventricular strain.

IMAGING STUDIES

- Chest x-ray may be normal; suggestive findings include elevated diaphragm, pleural effusion, dilation of pulmonary artery, infiltrate or consolidation, abrupt vessel cut-off, or atelectasis. A wedge-shaped consolidation in the middle and lower lobes is suggestive of a pulmonary infarction and is known as "Hampton's hump."
- Lung scan (in patient with normal chest x-ray examination):
  1. A normal lung scan rules out PE.
  2. A ventilation-perfusion mismatch is suggestive of PE, and a lung scan interpretation of high probability is confirmatory.
  3. If the clinical suspicion of PE is high and the lung scan is interpreted as low probability, moderate probability, or indeterminate, a pulmonary arteriogram is diagnostic; a positive arteriogram confirms diagnosis; a positive compressive duplex ultrasonography for DVT obviates the need for an arteriogram, because treatment with IV anticoagulants is indicated in these patients; the overall sensitivity of compressive ultrasonography for DVT in patients with PE is 29%, specificity

97%; adding ultrasonography in patients with a nondiagnostic lung scan prevents 9% of angiographies; however, this improvement in efficacy is achieved at the cost of unnecessary anticoagulant therapy in 26% of patients who have false-positive ultrasonography results.

- Spiral CT is an excellent modality for diagnosing PE. It may be used in place of the lung scan and is favored in patients with baseline lung abnormalities on initial chest x-ray. It has the added advantage of detecting other pulmonary pathology that can mimic pulmonary embolism.
- Angiography: pulmonary angiography is the gold standard; however, it is invasive, expensive, and not readily available in some clinical settings. False-positive pulmonary angiograms may result from mediastinal disorders such as radiation fibrosis and tumors. CT angiography is an accurate, noninvasive tool in the diagnosis of PE at the main, lobar, and segmental pulmonary artery levels. A major advantage of CT angiography over standard pulmonary angiography is its ability to diagnose intrathoracic disease other than PE that may account for the patient's clinical picture. It is also less invasive, less costly, and more widely available. Its major shortcoming is its poor sensitivity for subsegmental emboli. Gadolinium-enhanced magnetic resonance angiography of the pulmonary arteries has a moderate sensitivity and high specificity for the diagnosis of PE; MRA is best reserved for selected patients when CT scan and/or lung scan are inconclusive and the risk of pulmonary angiography is high.

TREATMENT

Rx

NONPHARMACOLOGIC THERAPY

Correction of risk factors (see "Etiology") to prevent future PE

ACUTE GENERAL Rx

- Heparin by continuous infusion for at least 5 days; many experts recommend a larger initial IV heparin bolus (15,000 to 20,000 U) to block platelet aggregation and thrombi and subsequent release of vasoconstrictive substances.
- Thrombolytic agents (urokinase, tPA, streptokinase): provide rapid resolution of clots; thrombolytic agents are the treatment of choice in patients with massive PE who are hemodynamically unstable and with no contraindication to their use. The use of thrombolytic agents in the treatment of hemodynamically stable patients with acute submassive pulmonary embolism remains controversial. Use of the thrombolytic agents alteplase (100 mg IV over a 2-hr period) in normotensive patients with moderate or severe right ventricular dysfunction identified by echocardiography has been advocated by some physicians. Use of alteplase in conjunction with heparin has been shown to improve the clinical course of stable patients who have acute submassive PE without internal bleeding. Additional studies are needed to confirm these findings before recommending routine use of this therapeutic approach.
- Long-term treatment is generally carried out with warfarin therapy started on day 1 or 2 and given in a dose to maintain the INR at 2 to 3.
- If thrombolytics and anticoagulants are contraindicated (e.g., GI bleeding, recent CNS surgery, recent trauma) or if the patient continues to have recurrent PE despite anticoagulation therapy, vena caval interruption is indicated by transvenous placement of a Greenfield vena caval filter.
- Acute pulmonary artery embolectomy may be indicated in a patient with massive pulmonary emboli and refractory hypotension.

CHRONIC Rx

Elimination of risk factors (see "Etiology") and monitoring of warfarin dose with INR on a routine basis

DISPOSITION

- Mortality can be reduced to <10% by rapid and effective treatment.
- Mortality from recurrent pulmonary emboli is 8% with effective treatment and >30% in patients with untreated pulmonary emboli.

PEARLS & CONSIDERATIONS

!

COMMENTS

- In hemodynamically stable patients with pulmonary embolism, initial treatment with once-daily SC administration of the synthetic antithrombotic agent fondaparinux without monitoring has been reported to be at least as safe and as effective as adjusted-dose IV unfractionated heparin. Several other trials have also demonstrated that fixed-dose low molecular weight heparin is as effective and safe as dose-adjusted IV unfractionated heparin for the initial treatment of nonmassive PE.
- The duration of oral anticoagulant treatment is 6 mo in patients with reversible risk factors and indefinitely in patients with persistence of risk factors that caused the initial PE.
- For the diagnosis of PE, Wells et al have developed the following clinical prediction rules to determine the probability of PE, assigning a score to each finding:
  1. Clinical signs/symptoms of DVT (minimum of leg swelling and pain with palpation of the deep veins of the legs (score = 3.0)
  2. No alternate diagnosis likely or more likely than PE (score = 3.0)
  3. Heart rate >100/min (score = 1.5)
  4. Immobilization or surgery in last 4 wk (score = 1.5)
  5. Previous history of DVT or PE (score = 1.5)
  6. Hemoptysis (score = 1.0)
  7. Cancer actively treated within last 6 months (score = 1.0)
- Probability of PE is high if total score is >6, moderate if 2-6, and low if < 2

SUGGESTED READINGS

Agnelli G et al: Extended oral anticoagulant therapy after a first episode of pulmonary embolism, *Ann Intern Med* 139:19, 2003.

Fedullo PF, Tapson VF: The evaluation of suspected pulmonary embolism, *N Engl J Med* 349:1247, 2003.

Quinlan DJ et al: Low-molecular weight heparin compared with IV unfractionated heparin for treatment of pulmonary embolism, *Ann Intern Med* 140:175, 2004.

The Matisse Investigators: Subcutaneous fondaparinux versus IV unfractionated heparin in the initial treatment of pulmonary embolism, *N Engl J Med* 349:1695, 2003.

Wells PS et al: Use of a clinical model for safe management of patients with suspected PE, *Ann Intern Med* 129:997, 1998.

AUTHOR: **FRED F. FERRI, M.D.**

BASIC INFORMATION

DEFINITION

Pulmonary hypertension (PH) is abnormally elevated pressure in the arterial side of the pulmonary circulation, usually defined as mean pulmonary pressure >25 mm Hg at rest or greater than 30 mmHg with exercise. Sustained elevation in pulmonary arterial pressure due to increased pulmonary venous pressure, hypoxic pulmonary vasoconstriction, or increased flow is often referred to as secondary pulmonary hypertension.

SYNONYMS

Primary pulmonary hypertension (PPH)
Secondary pulmonary hypertension

ICD-9CM CODES
416.0 Primary pulmonary hypertension
416.8 Secondary pulmonary
    hypertension

EPIDEMIOLOGY & DEMOGRAPHICS

- Primary pulmonary hypertension (PPH) is rare, occurring in 2 cases per 1 million people per year, with an overall prevalence estimated at 1,300 per million.
- PPH is more common in women than men (1.7:1).
- Secondary pulmonary hypertension is more common than PPH.
- Secondary pulmonary hypertension is the common pathophysiologic mechanism leading to cor pulmonale in patients with underlying pulmonary disease (e.g., COPD, pulmonary embolism).

PHYSICAL FINDINGS & CLINICAL PRESENTATION

Primary pulmonary hypertension:
- PPH is insidious and may go undetected for years.
- Exertional dyspnea is the most common presenting symptom (60%).
- Fatigue and weakness.
- Syncope.
- Chest pain.
- Loud P2 component of the second heart sound.
- Right-sided S4.
- Jugular venous distention.
- Abdominal distention/ascites.
- Prominent parasternal (RV) impulse.
- Holosystolic tricuspid regurgitation murmur heard best along the left fourth parasternal line that increases in intensity with inspiration.
- Peripheral edema.

Secondary pulmonary hypertension:
- Similar to PPH but depends on the underlying cause (e.g., left-sided CHF, mitral stenosis, COPD).

ETIOLOGY

- The etiology of PPH is unknown. Most cases are sporadic, but there is a 6% to 12% familial incidence.
- PPH is associated with several known risk factors: portal hypertension and liver cirrhosis, appetite-suppressant drugs (fenfluramine), and HIV disease.
- Several genetic abnormalities have been associated with the familial form of PPH, many of which are mutations in the genes that code for members of the TGF-_ family of receptors (BMPR-II, ALK-1) on chromosome 2q33.
- Familial PPH is an autosomal-dominant disease with variable penetrance, affecting only about 10% to 20% of carriers.
- Several factors have been identified that play a role in the pathogenesis of PPH, including a genetic predisposition, endothelial cell dysfunction, abnormalities in vasomotor control, thrombotic obliteration of the vascular lumen, and vascular remodeling through cell proliferation and matrix production. An emerging theory involves abnormal membrane potassium channels modulating calcium kinetics.
- Secondary pulmonary hypertension is primarily caused by underlying pulmonary and cardiac conditions including:
  1. Pulmonary thromboembolic disease
  2. Chronic obstructive pulmonary disease (COPD)
  3. Interstitial lung disease
  4. Obstructive sleep disorder
  5. Neuromuscular diseases causing hypoventilation (e.g., ALS)
  6. Collagen-vascular disease (e.g., SLE, CREST, systemic sclerosis)
  7. Pulmonary venous disease
  8. Left ventricular failure resulting from hypertension, CAD, aortic stenosis, and cardiomyopathy
  9. Valvular heart disease (e.g., mitral stenosis, mitral regurgitation)
  10. Congenital heart disease with left-to-right shunting (e.g., ASD)

DIAGNOSIS (Dx)

- The normal pulmonary arterial systolic pressure ranges from 18 to 30 mm Hg and the diastolic pressure ranges from 4 to 12 mm Hg.
- PH is a hemodynamic diagnosis involving two stages: detection of elevated pressure in the pulmonary arteries, and characterization of this abnormality to determine its etiology by ruling out secondary causes.
- Right-heart catheterization must be performed in all patients suspected of having PH to establish the diagnosis and document pulmonary hemodynamics.

- Primary pulmonary hypertension is a diagnosis of exclusion; all secondary causes as mentioned under "Etiology" must be excluded.

DIFFERENTIAL DIAGNOSIS

The differential diagnosis is as listed under "Etiology."

WORKUP

- Screening for the presence of PH using Doppler echocardiography is warranted in individuals with a known predisposing genetic mutation or first-degree relative with idiopathic PPH, scleroderma, congenital heart disease with left-to-right shunt, or portal hypertension undergoing evaluation for orthotopic liver transplantation.
- The workup of a patient suspected of having PPH includes a detailed evaluation of the heart and lungs. Blood tests, chest x-ray, pulmonary function tests, CT scan of the chest, radionuclide studies of the heart and lungs, echocardiogram, electrocardiograms, pulmonary angiogram, and right- and left-heart catheterization are all required to exclude secondary causes of pulmonary hypertension.
- Once the diagnosis has been made, functional assessment should be undergone to determine disease prognosis and potential treatment options.
- The degree of functional impairment as assessed by the WHO classification system, and the 6-minute walk test is a useful way to monitor disease progression and assess response to treatment.

LABORATORY TESTS

- CBC is usually normal in PPH but may show secondary polycythemia.
- ABGs show low PO_2 and oxygen saturation.
- PFT is done to exclude obstructive or restrictive lung disease.
- Overnight oximetry and sleep study to rule out sleep apnea/hypopnea.
- ECG may show evidence of both right atrial enlargement (tall P wave >2.5 mV in leads II, III, aVF) and right ventricular enlargement (right axis deviation >100 and R wave > S wave in lead V1).
- Other blood tests: ANA titer to screen for underlying connective tissue disease, HIV serology, liver function tests, and antiphospholipid antibodies.
- Assessment of exercise capacity is a key part of the evaluation of PH in characterizing the disease and determining prognosis and treatment options. The 6-minute walk test and cardiopulmonary exercise testing with gas exchange measurements are the most commonly used methods of assessment.

IMAGING STUDIES

- Chest x-ray shows enlargement of the main and hilar pulmonary arteries with rapid tapering of the distal vessels (Fig. 1-34). Right ventricular enlargement may be evident on lateral films.
- Lung perfusion scan (V/Q scan) aids in excluding chronic pulmonary embolism.
- Transthoracic Doppler echocardiogram including M-mode, 2 D, pulse, continuous and color Doppler assesses ventricular function, excludes significant valvular pathology, and visualizes abnormal shunting of blood between heart chambers if present. It also provides an estimate of pulmonary artery systolic pressure that has been shown by most studies to correlate well (0.57 to 0.93) with pressures measured by right-heart catheterization.
- Pulmonary angiogram is done in patients with suspicious V/Q scans.
- Cardiac catheterization is performed to directly measure pulmonary artery pressures and to detect any shunting of blood.

TREATMENT   Rx

NONPHARMACOLOGIC THERAPY

- Oxygen therapy to improve alveolar oxygen flow in both primary and secondary pulmonary hypertension
- Avoidance of vigorous exercise
- Chest physiotherapy

ACUTE GENERAL Rx

- PPH
  1. Diuretics (e.g., furosemide 40-80 mg qd) improve dyspnea and peripheral edema.
  2. Digoxin 0.25 mg qd has been used in patients with PPH.
  3. Vasodilator treatment is usually done with hemodynamic monitoring and includes IV adenosine, prostacyclin, or nitric oxide.
- Secondary pulmonary hypertension treatment is aimed at the underlying cause (see specific disease in text for treatment).

CHRONIC Rx

- Chronic anticoagulation with warfarin is recommended to prevent thromboses and has been shown to prolong life in patients with PPH.
- Calcium channel blockers may alleviate pulmonary vasoconstriction and prolong life in about 20% of patients with PPH.
- Continuous infusion of epoprostenol, or prostacyclin, a short-acting vasodilator and inhibitor of platelet aggregation, improves exercise capacity, quality of life, hemodynamics, and long-term survival in patients with WHO class III or IV function.
- Inhaled aerosolized prostacyclin, iloprost, 2.5 or 5.0 μg taken 6 to 9 times per day improves exercise capacity, NYHA class, and clinical deterioration in patients with primary pulmonary hypertension and selected forms of nonprimary pulmonary hypertension.
- The endothelin-receptor antagonist bosentan taken orally at a dose of 80-160 mg twice daily has been approved for the treatment of PPH and scleroderma pulmonary hypertension showing improvement in clinical class and exercise capacity. Newer selective and nonselective endothelin receptor antagonists are undergoing clinical trials.
- Combination therapy using inhaled iloprost taken 1 hour before oral sildenafil 12.5 or 50 mg causes pulmonary vasodilations and, pending future trials, may be considered as treatment for pulmonary hypertension.
- Lung transplantation and heart-lung transplantation are other options in end-stage class IV patients.
- Lung transplant recipients with PPH had survival rates of 73% at 1 yr, 55% at 3 yr, and 45% at 5 yr.

DISPOSITION

- The 6-min walk test is predictive of survival in patients with idiopathic PPH. Desaturation >10% during the test increases mortality risk 2.9 times over a median follow-up of 26 mo.

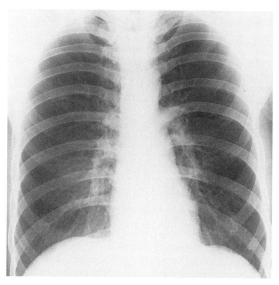

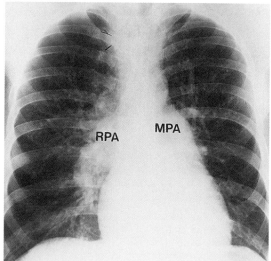

FIGURE 1-34 Progressive pulmonary arterial hypertension. This patient initially presented with a relatively normal chest radiograph **(A)**. However, several years later **(B)**, there is increasing heart size as well as marked dilation of the main pulmonary artery *(MPA)* and right pulmonary artery *(RPA)*. Rapid tapering of the arteries as they proceed peripherally is suggestive of pulmonary hypertension and is sometimes referred to as pruning. (From Mettler FA [ed]: *Primary care radiology,* Philadelphia, 2000, WB Saunders.)

- The actual 6-min walk distance on chronic epoprostenol treatment is more predictive of survival than the change in 6-min walk distance before and after treatment.
- WHO Class II and III patients with PPH have a mean survival of 3.5 yr.
- WHO Class IV patients have a mean survival of 6 mo.
- Logistic regression equations have been reported to predict survival or death within 1, 2, or 3 yr after diagnosis in patients with PPH.

REFERRAL

If the diagnosis of PPH is suspected, a consultation with a pulmonary specialist is recommended. Secondary causes of pulmonary hypertension may require consultations with rheumatology, neurology, and cardiology.

PEARLS & CONSIDERATIONS

COMMENTS

- The exertional dyspnea of PH is typically described by patients as being relentlessly progressive over several months to a year, often out of proportion to, or in the absence of, underlying heart or lung disease.

- Chest x-ray may reveal evidence of interstitial fluid within the lungs in cases of secondary pulmonary hypertension. PPH is not associated with infiltrates on CXR.
- Factors contributing to pulmonary arterial hypertension are:
  1. Alveolar hypoxia
  2. Acidosis
  3. Thromboemboli occluding arterial blood vessels (e.g., pulmonary embolism)
  4. Scarring or destruction of alveolar walls (e.g., COPD, infiltrative disease)
  5. Primary thickening of arterial walls as occurs in PPH
- RVSP as estimated by echocardiography is not a very good indicator of the presence of PH, because RVSP increases with age and BMI. Athletically conditioned men also have a higher resting RVSP, and thus these measurements can be misleading.
- Abrupt development of pulmonary edema during acute vasodilator testing suggests pulmonary veno-occlusive disease or pulmonary capillary hemangiomatosis and is a contraindication to chronic vasodilator treatment.

SUGGESTED READINGS

Barst RJ et al: Diagnosis and differential assessment of pulmonary arterial hypertension, *J Am Coll Cardiol* 43:40S, 2004.

Chatterjee K, De Marco T, Alpert JS: Pulmonary hypertension: hemodynamic diagnosis and management, *Arch Intern Med* 162:1925, 2002.

Ghofrani HA et al: Combination therapy with oral sildenafil and inhaled iloprost for severe pulmonary hypertension, *Ann Intern Med* 136:515, 2002.

Krowka MJ: Pulmonary hypertension: diagnosis and therapeutics, *Mayo Clin Proc* 75:625, 2000.

McLaughlin VV et al: Prognosis of pulmonary arterial hypertension: ACCP evidence-based clinical practice guidelines, *Chest* 1126:78S, 2004.

Nauser T, Stites S: Diagnosis and treatment of pulmonary hypertension, *Am Fam Physician* 63:1789, 2001.

Olschewski H et al: Inhaled iloprost for severe pulmonary hypertension, *N Engl J Med* 347:322, 2002.

Rubin LJ et al: Bosentan therapy for pulmonary arterial hypertension, *N Engl J Med* 346:896, 2002.

AUTHORS: **JASON IANNUCCILLI, M.D.,** and **PETER PETROPOULOS, M.D.**

BASIC INFORMATION

DEFINITION

Renal cell adenocarcinoma (RCA) is a primary adenocarcinoma originating in the renal parenchyma from the malignant transformation of proximal renal tubular epithelial cells.

SYNONYMS

Hypernephroma
Clear cell carcinoma of the kidney
Grawitz tumor

ICD-9CM CODES
189.0 Adenocarcinoma of kidney
189.1 (Renal pelvis)

EPIDEMIOLOGY & DEMOGRAPHICS

INCIDENCE: Approximately 1:10,000 persons/yr (3% of all adult malignancies)
AGE: Peak in age 50 to 70 yr
SEX: Male:female ratio of 2:1

PHYSICAL FINDINGS & CLINICAL PRESENTATION

Presenting findings in RCA patients:

Hematuria	50% to 60%
Elevated erythrocyte sedimentation rate	50% to 60%
Abdominal mass	25% to 45%
Anemia	20% to 40%
Flank pain	35% to 40%
Hypertension	20% to 40%
Weight loss	30% to 35%
Fever	5% to 15%
Hepatic dysfunction	10% to 15%
Classic triad (hematuria, abdominal mass, flank pain)	5% to 10%
Hypercalcemia	3% to 6%
Erythrocytosis	3% to 4%
Varicocele	2% to 3%

ETIOLOGY

Hereditary forms
- Familial renal carcinoma
- Renal carcinoma associated with von Hippel-Lindau disease
- Hereditary papillary renal cell carcinoma

Risk factors
- Cigarette smoking
- Obesity
- Use of diuretics
- Phenacetin-containing analgesics
- Asbestos exposure
- Gasoline and other petroleum products
- Lead
- Cadmium
- Thorotrast
- Role of the VHL gene located on chromosome 3

DIAGNOSIS

DIFFERENTIAL DIAGNOSIS

- Transitional cell carcinomas of the renal pelvis (8% of all renal cancers)
- Wilms' tumor
- Other rare primary renal carcinomas and sarcomas
- Renal cysts
- All causes of hematuria (see Section II)
- Retroperitoneal tumors

WORKUP

- Laboratory tests and imaging studies

LABORATORY TESTS

- CBC: anemia or erythrocytosis
- Elevated sedimentation rate
- Nonmetastatic hepatic dysfunction with elevated alkaline phosphatase, prolonged prothrombin time, and hypoalbuminemia
- Hypercalcemia (secondary to parathyroid related protein)
- Other: elevated ferritin, elevated insulin and glucagon levels, elevated alpha-fetoprotein, and elevated beta-human chorionic gonadotropin

IMAGING STUDIES

- Intravenous pyelography (IVP)
- Renal ultrasound
- Abdominal CT scan with contrast (Fig. 1-35)
- MRI
- Renal arteriogram

STAGING

See Table 1-13.

COMMON SITES OF METASTASES

Lung	50% to 60%
Bone	30% to 40%
Regional nodes	15% to 30%
Main renal vein	15% to 20%
Perirenal fat	10% to 20%
Adrenal (ipsilateral)	10% to 15%
Vena cava	10% to 15%
Brain	10% to 15%
Adjacent organs (colon, pancreas)	10%
Kidney (contralateral)	2%

TREATMENT **Rx**

- Surgery
  Surgical nephrectomy is the only effective management for stages I, II, and some stage III tumors.
  Various forms of partial nephrectomy may be available for patients with bilateral cancers or with a solitary kidney.
  The role of nephrectomy in patients with metastatic renal cell carcinoma is controversial and should probably be reserved for patients who have a solitary metastasis amenable to surgical resection.
- Angioinfarction (for palliation)
- Radiotherapy (for palliation)
- Chemotherapy (only 5% response rate)

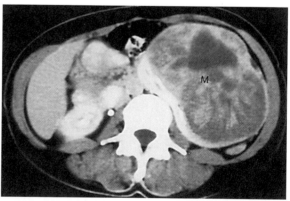

FIGURE 1-35 Large renal cell carcinoma. Large mass *(M)* containing areas of high enhancement, low enhancement, and necrosis. (From Stein JH [ed]: *Internal medicine,* ed 5, St Louis, 1998, Mosby.)

- Hormonal therapy (high-dose progesterone may achieve a 15% to 20% response rate)
- Immunotherapy (interleukin-2 may achieve a 15% to 30% response rate; alpha, beta, and gamma interferons are somewhat less effective; for example, interferon alfa-2b increased postnephrectomy median survival by 30% in one recent trial)
- Antivascular endothelial growth factor antibody Bevacizumab slows disease progression in metastatic renal cancer.

PROGNOSIS

Prognosis of surgically treated patients

TNM stage	5-year survival (%)
I	95
II	88
III (renal vein or vena cava)	50 to 60
III (nodal involvement)	15 to 25
IV	5 to 20

REFERRAL

To urologist

SUGGESTED READINGS

Curti BD: Renal cell carcinoma, *JAMA* 292:97, 2004.

Flanigan RC et al: Nephrectomy followed by interferon alfa-2b compared with interferon alfa-2b alone for metastatic renal-cell cancer, *N Engl J Med* 345:1655, 2002.

Jennings SB, Linehan WM: Renal, perirenal, and ureteral neoplasms. In Gillenwater JY et al: *Adult and Pediatric Urology,* ed 3, St Louis, 1996, Mosby.

Yang CJ: A randomized trial of Bevacizumab, an anti-vascular endothelial growth factor antibody, for metastatic renal cancer, *N Engl J Med* 349:427, 2003.

AUTHOR: **TOM J. WACHTEL, M.D.**

TABLE 1-13 Comparison of Conventional and TNM Staging Classification of RCC

Robson Stage	T	N	M
I: Tumor confined by capsule	T_1 (tumor 2.5 cm or less) T_2 (tumor >2.5 cm, limited to kidney)		
II: Tumor extension to perirenal fat or ipsilateral adrenal but confined by Gerota's fascia	T_3a (tumor invades adrenal gland or perinephric fat but not beyond Gerota's fascia)		
IIIa: Renal vein or inferior vena caval involvement	T_3b (renal vein or caval involvement below diaphragm) T_3c (caval involvement above diaphragm)	N_0 (nodes negative)	M_0 (no distant metastases)
IIIb: Lymphatic involvement	T_{1-4}	N_1 (single lymph node 2 cm or less) N_2 (single node between 2 and 5 cm, or multiple nodes <5 cm) N3 (single or multiple nodes >5 cm)	
IIIc: Combination of IIIa and IIIb	$T_{3, 4}$		
IVa: Spread to contiguous organs except ipsilateral adrenal	T_4 (tumor extends beyond Gerota's fascia)		
IVb: Distant metastases	T_{1-4}		M_1 (distant metastases)

BASIC INFORMATION

DEFINITION

Acute renal failure (ARF) is the rapid impairment in renal function resulting in retention of products in the blood that are normally excreted by the kidneys.

SYNONYMS

ARF

ICD-9CM CODES
584.9 Acute renal failure, unspecified

EPIDEMIOLOGY & DEMOGRAPHICS

- ARF requiring dialysis develops in 5/100,000 persons annually.
- >10% of ICU patients develop ARF.
- >40% of hospital ARF is iatrogenic.
- The most common cause of ARF in hospitalized patients is intrinsic renal failure caused by acute tubular necrosis (ATN).
- Acute renal failure occurs in 20% of patients with moderate sepsis and over 50% of patients with septic shock and positive blood cultures.

PHYSICAL FINDINGS & CLINICAL PRESENTATION

- The physical examination should focus on volume status. The physical findings noted below vary with the duration and rapidity of onset of renal failure
- Peripheral edema
- Skin pallor, ecchymoses
- Oliguria (however, patients can have nonoliguric renal failure), anuria
- Delirium, lethargy, myoclonus, seizures
- Back pain, fasciculations, muscle cramps
- Tachypnea, tachycardia
- Weakness, anorexia, generalized malaise, nausea

ETIOLOGY

- Prerenal: inadequate perfusion caused by hypovolemia, CHF, cirrhosis, sepsis. Sixty percent of community-acquired cases of ARF are due to prerenal conditions.
- Postrenal: outlet obstruction from prostatic enlargement, ureteral obstruction (stones), bilateral renal vein occlusion. Postrenal causes account for 5% to 15% of community-acquired ARF.
- Intrinsic renal: glomerulonephritis, acute tubular necrosis, drug toxicity, contrast nephropathy.
- Causes of acute renal failure are described in Section II.

DIAGNOSIS

DIFFERENTIAL DIAGNOSIS

Refer to "Etiology."

WORKUP

A thorough review of the patient's history is necessary to identify contributing factors (e.g., nephrotoxin exposure, hypertension, diabetes mellitus). Laboratory evaluation to quantify degree of abnormality; radiographic studies to exclude prerenal and postrenal factors. Categorization of renal failure into oliguric (urinary output <400 ml/day) or nonoliguric is important. Anuria is common in obstructive uropathy and acute cortical necrosis.

LABORATORY TESTS

- Elevated serum creatinine: the rate of rise of creatinine is approximately 1 mg/dl/day in complete renal failure.
- Elevated BUN: BUN/creatinine ratio is >20:1 in prerenal azotemia, postrenal azotemia, and acute glomerulonephritis; it is <20:1 in acute interstitial nephritis and acute tubular necrosis (Table 1-14).
- Electrolytes (potassium, phosphate) are elevated; bicarbonate level and calcium are decreased.
- CBC may reveal anemia because of decreased erythropoietin production, hemoconcentration, or hemolysis.
- Urinalysis may reveal the presence of hematuria (GN), proteinuria (nephrotic syndrome), casts (e.g., granular casts in ATN, RBC casts in acute GN, WBC casts in acute interstitial nephritis), eosinophiluria (acute interstitial nephritis).
- Urinary sodium and urinary creatinine should also be obtained to calculate the fractional excretion of sodium (FE_{Na}) (FE_{Na} = Urine sodium/plasma sodium × Plasma creatinine/urine creatinine × 100). The fractional excretion of sodium is <1 in prerenal failure, >1 in intrinsic renal failure in patients with urine output <400 ml/day.
- Urinary osmolarity is 250 to 300 mOsm/kg in ATN, <400 mOsm/kg in postrenal azotemia, and >500 mOsm/kg in prerenal azotemia and acute glomerulonephritis (Table 1-15).
- Additional useful studies are blood cultures for patients suspected of sepsis, LFTs, immunoglobulins, and protein electrophoresis in patients

TABLE 1-14 Serum and Radiographic Abnormalities in Renal Failure

	Prerenal	Postrenal (Acute)	Intrinsic Renal (Acute)	Intrinsic Renal (Chronic)
BUN	↑10:1 > Cr	↑ 20-40/d	↑ 20-40/d	Stable, ↑ varies with protein intake
Serum creatinine	N/moderate ↑	↑ 2-4/d	↑ 2-4/d	Stable ↑ (production equals excretion)
Serum potassium	N/moderate ↑	↑ varies with urinary volume	↑↑ (particularly when patient is oliguric) ↑↑↑ with rhabdomyolysis	Normal until end stage, unless tubular dysfunction (type 4 RTA)
Serum phosphorus	N/moderate ↑	Moderate ↑ ↑↑ with rhabdomyolysis	↑ Poor correlation with duration of renal disease	Becomes significantly elevated when serum creatinine level surpasses 3 mg/dl
Serum calcium	N	N/↓ with PO_4^{-3} retention	↓ (poor correlation with duration of renal failure)	Usually ↓
Renal size				
By ultrasound	N/↑	↑ and dilated calyces	N/↑	↓ and with ↑ echogenicity
FE_{Na}*	<1	<1 → 1	>1	>1

From Kiss B: Renal failure. In Ferri FF (ed): *Practical guide to the care of the medical patient*, ed 6, St Louis, 2004, Mosby.
↑, Increase; ↓, decrease; ↑↑, large increase; *Cr*, creatinine; *N*, normal; *Na*, sodium; *P*, plasma; *RTA*, renal tubular acidosis; *U*, urine.
*$FE_{Na} = U_{Na}/P_{Na}U_{Cr}/P_{cr} \times 100$.

suspected of myeloma, creatinine kinase in patients with suspected rhabdomyolysis.

- Renal biopsy may be indicated in patients with intrinsic renal failure when considering specific therapy; major uses of renal biopsy are differential diagnosis of nephrotic syndrome, separation of lupus vasculitis from other vasculitis and lupus membranous from idiopathic membranous, confirmation of hereditary nephropathies on the basis of the ultrastructure, diagnosis of rapidly progressing glomerulonephritis, separation of allergic interstitial nephritis from ATN, separation of primary glomerulonephritis syndromes. The biopsy may be performed percutaneously or by open method. The percutaneous approach is favored and generally yields adequate tissue in >90% of cases. Open biopsy is generally reserved for uncooperative patients, those with solitary kidney, and patients at risk for uncontrolled bleeding.

IMAGING STUDIES

- Chest x ray is useful to evaluate for CHF and for pulmonary renal syndromes (Goodpasture's syndrome, Wegener's granulomatosis).
- Ultrasound of kidneys is used to evaluate for kidney size (useful to distinguish ARF from CRF), to evaluate for the presence of obstruction, and to evaluate renal vascular status (with Doppler evaluation).

- Anterograde and/or retrograde pyelogram can be used for ruling out obstruction; useful in patients at high risk of obstruction.

TREATMENT

Rx

NONPHARMACOLOGIC THERAPY

- Stop all nephrotoxic medications
- Dietary modification to supply adequate calories while minimizing accumulation of toxins; appropriate control of fluid balance. Physicians should recommend a nutrition program with an energy prescription of 120 to 150 kJ/kg per day and restriction of potassium (60 mEq/day), sodium (90 mEq/day), and phosphorus (800 mg/day). Ideal protein supplementation ranges from 0.6 to 1.4 g/kg depending on whether dialysis is required
- Daily weight
- Modifications of dosage of renally excreted drugs

ACUTE GENERAL Rx

Treatment is variable with etiology of ARF:

- Prerenal: IV volume expansion in hypovolemic patients
- Intrinsic renal: discontinuation of any potential toxins and treatment of condition causing the renal failure
- Postrenal: removal of obstruction

CHRONIC Rx

- Monitoring of renal function and electrolytes.
- Prevention of further insults to the kidneys with proper hydration, especially before contrast studies, and avoidance of nephrotoxic agents. Hydration with sodium bicarbonate (addition of 154 ml of 1000 mEq/L sodium bicarbonate to 846 mL of 5% dextrose in water) before contrast exposure is more effective than hydration with sodium chloride for prophylaxis of contrast-induced renal failure. After appropriate clinical evaluation and measurement of blood pressure, patients should receive an initial IV bolus of 3 ml/kg/hr for 1 hr immediately before radiocontrast injection and the same fluid at a rate of 1 ml/kg/hr during the contrast exposure and for 6 hr after the procedure.
- Refer to topic on chronic renal failure for indications for initiation of dialysis. Daily hemodialysis is superior to every-other-day hemodialysis in patients with acute tubular necrosis and ARF.

DISPOSITION

- Prognosis is variable depending on the etiology of the renal failure, degree of renal failure, multiorgan involvement, and patient's age.
- Renal function recovery (ability to discontinue dialysis) varies from 50% to 75% in survivors of ARF.

TABLE 1-15   Urinary Abnormalities in Renal Failure

	Prerenal	Postrenal (Acute)	Intrinsic Renal (Acute)	Intrinsic Renal (Chronic)
Urinary volume	↓	Absent-to-wide fluctuation	Oliguric or nonoliguric	1000 ml + until end stage
Urinary creatinine	↑ (U/P Cr ±40)	↓ (U/P Cr ±20)	↓ (U/P Cr <20)	↓ (U/P Cr <20)
Osmolarity	↑ (±400 mOsm/kg)	(<350 mOsm/kg)	(<350 mOsm/kg)	(<350 mOsm/kg)
Degree of proteinuria	Minimum	Absent	Varies with cause of renal failure: Modest with ATN Nephrotic range common with acute glomerulopathies, usually <2 g/24 hr with interstitial disease*	Varies with cause of renal disease (from 1-2 g/d to nephrotic range)
Urinary sediment	Negative, or occasional hyaline cast	Negative or hematuria with stones or papillary necrosis Pyuria with infectious prostatic disease	ATN: muddy brown Interstitial nephritis: lymphocytes, eosinophils (in stained preparations), and WBC casts RPGN: RBC casts Nephrosis: oval fat bodies	Broad casts with variable renal "residual" acute findings

From Kiss B: Renal failure. In Ferri FF (ed): *Practical guide to the care of the medical patient*, ed 6, St Louis, 2004, Mosby.

↑, Increased; ↓, decreased; *ATN*, acute tubular necrosis; clearance = $\dfrac{\text{Urinary concentration} \times \text{Urinary volume}}{\text{Plasma concentration}}$ *Cr*, creatinine; *RBC*, red blood cell;

RPGN, rapidly progressive glomerulonephritis; *U/P*, urine/plasma; *WBC*, white blood cell.

- Overall mortality rate in ARF is nearly 50%, varying from 60% in patients with ATN to 35% in patients with prerenal or postrenal ARF.
- The combination of acute renal failure and sepsis is associated with a 70% mortality rate.

REFERRAL

- Nephrology consultation is recommended in renal failure.
- General indications for initiation of dialysis are:
  1. Florid symptoms of uremia (encephalopathy, pericarditis)
  2. Severe volume overload
  3. Severe acid-base imbalance
  4. Significant derangement in electrolyte concentrations (e.g., hyperkalemia, hyponatremia)
- Surgical consult may be necessary in patients with obstruction.

PEARLS & CONSIDERATIONS

COMMENTS

- It is important for physicians to recognize the growing list of medications that can result in ARF.

SUGGESTED READINGS

Albright RC: Acute renal failure: a practical update, *Mayo Clin Proc* 76:67, 2001.

Kellum JA, Decker JM: Use of dopamine in acute renal failure: a meta analysis, *Crit Care Med* 29:1526, 2001.

Klassen PS et al: Association between pulse pressure and mortality in patients undergoing maintenance hemodialysis, *JAMA* 287:1548, 2002.

Merten GJ et al: Prevention of contrast-induced nephropathy with sodium bicarbonate, *JAMA* 291:2328, 2004.

Nally JV: Acute renal failure in hospitalized patients, *Cleve Clin J Med* 69:569, 2002.

Schiffel H et al: Daily hemodialysis and the outcome of acute renal failure, *N Engl J Med* 346:305, 2002.

Schrier RW, Wang W: Acute renal failure and sepsis, *N Engl J Med* 351:159, 2004.

AUTHOR: **FRED F. FERRI, M.D.**

BASIC INFORMATION

DEFINITION

Chronic renal failure (CRF) is a progressive decrease in renal function (CFR <60 ml/min for ≥3 mo) with subsequent accumulation of waste products in the blood, electrolyte abnormalities, and anemia.

SYNONYMS

CRF
End-stage renal disease

ICD-9CM CODES
585 Chronic renal failure

EPIDEMIOLOGY & DEMOGRAPHICS

- The number of patients with ESRD is increasing at the rate of 7% to 9%/yr in the U.S. Each year 2/10,000 persons develop end-stage CRF.
- In the U.S., >250,000/yr receive dialysis treatment for ESRD.

PHYSICAL FINDINGS & CLINICAL PRESENTATION

- Skin pallor, ecchymoses
- Edema
- Hypertension
- Emotional lability and depression
- The clinical presentation varies with the degree of renal failure and its underlying etiology. Common symptoms are generalized fatigue, nausea, anorexia, pruritus, insomnia, taste disturbances

ETIOLOGY

- Diabetes (37%), hypertension (30%), chronic glomerulonephritis (12%)
- Polycystic kidney disease
- Tubular interstitial nephritis (e.g., drug hypersensitivity, analgesic nephropathy), obstructive nephropathies (e.g., nephrolithiasis, prostatic disease)
- Vascular diseases (renal artery stenosis, hypertensive nephrosclerosis)

DIAGNOSIS

Dx

- CRF is primarily distinguished from ARF by the duration (progression over several months).
- Sonographic evaluation of the kidneys reveals smaller kidneys with increased echogenicity in CRF.

WORKUP

- Laboratory evaluation and imaging studies should be aimed at identifying reversible causes of acute decrements in GFR (e.g., volume depletion, urinary tract obstruction, CHF) superimposed on chronic renal disease

- Kidney biopsy: generally not performed in patients with small kidneys or with advanced disease
- The glomerular filtration rate is the best overall indicator of kidney function. It can be estimated using prediction equations that take into account the serum creatinine level and some or all of specific variables (body size, age, sex, race). GFR calculators are available on the National Kidney Foundation Web site (http://www.kidney.org/kls/professionals/gfr_calculator.cfm)

LABORATORY TESTS

- Elevated BUN, creatinine, creatinine clearance
- Urinalysis: may reveal proteinuria, RBC casts
- Serum chemistry: elevated BUN and creatinine, hyperkalemia, hyperuricemia, hypocalcemia, hyperphosphatemia, hyperglycemia, decreased bicarbonate
- Measure urinary protein excretion. The finding of a ratio of protein to creatinine of >1000 mg/g suggests the presence of glomerular disease
- Special studies: serum and urine immunoelectrophoresis (in suspected multiple myeloma), ANA (in suspected SLE)

IMAGING STUDIES

Ultrasound of kidneys to measure kidney size and to rule out obstruction

TREATMENT

Rx

NONPHARMACOLOGIC THERAPY

- Provide adequate nutrition and calories (147 to 168 kJ/kg/day in energy intake, chiefly from carbohydrate and polyunsaturated fats). Referral to a dietician for nutritional therapy for patients with GFR <50 ml/1.73 m² is recommended and is now a covered service by Medicare.
- Restrict sodium (approximately 100 mmol/day), potassium (≤60 mmol/day), and phosphate (<800 mg/day).
- Adjust drug doses to correct for prolonged half-lives.
- Restrict fluid if significant edema is present.
- Protein restriction (≤0.8 g/kg/day) may slow deterioration of renal function; however, recent studies have not confirmed this benefit. There is insufficient evidence to recommend or advise against routine restriction of protein intake.

- Resistance exercise training can preserve lean body mass, nutritional status, and muscle function in patients with moderate chronic kidney disease.
- Avoid radiocontrast agents.
- Smoking cessation.
- Initiate hemodialysis or peritoneal dialysis (see "General Rx").
- Prompt to nephrologist is essential. Late evaluation of patients with chronic renal disease is associated with greater burden and severity of comorbid disease and shorter survival.
- Kidney transplantation in selected patients.

GENERAL Rx

- ACE inhibitors, ARBs, and nondihydropyridine calcium channel blockers (diltiazem or verapamil) are useful in reducing proteinuria and slowing the progression of chronic renal disease, especially in hypertensive diabetic patients. A systolic blood pressure between 110 and 129 mm Hg may be beneficial in patients with urine protein excretion >1.0 g/day. Systolic BP <110 mm Hg may be associated with a higher risk for kidney disease progression.
- Initiation of dialysis
  1. Urgent indications: uremic pericarditis, neuropathy, neuromuscular abnormalities, CHF, hyperkalemia, seizures.
  2. Judgmental indications: creatinine clearance 10 to 15 ml/min; progressive anorexia, weight loss, reversal of sleep pattern, pruritus, uncontrolled fluid gain with hypertension and signs of CHF.
- Erythropoietin for anemia: 2000 to 3000 U three times a week IV/SC to maintain Hct 30% to 33%.
- Diuretics for significant fluid overload (loop diuretics are preferred).
- Correction of hypertension to at least 130/85 mm Hg with ACE inhibitors (avoid in patients with significant hyperkalemia), ARBs, and/or nondihydropyridene calcium channel blockers (verapamil, diltiazem) can be used in patients intolerant to ACE inhibitors or when other agents are needed to control blood pressure.
- Correction of electrolyte abnormalities (e.g., calcium chloride, glucose, sodium polystyrene sulfonate for hyperkalemia), sodium bicarbonate in patients with severe metabolic acidosis.
- Lipid-lowering agents in patients with dyslipidemia, target LDL cholesterol is <100 mg/dl.

- Control of renal osteodystrophy with calcium supplementation and vitamin D. Starting dose of calcium carbonate is 0.5 g with each meal, increased until the serum phosphorus concentration is normalized (most patients require 5 to 10 g/day). Calcitriol 0.125 to 0.25 μg/day PO is effective in increasing serum calcium concentration. Paricalcitol, a new vitamin-D analogue has been reported as more effective than calcitriol in lessening the elevations in serum calcium and phosphorus levels.
- Sevelamer (Renagel) is a useful phosphate binder to reduce serum phosphate levels.

DISPOSITION

- Prognosis is influenced by comorbidity of multisystem diseases.
- Kidney transplantation in selected patients improves survival. The 2-yr kidney graft survival rate for living related donor transplantations is >80%, whereas the 2-yr graft survival rate for cadaveric donor transplantation is approximately 70%.

SUGGESTED READINGS

Jafar TH et al: Progression of chronic kidney disease: the role of blood pressure control, proteinuria, and angiotensin-converting enzyme inhibition, *Ann Intern Med* 139:244, 2003.

Johnson CA et al: Clinical practice guidelines for chronic kidney disease in adults, *Am Fam Physician* 70:869, 2004.

Kinchen KS et al: The timing of specialist evaluation in chronic kidney disease and mortality, *Ann Intern Med* 137:479, 2003.

Levey AS: Nondiabetic kidney disease, *N Engl J Med* 347:1505, 2002.

Lewey AS et al: National Kidney Foundation practice guidelines for chronic kidney disease: evaluation, classification, and stratification, *Ann Intern Med* 139:137, 2003.

Lewinsky NG: Specialist evaluation in chronic kidney disease: too little too late, *Ann Intern Med* 137:542, 2002.

Remuzzi G et al: Chronic renal diseases: renoprotective benefits of renin-angiotensin system inhibition, *Ann Intern Med* 136:604, 2002.

Yu HT: Progression of chronic renal failure, *Arch Intern Med* 163:1417, 2003.

AUTHOR: **FRED F. FERRI, M.D.**

BASIC INFORMATION (i)

DEFINITION

Restless legs syndrome is a primary neurologic disorder of unknown cause that manifests with both sensory and motor symptoms usually involving the lower extremities and disrupting sleep.

SYNONYMS

"Crazy legs" (lay term)
Nocturnal myoclonus

ICD-9CM CODES
333.99 Nocturnal myoclonus

EPIDEMIOLOGY & DEMOGRAPHICS

PREVALENCE: 5% to 15%
DEMOGRAPHICS: Age 2 yr, with no upper limit
- Age 30 to 79: 10%
- Age 80 and above: 19%
- Prevalence increases with age (may explain a slight female overrepresentation)
- Symptoms worsen with age

PHYSICAL FINDINGS & CLINICAL PRESENTATION

- Sensory nocturnal complaints usually affecting both lower extremities:
  - Crawly feeling or fizzle under the skin
  - Itching under the skin
  - Pain or ache
  - Electric shocks
  - Irresistible urge to move the symptomatic leg
- Other words used by patients to describe the leg symptoms: creeping, burning, searing, tugging, pulling, drawing, like water flowing, worms or bugs under the skin, restless, indescribable.

- Consistent symptom relief or improvement with leg movement or walking.
- Sleep disruption.
- Leg movements during sleep may occur but are not the prevailing complaint (unlike the urge to move). These movements are short bursts lasting <5 sec.
- Physical examination is normal.

ETIOLOGY

- Unknown/idiopathic
- Hereditary (30% to 60%)
- Associated with iron deficiency
- Associated with renal failure (end-stage)
- Associated with peripheral neuropathy or radiculopathy
- Associated with rheumatologic conditions (rheumatoid arthritis, fibromyalgia)
- Medication induced (selective serotonin reuptake inhibitors)

DIAGNOSIS (Dx)

DIFFERENTIAL DIAGNOSIS

- Periodic limb movement disorder (PLMD) (repetitive limb movements [lower extremities > upper extremities] occurring during sleep; associated with arousals from sleep and daytime sleeping; patient is typically unaware, but bed partner reports restlessness or kicking during sleep)
- Peripheral neuropathy and radiculopathy
- Anxiety and mood disorders
- Chronic fatigue
- Other sleep disorders
- Neuroleptic-induced akathisia
- Dyskinesias while awake
- Nocturnal leg cramps with or without peripheral artery disease

WORKUP

- History is typically diagnostic with sensitivity and specificity both >90%
- Sleep logs
- Polysomnography
- Ambulatory recording of leg activity
- CBC, iron, TIBC

TREATMENT (Rx)

- Dopaminergic drugs are first line: levodopa/carbidopa (Sinemet), pergolide, ropinirole, or pramipexole
- Benzodiazepines
- Trazodone
- Opioids
- Gabapentin (Neurontin)

PROGNOSIS

Tendency to worsen with age

SUGGESTED READINGS

Allen RP: Restless legs syndrome: epidemiology and diagnosis, *Med Behav* 1:36, 1998.
Earley CJ: Restless legs syndrome, *N Engl J Med* 348:2103, 2003.
Lin SC et al: Effect of pramipexole in treatment of resistant restless legs syndrome, *Mayo Clin Proc* 73:497, 1998.
National Heart, Lung, and Blood Institute Working Group on Restless Legs Syndrome: Restless legs syndrome: detection and management in primary care, *Am Fam Physician* 62:108, 2000.
Phillips B et al: Epidemiology of restless legs symptoms in adults, *Arch Intern Med* 160:2137, 2000.

AUTHOR: **TOM J. WACHTEL, M.D.**

BASIC INFORMATION

DEFINITION

Allergic rhinitis is an inflammatory disorder involving the upper respiratory tract characterized by itching of the eyes, nose, and palate and nasal congestion. It can further be classified as seasonal if this complex of symptoms occurs at a particular time of the year or perennial if the symptoms occur year-round. Common seasonal allergens include tree, grass, weed, pollen, fungi, and molds. Perennial rhinitis is often caused by such allergens as dust mites, cockroaches, animal proteins, and fungi.

ICD-9CM CODES
472.0 Rhinitis
473.9 Sinusitis

EPIDEMIOLOGY & DEMOGRAPHICS

PREVALENCE IN U.S.: Studies estimate the prevalence to be between 9% and 40% of the population.

PHYSICAL FINDINGS & CLINICAL PRESENTATION

- Patients can present with any combination of the following: postnasal drip, maxillary and frontal sinus pressure, pharyngitis, cough, watery eyes, itch, vertigo, sneeze, and nasal congestion.
- In patients with active rhinitis the nasal mucosa must be visualized to evaluate nasal anatomy for discharge, polyps, tumors, and intact mucosa.

DIAGNOSIS

DIFFERENTIAL DIAGNOSIS

In general history can differentiate allergic rhinitis from the following: infectious rhinitis, vasomotor rhinitis (idiopathic), occupational rhinitis, and rhinitis medicamentosa.

TREATMENT

NONPHARMACOLOGIC THERAPY

Preventive measures include allergen avoidance and environmental measures. Identifying allergens may be difficult but in most cases can be identified by history alone. Use of bed covers impermeable to dust mite allergens has not been shown to alleviate rhinitis. Measures that have been successful in previous research include maintaining the humidity at no greater than 50% and hot water washing of bedding once per week. HEPA filters may reduce animal and dust allergens, but do not control symptoms.

INTRANSAL Rx

Intranasal corticosteroid therapy is considered first line therapy for allergic rhinitis because of its limited side effect profile and significantly greater relief of nasal symptoms, sneezing, itch, and postnasal drip than oral antihistamines. Azelastine, a topical intranasal second-generation antihistamine, is also efficacious in relief of the total allergic symptom profile including rhinorrhea, sneezing, postnasal drip, itchy eyes/ears/throat, and nasal congestion, but is believed to be less effective than intranasal corticosteroids. In several randomized trials monotherapy with azelastine was as effective as dual therapy of azelastine plus loratadine or fexofenadine. Intranasal decongestant therapy prepared with a topical α-adrenergic agonist (e.g., oxymetazoline) reduces nasal congestion but should be avoided due to risk of nasal hyperreactivity and rebound swelling. Any usage should be limited to 3 days.

ORAL Rx

- First-generation oral antihistamines should be avoided due to their anticholinergic and sedating effects. They also have a negative impact on cognitive function. The second-generation oral antihistamines (loratadine, desloratadine, fexofenadine) are less sedating than the first-generation medications and are effective in relief of sneezing, rhinorrhea, and itch. The second-generation certerzidine may be more effective in relieving the symptoms of sneezing, rhinorrhea, and itch but is associated with more sedation than other second-generation oral antihistamines. In general the second-generation medications are minimally effective against nasal congestion.

- Short-term (i.e., 3 to 4 days) over-the-counter therapy for nasal congestion is commonly advised with pseudoephedrine, which increases pulse pressure and systolic blood pressure and should be avoided in persons with coronary artery disease and hypertension. Pseudoephedrine also tightens the urinary bladder outlet and can worsen lower urinary tract symptoms in men with benign prostatic hypertrophy. An additive effect on the lower urinary tract is seen with the combination of decongestant and antihistamine.

REFERRAL

Patients with symptoms not amenable to medical treatment should be evaluated by allergist/immunologist for allergen identification and possibly immunotherapy. An ENT specialist should evaluate patients with suspected or visualized structural abnormality when anterior rhinoscopy is required for possible biopsy or surgery.

PEARLS & CONSIDERATIONS

COMMENTS

- Nasal inflammation can lead to obstruction of the osteomeatal complex, predisposing patients to as many as 30% and 80% of acute and chronic bacterial infections of the sinuses, respectively.
- In the elderly, systemic treatments should be reserved for patients who fail intranasal therapy.
- Patients who have a history of upper respiratory tract symptoms at the same time of the year probably have allergic rhinosinusitis rather than infection.

SUGGESTED READINGS

Berger WE: Weighing the pros and cons of a wide array of therapies: how to get your patient's allergic rhinitis under control, *J Resp Dis* 26:150-161, 2005.

Dykewicz MS: Rhinitis and sinusitis, *J Allergy Clin Immuno* 111:S520-S529, 2003.

Kaszuba SM, Baroody FM, DeTineo M: Superiority of intranasal corticosteroids compared with an oral antihistamine in the as-needed treatment of seasonal allergic rhinitis, *Arch Int Med* 161:2581-2592, 2001.

AUTHOR: **MICHAEL P. GERARDO, D.O., M.P.H.**

BASIC INFORMATION

DEFINITION

Rotator cuff syndrome refers to a spectrum of afflictions involving the tendons of the rotator cuff (primarily the supraspinatus), ranging from simple strains and tendinitis to complete rupture with cuff-tear arthropathy.

SYNONYMS

Impingement syndrome
Painful arc syndrome
Internal derangement of the subacromial joint
Supraspinatus syndrome

ICD-9CM CODES
726.10 Rotator cuff syndrome
727.61 Rotator cuff rupture

EPIDEMIOLOGY & DEMOGRAPHICS

PREVALENCE: 5% to 10% of the general population
PREDOMINANT AGE: Uncommon under 20 yr of age
PREDOMINANT SEX: More common in males than females

PHYSICAL FINDINGS & CLINICAL PRESENTATION

- Pain, often at night
- Rotator cuff tenderness
- Referred pain down deltoid, especially with abduction between 70 and 120 degrees ("the painful arc") (Fig. 1-36)
- Weakness in abduction or forward flexion
- Increased pain with overhead activities
- Atrophy in long-standing cases of complete tear
- Positive "drop-arm" test (weakness of abduction against downward pressure at 90°)

ETIOLOGY

- Microtrauma from repetitive use
- Abnormally shaped acromion
- Shoulder instability
- Worsening of process by the overhead throwing motion

DIAGNOSIS

DIFFERENTIAL DIAGNOSIS

- Shoulder instability
- Degenerative arthritis
- Cervical radiculopathy
- Avascular necrosis
- Suprascapular nerve entrapment

WORKUP

- In chronic tendinitis, clinical findings similar to those seen in partial rupture
- Even with complete rupture, may have full, active range of motion in shoulder

IMAGING STUDIES

- Plain radiography
- Ultrasonography may be useful but only in diagnosing moderately large tears
- MRI to evaluate full- or partial-thickness tears, chronic tendinitis, and other causes of shoulder pain
- Since MRI, arthrography is rarely used

TREATMENT

ACUTE GENERAL Rx

- Rest to avoid overhead activity
- Ice or heat for comfort
- Carefully supervised program of stretching and strengthening
- Medication: NSAIDs, subacromial corticosteroid injection (once or twice at 2 wk intervals)

DISPOSITION

- All forms are likely to respond to non-surgical management.
- Even many complete rotator cuff tears have minimal pain and little loss of function.

REFERRAL

For orthopedic consultation in cases that fail to respond to medical management or in which rotator cuff tear is suspected

PEARLS & CONSIDERATIONS

COMMENTS

- There is considerable disagreement regarding the likelihood of recovery once a significant rotator cuff rupture has developed.
- Indications for surgery vary among surgeons.
- Injection is contraindicated in the presence of local infection.

SUGGESTED READINGS

Biberthaler P et al: Microcirculation associated with degenerative rotator cuff lesions, *J Bone Joint Surg* 85A:475, 2003.

Gorski JM, Schwartz LH: Shoulder impingement presenting as neck pain, *J Bone Joint Surg* 85:635, 2003.

Green A: Chronic massive rotator cuff tears: evaluation and management, *J Am Acad Orthop Surg* 11:321, 2003.

Tashjian RZ et al: The effect of comorbidity on self-assessed function in patients with chronic rotator cuff tears, *J Bone Joint Surg* 86A:355, 2004.

Teefey SA et al: Detection and quantification of rotator cuff tears, *J Bone Joint Surg* 86A:708, 2004.

Wendelboe AM et al: Associations between body mass index and surgery for rotator cuff tendinitis, *J Bone Joint Surg* 86A:743, 2004.

AUTHOR: **LONNIE R. MERCIER, M.D.**

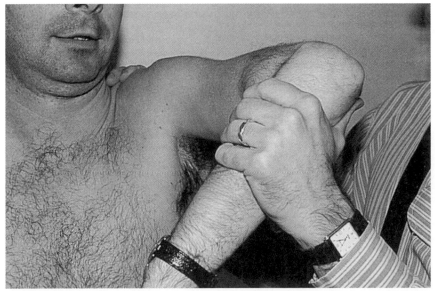

FIGURE 1-36 Rotator cuff lesions are often accompanied by painful impingement of the upwardly subluxating humerus onto the acromion. Evidence for this as a cause of pain is elicited by impingement tests, for example, by forced, passive, internal rotation and abduction of the shoulder, as shown here. (From Klippel J, Dieppe P, Ferri F [eds]: *Primary care rheumatology*, London, 1999, Mosby.)

BASIC INFORMATION

DEFINITION

Scabies is a contagious disease caused by the mite *Sarcoptes scabiei*.

ICD-9CM CODES
133.0 Scabies

EPIDEMIOLOGY & DEMOGRAPHICS

- Scabies is generally acquired by sleeping with or in the bedding of infested individuals.
- It is generally associated with poor living conditions and is also common in hospitals and nursing homes.

PHYSICAL FINDINGS & CLINICAL PRESENTATION

- Primary lesions are caused when the female mite burrows within the stratum corneum, laying eggs within the tract she leaves behind; burrows (linear or serpiginous tracts) end with a minute papule or vesicle.
- Primary lesions are most commonly found in the web spaces of the hands, wrists, buttocks, scrotum, penis, breasts, axillae, and knees.
- Secondary lesions result from scratching or infection.
- Intense pruritus, especially nocturnal, is common; it is caused by an acquired sensitivity to the mite or fecal pellets and is usually noted 1 to 4 wk after the primary infestation.
- Examination of the skin may reveal burrows, tiny vesicles, excoriations, inflammatory papules.
- Widespread and crusted lesions (Norwegian or crusted scabies) may be seen in elderly and immunocompromised patients.

ETIOLOGY

Human scabies is caused by the mite *Sarcoptes scabiei,* var. *hominis* (Fig. 1-37).

DIAGNOSIS

DIFFERENTIAL DIAGNOSIS

- Pediculosis
- Atopic dermatitis
- Flea bites
- Seborrheic dermatitis
- Dermatitis herpetiformis
- Contact dermatitis
- Nummular eczema
- Syphilis
- Other insect infestation

WORKUP

Diagnosis is made on the clinical presentation and on the demonstration of mites, eggs, or mite feces.

LABORATORY TESTS

- Microscopic demonstration of the organism, feces, or eggs: a drop of mineral oil may be placed over the suspected lesion before removal; the scrapings are transferred directly to a glass slide; a drop of potassium hydroxide is added and a cover slip is applied.
- Skin biopsy is rarely necessary to make the diagnosis.

TREATMENT

NONPHARMACOLOGIC THERAPY

Clothing, underwear, and towels used in the 48 hr before treatment must be laundered.

ACUTE GENERAL Rx

- Following a warm bath or shower, Lindane (Kwell, Scabene) lotion should be applied to all skin surfaces below the neck (can be applied to the face if area is infested); it should be washed off 8-12 hr after application. Repeat application 1 wk later is usually sufficient to eradicate infestation.
- Pruritus generally abates 24-48 hr after treatment, but it can last up to 2 wk; oral antihistamines are effective in decreasing postscabietic pruritus.
- Topical corticosteroid creams may hasten the resolution of secondary eczematous dermatitis.
- If the patient is a resident of an extended care facility, it is important to educate the patients, staff, family, and frequent visitors about scabies and the need to have full cooperation in treatment. Scabicide should be applied to all patients, staff, and frequent visitors, whether symptomatic or not; symptomatic family members of staff and visitors should also receive treatment.
- Permethrin 5% cream (Elimite) is also effective with usually one treatment; it should be massaged into the skin from head to soles of feet; remove 8-14 hr later by washing. If living mites are present after 14 days, treat again.
- A single dose (150-200 mg/kg in 6-mg tablets) of ivermectin, an antihelmintic agent, is as effective as topical lindane for the treatment of scabies. It is the best treatment for generalized crusted scabies.

DISPOSITION

Refractory cases usually are seen with immunocompromised hosts or patients with underlying skin diseases.

PEARLS & CONSIDERATIONS

COMMENTS

- Sexual partners should be notified and treated.

SUGGESTED READINGS

Fawcett RS: Ivermectin use in scabies, *Am Fam Physician* 68:1089, 2003.
Flinders DC, DeSchweinitz P: Pediculosis and scabies, *Am Fam Physician* 341:8, 2004.

AUTHOR: **FRED F. FERRI, M.D.**

FIGURE 1-37 Scabies organism in a wet mount preparation. (From Mandell GL: *Mandell, Douglas, and Bennett's principles and practice of infectious diseases,* ed 5, New York, 2000, Churchill Livingstone.)

BASIC INFORMATION

DEFINITION

Generalized tonic-clonic seizures

- Generalized tonic-clonic seizures are marked by paroxysmal hypersynchronous neuronal activity involving both cerebral hemispheres resulting in loss of consciousness with tonic muscle contraction followed by rhythmic clonic contractions. The seizure may start focally in one region or hemisphere of the brain with subsequent secondary generalization.

Partial seizures

- In partial seizures, the onset of abnormal electrical activity originates in a focal region or lobe of the brain. Clinical manifestations may involve sensory, motor, autonomic, or psychic symptoms. Consciousness may be preserved (simple partial seizures) or impaired (complex partial seizures).

SYNONYMS

Epilepsy
Convulsive disorders

ICD-9CM CODES
345.1 Generalized convulsive epilepsy
345.4 Partial epilepsy, with impairment of consciousness
345.5 Partial epilepsy, without impairment of consciousness

EPIDEMIOLOGY & DEMOGRAPHICS

INCIDENCE (IN U.S.): 100 cases/100,000 persons/yr
PREVALENCE (IN U.S.): Approximately 6.5 cases/1000 persons for all types of epilepsy
PREDOMINANT SEX: Males slightly higher than females
GENETICS: Genetic predisposition exists for the idiopathic generalized epilepsies

PHYSICAL FINDINGS & CLINICAL PRESENTATION

The hallmark for a seizure is typically its unpredictable occurrence as a spell.
1. Generalized tonic-clonic seizure (described as grand mal seizure in outdated texts)
   - Sequence of motor events during the seizure typically includes widespread tonic muscle contraction evolving to clonic jerking.
   - Typically associated with postictal confusion lasting up to several hours.
   - May be associated with tongue, cheek, or lip biting or urinary incontinence.
   - Generally normal neurologic examination. Focal deficits may be found in patients with an underlying lesion causing the seizures.
   - Rarely postictal neurologic deficits may be seen in the absence of specific brain lesions; they resolve in less than 48 hours.
   - Postictal fever usually resolves in 24 to 48 hours if there is no comorbid infection.
   - Aspiration pneumonitis is more common in the elderly as a complication.
2. Partial seizure
   - Clinical presentation is varied and depends on the site of origin of the abnormal electrical discharges.
   - Symptoms of simple partial seizures can include focal motor or sensory symptoms; language disturbance; olfactory, visual, or auditory hallucinations; visceral sensations, or fear or panic.
   - With complex partial seizures, there is a loss or reduction of awareness. This may be preceded by an aura. There may be associated automatisms or alterations in behavior.
   - There may be a "march" or progression of symptoms over seconds to minutes as the ictal focus spreads along the cortex.
   - Neurologic examination ranges from normal to focal neurologic deficits, depending on underlying cause.

ETIOLOGY

- Seizures are a symptom of an underlying abnormality affecting the CNS, not a disease.
- Etiology of seizures can be divided into idiopathic, symptomatic, or cryptogenic causes.
- With idiopathic generalized tonic-clonic seizures, there is a postulated inherited basis for the disorder. They can continue over the patient's lifetime.
- Symptomatic generalized tonic-clonic seizures and most partial seizures result from an underlying cause such as metabolic or toxic abnormalities (including medications), stroke, vascular malformations, CNS infection, brain tumor, and trauma.
- Cryptogenic seizures are those without a clear underlying cause (rare onset in the elderly).

DIAGNOSIS

- Differential diagnosis of generalized seizures
  - Syncope especially when the event was unwitnessed
  - Psychogenic events
- Differential diagnosis of partial seizures
  - Migraine
  - TIA
  - Presyncope
  - Psychogenic phenomena
- See Seizure in Section II.

LABORATORY TESTS

- Glucose, bun, creatinine, electrolytes
- CBC
- ALT, alkaline phosphatase
- Calcium, phosphorus, magnesium
- Oxygen saturation
- When appropriate alcohol level and toxicology screen
- Lumbar puncture as indicated by history and physical examination
- EEG: most valuable diagnostic tool for identifying seizure type and predicting the likelihood of recurrence

IMAGING STUDIES

- MRI with contrast: modality of choice because of its high sensitivity for stroke, tumor, abscess, atrophy, and vascular malformations
- CT scan without contrast if hemorrhage is suspected

TREATMENT Rx

NONPHARMACOLOGIC THERAPY

Avoid sleep deprivation or environmental precipitants (e.g., photosensitive epilepsy).

ACUTE GENERAL Rx

- Single seizures lasting <5 min generally require no acute pharmacologic intervention.
- Status epilepticus: >30 min of continuous seizure activity or sequential seizures without full recovery of consciousness between seizures.
  - Maintain/protect airway.
  - Give oxygen.
  - Monitor/maintain vital signs.
  - Gain IV access.
  - Lorazepam 0.1 mg/kg IV at 2 mg/min.
  - If ineffective, give phosphenytoin 20 mg IV at 150 mg/min or phenytoin at 50 mg/min.
  - If still ineffective, use phenobarbital 20 mg/kg IV at 100 mg/min.
  - Thiamine and hypertonic glucose, both IV, are usually administered.
- See Table 1-16.

ACUTE Rx

- Generalized tonic-clonic seizures
  - Sodium valproate and phenytoin are appropriate first line therapeutic agents.
  - Newer agents such as lamotrigine and topiramate may be better tolerated.
  - For each patient, anticonvulsant choice is influenced by factors such as effectiveness, cost, adverse effects,

ease of administration, and type of epilepsy syndrome if present.

- A single seizure with an identifiable and easily correctable provoking factor (e.g., hyponatremia) does not warrant long-term use of anticonvulsants.
- Partial seizures
  - Carbamazepine or phenytoin are common first line therapeutic agents.
  - Sodium valproate may also be effective.
  - Newer agents such as lamotrigine or oxcarbazepine may be better tolerated, but they are more expensive.

DISPOSITION

- Varies with underlying etiology.
- Approximately 70% of patients are controlled with medication.

REFERRAL

If uncertain about diagnosis or patient fails to respond to appropriate medication, refer to a neurologist or epilepsy specialist for further evaluation. In addition, some types of partial seizures, particularly temporal lobe epilepsy, are amenable to surgical resection.

PEARLS & CONSIDERATIONS

CAUTION

EEG is normal in as many as 50% of patients; thus diagnosis is primarily by history. Usually, a single seizure is not treated with chronic anticonvulsants.

COMMENTS

- Patient education information can be obtained from the Epilepsy Foundation of America, 4351 Garden City Drive, Landover, MD 20785; phone: (800) EFA-1000.

SUGGESTED READINGS

Browne TR, Holmes GL: Epilepsy, *N Engl J Med* 344:1145, 2001.
Chabolla DR: Characteristics of the epilepsies, *Mayo Clin Proc* 77:981, 2002.
Torres MR, Ahern GL, Labiner DM: Seizures and epilepsy: an approach to diagnosis and management, *JCOM* 12:103-115, 2005.
Wiebe S et al: A randomized controlled trial of surgery for temporal-lobe epilepsy, *N Engl J Med* 345:311, 2001.

AUTHORS: **JOHN E. CROOM, M.D., PH.D.,** with revisions by **TOM J. WACHTEL, M.D.**

TABLE 1-16 Drug of Choice in Treatment of Epilepsy

Seizure Type	Drug of Choice
Generalized tonic-clonic, simple, and complex partial	Phenytoin, valproic acid
	Carbamazepine, phenobarbital
	Levetiracetam, zonisamide
Absence	Ethosuximide
	Valproic acid
Temporal epilepsy	Phenytoin, gabapentin

	Newer Drugs
Generalized tonic-clonic, simple, partial, and complex partial	Lamotrigine
	Tiagabine
	Topiramate
	Zonisamide
	Oxcarbazepine
	Levetiracetam
	Gabapentin

From Ferri F (ed): *Ferri's Clinical Advisor: Instant Diagnosis and Treatment,* Philadelphia, 2005, Mosby.

BASIC INFORMATION

DEFINITION

Sexual dysfunction implies persistent or recurrent difficulty involving the social, psychological, cognitive, hormonal, or physical functional aspects of sexual response.

SYNONYMS

Impotence
Frigidity

ICD-9CM CODES
V417.0 Sexual function problem
607.84 Impotence
625.0 Dyspareunia
602.71 Inhibited sexual desire

EPIDEMIOLOGY & DEMOGRAPHICS

Normal sexual function extends throughout the life span though there appears to be a linear trend toward reduced frequency of sexual encounters as people age.

PHYSICAL FINDINGS & CLINICAL PRESENTATION

MALE CLINICAL PRESENTATION
- Libido dysfunction
- Erectile dysfunction
- Ejaculatory dysfunction
- Interpersonal conflict

MALE PHYSICAL PRESENTATION
- Neuropathy
  - Impaired response to Valsalva maneuver
  - Absent bulbocavernous or cremasteric reflexes
- Peyronie's disease
- Hypogonadism

FEMALE CLINICAL PRESENTATION
- Libido dysfunction
- Sexual arousal disorder
- Orgasmic disorder
- Sexual pain disorder
- Interpersonal conflict

FEMAL PHYSICAL PRESENTATION
- Gynecologic tumors
- Interstitial cystitis
- Retroverted uterus
- Vaginal atrophy
- Vulvar or vaginal infection

ETIOLOGY
- Testosterone deficiency
- Hypogonadism
- Urinary incontinence
- Chronic pain
- Interpersonal conflict
- Males: vascular insufficiency
- Females: dyspareunia and vaginal dryness

DIAGNOSIS

DIFFERENTIAL DIAGNOSIS
- Hormonal:
  - Low testosterone
  - Diabetes mellitus
  - Thyroid disorders
- Psychological:
  - Interpersonal conflict
  - History of sexual abuse
  - Depression
- Physical nongonadal:
  - Osteoarthritis
  - Pelvic fracture
  - Cardiac disorders
  - Urinary incontinence
  - Postoperative (ostomy, mastectomy, hysterectomy)
- Physical gonadal:
  - Vaginal atrophy
  - Testicular atrophy
  - Scar tissue
- Medication induced:
  - Antidepressants
  - Antihypertensives

WORKUP
- Sexual history with emphasis on interpersonal relations
- Physical examination with emphasis on musculoskeletal function, gonadal atrophy, and cardiovascular status
- Medication review

LABORATORY TESTS
- Total and bioavailable testosterone
- Blood sugar
- Thyroid stimulating hormone
- Luteinizing hormone
- Prolactin

IMAGING STUDIES
Penile to brachial pressure index

TREATMENT

NONPHARMACOLOGIC THERAPY
- Psychological counseling
- Vacuum tumescent device (penile and clitoral devices FDA approved)
- Penile implant
- Pelvic relaxation exercises

ACUTE GENERAL Rx

MALE
- Testosterone replacement therapy
- Phosphodiesterase inhibitors (sildenafil, vardenafil, tadalafil)
- Yohimbine
- Intracavernous injection (papaverine, prostaglandin E1, pentolaine)

FEMALE
- Estrogen replacement therapy
- Testosterone supplementation
- Water soluble lubricants

DISPOSITION

Patients benefit from regular follow-up and reassurance.

REFERRAL

Individual and couple psychotherapy and counseling

PEARLS & CONSIDERATIONS

COMMENTS
- Normal sexual function is a meaningful part of a person's function throughout his or her life span.
- Resolving the sexual dysfunction of one partner may create new interpersonal conflict.
- Normal sexual relations are not always between male and female spouses, and the patient's sexual partner is not always the obvious person.

PREVENTION

Physical exercise and screening

SUGGESTED READINGS

Gott M, Hinchliff S: Barriers to seeking treatment for sexual problems in primary care: a qualitative study with older people, *Fam Pract* 20:690-695, 2003.

Hazzard WR: *Principles of Geriatric Medicine and Gerontology*, New York, 2002, McGraw-Hill Professional, pp 1312-1323.

MayoClinic.com: Intimacy and aging: tips for sexual health and happiness, www.mayoclinic.com

AUTHOR: **JOHN A. STOUKIDES, M.D., R.PH.**

BASIC INFORMATION

DEFINITION

Sick sinus syndrome is a group of cardiac rhythm disturbances characterized by abnormalities of the sinus node including (1) sinus bradycardia, (2) sinus arrest or exit block, (3) combinations of sinoatrial or atrioventricular conduction defects, and (4) supraventricular tachyarrhythmias. These abnormalities may coexist in a single patient so that a patient may have episodes of bradycardia and episodes of tachycardia.

SYNONYMS

Bradycardia-tachycardia syndrome

ICD-9CM CODES

427.81 Sick sinus syndrome

EPIDEMIOLOGY & DEMOGRAPHICS

- Typically associated with ischemic heart disease but may occur in the presence of a normal heart

PHYSICAL FINDINGS & CLINICAL PRESENTATION

- Lightheadedness, dizziness, syncope, palpitation
- Arterial embolization (e.g., stroke) associated with atrial fibrillation
- Physical examination may be normal or reveal abnormalities (e.g., heart murmurs or gallop sounds) associated with the underlying heart disease

ETIOLOGY

- Fibrosis or fatty infiltration involving the sinus node, atrioventricular node, the His bundle, or its branches
- In addition, inflammatory or degenerative changes of the nerves and ganglia surrounding the sinus nodes and other sclerodegenerative changes may be found

DIAGNOSIS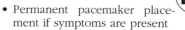

DIFFERENTIAL DIAGNOSIS

- Bradycardia: atrioventricular block
- Tachycardia: atrial fibrillation
- Atrial flutter
- Paroxysmal atrial tachycardia
- Sinus tachycardia
- Syncope (see "Syncope" in Section I)

WORKUP

- ECG
- Ambulatory cardiac rhythm monitoring
- 24-hour ambulatory ECG (Holter) (Fig. 1-38)
- Event recorder
- Electrophysiologic testing including sinus nodal recovery time and sino-atrial conduction time

TREATMENT   **Rx**

- Permanent pacemaker placement if symptoms are present
- The drug treatment of the tachycardia (e.g., with digitalis or calcium channel blockers) may worsen or bring out the bradycardia and become the reason for pacemaker requirement

REFERRAL

To cardiologist

SUGGESTED READING

Zipes DP, Olgin JE: Sick sinus syndrome. In Braunwald E (ed): *Heart Disease: A Textbook of Cardiovascular Medicine*, ed 6, Philadelphia, 2001, WB Saunders.

AUTHOR: **TOM J. WACHTEL, M.D.**

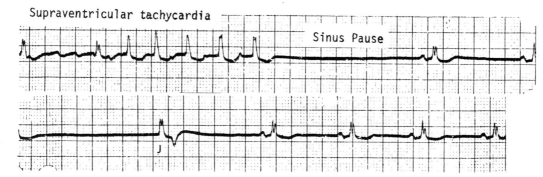

FIGURE 1-38   Brady-tachy (sick sinus) syndrome. This rhythm strip shows a narrow-complex tachycardia (probably atrial flutter) followed by a sinus pause, an AV junctional escape beat *(J)*, and then sinus rhythm. (From Goldberger AL: *Clinical electrocardiography,* ed 5, St Louis, 1994, Mosby.)

BASIC INFORMATION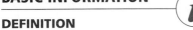

DEFINITION

Sjögren's syndrome (SS) is an autoimmune disorder characterized by lymphocytic and plasma cell infiltration and destruction of salivary and lacrimal glands with subsequent diminished lacrimal and salivary gland secretions.

- *Primary:* dry mouth (xerostomia) and dry eyes (xerophthalmia) develop as isolated entities.
- *Secondary:* associated with other disorders.

SYNONYMS

SS
Sicca syndrome

ICD-9CM CODES
710.2 Sjögren's syndrome

EPIDEMIOLOGY & DEMOGRAPHICS

INCIDENCE/PREVALENCE: 1 case/2500 persons; secondary SS is just as common and can affect up to one third of SLE patients and nearly 20% of RA patients.
PREDOMINANT AGE: Peak incidence is in the sixth decade.
PREDOMINANT SEX: Female > male

PHYSICAL FINDINGS & CLINICAL PRESENTATION

- Dry mouth with dry lips (cheilosis), erythema of tongue (Fig. 1-39), and other mucosal surfaces, carious teeth
- Dry eyes (conjunctival injection, decreased luster, and irregularity of the corneal light reflex)
- Possible salivary gland enlargement and dysfunction with subsequent difficulty in chewing and swallowing food and in speaking without frequent water intake

- Purpura (nonthrombocytopenic, hyperglobulinemic, vasculitic) may be present
- Evidence of associated conditions (e.g., RA or other connective disease, lymphoma, hypothyroidism, COPD, trigeminal neuropathy, chronic liver disease, polymyopathy)

ETIOLOGY

Autoimmune disorder

DIAGNOSIS

DIFFERENTIAL DIAGNOSIS

- Medication-related dryness (e.g., anticholinergics)
- Age-related exocrine gland dysfunction
- Mouth breathing
- Anxiety
- Other: sarcoidosis, primary salivary hypofunction, radiation injury, amyloidosis

WORKUP

Workup involves the demonstration of the following criteria for diagnosis of primary and secondary Sjögren's syndrome:
PRIMARY:
- Symptoms and objective signs of ocular dryness:
  1. Schirmer's test: <8 mm wetting per 5 min
  2. Positive rose bengal or fluorescein staining of cornea and conjunctiva to demonstrate keratoconjunctivitis sicca
- Symptoms and objective signs of dry mouth:
  1. Decreased parotid flow using Lashley cups or other methods
  2. Abnormal biopsy result of minor salivary gland (focus score >2 based on average of four assessable lobules)

- Evidence of systemic autoimmune disorder:
  1. Elevated titer of rheumatoid factor >1:320
  2. Elevated titer of ANA >1:320
  3. Presence of anti-SS A (Ro) or anti-SS B (La) antibodies
SECONDARY:
- Characteristic signs and symptoms of SS (described in "Physical Findings")
- Clinical features sufficient to allow a diagnosis of RA, SLE, polymyositis, or scleroderma

LABORATORY TESTS

- Positive ANA (>60% of patients) with autoantibodies anti-SS A and anti-SS B may be present.
- Additional laboratory abnormalities may include elevated ESR, anemia (normochromic, normocytic), abnormal liver function studies, elevated serum β_2 microglobulin levels, rheumatoid factor.
- A definite diagnosis SS can be made with a salivary gland biopsy.

TREATMENT

NONPHARMACOLOGIC THERAPY

- Adequate fluid replacement
- Proper oral hygiene to reduce the incidence of caries

ACUTE GENERAL Rx

- Use artificial tears frequently.
- Pilocarpine 5 mg PO qid is useful to improve dryness. A cyclosporine 0.05% ophthalmic emulsion (Restasis) may also be useful for dry eyes. Recommended dose is one drop bid in both eyes.
- Cevimeline (Evoxac), a cholinergic agent with muscarinic agonist activity, 30 mg PO tid is effective for the treatment of dry mouth in patients with Sjögren's syndrome.

CHRONIC Rx

Periodic dental and ophthalmology evaluations to screen for complications

PEARLS & CONSIDERATIONS

COMMENTS

Unusual presentations of SS may occur in association with polymyalgia rheumatica, chronic fatigue syndrome, FUO, and inflammatory myositis.

SUGGESTED READING

Kassan SS, Moutsopoulos HM: Clinical manifestations and early diagnosis of Sjögren syndrome, *Arch Intern Med* 164:1275, 2004.

AUTHOR: **FRED F. FERRI, M.D.**

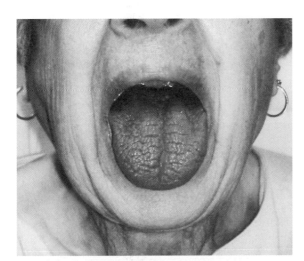

FIGURE 1-39 **"Crocodile tongue" in SS patient.** (From Noble J: *Primary care medicine,* ed 3, St Louis, 2001, Mosby.)

BASIC INFORMATION

DEFINITION

The American Academy of Sleep Disorders defines obstructive sleep apnea as "characterized by repetitive episodes of upper airway obstruction that occur during sleep, usually associated with a reduction in blood oxygen saturation."

SYNONYMS

Sleep apnea syndrome
Obstructive sleep apnea-hypopnea syndrome

ICD-9CM CODE
780.53 Obstructive sleep apnea syndrome

EPIDEMIOLOGY & DEMOGRAPHICS

Obstructive sleep apnea (OSA) occurs most frequently in 40- to 65-year-old men (4%) and women (2%). The prevalence is higher in obese and hypertensive individuals.

PHYSICAL FINDINGS & CLINICAL PRESENTATION

- Systemic hypertension
- History of snoring, witnessed apneas, and excessive daytime somnolence
- Obesity with body mass index >27 kg/m², neck circumference >43 cm (17″) in men
- Working memory impairment, inability to concentrate, short tempered
- Examination of oropharynx may reveal erythema caused by snoring and narrowing secondary to large tonsils, pendulous uvula, excessive soft tissue, prominent tongue and retrognathia
- Patient's bed partner may report loud snoring, episodic choking sounds, disrupted sleep with repetitive arousals, thrashing movements of extremities during sleep
- Decreased libido, mood swings, depression, and chronic fatigue

ETIOLOGY

Narrowing of upper airway secondary to:
- Obesity
- Macroglossia
- Tonsillar and adenoid hypertrophy
- Micrognathia
- Muscular weakness
- Use of alcohol or sedatives at bedtime

DIAGNOSIS

DIFFERENTIAL DIAGNOSIS

- Excessive Daytime Somnolence
  Inadequate sleep time
  Pulmonary disease
  Parkinsonism
  Sleep-related epilepsy
  Narcolepsy
  Hypothyroidism
- Sleep Fragmentation
  Sleep-related asthma
  Sleep-related GERD
  Periodic limb movement disorder
  Parasomnias
  Psychophysiologic insomnia
  Panic disorder
  Narcolepsy

WORKUP

- Medical history should include questions about snoring, witnessed apneas, and excessive daytime sleepiness. Additional history concerning morning headaches, alcohol intake, weight gain, and mood/personality changes also may help to implicate apnea.
- Sleep apnea can be confirmed by overnight polysomnography (gold standard). Testing is performed during the patient's habitual sleep hours and ideally includes all stages of sleep and body positions. Patients with sleep apnea have >5 apneic/hypopneic episodes per hour (termed respiratory disturbance index, or RDI) with desaturations of at least 4% by oximetry or coincidental arousals. Overnight oximetry tests can suggest the presence of sleep apnea but are not sufficient to rule out sleep apnea.
- Portable monitors that measure RDI are available but they lack the EEG, EMG, and technical observations necessary to diagnose sleep apnea with reliable accuracy. The use of such devices is usually related to limited availability of polysomnography.

LABORATORY TESTS

- TSH level is indicated in suspected hypothyroidism.
- CBC (with iron studies) is indicated for detecting anemia.
- Pulmonary function tests are indicated for detecting related pulmonary disorders.
- ECG is indicated for detecting related heart disease (e.g., CHF and arrhythmias).

IMAGING STUDIES

Radiography of soft tissues in the neck in patients with suspected anatomic abnormalities

TREATMENT

NONPHARMACOLOGIC THERAPY

- Weight loss in overweight patients including bariatric surgery
- Avoidance of sedating medications and alcohol
- Sleep hygiene training
- Elimination of the supine sleeping position
- For mild obstructive sleep apnea in select patient populations (e.g., retrognathia) an oral appliance (constructed by a qualified dentist) may be useful to push the mandible forward
- Uvulopalatopharyngoplasty (UPPP, both standard and laser-assisted [LAUP]) in patients with significant obstruction of retropalatal airway
- Nasal septoplasty in patients with nasoseptal deformity

ACUTE GENERAL Rx

- Nighttime treatment with continuous positive airway pressure (CPAP) provides immediate resolution of sleep apnea. Symptoms of excessive daytime somnolence may linger and necessitate further investigation or medical therapy
- Tracheostomy: reserved for life-threatening cases that are unresponsive to other treatments
- Nasal steroids in allergy or sinusitis patients

CHRONIC Rx

- CPAP therapy
- Weight loss

DISPOSITION

- Most patients improve with weight loss and CPAP.
- Overall success rate for UPPP is about 40% for snoring; likely less effective for apnea.
- Weight loss over time may reduce the need for CPAP pressure or obviate its use entirely.

REFERRAL

- Sleep physician for proper study type(s) and/or complex symptoms
- Surgical referral for patients unresponsive to weight loss and CPAP
- Dental referral for oral devices

PEARLS & CONSIDERATIONS

- In a primary care setting, patients with high risk of sleep apnea are those who meet two of the following three criteria: (1) snoring, (2) persistent daytime sleepiness or drowsiness while driving, (3) obesity or hypertension.
- Some patients with sleep apnea experience nocturnal dysrhythmias (bradycardia, paroxysmal tachyarrhythmias). In cardiac patients, trials using atrial overdrive pacing have demonstrated a significant reduction in the number of episodes of sleep apnea without reduction in the total sleep time.

- The use of vagal nerve stimulators (VNS) in epilepsy patients has been associated with an increase in apneas and hypopneas. VNS-related respiratory events may be reduced by altering VNS stimulation parameters or by initiating CPAP.

SUGGESTED READINGS

American Academy of Pediatrics: Clinical practice guideline: diagnosis and management of childhood obstructive sleep apnea syndrome, *Pediatrics* 109:704, 2002.

Arens, R: Obstructive sleep apnea in childhood, clinical features. In Loughlin G, Carroll J, Marcus C (eds): *Sleep and Breathing in Children,* New York, 2000, Marcel Dekker.

Chervin RD et al: Inattention, hyperactivity and symptoms of sleep-disordered breathing, *Pediatrics* 109:449, 2002.

Flemons WW: Obstructive sleep apnea, *N Engl J Med* 347:498, 2002.

Garrigue A et al: Benefit of atrial pacing in sleep apnea syndrome, *N Engl J Med* 346:404, 2002.

Marzec M et al: Effects of vagal nerve stimulation on sleep-related breathing in epilepsy patients, *Epilepsia* 44:930, 2003.

Partinen M, Hublin C: Epidemiology of sleep disorders. In Kryger M, Roth T, Dement W (eds): *Principles and Practice of Sleep Medicine,* ed 3, Philadelphia, 2000, WB Saunders.

Schroeder BM: Obstructive sleep apnea syndrome in children, *Am Fam Physician* 66:1338, 2002.

The International Classification of Sleep Disorders Revised, Diagnostic and Coding Manual. American Academy of Sleep Medicine, 2000.

AUTHOR: **J.S. DURMER, M.D., PH.D.**

BASIC INFORMATION

DEFINITION

Spinal stenosis is the pathologic condition compressing or narrowing the spinal canal, nerve root canal, or intervertebral foramina.

SYNONYMS

Central spinal stenosis
Lateral spinal stenosis
Spondylosis

ICD-9CM CODES

724.02 Spinal stenosis lumbar, lumbosacral

EPIDEMIOLOGY & DEMOGRAPHICS

- More common in the elderly.
- More than 30,000 patients underwent surgery for spinal stenosis in 1994.

CLINICAL PRESENTATION & PHYSICAL FINDINGS

- Neurogenic claudication: leg, buttock, or back pain precipitated by walking and relieved by sitting. The relief by sitting is the reason that the term *pseudoclaudication* is used sometimes. The mechanism of relief, however, is flexion of the spine. Look for the "shopping cart sign." Ask the patient to pay attention for symptom relief by bending forward.
- Radicular leg pain
- Paresthesias
- Difficulty standing or lying in an erect position
- Decreased lumbar extension
- Normal peripheral pulses
- Positive Romberg
- Wide-based gait
- Reduced knee and ankle reflex
- Urine incontinence

ETIOLOGY

- Degenerative (hypertrophy of the articular processes, disk degeneration, ligamentum flavum hypertrophy, spondylolisthesis)
- Fracture/trauma
- Postoperative (postlaminectomy)
- Paget's disease
- Ankylosing spondylitis
- Tumors
- Acromegaly

DIAGNOSIS **Dx**

DIFFERENTIAL DIAGNOSIS

Spinal stenosis must be differentiated from other common causes of back and leg pain; osteoarthritis of the knee or hip, osteomyelitis, epidural abscess, metastatic tumors, multiple myeloma, intermittent claudication secondary to peripheral vascular disease, neuropathy, scoliosis, herniated nucleus pulposus, spondylolisthesis, acute cauda equina syndrome, ankylosing spondylitis, Reiter's syndrome, fibromyalgia.

WORKUP

The workup of spinal stenosis consists of a detailed history, physical examination, and specific imaging studies.

IMAGING STUDIES

- Lumbar spine film.
- CT scan of the lumbosacral spine: sensitivity (75% to 85%), specificity (80%).
- MRI of the lumbosacral spine: sensitivity (80% to 90%), specificity (95%).
- Myelogram: sensitivity (77%), specificity (72%). Absolute stenosis is defined as the anterior-posterior (AP) diameter of the spinal canal <10 mm. Relative stenosis: 10-12 mm AP diameter.
- CT and MRI can visualize both the central and lateral canals.

Electromyography (EMG) and nerve conduction velocity (NCV) are additional studies that may be useful in differentiating peripheral neuropathy from lumbar spinal stenosis.

TREATMENT **Rx**

NONPHARMACOLOGIC THERAPY

- Physiotherapy
- Lumbar corsets
- Back exercises
- Abdominal muscle strengthening
- Aquatic exercises

ACUTE GENERAL Rx

- Surgery is indicated in patients with significant compression of nerve roots as determined by MRI or CT and incapacitating symptoms limiting activities of daily living or bladder and bowel incontinence. However, because the severity of symptoms varies over time, medical treatment should usually precede surgery in the absence of nerve root compression.

- Surgical procedures include decompressive laminectomy, arthrodesis, hemilaminectomy, and medial facetectomy.

CHRONIC Rx

- Conservative therapy with NSAIDs (ibuprofen 800 mg PO tid, naproxen 500 mg PO bid) should be tried for symptomatic relief in addition to acetaminophen 1 g PO qid.
- Epidural steroid injections may provide temporary relief.

DISPOSITION

- Approximately 20% of patients having surgery require repeat surgery within 10 yr. Nearly one third of the patients continue to experience pain.
- The natural history of spinal stenosis is one of slow progression. In some cases symptoms improve. Although not very common, cord compression with resultant bowel and bladder incontinence and paresis can occur.

REFERRAL

- Patients who have spinal stenosis unresponsive to medical treatment, and patients with symptomatic radiculopathy should be referred to an orthopedic surgeon specializing in back surgery or to a neurosurgeon.
- Pain clinic referrals can be made if surgery is contraindicated or if the patient does not want surgery.

PEARLS & CONSIDERATIONS

COMMENTS

Approximately one third of the patients with neurogenic claudication have coexisting peripheral vascular disease.

SUGGESTED READINGS

Fritz JM et al: Lumbar spinal stenosis: a review of current concepts in evaluation, management, and outcome measurements, *Arch Phys Med Rehabil* 79:700, 1998.
Schonstrom N, Willen J: Imaging lumbar spinal stenosis, *Radiol Clin North Am* 39(1):31, 2001.
Sheehan JM, Shaffrey CI, Jane JA: Degenerative lumbar stenosis: the neurosurgical perspective, *Clin Orthop* 384:61, 2001.
Snyder DL, Doggett D, Turkelson C: Treatment of degenerative lumbar spinal stenosis, *Am Fam Physician* 70:517-520, 2004.

AUTHORS: **PETER PETROPOULOS, M.D.,** with minor revisions by **TOM J. WACHTEL, M.D.**

BASIC INFORMATION

DEFINITION

Squamous cell carcinoma (SCC) is a malignant tumor of the skin arising in the epithelium.

SYNONYMS

SCC
Skin cancer

ICD-9CM CODES
173.9 Skin neoplasm, site unspecified

EPIDEMIOLOGY & DEMOGRAPHICS

- SCC is the second most common cutaneous malignancy, comprising 20% of all cases of nonmelanoma skin cancer.
- Incidence is highest in lower latitudes (e.g., southern U.S., Australia).
- Male:female ratio of 2:1.
- Incidence increases with age and sun exposure.
- Average age at diagnosis is 66 yr.

PHYSICAL FINDINGS & CLINICAL PRESENTATION

- SCC commonly affects scalp, neck region, back of hands, superior surface of the pinna, and the lip.
- The lesion may have a scaly, erythematous macule or plaque.
- Telangiectasia, central ulceration may also be present (Fig. 1-40).
- Most SCC present as exophytic lesions that grow over a period of months.

ETIOLOGY

Risk factors include UVB radiation and immunosuppression (renal transplant recipients have a threefold increased risk).

DIAGNOSIS **Dx**

DIFFERENTIAL DIAGNOSIS

- Keratoacanthomas
- Actinic keratosis
- Amelanotic melanoma
- Basal cell carcinoma
- Benign tumors
- Healing traumatic wounds
- Spindle cell tumors
- Warts

WORKUP

Diagnosis is made with full-thickness skin biopsy (incisional or excisional).

TREATMENT **Rx**

ACUTE GENERAL Rx

- Electrodesiccation and curettage for small SCCs (<2 cm in diameter), superficial tumors and lesions located in extremity and trunk.
- Tumors thinner than 4 mm can be managed by simple local removal.
- Lesions between 4 and 8 mm thick or those with deep dermal invasion should be excised.
- Tumors penetrating the dermis can be treated with several modalities, including excision and Mohs' surgery, radiation therapy, and chemotherapy.

- Metastatic SCC (rare) can be treated with cryotherapy and combination of chemotherapy using 13-*cis*-retinoic acid and interferon α-2A.

DISPOSITION

- Survival is related to size, location, degree of differentiation, immunologic status of the patient, depth of invasion, and presence of metastases. Risk factors for metastasis include lesions on the lip or ear, increasing lesion depth, and poor cell differentiation.
- Patients whose tumors penetrate through the dermis or exceed 8 mm in thickness are at risk of tumor recurrence.
- The most common metastatic locations are regional lymph nodes, liver, and lung.
- Tumors on the scalp, forehead, ears, nose, and lips also carry a higher risk.
- SCCs originating in the lip and pinna metastasize in 10% to 20% of cases.
- Five-year survival for metastatic squamous cell carcinoma is 34%.

REFERRAL

Oncology referral for metastatic SCC

PEARLS & CONSIDERATIONS

COMMENTS

SCC arising in areas of prior radiation, thermal injury, and areas of chronic ulcers or chronic draining sinuses are more aggressive and have a higher frequency of metastases than those originating in actinic damaged skin.

AUTHOR: **FRED F. FERRI, M.D.**

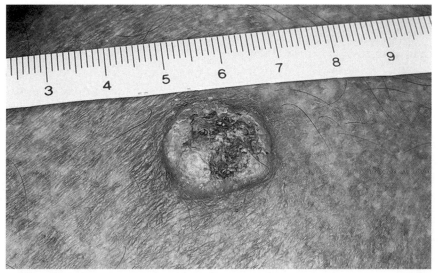

FIGURE 1-40 Squamous cell carcinoma. Nodular hyperkeratotic lesion with central erosion. (From Noble J et al: *Textbook of primary care medicine*, ed 3, St Louis, 2001, Mosby.)

BASIC INFORMATION

DEFINITION

Stasis dermatitis refers to an inflammatory skin disease of the lower extremities, commonly seen in patients with chronic venous insufficiency (Fig. 1-41).

ICD-9CM CODES
459.81 Stasis dermatitis

EPIDEMIOLOGY & DEMOGRAPHICS

- Stasis dermatitis occurs more frequently in the elderly
- Rarely seen before the age of 50 yr
- Estimated to occur in up to 6% to 7% of the patients >50 yr
- Occurs in women more often than men, perhaps related to lower extremity venous impairment aggravated through pregnancy

PHYSICAL FINDINGS & CLINICAL PRESENTATION

- Insidious onset
- Pruritus
- Chronic edema usually described as "brawny" edema as stasis dermatitis pathologically is associated with dermal fibrosis
- Erythema
- Scaly
- Eczematous patches
- Commonly located over the medial malleolus
- Progressive pigment changes can occur as a result of extravasation of red blood cells and hemosiderin deposition within the cutaneous tissue.
- Secondary infections can occur

ETIOLOGY

- Stasis dermatitis is thought to occur as a direct result from any insult or injury of the lower extremity venous system leading to venous insufficiency including:
  1. Deep vein thrombosis
  2. Trauma
  3. Pregnancy
  4. Vein stripping
  5. Vein harvesting in patients requiring coronary artery bypass grafting (CABG)

- Venous insufficiency subsequently results in venous hypertension, causing skin inflammation and the aforementioned physical findings and clinical presentation.

DIAGNOSIS (Dx)

The diagnosis of stasis dermatitis is primarily made by a detailed history and physical examination.

DIFFERENTIAL DIAGNOSIS

- Contact dermatitis
- Atopic dermatitis
- Cellulitis
- Tinea dermatophyte infection
- Pretibial myxedema
- Nummular eczema
- Lichen simplex chronicus
- Xerosis
- Asteatotic eczema
- Deep vein thrombosis

WORKUP

The workup of a patient with stasis dermatitis is directed at excluding potential life-threatening causes (e.g., deep vein thrombosis) and complications (e.g., cellulites and sepsis).

LABORATORY TESTS

Blood tests are generally not very helpful unless a secondary infection is present.

IMAGING STUDIES

- X-rays, CT scans, and MRIs are generally not very helpful.
- Doppler studies are indicated in any patient suspected of having a deep vein thrombosis.

TREATMENT (Rx)

NONPHARMACOLOGIC THERAPY

- Leg elevation
- Compression stocking with a gradient of at least 30-40 mm Hg
- For weeping skin lesions, wet to dry dressing changes are helpful

ACUTE GENERAL Rx

- In patients with acute stasis dermatitis, a compression (Unna) boot can be applied. An Unna boot consists of a roll

of gauze that is saturated with zinc oxide ointment supported with an elastic wrap. Unna boots are most effective for ambulatory patients. Nonambulatory patients do better with compression devices (elastic or pneumatic).
- Topical corticosteroid creams or ointments (e.g., triamcinolone 0.1% bid) are used frequently to help reduce inflammation and itching.
- Secondary infections should be treated with appropriate antibiotics. Most secondary infections are the result of *Staphylococcus* or *Streptococcus* organisms.

CHRONIC Rx

- Patients with chronic stasis dermatitis can be treated with topical emollients (e.g., white petrolatum, lanolin, Eucerin).
- Topical dressings (e.g., DuoDerm) are effective in the treatment of chronic venous stasis ulcers.

DISPOSITION

- The mainstay of treatment of stasis dermatitis is to control leg edema and prevent venous stasis ulcers from developing.
- Chronic venous stasis ulcers may take months to heal and may require skin grafting.

REFERRAL

- Dermatology referral is made if the diagnosis is unclear.
- Vascular surgery referral is made for assistance in the management of chronic venous insufficiency and chronic venous stasis ulcers.

PEARLS & CONSIDERATIONS (!)

COMMENTS

- Inflammatory skin changes from stasis dermatitis are thought to result from poor oxygen perfusion to the lower-extremity skin tissue. Various theories, including venous pooling, arteriovenous shunting, increased venous hydrostatic pressure affecting microcirculation, fibrin barriers preventing oxygen diffusion, and leukocyte trapping with resultant microvascular damage, have all been hypothesized as causes of stasis dermatitis.
- Diuretic use should be avoided or limited to intermittent short courses.

SUGGESTED READINGS

Flugman SL et al: Stasis dermatitis, www.emedicine.com.
Yuwono HS: Diagnosis and treatment in the management of chronic venous insufficiency, *Clin Hemorheol Microcirc* 23(2-4):233, 2000.

AUTHOR: **PETER PETROPOULOS, M.D.**

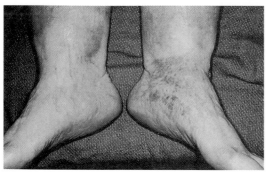

FIGURE 1-41 Moderate stasis dermatitis with hyperpigmentation and bilateral venous insufficiency. (Courtesy Department of Dermatology, University of North Carolina at Chapel Hill. From Goldstein BG, Goldstein AO: *Practical dermatology,* ed 2, St Louis, 1997, Mosby.)

BASIC INFORMATION

DEFINITION

Stroke describes acute brain injury caused by decreased blood supply or hemorrhage.

SYNONYMS

Cerebrovascular accident (CVA)

ICD-9CM CODES
436 Acute stroke

EPIDEMIOLOGY & DEMOGRAPHICS

INCIDENCE (IN U.S.):
- Occurs in 10 to 20/100,000 persons >65 yr of age

PREVALENCE (IN U.S.): Estimated at 2 million persons

PREDOMINANT SEX: Incidence is 30% higher in males

PREDOMINANT AGE: 60+ yr

PEAK INCIDENCE: 80-84 yr

PHYSICAL FINDINGS & CLINICAL PRESENTATION

Motor and/or sensory and/or cognitive deficits, depending on distribution and extent of involved vascular territory. More common manifestations include contralateral motor weakness or sensory loss, as well as language difficulties (aphasia; predominantly left-sided lesions) and visuospatial/neglect phenomena (predominantly right-sided lesions). Onset is usually sudden; however, this depends on specific etiology (Table 1-17).

ETIOLOGY

- 70%-80% are caused by ischemic infarcts; 20%-30% are hemorrhagic.
- 80% of ischemic infarcts are from occlusion of large or small vessels caused by atherosclerotic vascular disease (due to hypertension, hyperlipidemia, tobacco abuse), 15% are caused by cardiac embolism, 5% are from other causes, including hypercoagulable states and vasculitis.

- Small vessel occlusion is most often caused by lipohyalinosis precipitated by chronic hypertension.
- Risk factors for ischemic stroke are described in Box 1-4.

DIAGNOSIS

DIFFERENTIAL DIAGNOSIS

- TIA (Transient ischemic attack, traditionally defined as focal neurologic deficits lasting <24 hr [usually lasting <60 min])
- Migraine
- Seizure
- Mass lesion

WORKUP

- Thorough history and physical examination, including detailed neurologic and cardiovascular evaluation to identify vascular territory and likely etiology (Table 1-17). Infectious, toxic, and metabolic causes should be excluded because each may cause clinical deterioration of old stroke symptoms.
- Cardiac: mandatory ECG, telemetry, consider serial cardiac enzymes; transthoracic and/or transesophageal echocardiography Holter monitor should be seriously considered especially in setting of suspected embolic etiology. Carotid Doppler should be performed in cases of embolic stroke to anterior or middle cerebral artery territory.

LABORATORY TESTS

- CBC
- Platelet count
- PT (INR)
- PTT
- BUN, creatinine
- Lipid panel
- Glucose
- Electrolytes
- Urinalysis
- Additional tests, depending on suspected etiology (in younger patients; e.g., coagulopathies)

IMAGING STUDIES

- CT scan without contrast to distinguish hemorrhage from infarct (Figs. 1-42 and 1-43)
- An MRI is superior to CT in identifying abnormalities in the posterior fossa and, in particular, lacunar (small vessel) infarcts. Diffusion weighted imag-

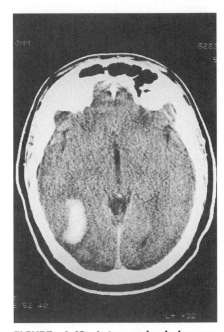

FIGURE 1-42 Intracerebral hemorrhage. Noncontrast CT scan demonstrates an intracerebral hemorrhage in the right occipital lobe. (From Specht N [ed]: *Practical guide to diagnostic imaging,* St Louis, 1998, Mosby.)

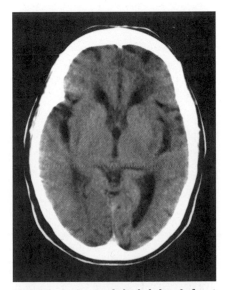

FIGURE 1-43 Occipital lobe infarct (posterior cerebral artery territory). Note the large right occipital hypodensity with mass effect caused by infarction and subsequent edema. (From Cwinn AA, Grahovac SZ [eds]: *Emergency CT scans of the head: a practical atlas,* St Louis, 1998, Mosby.)

BOX 1-4 Risk Factors for Ischemic Stroke

Diabetes
Hypertension
Smoking
Family history of premature vascular disease
Hyperlipidemia
Atrial fibrillation
History of transient ischemic attack (TIA)
History of recent myocardial infarction
History of congestive heart failure (left ventricular [LV] ejection fraction, 25%)
Drugs (sympathomimetics, oral contraceptive pill, cocaine)

From Andreoli TE (ed): *Cecil essentials of medicine,* ed 5, Philadelphia, 2001, WB Saunders.

TABLE 1-17 Neurologic Signs Associated with Cerebrovascular Accident by Location

Artery Affected	Neurologic Signs
Internal Carotid Artery	
(Supplies the cerebral hemispheres and diencephalon by the ophthalmic and ipsilateral hemisphere arteries)	Occasional unilateral blindness Severe contralateral hemiplegia, hemianesthesia, and hemianopia Profound aphasia if left hemisphere involved
Middle Cerebral Artery	
(Supplies structures of higher cerebral processes of communication; language interpretation; perception and interpretation of space, sensation, form, and voluntary movement)	Alterations in communication, cognition, mobility, and sensation Homonymous hemianopia Contralateral hemiplegia or hemiparesis
Anterior Cerebral Artery	
(Supplies medial surfaces and upper convexities of frontal and parietal lobes and medial surface of hemisphere, which includes motor and somesthetic cortex serving the legs)	Emotional lability Confusion, amnesia, personality changes Urinary incontinence Impaired mobility, with weakness greater in lower extremities than in upper
Posterior Cerebral Artery	
(Supplies medial and inferior temporal lobes, medial occipital lobe, thalamus, posterior hypothalamus, and visual receptive area)	Homonymous hemianopia Hemianesthesia Cortical blindness Memory deficits
Vertebral or Basilar Arteries	
(Supply the brainstem and cerebellum) Incomplete occlusion	Drop attacks Unilateral and bilateral weakness of extremities Diplopia, homonymous hemianopia Nausea, vertigo, tinnitus, and syncope Dysphagia Dysarthria Sometimes confusion and drowsiness
Anterior portion of pons	"Locked-in" syndrome—no movement except eyelids; sensation and consciousness preserved
Complete occlusion or hemorrhage	Coma Miotic pupils Decerebrate rigidity Respiratory and circulatory abnormalities Death
Posterior Inferior Cerebellar Artery	
(Supplies the lateral and posterior portion of the medulla)	Wallenberg syndrome Dysphagia, dysphonia Ipsilateral anesthesia of face and cornea for pain and temperature (touch preserved) Ipsilateral Horner syndrome Contralateral loss of pain and temperature sensation in trunk and extremities Ipsilateral decompensation of movement (cerebellar signs)
Anterior Inferior and Superior Cerebellar Arteries	
(Supply the cerebellum)	Difficulty in articulation, swallowing, gross movements of limbs; nystagmus (cerebellar signs)
Anterior Spinal Artery	
(Supplies the anterior spinal cord)	Flaccid paralysis, below level of lesion Loss of pain, touch, temperature sensation (proprioception preserved, sensory level)
Posterior Spinal Artery	
(Supplies the posterior spinal cord)	Sensory loss, particularly proprioception, vibration, touch, and pressure (movement preserved)

Adapted from Seidel HM (ed): *Mosby's guide to physical examination*, ed 4, St Louis, 1999, Mosby.

ing (DWI) is best to determine hyper-acute ischemia (positive within 15-30 min of symptom onset). MRA is recommended to help identify vascular pathology (e.g., extent of intracranial atherosclerosis or vascular distribution of ischemia)

- In select cases (e.g., hemorrhagic stroke), conventional angiography may identify aneurysms or other vascular malformations

TREATMENT

NONPHARMACOLOGIC THERAPY

- To prevent pulmonary emboli, above-the-knee elastic stockings, pneumatic boots, or SQ heparin if nonhemorrhagic etiology and patient is immobile in bed
- Carotid endarterectomy (CEA) is recommended in patients with carotid territory stroke associated with 70% to 99% ipsilateral carotid stenosis, performed by an experienced surgeon who has demonstrated low morbidity and mortality
- Modification of risk factors (e.g., smoking cessation, exercise, diet)

ACUTE GENERAL Rx

- Box 1-5 describes initial considerations for patients with stroke.
- Judicious control of blood pressure; patients with chronic hypertension may extend the area of infarction if the blood pressure is lowered into the "normal" range. It is best not to lower blood pressure too aggressively in the acute setting unless it is very markedly elevated. Adequate hydration and bed rest (e.g., head of bed down in pressure dependent ischemia vs. head of bed up if patient is aspiration risk). Tight glycemic control is also recommended (e.g., sliding scale insulin).
- Patients presenting <3 hr after onset of a nonhemorrhagic stroke, thrombolytic therapy in a specialized stroke center is beneficial in selected populations.

ACUTE SPECIFIC Rx

- Depends on several factors, including etiology, vascular territory involved, risk factors, and elapsed time from symptom onset to arrival at hospital.
- Box 1-6 describes criteria for thrombolytic therapy in patients with thromboembolic stroke (IV tPA inclusion criteria include clearly defined symptom onset within 3 hr of onset of treatment, measurable deficit with NIH Stroke Scale >4, and no evidence for bleed on neuroimaging).
- If atrial fibrillation and/or a cardiac mural thrombus is found on echocardiography, heparin may be considered.
- If a subarachnoid or intracerebral hemorrhage is found on CT, MR angiography and/or cerebral angiography may be indicated to identify aneurysm. If no aneurysm is found and clot is expanding, neurosurgical evacuation of clot may be attempted, but outcomes are generally poor.
- In select cases of patients presenting >3 hr but <6 hr, an *interventional* neuroradiologist or neurosurgeon may be able to offer either direct injection of a clot-busting agent (such as intraarterial tPA) or direct extraction of the clot (e.g., FDA approved Merci Retrieval System). However, this remains investigational and has yet to be well studied in the setting of a controlled trial. Intracranial angioplasty/stenting may also be a consideration.

BOX 1-5   Initial Considerations for Patients with Strokes

Initial care
    Stabilize the patient, secure the airway, and provide adequate oxygenation
    Assess level of consciousness, language, visual fields, eye movements, and pupillary movements
    Obtain history and perform physical examination
    Perform CT of head without contrast
    Obtain CBC with platelets and differential, electrolytes, creatinine, BUN, glucose, PT/PTT, arterial blood gas, or oxygen saturation
    Consider a toxicology screen
    Consider special coagulation studies such as antiphospholipid antibodies, factor V Leiden assay, protein C and protein S,
        antithrombin III, ANA, fibrinogen, RPR, homocysteine, serum protein electrophoresis
Consider acute intervention with t-PA if symptoms for less than 3 hr
Consider the following with admission orders
    Transthoracic echocardiogram (consider transesophageal echocardiogram if transthoracic echocardiogram is equivocal or there is a
        high suspicion of cardiogenic thromboembolism)
    Carotid duplex ultrasonography
    Telemetry
    Supplemental oxygen and appropriate oxygen saturation monitoring
    Antiplatelet therapy
    Fluid restriction if infarct is large, to reduce cerebral edema
    Close monitoring of intake and output
    Regular determinations of blood glucose levels to avoid hyperglycemia
    NPO if there are concerns about the pharyngeal reflex pending swallowing evaluation
    Elevate the head of the bed 20-30 degrees to reduce cerebral edema
    Bed rest for the first 24 hr with fall precautions, then advance as appropriate
    Vital signs and neurologic checks every 2 hr times four until stable
    Prophylaxis for DVT if immobile (elastic stockings at a minimum)
    Speech therapy consultation to evaluate swallowing
    Neurology, physical therapy, occupational therapy, nutrition, and social services consultations

From Rakel RE (ed): *Principles of family practice*, ed 6, Philadelphia, 2002, WB Saunders.
ANA, Antinuclear antibodies; *BUN,* blood urea nitrogen; *CBC,* complete blood count; *CT,* computed tomography; *DVT,* deep vein thrombosis; *NPO,* nothing by mouth; *PT/PTT,* prothrombin time/partial thromboplastin time; *RPR,* rapid plasma reagin; *t-PA,* tissue plasminogen activator.

CHRONIC Rx

- Antiplatelet therapy (aspirin, dipyridamole/aspirin [Aggrenox], clopidogrel [Plavix], or ticlopidine) reduces the risk of subsequent stroke.
- If patient presents with first TIA/stroke and was on no prior antiplatelet agent, aspirin (325 mg vs. 81 mg each day) is usually chosen initially. If a TIA occurs while on aspirin, the patient should be switched to dipyridamole/aspirin or clopidogrel.
- Warfarin is usually reserved for patients with cardioembolic stroke as well as for patients with atrial fibrillation.

DISPOSITION

Prognosis depends on severity of deficits, etiology, and other concurrent medical/surgical illness. A polymodality physical medicine and rehabilitative approach is an integral part of poststroke recovery. This includes physical, occupational, and speech therapy individualized depending on deficits.

REFERRAL

- Neurology/neurosurgical referral depending on etiology and resources available; depending on time of symptom onset, transfer of patient to institution able to provide more specific acute treatment can be considered.
- Vascular surgery if patient is candidate for CEA. If not a surgical candidate and endovascular treatment is available, refer to interventional neuroradiologist for carotid stenting.

SUGGESTED READINGS

American Heart Association Scientific Statement: Primary prevention of ischemic stroke: a statement for health care professionals from the stroke council of the American Heart Association, *Circulation* 103:167, 2001.

Barnett HJM: A modern approach to posterior circulation ischemic stroke, *Arch Neurol* 59:359, 2002.

Benevante D, Hart RG: Stroke: management of acute ischemic stroke, *Am Fam Physician* 59:2828, 1999.

Caplan LR: Stroke treatment: promising but still struggling, *JAMA* 279:1304, 1998.

Diener HC et al: Aspirin and clopidogrel compared with clopidogrel alone after recent ischaemic stroke or transient ischaemic attack in high-risk patients (MATCH): randomised, double-blind, placebo-controlled trial, *Lancet* 364(9431):331, 2004.

Endovascular versus surgical treatment in patients with carotid stenosis in the Carotid and Vertebral Artery Transluminal Angioplasty Study (CAVATAS): a randomised trial, *Lancet* 357(9270):1729, 2001.

Green DM et al: Serum potassium level and dietary potassium intake as risk factors for stroke, *Neurology* 59:314, 2002.

Halperin JL, Fuster V: Patent foramen ovale and recurrent stroke: another paradoxical twist, *Circulation* 105:2580, 2002.

Meschia JF et al: Thrombolytic treatment of acute ischemic stroke, *Mayo Clin Proc* 77:542, 2002.

Qureshi A et al: Spontaneous intracranial hemorrhage, *N Engl J Med* 344:1450, 2001.

Sacco RL et al: High-density lipoprotein cholesterol and ischemic stroke in the elderly, *JAMA* 285:2729, 2001.

Strauss SE et al: New evidence for stroke prevention, clinical applications and scientific review, *JAMA* 288:1388, 2002.

AUTHOR: **RICHARD S. ISAACSON, M.D.**

BOX 1-6   Criteria for Tissue Plasminogen Activator (alteplase [Activase]) Use in Patients with Thromboembolic Stroke

Criteria for considering t-PA as a treatment option
  Noncontrast CT without evidence of hemorrhage
  Time since onset of symptoms clearly <3 hr before t-PA administration would begin
Criteria for excluding t-PA as a treatment option
Historical and clinical findings
  Clinical presentation suggests subarachnoid hemorrhage, even if CT is normal
    Sudden, severe headache, often with loss of consciousness at onset
    Vomiting common
  Active internal bleeding, increased risk of bleeding, or known bleeding diathesis, including:
    Recent use of warfarin with a prolonged international normalized ratio (INR)—some would add current use of warfarin regardless of INR
    Use of heparin within 48 hr with a prolonged aPTT
    Platelet count <100,000/mm3
    History of intracranial hemorrhage
    Known arteriovenous malformation or aneurysm
    GI or GU bleeding within the past 21 days
    Arterial puncture within the past 7 days
  Recent lumbar puncture
  Stroke, intracranial surgery, or head trauma within the previous 3 mo
  Major surgery or serious trauma within the preceding 14 days
  Persistent systolic blood pressure >185 mm Hg or diastolic blood pressure >110 mm Hg
  Seizure at stroke onset
  Rapidly improving neurologic signs
  Isolated, mild neurologic deficits
  Acute myocardial infarction
  Post–myocardial infarction pericarditis
  Blood glucose >50 mg/dl or <400 mg/dl
CT findings
  Evidence of intracranial hemorrhage
  Hypodensity or effacement of the sulci in 1/3 of the territory of the middle cerebral artery

From Rakel RE (ed): *Principles of family practice*, ed 6, Philadelphia, 2002, WB Saunders.
aPTT, Activated partial thromboplastin time; *CT,* computed tomography; *GI,* gastrointestinal; *GU,* genitourinary; *t-PA,* tissue plasminogen activator.

BASIC INFORMATION

DEFINITION

A subdural hematoma is bleeding into the subdural space, caused by rupture of bridging veins between the brain and venous sinuses.

ICD-9CM CODES
432.1 Subdural hematoma

EPIDEMIOLOGY & DEMOGRAPHICS

Nearly all cases are caused by trauma, although the trauma may be quite trivial and easily overlooked. Victims are commonly at the extremes of age. Coagulation abnormalities, especially use of anticoagulation in the elderly, is a significant risk factor.

PHYSICAL FINDINGS & CLINICAL PRESENTATION

- Vague headache, often worse in morning than evening.
- Some apathy, confusion, and clouding of consciousness is common, although frank coma may complicate late cases. Chronic subdural hematomas may cause a dementia picture.
- Neurologic symptoms may be transient, simulating TIA.
- Almost any sign of cortical dysfunction may occur, including hemiparesis, sensory deficits, or language abnormalities, depending on which part of the cortex the hematoma presses on.
- New-onset seizures should raise the index of suspicion.

ETIOLOGY

Traumatic rupture of cortical bridging veins, especially where stretched by underlying cerebral atrophy.

DIAGNOSIS

DIFFERENTIAL DIAGNOSIS

- Epidural hematoma
- Subarachnoid hemorrhage
- Mass lesion (e.g., tumor)
- Ischemic stroke
- Intraparenchymal hemorrhage

WORKUP

- CT scan is sensitive for diagnosis and should be performed in a timely fashion (Fig. 1-44).
- Hematocrit, platelet count, PTT, and PT/INR should be routinely checked.

TREATMENT **Rx**

NONPHARMACOLOGIC THERAPY

Small subdural hematomas may be left untreated and the patient observed, but if there is an underlying cause, such as anticoagulation, this should be rapidly corrected to prevent further accumulation of blood.

ACUTE THERAPY

- Neurosurgical drainage of blood from subdural space via burr hole is the definitive procedure, although it is common for the hematoma to reaccumulate.

- There is an increased risk of seizures, which should be treated appropriately if they arise.
- Reverse anticoagulation where appropriate.

DISPOSITION

Referral to neurosurgery for possible evacuation

PEARLS & CONSIDERATIONS **!**

- The elderly are particularly susceptible to subdural hematomas because of cerebral atrophy, which stretches subdural veins, and because of fall risk.
- Relatively minor trauma may cause a subdural hematoma.
- Caution should be taken in interpreting CT findings in the subacute stage, where blood appears as isodense to brain, and therefore the distance from the cortical sulci to the skull needs to be evaluated.

SUGGESTED READINGS
Chen JC, Levy ML: Causes, epidemiology, and risk factors of chronic subdural hematoma, *Neurosurg Clin N Am* 11(3):399, 2000.
Voelker JL: Nonoperative treatment of chronic subdural hematoma, *Neurosurg Clin N Am* 11(3):507, 2000.

AUTHOR: **DANIEL MATTSON, M.D., M.SC.(MED.)**

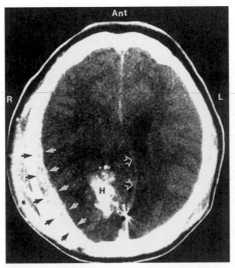
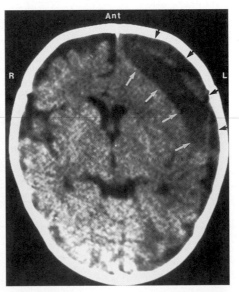

FIGURE 1-44 Subdural hematomas. A noncontrasted computed tomography scan of an acute subdural hematoma **(A)** shows a crescentic area of increased density in the right posterior parietal region between the brain and the skull *(black and white arrows)*. An area of intraparenchymal hemorrhage *(H)* is also seen; a chronic subdural hematoma for a different patient is shown in **(B)**. There is an area of decreased density in the left frontoparietal region *(arrows)* effacing the sulci, compressing the anterior horn of the left lateral ventricle, and shifting the midline somewhat to the right. (From Mettler FA [ed]: *Primary care radiology,* Philadelphia, 2000, WB Saunders.)

BASIC INFORMATION

DEFINITION

Syncope is the temporary loss of consciousness resulting from an acute global reduction in cerebral blood flow.

ICD-9CM CODES
720.2 Syncope

EPIDEMIOLOGY & DEMOGRAPHICS

- Syncope accounts for 3% to 5% of emergency room visits.
- 30% of the adult population will experience at least one syncopal episode during their lifetime.
- Incidence of syncope is highest in elderly men and young women.

PHYSICAL FINDINGS & CLINICAL PRESENTATION

- Blood pressure: if low, consider orthostatic hypotension; if unequal in both arms (difference >20 mm Hg), consider subclavian steal or dissecting aneurysm. (NOTE: Blood pressure and heart rate should be recorded in the supine and standing positions.) If there is drop in BP but no change in HR, the patient may be on a beta blocker or may have an autonomic neuropathy.
- Pulse: if patient has tachycardia, bradycardia, or irregular rhythm, consider arrhythmia.
- Heart: if there are murmurs present suggestive of AS or IHSS, consider syncope secondary to left ventricular outflow obstruction; if there are JVD and distal heart sounds, consider cardiac tamponade.
- Carotid sinus pressure: can be diagnostic if it reproduces symptoms and other causes are excluded; a pause >3 sec or a systolic BP drop >50 mm Hg without symptoms or <30 mm Hg with symptoms when sinus pressure is applied separately on each side for <5 sec is considered abnormal. This test should be avoided in patients with carotid bruits or cerebrovascular disease; ECG monitoring, IV access, and bedside atropine should be available when carotid sinus pressure is applied.

ETIOLOGY

- Neurally mediated syncope
  1. Psychophysiologic (emotional upset, panic disorders, hysteria)
  2. Visceral reflex (micturition, defecation, food ingestion, coughing, ventricular contraction; glossopharyngeal neuralgia)
  3. Carotid sinus pressure
  4. Reduction of venous return caused by Valsalva maneuver
- Orthostatic hypotension
  1. Hypovolemia
  2. Vasodilator medications

  3. Autonomic neuropathy (diabetes, amyloid, Parkinson's disease, multisystem atrophy)
  4. Pheochromocytoma
  5. Carcinoid syndrome
- Cardiac
  1. Reduced cardiac output
     a. Left ventricular outflow obstruction (aortic stenosis, hypertrophic cardiomyopathy)
     b. Obstruction to pulmonary flow (pulmonary embolism, pulmonic stenosis, primary pulmonary hypertension)
     c. MI with pump failure
     d. Cardiac tamponade
     e. Mitral stenosis
     f. Reduction of venous return (atrial myxoma, valve thrombus)
     g. β-blockers
  2. Arrhythmias or asystole
     a. Extreme tachycardia (>160 to 180 bpm)
     b. Severe bradycardia (<30 to 40 bpm)
     c. Sick sinus syndrome
     d. AV block (second- or third-degree)
     e. Ventricular tachycardia or fibrillation
     f. Long QT syndrome
     g. Pacemaker malfunction
     h. Psychotropic medications and beta blockers
  3. Other causes
     a. Hypoxia
     b. Hypoglycemia
     c. Anemia
     d. Hyperventilation

DIAGNOSIS

Dx

DIFFERENTIAL DIAGNOSIS

1. Seizure (see "Workup")
2. Vertebrobasilar TIA usually manifests as diplopia, vertigo, ataxia but not loss of consciousness. Isolated syncopal episodes without accompanying neurologic symptoms are unlikely to be a TIA
3. Recreational drugs/alcohol
4. Psychologic stress

WORKUP

The history is crucial to diagnosing the cause of syncope and may suggest a diagnosis that can be evaluated with directed testing:

- Sudden loss of consciousness: consider cardiac arrhythmias.
- Gradual loss of consciousness: consider orthostatic hypotension, vasodepressor syncope, hypoglycemia.
- History of aura before loss of consciousness (LOC) or prolonged confusion (>1 min), amnesia, or lethargy after LOC suggests seizure rather than syncope.

- Patient's activity at the time of syncope:
  1. Micturition, coughing, defecation: consider syncope secondary to decreased venous return.
  2. Turning head or while shaving: consider carotid sinus syndrome.
  3. Physical exertion in a patient with murmur: consider aortic stenosis.
  4. Arm exercise: consider subclavian steal syndrome.
  5. Assuming an upright position: consider orthostatic hypotension.
  6. Postprandial syncope
- Associated events:
  1. Chest pain: consider MI, pulmonary embolism.
  2. Palpitations: consider arrhythmias.
  3. Incontinence (urine or fecal) and tongue biting are associated with seizure or syncope.
  4. Brief, transient shaking after LOC may represent myoclonus from global cerebral hypoperfusion and not seizures. However, sustained tonic/clonic muscle action is more suggestive of seizure.
  5. Focal neurologic symptoms or signs point to a neurologic event such as a seizure with residual deficits (e.g., Todd's paralysis) or cerebral ischemic injury.
  6. Psychologic stress: syncope may be vasovagal.
- Review current medications, particularly antihypertensive and psychotropic drugs.

LABORATORY TESTS

Routine blood tests rarely yield diagnostically useful information and should be done only if they are specifically suggested by the results of the history and physical examination. The following are commonly ordered tests.
- CBC to rule out anemia, infection
- Electrolytes, BUN, creatinine, magnesium, calcium to rule out electrolyte abnormalities and evaluate fluid status
- Serum glucose level
- Cardiac isoenzymes should be obtained if the patient gives a history of chest pain before the syncopal episode
- ABGs to rule out pulmonary embolus, hyperventilation (when suspected)
- Evaluate drug and alcohol levels when suspecting toxicity

IMAGING STUDIES

- Echocardiogram is useful in patients with a heart murmur to rule out AS, IHSS, or atrial myxoma.
- If seizure is suspected, CT scan and/or MRI of the head and EEG may be useful.
- If head trauma or neurologic signs on examination, CT or MRI may be helpful.

- If pulmonary embolism is suspected, ventilation-perfusion scan should be done.
- If arrhythmias are suspected, a 24-hr Holter monitor and admission to a telemetry unit is appropriate. Generally, Holter monitoring is rarely useful, revealing a cause for syncope in <3% of cases. Loop recorders that can be activated after syncopal episode to retrieve information about the cardiac rhythm during the preceding 4 min add considerable diagnostic yield in patients with unexplained syncope.
- Implantable cardiac monitors that function as permanent loop recorders or implantable cardioverter-defibrillators, which are placed subcutaneously in the pectoral region with the patient under local anesthesia, are useful in patients with cardiac syncope.
- Electrophysiologic studies may be indicated in patients with structural heart disease and/or recurrent syncope.
- ECG to rule out arrhythmias; may be diagnostic in 5% to 10% of patients.

TILT-TABLE TESTING

- Useful to support a diagnosis of neurally mediated syncope. Patients older than age 50 should have stress testing before tilt-table testing. Positive results would preclude tilt-table testing.
- Indicated in patients with recurrent episodes of unexplained syncope as well as for patients in high-risk occupations (e.g., pilots, bus drivers) (Fig. 1-45). The test is also useful for identifying patients with prominent bradycardic response who may benefit from implantation of a permanent pacemaker.
- It is performed by keeping the patient in an upright posture on a tilt table with footboard support. The angle of the tilt table varies from 60 to 80 degrees. The duration of upright posture during tilt-table testing varies from 25 to 45 min.
- The hallmark of neurally mediated syncope is severe hypotension associated with a paradoxical bradycardia triggered by a specific stimulus. The diagnosis of neurally mediated syncope is likely if upright tilt testing reproduces these hemodynamic changes in <15 min and causes presyncope or syncope.

PSYCHIATRIC EVALUATION

- Generalized anxiety disorder, pain disorder, and major depression predispose patients to neurally mediated reactions and may result in syncope.
- Alcohol and drug dependence can also lead to syncope.

TREATMENT

NONPHARMACOLOGIC THERAPY

- Ensure proper hydration; consider TED stockings and salt tablets.
- Eliminate medications that may induce hypotension.

ACUTE GENERAL Rx

- Varies with the underlying etiology of syncope (e.g., pacemaker in patients with syncope secondary to complete heart block)
- Syncope caused by orthostatic hypotension is treated with volume replacement in patients with intravascular volume depletion. Also consider midodrine to promote venous return via adrenergic-mediated vasoconstriction and Florinef for its mineralocorticoid effects to increase intravascular volume

DISPOSITION

Prognosis varies with the age of the patient and the etiology of the syncope. Generally:

- Benign prognosis (very low 1-yr morbidity) in patients age <70 yr and having vasovagal/psychogenic syncope or syncope of unknown cause
- Poor prognosis (high mortality and morbidity) in patients with cardiac syncope
- Patients with the following risk factors have a higher 1-yr mortality: abnormal ECG, history of ventricular arrhythmia, history of CHF

REFERRAL

Hospital admission in elderly patients without prior history of syncope or unknown etiology of their syncope and in any patients suspected of having cardiac syncope.

PEARLS & CONSIDERATIONS (!)

COMMENTS

- Section III, Syncope, describes an algorithmic approach to the patient.
- The etiology of syncope is identified in <50% of cases during the initial evaluation.
- A thorough history and physical examination are the most productive means of establishing a diagnosis in patients with syncope.

SUGGESTED READINGS

Fenton AM et al: Vasovagal syncope, *Ann Intern Med* 133:722, 2000.
Kapoor WN: Syncope, *N Engl J Med* 343:1856, 2000.
Menozzi C et al: Mechanism of syncope in patients with heart disease and negative electrophysiologic test, *Circulation* 105:2741, 2002.
Soteriades ES et al: Incidence and prognosis of syncope, *N Engl J Med* 347:878, 2002.

AUTHOR: **SEAN I. SAVITZ, M.D.**

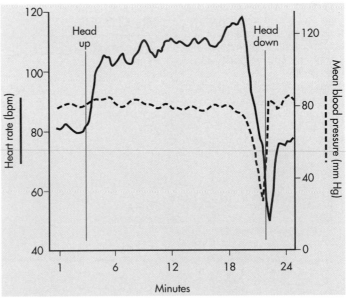

FIGURE 1-45 Head-up tilt test performed on an 18-year-old woman with a history of syncope associated with pain, preceded by a prodrome of dizziness, graying vision, and diaphoresis. A similar prodrome preceded syncope during the test. Note the precipitous, nearly simultaneous, decline of heart rate and blood pressure after an initial rise in heart rate. Vital signs returned to normal rapidly after the head was lowered. (Courtesy Robert F. Sprung, University of Utah. In Goldman L, Ausiello D [eds]: *Cecil textbook of medicine*, ed 22, Philadelphia, 2004, WB Saunders.)

BASIC INFORMATION

DEFINITION

Tardive dyskinesia (TD) is a syndrome of involuntary movements associated with the long-term use of antipsychotic medication, particularly dopamine-blocking neuroleptics. Patients usually exhibit rapid, repetitive, stereotypic movements mostly involving the oral, buccal, and lingual areas.

ICD-9CM CODES

333.82 Tardive dyskinesia

EPIDEMIOLOGY & DEMOGRAPHICS

- The disorder is caused by dopamine-blocking neuroleptics (e.g., Haldol). The incidence is declining with the use of newer generation antipsychotics.
- At least 20% of patients treated with standard neuroleptic drugs are affected with TD, and approximately 5% are expected to develop TD with each year of neuroleptic treatment.
- The risk is greatest in the early years of exposure.
- Higher incidence and lower remission rates are seen in older persons.

PHYSICAL FINDINGS & CLINICAL PRESENTATION

- Typically appears with the reduction or withdrawal of the antipsychotics
- Characterized by:
  1. TD primarily involves the tongue, lips, and jaw. A combination of tongue twisting and protrusion, lip smacking and puckering, and chewing movements in a repetitive and stereotypic fashion is often observed.
  2. Slow, writhing movements of the arms and legs
  3. Symptoms subside when the antipsychotic is reintroduced

4. The involuntary mouth movements in TD may be voluntarily suppressed by patients. They are also suppressed by voluntary actions such as putting food in the mouth or talking.

ETIOLOGY

Tardive dyskinesia results from chronic exposure to dopamine receptor blocking agents—drugs primarily used to treat psychosis. TD has not been reported with dopamine depleters (such as reserpine) and are seldom reported with atypical antipsychotic drugs such as clozapine. Some drugs for nausea (such as metoclopramide and prochlorperazine) and depression (such as amoxapine) can also cause TD.

DIAGNOSIS

DIFFERENTIAL DIAGNOSIS

- Huntington's chorea
- Excessive treatment with L-dopa

WORKUP

- Complete neuropsychiatric history (including medication history) and examination.
- If presentation atypical, consider evaluation with CBC, serum electrolytes, thyroid function tests, serum ceruloplasmin, and connective tissue disease screen.

IMAGING STUDIES

Brain imaging normal in TD.

TREATMENT

NONPHARMACOLOGIC THERAPY

None

PHARMACOLOGIC THERAPY

- Treatment predicated on prevention—limiting the indications for neuroleptics and using the lowest effective dose and withdrawn when feasible.
- Use atypical antipsychotics if possible. Clozapine and quetiapine have the lowest reported incidence of TD.

CHRONIC Rx

- Benzodiazapines and vitamin E may be helpful but controlled trial evidence is weak.
- Clozapine, olanzapine and amisulpride may be of symptomatic help, but long-term efficacy is unproven.

REFERRAL

Movement disorder specialist if symptoms are severe

PEARLS & CONSIDERATIONS

Only as a last resort, for persistent, disabling, and treatment-resistant TD, should neuroleptics be resumed to treat TD in the absence of active psychosis.

SUGGESTED READINGS

Casey DE: Pathophysiology of antipsychotic drug-induced movement disorders, *J Clin Psychiatry* 65(suppl9):25, 2004.

Fernandez HH, Friedman JH: Classification and treatment of tardive syndromes, *Neurologist* 9(1):16, 2003.

McGrath JJ, Soares KV: Miscellaneous treatments for neuroleptic-induced tardive dyskinesia, *Cochrane Database Syst Rev* (2):CD000208, 2003.

AUTHOR: **MITCHELL D. FELDMAN, M.D., M.PHIL.**

BASIC INFORMATION

DEFINITION

Tarsal tunnel syndrome is a rare entrapment neuropathy that develops as a result of compression of the posterior tibial nerve in the tunnel formed by the flexor retinaculum behind the medial malleolus of the ankle (Fig. 1-46).

ICD-9CM CODES
355.5 Tarsal tunnel syndrome

EPIDEMIOLOGY & DEMOGRAPHICS

PREVALENCE: Unknown
PREDOMINANT SEX: Female = male

PHYSICAL FINDINGS & CLINICAL PRESENTATION

- Neuritic symptoms along the course of the posterior tibial nerve in the sole and heel
- Swelling over tarsal tunnel
- Possible positive Tinel's sign
- Possible reproduction of symptoms with sustained eversion of hindfoot or digital compression of tunnel
- Sensory and motor changes unusual

ETIOLOGY

Space-occupying lesions (ganglia, varicosities, lipomas, synovial hypertrophy)

DIAGNOSIS **Dx**

DIFFERENTIAL DIAGNOSIS

- Plantar fasciitis
- Peripheral neuropathy
- Proximal radiculopathy
- Local tendinitis
- Peripheral vascular disease
- Morton's neuroma

ELECTRICAL STUDIES

Electrodiagnostic testing is often inconclusive. Delayed sensory conduction or increased motor latency may be seen.

TREATMENT

- NSAIDs
- Immobilization for 4-6 wk with ankle orthosis or fracture cast boot
- Medial heel wedge or orthotic to minimize heel eversion
- Local steroid injection into tunnel (avoiding the posterior tibial nerve) if symptoms persist

REFERRAL

For surgical decompression if needed. Results of surgery are mixed unless an obvious compressive lesion is found.

SUGGESTED READINGS

Aldridge T: Diagnosing heel pain in adults, *Am Fam Physician* 70:332, 2004.

Gorter K et al: Variation in diagnosis and management of common foot problems by GPs, *Fam Pract* 18(6):569, 2001.

Labib SA et al: Heel pain triad (HPT): the combination of plantar fasciitis, posterior tibial tendon dysfunction and tarsal tunnel syndrome, *Foot Ankle Int* 23(3):212, 2002.

Mizel MS et al: Evaluation and treatment of chronic ankle pain, *Instr Course Lect* 53:311, 2004.

Mondelli M, Morana P, Padua L: An electrophysiological severity scale in tarsal tunnel syndrome, *Acta Neurol Scand* 109:284, 2004.

Pecina M: Diagnostic tests for tarsal tunnel syndrome, *J Bone Joint Surg Am* 84-A(9):1714, 2002.

AUTHOR: **LONNIE R. MERCIER, M.D.**

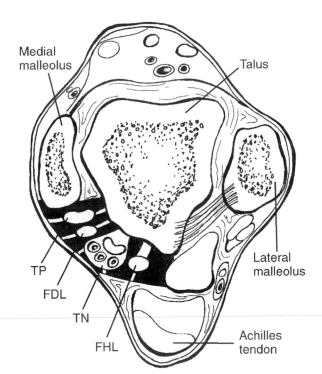

FIGURE 1-46 Anatomy of tarsal tunnel syndrome. Transverse view of ankle. *FDL,* Flexor digitorum longus; *FHL,* flexor hallucis longus tendon; *TN,* tibial nerve (single contour), posterior tibial artery, veins; *TP,* tibialis posterior tendon. Tendons and neurovascular elements are included into individual fibrous septa that connect periosteum with the deep fascia. (From Canoso J: *Rheumatology in primary care,* Philadelphia, 1997, WB Saunders.)

BASIC INFORMATION

DEFINITION

The biceps muscle has two heads:
- The short head arises from the tip of the coracoid process of the scapula with the coracobrachialis.
- The long head arises from the supraglenoid tubercle of the scapula and runs through the intertubercular groove between the greater and lesser tubercles of the humerus.
- The two heads join in the distal arm to form one strong tendon, which inserts on the radial tuberosity on the upper end of the radius.
- Tendinitis results from a repetitive stress leading to microscopic tears in the tendon that can generate an inflammatory response.
- Tenosynovitis occurs as a result of a direct injury or irritation in which the tendon rubs over a bony prominence and produces inflammation of the tendon sheath.
- Tendinosis refers to degenerative change in the tendon. Tendinitis, tenosynovitis, and tendinosis often coexist.

SYNONYMS

Tendinitis

ICD-9CM CODES

EPIDEMIOLOGY & DEMOGRAPHICS

Shoulder pain is common in all age groups and in both sexes, but the incidence of bicipital tendinitis is unknown and cases are often misclassified as rotator cuff tendinitis and vice versa.

PHYSICAL FINDINGS & CLINICAL PRESENTATION

- Patients with bicipital tendinitis typically describe pain in the region of the anterior shoulder, which may radiate to the elbow.
- The pain is aggravated by shoulder flexion, forearm supination, or elbow flexion. The pain may be exacerbated by beginning the activity but improves as the activity continues. The pain then may return after the patient ceases the activity.

- Physical examination reveals tenderness localized over the bicipital groove. Active shoulder abduction, flexion, and internal rotation aggravate the pain.
- Flexion against resistance: with the forearm in the supinated position and the elbow fully extended the patient attempts to flex the arm (forward flexion at the shoulder) against the resistance provided by the examiner. Tenderness in the bicipital groove is considered a positive test result and is indicative of bicipital tendinitis.

ETIOLOGY

- The biceps tendon is susceptible to overuse injuries, especially in individuals performing repetitive lifting activities. Degenerative changes associated with aging predispose the elderly patient to injury.
- Known causes of bicipital tendinitis include the following:
  - Poor lifting techniques
  - Chronic repetitive upper extremity activities
  - Lack of flexibility
  - Anatomic abnormalities
- Often no specific cause can be identified.

DIAGNOSIS

DIFFERENTIAL DIAGNOSIS

- Myofascial pain
- Rotator cuff disease or injury
- Adhesive capsulitis
- Brachial neuritis
- Cervical radiculopathy
- Musculocutaneous neuropathy
- Shoulder instability
- Acromioclavicular injury or arthritis

WORKUP

The history and physical examination are usually sufficient to make the diagnosis of bicipital tendinitis. Local anesthetic infiltration of the region of the bicipital groove may help make the diagnosis.
- Electromyography or nerve conduction studies to rule out neuropathy and radiculopathy.
- Ultrasound or MRI may assist to rule out other shoulder pathology (e.g., rotator cuff tear).

TREATMENT

NONPHARMACOLOGIC THERAPY

- Avoid activity that aggravates the condition.
- Physical therapy:
  - If there is no shoulder instability, perform gradual stretching of biceps and anterior shoulder capsule.
  - Circumduction, pendulum, two-hand rod swinging, and lateral and front finger wall walking may begin as symptoms abate.
  - Perform progressive resistance exercises as soon as symptoms subside.
  - Apply moist heat to help facilitate stretching and reduce pain.
  - Physical therapy should involve soft tissue therapy with massage.
  - Electrical stimulation or ultrasound may be beneficial if symptoms interfere with therapeutic exercise.

PHARMACOLOGIC THERAPY

- Nonsteroidal antiinflammatory drugs.
- Topical capsaicin (0.075% strength applied tid).
- Injection with anesthetic (e.g., 1.5 cc of lidocaine 1% or 2%) and corticosteroid (e.g., triamcinolone 20 to 40 mg) into the biceps tendon sheath in the intertubercular groove. May be repeated on a 4-week basis.
- Myofascial trigger point injections with dilute local anesthetic in the parascapular muscles may be beneficial.
- Surgery may be required in refractory cases with persistent pain that has not responded to any other treatments. Surgery often involves decompression of the musculotendinous structure through tenolysis under arthroscopy or using an open surgical technique.

SUGGESTED READINGS

Barr KP: Rotator cuff disease, *Phys Med Rehabil Clin N Am* 15(2):475-491, 2004.

Mehta S, Gimbel JA, Soslowsky LJ: Etiologic and pathogenetic factors for rotator cuff tendinopathy, *Clin Sports Med* 22(4):791-812, 2003.

AUTHOR: **TOM J. WACHTEL, M.D.**

BASIC INFORMATION

DEFINITION

Superficial thrombophlebitis is inflammatory thrombosis in subcutaneous veins.

SYNONYMS

Phlebitis

ICD-9CM CODES
451.0 Thrombophlebitis, superficial

EPIDEMIOLOGY & DEMOGRAPHICS

- 20% of superficial thrombophlebitis cases are associated with occult DVT.
- Catheter-related thrombophlebitis incidence is 100:100,000.

PHYSICAL FINDINGS & CLINICAL PRESENTATION

- Subcutaneous vein is palpable, tender; tender cord is present with erythema and edema of the overlying skin and subcutaneous tissue.
- Induration, redness, and tenderness are localized along the course of the vein. This linear appearance rather than circular appearance is useful to distinguish thrombophlebitis from other conditions (cellulitis, erythema nodosum).
- There is no significant swelling of the limb (superficial thrombophlebitis generally does not produce swelling of the limb).
- Low-grade fever may be present. High fever and chills are suggestive of septic phlebitis.

ETIOLOGY

- Trauma to preexisting varices
- Intravenous cannulation of veins (most common cause)
- Abdominal cancer (e.g., carcinoma of pancreas)
- Infection (*Staphylococcus* is the most common pathogen)
- Hypercoagulable state
- DVT

DIAGNOSIS

DIFFERENTIAL DIAGNOSIS

- Lymphangitis
- Cellulitis
- Erythema nodosum
- Panniculitis
- Kaposi's sarcoma

WORKUP

Laboratory evaluation to exclude infectious etiology and imaging studies to rule out DVT in suspected cases

LABORATORY TESTS

CBC with differential, blood cultures, culture of IV catheter tip (when secondary to intravenous cannulation)

IMAGING STUDIES

- Serial ultrasound or venography in patients with suspected DVT
- CT scan of abdomen in patients with suspected malignancy (Trousseau's syndrome: recurrent migratory thrombophlebitis)

TREATMENT

NONPHARMACOLOGIC THERAPY

- Warm, moist compresses
- It is not necessary to restrict activity; however, if there is extensive thrombophlebitis, bed rest with the leg elevated will limit the thrombosis and improve symptoms.

ACUTE GENERAL Rx

- NSAIDs to relieve symptoms
- Treatment of septic thrombophlebitis with antibiotics with adequate coverage of *Staphylococcus*
- Ligation and division of the superficial vein at the junction to avoid propagation of the clot in the deep venous system when the thrombophlebitis progresses toward the junction of the involved superficial vein with deep veins

DISPOSITION

Clinical improvement within 7-10 days

REFERRAL

Surgical referral in selected cases (see "Acute General Rx")

PEARLS & CONSIDERATIONS

COMMENTS

- Patients with positive cultures should be evaluated and treated for endocarditis.
- Septic thrombophlebitis is more common in IV drug addicts.

AUTHOR: **FRED F. FERRI, M.D.**

BASIC INFORMATION

DEFINITION

Deep vein thrombosis (DVT) is the development of thrombi in the deep veins of the extremities or pelvis.

SYNONYMS

DVT
Deep venous thrombophlebitis

ICD-9CM CODES

451.1 Thrombosis of deep vessels of lower extremities
451.83 Thrombosis of deep veins of upper extremities
541.9 Deep vein thrombosis of unspecified site

EPIDEMIOLOGY & DEMOGRAPHICS

- Annual incidence in urban population is 1.6 cases/1000 persons.
- The risk of recurrent thromboembolism is higher among men than women.

PHYSICAL FINDINGS & CLINICAL PRESENTATION

- Pain and swelling of the affected extremity
- In lower extremity DVT, leg pain on dorsiflexion of the foot (Homans' sign)
- Physical examination may be unremarkable

ETIOLOGY

The etiology is often multifactorial (prolonged stasis, coagulation abnormalities, vessel wall trauma). The following are risk factors for DVT:

- Prolonged immobilization (≥3 days)
- Postoperative state
- Trauma to pelvis and lower extremities
- High-dose estrogen therapy; conjugated equine estrogen but not esterified estrogen is associated wtih increased risk of DVT; estrogen plus progestin is associated with doubling the risk of venous thrombosis
- Visceral cancer (lung, pancreas, alimentary tract, GU tract)
- Age >60 yr
- History of thromboembolic disease
- Hematologic disorders (e.g., antithrombin III deficiency, protein C deficiency, protein S deficiency, heparin cofactor II deficiency, sticky platelet syndrome, G20210A prothrombin mutation, lupus anticoagulant, dysfibrinogenemias, anticardiolipin antibody, hyperhomocystinemia, concurrent homocystinuria, high levels of factors VIII, XI, and factor V Leiden mutation)
- Obesity, CHF
- Surgery, fracture, or injury involving lower leg or pelvis
- Surgery requiring >30 min of anesthesia
- Gynecologic surgery (particularly gynecologic cancer surgery)
- Recent travel (within 2 wk, lasting >4 hr)
- Smoking and abdominal obesity
- Central venous catheter or pacemaker insertion
- Superficial vein thrombosis, varicose veins

DIAGNOSIS

DIFFERENTIAL DIAGNOSIS

- Postphlebitic syndrome
- Superficial thrombophlebitis
- Ruptured Baker's cyst
- Cellulitis, lymphangitis, Achilles tendinitis
- Hematoma
- Muscle or soft tissue injury, stress fracture
- Varicose veins, lymphedema
- Arterial insufficiency
- Abscess
- Claudication
- Venous stasis

WORKUP

The clinical diagnosis of DVT is inaccurate. Pain, tenderness, swelling, or color changes are not specific for DVT. Compression ultrasonography is preferred as the initial study to diagnose DVT. An initial negative test should be repeated after 5 days (if the clinical suspicion of DVT persists) to detect propagation of any thrombosis to the proximal veins. Comprehensive ultrasonography is a more extensive test, which examines the deep veins from the inguinal ligament to the level of the malleolus. Recent literature reports indicate that it may be safe to withhold anticoagulation after negative results on comprehensive duplex ultrasonography in patients with a suspected first episode of symptomatic DVT of the leg.

LABORATORY TESTS

- Laboratory tests are not specific for DVT. Baseline PT (INR), PTT, and platelet count should be obtained on all patients before starting anticoagulation.
- Use of D-dimer assay by ELISA may be useful in the management of suspected DVT. The combination of a normal D-dimer study on presentation together with a normal compression venous ultrasound is useful to exclude DVT and generally eliminate the need to do repeat ultrasound at 5-7 days. Recent trials indicate that DVT can be ruled out in patients who are clinically unlikely to have DVT and who have a negative D-dimer test. Compressive ul-

trasonography can be safely omitted in such patients.
- Laboratory evaluation of patients with recurrent thrombosis without obvious causes and those with a family history of thrombosis should include protein S, protein C, fibrinogen, antithrombin III level, lupus anticoagulant, anticardiolipin antibodies, factor V Leiden, factor VIII, factor IX, and plasma homocysteine levels.

IMAGING STUDIES

- Compression ultrasonography is generally preferred as the initial study because it is noninvasive and can be repeated serially (useful to monitor suspected acute DVT); it offers good sensitivity for detecting proximal vein thrombosis (in the popliteal or femoral vein). Its disadvantages are poor visualization of deep iliac and pelvic veins and poor sensitivity in isolated or nonocclusive calf vein thrombi.
- Contrast venography is the gold standard for evaluation of DVT of the lower extremity. It is, however, invasive and painful. Additional disadvantages are the increased risk of phlebitis, new thrombosis, renal failure, and hypersensitivity reaction to contrast media; it also gives poor visualization of deep femoral vein in the thigh and internal iliac vein and its tributaries.
- Magnetic resonance direct thrombus imaging (MRDTI) is an accurate noninvasive test for diagnosis of DVT. Current limitations are its cost and lack of widespread availability.

TREATMENT

NONPHARMACOLOGIC THERAPY

- Initial bed rest for 1-4 days followed by gradual resumption of normal activity
- Patient education on anticoagulant therapy and associated risks

ACUTE GENERAL Rx

- Traditional treatment consists of IV unfractionated heparin for 4 to 7 days followed by warfarin therapy. Low–molecular-weight heparin enoxaparin (Lovenox) is also effective for initial management of DVT and allows outpatient treatment. Recommended dose is 1 mg/kg q12h SC and continued for a minimum of 5 days and until a therapeutic INR (2-3) has been achieved with warfarin. Once-daily fondaparinux (Arixtra), a synthetic analog of heparin, is also as effective and safe as twice daily enoxaparin in the initial treatment of patients with symptomatic

DVT. Warfarin therapy should be initiated when appropriate (immediately or within 72 hr of initiation of heparin). A 5 mg loading dose of warfarin is recommended in inpatients because it produces less excess anticoagulation than does a 10 mg dose; the smaller dose also avoids the development of a potential hypercoagulable state caused by precipitous decreases in levels of protein C during the first 36 hr of warfarin therapy. In the outpatient setting, a warfarin nomogram using 10 mg loading doses may be more effective in reaching a therapeutic INR.

- Low–molecular-weight heparin, when used, should be overlapped with warfarin for at least 5 days and until the INR has exceeded 2 for 2 consecutive days.
- Exclusions from outpatient treatment of DVT include patients with potential high complication risk (e.g., hemoglobin <7, platelet count <75,000, guaiac-positive stool, recent CVA or noncutaneous surgery, noncompliance).
- Insertion of an inferior vena cava filter to prevent pulmonary embolism is recommended in patients with contraindications to anticoagulation.
- Thrombolytic therapy (streptokinase) can be used in rare cases (unless contraindicated) in patients with extensive iliofemoral venous thrombosis and a low risk of bleeding.

CHRONIC Rx

- Conventional-intensity warfarin therapy is more effective than low-intensity warfarin therapy for the long term prevention of recurrent DVT. The low-intensity warfarin regimen does not reduce the risk of clinically important bleeding.
- The optimal duration of anticoagulant therapy varies with the cause of DVT and the patient's risk factors:
1. Therapy for 3-6 mo is generally satisfactory in patients with reversible risk factors (low-risk group).
2. Anticoagulation for at least 6 mo is recommended for patients with idiopathic venous thrombosis or medical risk factors for DVT (intermediate-risk group)
3. Indefinite anticoagulation is necessary in patients with DVT associated with active cancer; long-term anticoagulation is also indicated in patients with inherited thrombophilia (e.g., deficiency of protein C or S antibody), antiphospholipid, and those with recurrent episodes of idiopathic DVT (high-risk group).

- Measurement of D-dimer after withdrawal of oral anticoagulation may be useful to estimate the risk of recurrence. Patients with a first spontaneous DVT and a D-dimer level <250 μg/ml after withdrawal of oral anticoagulation have a low risk of DVT recurrence.

PEARLS & CONSIDERATIONS

COMMENTS

- When using heparin, there is a risk of heparin-induced thrombocytopenia (with unfractionated more so than with LMWH). Platelet count should be obtained initially and repeated every 3 days while on heparin.
- Prophylaxis of DVT is recommended in all patients at risk (e.g., low–molecular-weight heparin [enoxaparin 30 mg SC bid] after major trauma, post surgery of hip and knee; enoxaparin 40 mg SC qd post–abdominal surgery in patients with moderate to high DVT risk; gradient elastic stockings alone or in combination with intermittent pneumatic compression [IPC] boots following neurosurgery).
- Ximelagatran is an oral direct thrombin inhibitor. For prophylaxis of venous thromboembolism, ximelagatran 24 mg PO bid started the morning after total knee arthroplasty is well tolerated and at least as effective as warfarin, but it does not require coagulation monitoring or dose adjustment.
- Fondaparinux (Arixtra), a synthetic analog of heparin, can also be used for prevention of DVT after hip fracture surgery, hip replacement, or knee replacement. Initial dose is 2.5 mg SC given 6 to 8 hr postoperatively and continued daily. Its bleeding risk is similar to enoxaparin; however, it is more effective in preventing DVT.
- The risk of recurrent venous thromboembolism in heterozygous carriers of factor V Leiden and a first spontaneous venous thromboembolism is similar to that of noncarriers of factor V Leiden; therefore heterozygous patients should receive secondary thromboprophylaxis for a similar length of time as patients without factor V Leiden.
- Approximately 20%-50% of patients with DVT develop postthrombotic syndrome characterized by leg edema, pain, venous ectasia, skin induration, and ulceration.

- Exercise following DVT is reasonable because it improves flexibility of the affected leg and does not increase symptoms in patients with postthrombotic syndrome.

SUGGESTED READINGS

Baarslag et al: Prospective study of color duplex ultrasonography compared with contrast venography in patients suspected of having deep venous thrombosis of the upper extremities, *Ann Intern Med* 136:865, 2002.

Bates SM, Ginsberg JS: Treatment of deep-vein thrombosis, *N Engl J Med* 351:268, 2004.

Berquist D et al: Duration of prophylaxis against venous thromboembolism with enoxaparin after surgery for cancer, *N Engl J Med* 346:975, 2002.

Eichinger S et al: D-Dimer levels and risk of recurrent venous thromboembolism, *JAMA* 290:1071, 2003.

Francis CW et al: Ximelagatran versus warfarin for the prevention of venous thromboembolism after total knee arthroplasty, *Ann Intern Med* 137:648, 2002.

Fraser DG et al: Diagnosis of lower-limb deep venous thrombosis: a prospective blinded study of magnetic resonance direct thrombus imaging, *Ann Intern Med* 136:89, 2002.

Kahn SR et al: Acute effects of exercise in patients with previous DVT: impact of the post-thrombotic syndrome, *Chest* 123:399, 2003.

Kelly et al: Plasma D-Dimers in the diagnosis of venous thromboembolism, *Arch Intern Med* 162:747, 2002.

Kovacs MJ et al: Comparison of 10-mg and 5mg warfarin initiation nomograms together with low-molecular-weight heparin for outpatient treatment of acute venous thromboembolism. A randomized, double-blind, controlled trial, *Ann Intern Med* 138:714, 2003.

Kraaijenhagen RA et al: Simplification of the diagnostic management of suspected deep vein thrombosis, *Arch Intern Med* 162:907, 2002.

Meyer G et al: Comparison of low-molecular-weight heparin and warfarin for the secondary prevention of venous thromboembolism in patients with cancer, *Arch Intern Med* 162:1729, 2002.

Schulman S et al: Secondary prevention of venous thromboembolism with the oral direct thrombin inhibitor ximelagran, *N Engl J Med* 349:1713, 2003.

Stevens SM et al: Withholding anticoagulation after a negative result on duplex ultrasonography for suspected symptomatic deep venous thrombosis, *Ann Intern Med* 140:985, 2004.

Wells PS et al: Evaluation of d-dimer in the diagnosis of suspected deep vein thrombosis, *N Engl J Med* 349:1227, 2003.

AUTHOR: **FRED F. FERRI, M.D.**

BASIC INFORMATION

DEFINITION

A thyroid nodule is an abnormality found on physical examination of the thyroid gland; nodules can be benign (70%) or malignant.

ICD-9CM CODES
241.0 Nodule, thyroid

EPIDEMIOLOGY & DEMOGRAPHICS

- Palpable thyroid nodules occur in 4%-7% of the population.
- Thyroid nodules can be found in 50% of autopsies; however, only 1 in 10 is palpable.
- Malignancy is present in 5%-30% of palpable nodules.
- Incidence of thyroid nodules increases after 45 yr of age. They are found more frequently in women.
- History of prior head and neck irradiation increases the risk of thyroid cancer.
- Increased likelihood that nodule is malignant: nodule increasing in size or >2 cm, regional lymphadenopathy, fixation to adjacent tissues, symptoms of local invasion (dysphagia, hoarseness, neck pain, male sex, family history of thyroid cancer or polyposis [Gardner syndrome]).

PHYSICAL FINDINGS & CLINICAL PRESENTATION

- Palpable, firm, and nontender nodule in the thyroid area should prompt suspicion of carcinoma. Signs of metastasis are regional lymphadenopathy, inspiratory stridor.
- Signs and symptoms of thyrotoxicosis can be found in functioning nodules.

ETIOLOGY

- History of prior head and neck irradiation
- Family history of pheochromocytoma, carcinoma of the thyroid, and hyperparathyroidism (medullary carcinoma of the thyroid is a component of MEN-II)

DIAGNOSIS

DIFFERENTIAL DIAGNOSIS

- Thyroid carcinoma
- Multinodular goiter
- Thyroglossal duct cyst
- Epidermoid cyst
- Laryngocele
- Nonthyroid neck neoplasm
- Branchial cleft cyst

WORKUP

- Fine-needle aspiration (FNA) biopsy is the best diagnostic study; the accuracy can be >90%, but it is directly related to the level of experience of the physician and the cytopathologist interpreting the aspirate.
- FNA biopsy is less reliable with thyroid cystic lesions; surgical excision should be considered for most thyroid cysts not abolished by aspiration.
- A diagnostic approach to thyroid nodule is described in Section III.

LABORATORY TESTS

- TSH, T_4, and serum thyroglobulin levels should be obtained before thyroidectomy in patients with confirmed thyroid carcinoma on FNA biopsy.
- Serum calcitonin at random or after pentagastrin stimulation is useful when suspecting medullary carcinoma of the thyroid and in anyone with a family history of medullary thyroid carcinoma.

IMAGING STUDIES

- Thyroid ultrasound is done in some patients to evaluate the size of the thyroid and the number, composition (solid vs. cystic), and dimensions of the thyroid nodule; solid thyroid nodules have a higher incidence of malignancy, but cystic nodules can also be malignant.
- The introduction of high-resolution ultrasonography has made it possible to detect many nonpalpable nodules (incidentalomas) in the thyroid (found at autopsy in 30%-60% of cadavers). Most of these lesions are benign. For most patients with nonpalpable nodules that are incidentally detected by thyroid imaging, simple follow-up neck palpation is sufficient.
- Thyroid scan with technetium-99m pertechnetate:
  1. Classifies nodules as hyperfunctioning (hot), normally functioning (warm), or nonfunctioning (cold); cold nodules have a higher incidence of malignancy.
  2. Scan has difficulty evaluating nodules near the thyroid isthmus or at the periphery of the gland.
  3. Normal tissue over a nonfunctioning nodule might mask the nodule as "warm" or normally functioning.
- Both thyroid scan and ultrasound provide information about the risk of malignant neoplasia based on the characteristics of the thyroid nodule, but their value in the initial evaluation of a thyroid nodule is limited because neither provides a definite tissue diagnosis.

TREATMENT

GENERAL Rx

- Evaluation of results of FNA
  1. Normal cells: may repeat biopsy during present evaluation or reevaluate patient after 3-6 mo of suppressive therapy (l-thyroxine, prescribed in doses to suppress the TSH level to 0.1-0.5)
     a. Failure to regress indicates increased likelihood of malignancy.
     b. Reliance on repeat needle biopsy is preferable to routine surgery for nodules not responding to thyroxine.
  2. Malignant cells: surgery
  3. Hypercellularity: thyroid scan
     a. Hot nodule: ^{131}I therapy if the patient is hyperthyroid
     b. Warm or cold nodule: surgery (rule out follicular adenoma vs. carcinoma)

DISPOSITION

Variable with results of FNA biopsy.

REFERRAL

Surgical referral for FNA biopsy

PEARLS & CONSIDERATIONS

COMMENTS

- Most solid, benign nodules grow, therefore an increase in nodule volume alone is not a reliable predictor of malignancy.
- Surgery is indicated in hard or fixed nodule, presence of dysphagia or hoarseness, and rapidly growing solid masses regardless of "benign" results on FNA.
- Suppressive therapy of malignant thyroid nodules postoperatively with thyroxine is indicated. The use of suppressive therapy for benign solitary nodules is controversial.

SUGGESTED READINGS

Alexander EK et al: Natural history of benign solid and cystic thyroid nodules, *Ann Intern Med* 138:315, 2003.

Welker MJ, Orlov D: Thyroid nodules, *Am Fam Physician* 67:559, 2003.

AUTHOR: **FRED F. FERRI, M.D.**

BASIC INFORMATION

DEFINITION

Tinea corporis is a dermatophyte fungal infection caused by the genera *Trichophyton* or *Microsporum*.

SYNONYMS

Ringworm
Body ringworm
Tinea circinata

ICD-9CM CODES
110.5 Tinea corporis

EPIDEMIOLOGY & DEMOGRAPHICS

- The disease is more common in warm climates.
- There is no predominant age or sex.

PHYSICAL FINDINGS & CLINICAL PRESENTATION

- Typically appears as single or multiple annular lesions with an advancing scaly border; the margin is slightly raised, reddened, and may be pustular.
- The central area becomes hypopigmented and less scaly as the active border progresses outward (Fig. 1-47).
- The trunk and legs are primarily involved.
- Pruritus is variable.

- It is important to remember that recent topical corticosteroid use can significantly alter the appearance of the lesions.

ETIOLOGY

Trichophyton rubrum is the most common pathogen.

DIAGNOSIS

DIFFERENTIAL DIAGNOSIS

- Pityriasis rosea
- Erythema multiforme
- Psoriasis
- SLE
- Syphilis
- Nummular eczema
- Eczema
- Granuloma annulare
- Lyme disease
- Tinea versicolor
- Contact dermatitis

WORKUP

Diagnosis is usually made on clinical grounds. It can be confirmed by direct visualization under the microscope of a small fragment of the scale using wet mount preparation and potassium hydroxide solution; dermatophytes appear as translucent branching filaments (hyphae) with lines of separation appearing at irregular intervals.

LABORATORY TESTS

- Microscopic examination of hyphae
- Mycotic culture is usually not necessary
- Biopsy is indicated only when the diagnosis is uncertain and the patient has failed to respond to treatment

TREATMENT

NONPHARMACOLOGIC THERAPY

Affected areas should be kept clean and dry.

ACUTE GENERAL Rx

- Various creams are effective; the application area should include normal skin about 2 cm beyond the affected area:
  1. Miconazole 2% cream (Monistat-Derm) applied bid for 2 wk
  2. Clotrimazole 1% cream (Mycelex) applied and gently massaged into the affected areas and surrounding areas bid for up to 4 wk
  3. Naftifine 1% cream (Naftin) applied qd
  4. Econazole 1% (Spectazole) applied qd
- Systemic therapy is reserved for severe cases and is usually given up to 4 wk; commonly used agents:
  1. Ketoconazole (Nizoral), 200 mg qd
  2. Fluconazole (Diflucan), 200 mg qd
  3. Terbinafine (Lamisil), 250 mg qd

DISPOSITION

Majority of cases resolve without sequelae within 3-4 wk of therapy.

REFERRAL

Dermatology referral in patients with persistent or recurrent infections

SUGGESTED READINGS

Friedlander SF et al: Terbinafine in the treatment of trichophytin tinea capitis, *Pediatrics* 109:602, 2002.
Hainer BL: Dermatophyte infections, *Am Fam Physician* 67:101, 2003.
Weinstein A, Berman B: Topical treatment of common superficial tinea infections, *Am Fam Physician* 65:2095, 2002.

AUTHOR: **FRED F. FERRI, M.D.**

FIGURE 1-47   Annular lesion (tinea corporis). Note raised erythematous scaling border and central clearing. (From Noble J et al: *Textbook of primary care medicine,* ed 3, St Louis, 2001, Mosby.)

Section I

DISEASES AND DISORDERS

BASIC INFORMATION

DEFINITION

Tinea pedis is a dermatophyte infection of the feet.

SYNONYMS

Athlete's foot

ICD-CM CODES
110.4 Tinea pedis

EPIDEMIOLOGY & DEMOGRAPHICS

- Most common dermatophyte infection
- Increased incidence in hot humid weather. Occlusive footwear is a contributing factor
- More common in adult males

PHYSICAL FINDINGS & CLINICAL PRESENTATION

- Typical presentation is variable and ranges from erythematous scaling plaques (see Fig. 1-48) and isolated blisters to interdigital maceration.
- The infection usually starts in the interdigital spaces of the foot. Most infections are found in the toe webs or in the soles.
- Fourth or fifth toes are most commonly involved.

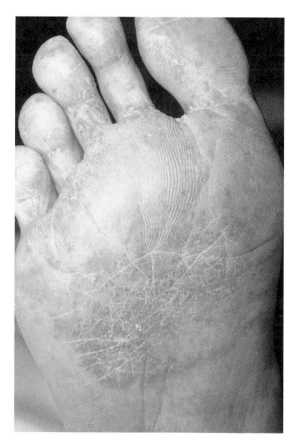

FIGURE 1-48 Tinea pedis. (From Goldstein BG, Goldstein AO: *Practical dermatology*, ed 2, St Louis, 1997, Mosby.)

- Pruritus is common and is most intense following removal of shoes and socks.
- Infection with *Tinea rubrum* often manifests with a moccasin distribution affecting the soles and lateral feet.

ETIOLOGY

Dermatophyte infection caused by *T. rubrum, T. mentagrophytes,* or less commonly *E. floccosum*

DIAGNOSIS **Dx**

DIFFERENTIAL DIAGNOSIS

- Contact dermatitis
- Toe web infection
- Eczema
- Psoriasis
- Keratolysis exfoliativa

WORKUP

- Diagnosis is usually made by clinical observation.
- Laboratory testing, when performed, generally consists of a simple potassium hydroxide (KOH) preparation with mycologic examination under a light microscope to confirm the presence of dermatophytes.

LABORATORY TESTS

- Microscopic examination of a scale or the roof of a blister with 10% KOH under low or medium power will reveal hyphae.
- Mycologic culture is rarely indicated in the diagnosis of tinea pedis.
- Biopsy is reserved for when the diagnosis remains in question after testing or failure to respond to treatment.

IMAGING STUDIES

None

TREATMENT

NONPHARMACOLOGIC THERAPY

- Keep infected area clean and dry. Aerate feet by using sandals when possible.
- Use 100% cotton socks rather than nylon socks to reduce moisture.
- Areas likely to become infected should be dried completely before being covered with clothes.

ACUTE GENERAL THERAPY

- Butenafine Hcl 1% (Mentax) cream applied bid for 1 wk or qd for 4 wk is effective in interdigital tinea pedis.
- Ciclopirox 0.77% (Loprox) cream applied bid for 4 wk is also effective.
- Clotrimazole 1% (Lotrimin AF) cream is an OTC treatment. It should be applied to affected and surrounding area bid for up to 4 wk.
- Naftifine (Naftin) 1% cream applied qd or gel applied bid for 4 wk also produces a significantly high cure rate.
- When using topical preparations, the application area should include normal skin about 2 cm beyond the affected area.
- Areas of maceration can be treated with Burow's solution soaks for 10-20 min bid followed by foot elevation.
- Oral agents (fluconazole 150 mg once/wk for 4 wk) can be used in combination with topical agents in resistant cases.

PEARLS & CONSIDERATIONS **!**

Combination therapy of antifungal and corticosteroid (clotrimazole/betamethasone [Lotrisone]) should only be used when the diagnosis of fungal infection is confirmed and inflammation is a significant issue.

SUGGESTED READING

Weinstein A, Berman B: Topical treatment of common superficial tinea infections, *Am Fam Physician* 65:2095, 2002.

AUTHOR: **FRED F. FERRI, M.D.**

BASIC INFORMATION

DEFINITION

Tinnitus is the false perception of sound in the absence of an acoustic stimulus.

SYNONYM

Ringing in the ear(s)

ICD-9CM CODES
388.30 Tinnitus

EPIDEMIOLOGY & DEMOGRAPHICS

- Prevalence: 45-65 yr old: 7% in men, 4% in women; above age 65: 10% in men, 5% in women
- More common in whites than in blacks
- More common in the southern U.S.
- Frequent association with hearing loss

SYMPTOMS (ALWAYS SUBJECTIVE)

- Ringing (35.5%)
- Buzzing (11.2%)
- Cricket-like (8.5%)
- Hissing (7.8%)
- Whistling (6.6%)
- Humming (5.3%)
- The pitch is high in most cases
- Tinnitus is reported to be unilateral (34%), bilateral with lateral dominance (44%), or equal in both ears (22%)
- Patients typically wait for several years before seeking medical attention
- Most patients report that the tinnitus is much louder subjectively than it is when matched with audible sounds

ETIOLOGY

OTOLOGIC:
- Noise-induced hearing loss
- Presbycusis
- Otosclerosis
- Otitis
- Ceruminosis
- Meniere's disease

NEUROLOGIC:
- Head and neck injury
- Multiple sclerosis
- Acoustic neuroma
- Other brain tumors

INFECTIONS:
- Otitis media
- Meningitis
- Lyme disease
- Syphilis

TOXIC (DRUGS):
- Aspirin
- NSAIDs
- Aminoglycosides
- Loop diuretics
- Vincristine

OTHER:
- Facial and dental disorders

DIAGNOSIS

DIFFERENTIAL DIAGNOSIS

- Objective tinnitus: hearing real sounds
  1. Pulsatile sounds: carotid stenosis, aortic valve disease, high cardiac output, arteriovenous malformations
  2. Muscular sounds: palatal myoclonus, spasm of stapedius or tensor tympani muscle
  3. Spontaneous autoacoustic emissions auditory hallucinations

WORKUP

- Description of the sound
  1. Constant or episodic
  2. Unilateral or bilateral
  3. Gradual or sudden onset
  4. Duration
  5. Hearing loss present or not
  6. Vertigo present or not
  7. Precipitating factors (e.g., background noise, alcohol, stress, sleep)
  8. Impact in daily life

PHYSICAL EXAMINATION

- Focus on head and neck
- Vital signs
- Signs of associated illnesses

LABORATORY

- CBC, FBS, creatinine, ALT, Alk Phos, TSH, lipids, ESR, Lyme titer
- Comprehensive audiologic evaluation
- In selected cases: brain magnetic resonance imaging with contrast

TREATMENT

- Prevent (further) hearing loss with appropriate ear protection and avoidance of noise exposure.
- Treat any identified etiologic factor and avoid ototoxic drugs
- Medications:
  1. Antiarrhythmic drugs (lidocaine, tocainide, flecainide) probably ineffective
  2. Benzodiazepines may help, but tinnitus recurs upon cessation of therapy
  3. Carbamazepine and other anticonvulsants are ineffective
  4. Antidepressants may be helpful and are worth a trial (most studies involve tricyclics)
  5. Gingko biloba may be helpful
- Acupuncture is ineffective
- Tinnitus retraining (habituation) may lead to improvement in as many as 75% of patients. Programs include counseling combined with low-level broadband noise exposure and usually take 1.5 years to complete
- Masking devices that cover up the unwanted sounds may be helpful in selected patients
- Surgical treatment is controversial
- Self-help groups (e.g., the American Tinnitus Association) provide useful information and support
- Patient education and reassurance

REFERRAL

ENT

SUGGESTED READINGS

Lockwood AH, Salvi RJ, Burkard RF: Tinnitus, *N Engl J Med* 347:904, 2002.
Noell CA, Meyeroff WL: Tinnitus: diagnosis and treatment of this elusive symptom, *Geriatrics* 58:28, 2003.

AUTHOR: **TOM J. WACHTEL, M.D.**

BASIC INFORMATION

DEFINITION

Transient ischemic attack (TIA) refers to a transient neurologic dysfunction caused by focal brain or retinal ischemia with symptoms typically lasting less than 60 min but always less than 24 hr and is followed by a full recovery of function. Acute brain ischemia is a medical emergency requiring prompt neurologic evaluation and potential intervention.

SYNONYMS

TIA

ICD-9CM CODES
435.9 Unspecified transient cerebral ischemia

EPIDEMIOLOGY & DEMOGRAPHICS

INCIDENCE (IN U.S.): 49 cases/100,000 persons/yr
PREDOMINANT SEX: Males > females
PEAK INCIDENCE: >60 yr

PHYSICAL FINDINGS & CLINICAL PRESENTATION

- During an episode, neurologic abnormalities are confined to discrete vascular territory.
- Typical carotid territory symptoms are ipsilateral monocular visual disturbance, contralateral homonymous hemianopsia, contralateral hemimotor or sensory dysfunction, and language dysfunction (dominant hemisphere) alone or in combination.
- Typical vertebrobasilar territory symptoms are binocular visual disturbance, vertigo, diplopia, dysphagia, dysarthria, and motor or sensory dysfunction involving the ipsilateral face and contralateral body.

ETIOLOGY

- Cardioembolic
- Large vessel atherothrombotic disease
- Lacunar disease
- Hypoperfusion with fixed arterial stenosis
- Hypercoagulable states

DIAGNOSIS Dx

DIFFERENTIAL DIAGNOSIS

- Hypoglycemia
- Seizures
- Migraine
- Subdural hemorrhage
- Mass lesions
- Vestibular disease
- Section II describes the differential diagnosis of neurologic deficits, focal and multifocal.

WORKUP

- Thorough history and physical examination
- Ancillary investigations including neuroimaging aimed at identifying the etiology quickly

LABORATORY TESTS

- CBC with platelets
- PT (INR) and PTT
- Glucose
- Lipid profile
- ESR (if clinical suspicion for infectious or inflammatory process)
- Urinalysis
- Chest x-ray
- ECG and consider cycling cardiac enzymes
- Other tests as dictated by suspected etiology

IMAGING STUDIES

- Head CT scan to exclude hemorrhage including a subdural hemorrhage
- MRI and MRA. (In several studies, MRI with diffusion-weighted imaging has identified early ischemic brain injury in up to 50% of patients with TIA.) MRA of the brain and neck can identify large vessel intracranial and extracranial stenoses, arteriovenous malformations, and aneurysms
- Carotid Doppler studies identify carotid stenosis; neck ultrasound can also visualize stenoses of the vertebrobasilar arteries
- Echocardiography if cardiac source is suspected
- Telemetry for hospitalized patients for at least 24 hr. May consider 24-hr Holter if patient is being discharged
- Four-vessel cerebral angiogram if considering carotid endarterectomy or carotid stent

TREATMENT Rx

NONPHARMACOLOGIC THERAPY

- Carotid endarterectomy for carotid territory TIA associated with an ipsilateral stenosis of 70%-99%: should be done by a surgeon who is experienced with and performs this procedure frequently. Carotid stenting is also being performed in patients who are not surgical candidates. Trials are comparing stenting versus surgery for carotid disease.
- Modification of risk factors including smoking cessation.

ACUTE GENERAL Rx

- Depends on etiology
- If the time of the onset of symptoms is clear, and there are significant deficits on neurologic examination, and brain hemorrhage has been ruled out, then the patient may be a candidate for thrombolytic therapy, but this should be discussed with a neurologist or a specialist in cerebrovascular disease.
- Acute anticoagulation: no data supporting benefits in the acute setting. Heparin is considered for new-onset atrial fibrillation and atherothrombotic carotid disease causing recurrent transient neurologic symptoms especially in the setting before carotid endarterectomy or carotid stenting. Also considered for basilar artery thrombosis given concern for progression to brainstem stroke with high morbidity and mortality.
- Section III, Transient Ischemic Attacks, describes a treatment algorithm.

CHRONIC Rx

- No data supporting the use of long-term anticoagulation in the management of TIA, although stroke patients with atrial fibrillation or demonstrated cardiac thrombi have been shown to benefit from long-term warfarin therapy.
- First line of treatment has traditionally been aspirin. No significant benefit of high-dose aspirin (up to 1500 mg/day) has been conclusively found over lower doses (75 mg to 325 mg/day). A baby aspirin (81 mg/day) is therefore appropriate.
- Also consider aspirin/dipyridamole extended-release capsules (Aggrenox, 1 capsule po bid) or Plavix as a first-line therapy. In a study of patients with TIA or stroke, Aggrenox reduced subsequent cerebrovascular events to a greater extent than either drug alone. Plavix is equally effective to aspirin in secondary prevention but the combination of aspirin and Plavix for patients with TIA or stroke causes more life threatening bleeding than Plavix alone. Recommend Aggrenox or oral anticoagulation for patients who continue to have TIAs while on aspirin (aspirin failures), but there are no data to support this recommendation.
- In patients with cerebrovascular disease, HMG-CoA reductase inhibitors (statins) have been shown to provide significant protection against subsequent vascular events such as MI and stroke even for LDLs <100. Consider starting a statin agent unless LDL is <70.

DISPOSITION

- According to one study, 10% to 20% of patients have a stroke in the next 90 days, and in 50% of these patients, stroke occurs in the first day or two after the TIA.
- Another study showed a stroke risk of 4.4% in the first month and 11.6% in the first year.
- The annual risk of myocardial infarction is 2.4%.
- One-year and 3-yr survival rates are 98% and 94%, respectively.

REFERRAL

Consider referring patients with TIA for an urgent neurologic evaluation and management.

PEARLS & CONSIDERATIONS

CAVEAT

Urgently evaluate all patients who present with symptoms suggestive of acute brain ischemia. Do not wait for symptoms to resolve to distinguish TIA versus stroke.

SUGGESTED READINGS

Alamowitch S et al: Risk, causes, and prevention of ischaemic stroke in elderly patients with symptomatic internal-carotid-artery stenosis, *Lancet* 357:1154, 2001.

Albers GW: A review of published TIA treatment recommendations, *Neurology* 62:S26, 2004.

Albers GW et al: Transient ischemic attack—proposal for a new definition, *N Engl J Med* 347:1713, 2002.

Albers GW et al: Antithrombotic and thrombolytic therapy for ischemic stroke, *Chest* 119:300S, 2001.

Algra A et al: Oral anticoagulants versus antiplatelet therapy for preventing further vascular events after transient ischaemic attack or minor stroke of presumed arterial origin, *Stroke* 34:234, 2003.

Diener HC et al: Aspirin and clopidrogrel compared with clopidogrel alone after recent ischemic stroke or transient ischaemic attack in high risk patients (MATCH): randomized, double-blind, placebo-controlled trial, *Lancet* 364:331, 2004.

Gorelick PB et al: Prevention of a first stroke, *JAMA* 281:1112, 1999.

Heart Protection Study Collaborative Group: MRC/BHF heart protection study of cholesterol lowering with simvastatin in 20,536 high-risk individuals: a randomized placebo-controlled trial, *Lancet* 360:7, 2002.

Johnston SC: Clinical practice. Transient ischemic attack, *N Engl J Med* 347:1687, 2002.

Sarasin FP, Gaspoz JM, Bounameaux H: Cost-effectiveness of new antiplatelet regimens used as secondary prevention of stroke or transient ischemic attack, *Arch Intern Med* 160(18):2773, 2000.

AUTHOR: **SEAN I. SAVITZ, M.D.**

BASIC INFORMATION

DEFINITION

Trigeminal neuralgia is a syndrome characterized by recurrent excruciating paroxysms of lancinating pain in the distribution of one or more divisions of the trigeminal (fifth) nerve.

SYNONYMS

Tic douloureux

ICD-9CM CODES

350.1 Trigeminal neuralgia

EPIDEMIOLOGY & DEMOGRAPHICS

INCIDENCE (IN U.S.): 3-5/100,000
PREVALENCE (IN U.S.): 155/1 million persons
PREDOMINANT SEX: Slight predominance of females to males
PEAK INCIDENCE: Median age 67 years
GENETICS: Uncommonly familial and possibly caused by underlying genetic etiology (see below in "Etiology" under "Rare causes")

PHYSICAL FINDINGS & CLINICAL PRESENTATION

- Each attack lasts only seconds but may cluster.
- Often, attacks are brought on by mild stimulation of trigger zones, located in the affected division of the fifth nerve. These triggers include light touching, eating, drinking, shaving, and draft of air.

ETIOLOGY

- It is thought that 80%-90% of cases are due to compression of the trigeminal nerve root at the cerebellopontine angle by an aberrant loop of artery or vein, and rarely a saccular aneurysm or arteriovenous malformation
- Compressive lesions such as schwannomas, epidermoid cysts, and meningiomas, also typically at the cerebellopontine angle

- Bony compression of the fifth nerve (e.g., from an osteoma or deformity resulting from osteogenesis imperfecta)
- Primary demyelinating disorders: multiple sclerosis (2%-4% of patients) and rarely Charcot-Marie-Tooth disease. In multiple sclerosis, usually there is a plaque of demyelination at the root entry zone of the fifth nerve in the pons
- Rare causes: (a) infiltrative disorders such as carcinomatous or amyloid deposits in the fifth nerve root, nerve proper, or ganglion; (b) familial occurrence has been reported in Charcot-Marie-Tooth disease

DIAGNOSIS

DIFFERENTIAL DIAGNOSIS

- Temporomandibular joint disease
- Rhinosinusitis
- Dental pathology
- The differential diagnosis of headache and facial pain is described in Section II.

WORKUP

MRI scans (CT scan with thin posterior fossa cuts if MRI not available) for all patients to exclude mass lesions or evidence of central demyelination as in multiple sclerosis

IMAGING STUDIES

See "Workup."

TREATMENT

NONPHARMACOLOGIC THERAPY

- In refractory cases, surgical options, including percutaneous radiofrequency gangliolysis and microvascular decompression
- Gamma-knife radiosurgery is an increasingly popular alternative to conventional surgery for trigeminal neuralgia

ACUTE GENERAL Rx

None, episodes are too brief

CHRONIC Rx

- Carbamazepine provides relief to at least 75% of patients. Begin with 100 mg bid and increase gradually as tolerated using a tid regimen.
- Alternatively may use gabapentin, 400 mg PO tid. Doses as high as 3600 mg/day are easily tolerated, but some patients experience sedation. Topiramate (Topamax) 25 mg qhs gradually titrated up to 100 mg bid is also effective.

DISPOSITION

Spontaneous remissions occur after months to years.

REFERRAL

If uncertain about diagnosis or if surgical treatment is necessary

PEARLS & CONSIDERATIONS

Even in patients with multiple sclerosis, a vascular compression may be the source of symptoms and thus may benefit from intervention such as surgery.

COMMENTS

Because prolonged remission may occur, drug tapering at yearly intervals is recommended.

SUGGESTED READINGS

Elias WJ, Burchiel KJ: Trigeminal neuralgia and other neuropathic pain syndromes of the head and face, *Curr Pain Headache Rep* 6(2):115, 2002.

Kitt CA et al. Trigeminal neuralgia: opportunities for research and treatment, *Pain* 85:3, 2000

Loeser JD: Tic douloureux, *Pain Res Manag* 6(3):156, 2001.

Love S, Coakham HB: Trigeminal neuralgia: pathology and pathogenesis, *Brain* 124(Pt 12):2347, 2001.

Maesawa S et al: Clinical outcomes after stereotactic radiosurgery for idiopathic trigeminal neuralgia, *J Neurosurg* 94:16, 2001.

AUTHOR: **U. SHIVRAJ SOHUR, M.D., PH.D.**

BASIC INFORMATION

DEFINITION

Digital stenosing tenosynovitis refers to an inflammatory process of the digital flexor tendon sheath.

SYNONYMS

Trigger finger

ICD-9CM CODES
727.03 Trigger finger (acquired)

EPIDEMIOLOGY & DEMOGRAPHICS

- Trigger finger can be found in all age groups but is commonly found in patients older than 45 yr
- More frequently affects females (4:1)
- Occupational risk groups: meat cutters, seamstresses, tailors, and dentists
- In adults the middle finger is most often affected (Fig. 1-49)

PHYSICAL FINDINGS & CLINICAL PRESENTATION

- Hand pain
- Painful triggering or snapping with flexion and extension of the affected digit
- Locking or loss of active digital extension is the most common symptom
- The digit possibly fixed in flexion (trapped or incarcerated)
- Usually affects one digit
- If more digits are involved, a systemic cause most likely present (e.g., diabetes, rheumatoid arthritis)
- A palpable tender nodule noted at the MCP joint of the affected digit
- Pain over the flexor tendon with resisted flexion
- Pain with passive stretching

ETIOLOGY

Trigger finger is described as being primary or secondary:
- Primary (idiopathic)
- Secondary
  1. Diabetes
  2. Rheumatoid arthritis
  3. Hypothyroidism
  4. Histiocytosis
  5. Amyloidosis
  6. Gout

DIAGNOSIS **Dx**

The diagnosis of trigger finger is usually made by the clinical historical presentation and by physical examination.

DIFFERENTIAL DIAGNOSIS

- Dupuytren's contracture
- De Quervain's tenosynovitis
- Acute digital tenosynovitis
- Proliferative tenosynovitis
- Carpal tunnel syndrome
- Flexion tendon rupture
- Trauma

WORKUP

If a secondary cause of trigger finger is suspected, a workup should be pursued.

LABORATORY TESTS

- CBC with differential
- Electrolytes, BUN, and creatinine
- Blood glucose
- Thyroid function tests
- Uric acid
- Rheumatoid factor

IMAGING STUDIES

X-ray studies are not very helpful unless a secondary cause has affected other organs (e.g., rheumatoid lung).

TREATMENT **Rx**

NONPHARMACOLOGIC THERAPY

Splinting can be tried early in the course but has been very successful.

ACUTE GENERAL Rx

- In primary idiopathic trigger finger steroid injection, 15-20 mg depomethylprednisolone acetate in 1 ml 1% Xylocaine has been used with success.
- Triamcinolone 10 mg with 1 ml of 1% Xylocaine is an alternative steroid choice to be used in patients who do not respond to the first injection.
- If symptoms do not resolve in 3 wk, a repeat injection can be tried.

CHRONIC Rx

- Surgical release is indicated in patients with refractory symptoms (e.g., locked digits) despite nonpharmacologic and acute treatment.
- Surgery is also indicated in patients with recurrent symptoms despite steroid injection therapy.

DISPOSITION

- Following steroid injection, symptoms usually resolve in 3-5 days, and locking resolves in 60% of the cases in 2-3 wk.
- If symptoms recur, a repeat steroid injection improves the symptoms in >80% of patients.
- Diabetic patients do not have the same success rate with steroid injections as the primary idiopathic group.

REFERRAL

If steroid injection therapy is considered, a rheumatology consult may be requested.

PEARLS & CONSIDERATIONS **!**

COMMENTS

If more than one digit is involved, a workup for a secondary systemic cause is in order.

SUGGESTED READINGS

Canoso JJ: Trigger finger. In *Rheumatology in Primary Care,* Philadelphia, 1997, Saunders.

Chin DH, Jones NF: Repetitive motion hand disorder, *J Calif Dent Assoc* 30(2):49, 2002.

Moore JS: Flexor tendon entrapment of the digits (trigger finger and trigger thumb), *J Occup Environ Med* 42(5):526, 2000.

Saldana MJ: Trigger digits: diagnosis and treatment, *J Am Acad Orthop Surg* 9(4):246, 2001.

AUTHOR: **PETER PETROPOULOS, M.D.**

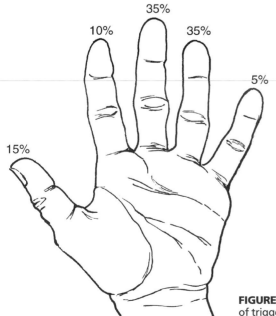

FIGURE 1-49 Trigger finger. Frequency of trigger finger according to digit in adults. (From Canoso J: *Rheumatology in primary care,* Philadelphia, 1997, WB Saunders.)

BASIC INFORMATION

DEFINITION

Trochanteric bursitis is a presumed inflammation or irritation of the gluteus maximus bursa or the bursa separating the greater trochanter from the gluteus medius and gluteus minimus (Fig. 1-50).

SYNONYMS

Greater trochanteric pain syndrome

ICD-9CM CODES
726.5 Bursitis trochanteric area

EPIDEMIOLOGY & DEMOGRAPHICS

- Trochanteric bursitis is commonly associated with other conditions:
  1. Osteoarthritis of the hip
  2. Lumbar spinal degenerative joint disease
  3. Rheumatoid arthritis
- Incidence peaks between the fourth and sixth decades of life but can occur at any age group
- Occurs in females > males (4:1)

PHYSICAL FINDINGS & CLINICAL PRESENTATION

- Hip pain is the most common complaint. The pain is chronic, intermittent, and located over the lateral thigh.
- Numbness can be present.
- Pain is precipitated with prolonged lying or standing on the affected side.
- Walking, climbing, and running exacerbate the pain.
- Point tenderness over the greater trochanter is noted.
- Pain is reproduced with resisted hip abduction.

ETIOLOGY

- The specific cause of trochanteric bursitis is not known although repetitive high-intensity use of the hip joint, trauma, infection (tuberculosis and bacterial), and crystal deposition can precipitate the disease.

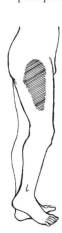

FIGURE 1-50 Typical location of pain in trochanteric bursitis syndrome. This is also a frequent pain radiation site for lumbar spine lesion, various nerve compression syndromes, and hip disease, particularly in osteonecrosis of the femoral head. (From Canoso J: *Rheumatology in primary care*, Philadelphia, 1997, WB Saunders.)

- Trochanteric bursitis can occur when other conditions such as osteoarthritis of the knee and hip and bunions of the feet cause changes in the patient's gait, placing varus stress on the hip joint.

DIAGNOSIS

A detailed physical examination and clinical presentation usually make the diagnosis of trochanteric bursitis. Laboratory tests and x-ray images are helpful adjunctive studies used to exclude other conditions either associated with or mimicking trochanteric bursitis.

DIFFERENTIAL DIAGNOSIS

- Osteoarthritis of the hip
- Osteonecrosis of the hip
- Stress fracture of the hip
- Osteoarthritis of the lumbar spine
- Fibromyalgia
- Iliopsoas bursitis
- Trochanteric tendonitis
- Gout
- Pseudogout
- Trauma
- Neuropathy

WORKUP

A workup is indicated if suspected associated conditions exist; otherwise treatment can be started on clinical grounds alone.

LABORATORY TESTS

CBC with differential may show elevated white count if infection is present.
ESR is elevated in an infectious process.
Uric acid may be elevated in patients with gout.

IMAGING STUDIES

- Plain x-rays of the hip are not very helpful in diagnosing trochanteric bursitis. Sometimes calcifications may be seen around the greater trochanter.
- Bone scan can be done but is usually not necessary.
- CT and MRI may show bursitis but are usually not warranted because it will not alter treatment.

TREATMENT

NONPHARMACOLOGIC THERAPY

- Heat 15-20 min four to six times per day
- Ultrasound therapy
- Rest
- Partial weight bearing
- Physical therapy to strengthen back, hip, and knee muscles

ACUTE GENERAL Rx

- NSAIDs, ibuprofen 800 mg PO tid, or naproxen 500 mg PO bid is used for pain relief.
- Acetaminophen 500-mg tablet, 1-2 tablets PO q6h prn can be used with NSAIDs or alternating with NSAIDs.
- Corticosteroid injection (30-40 mg depomethylprednisolone acetate mixed with 3 ml 1% Xylocaine)

CHRONIC Rx

Although rarely done, surgical removal of the bursa is possible for patients with refractory symptoms or infection.

DISPOSITION

- Most patients respond to NSAIDs and/or nonpharmacologic therapy.
- If steroid injection is used, approximately 70% of patients respond after the first injection and more than 90% respond to two injections.
- 25% of patients receiving steroid injection may develop a relapse.

REFERRAL

A rheumatology or orthopedics referral may be made if steroid injection therapy is needed or if the etiology is thought to be infectious.

PEARLS & CONSIDERATIONS

COMMENTS

- The absence of pain with flexion and extension differentiates trochanteric bursitis from degenerative joint disease of the hip.
- Localization of pain over the lateral thigh differentiates trochanteric bursitis from pain caused by meralgia paresthetica located over the anterolateral thigh and pain from osteoarthritis located over the inner thigh groin area.

SUGGESTED READINGS

Adkins SB, Figler RA: Hip pain in athletes, *Am Fam Physician* 61(7):2109, 2000.
Canoso JJ: Hip pain. In Canoso JJ, Kersey R (eds): *Rheumatology in primary care*. Philadelphia, 1997, WB Saunders.

AUTHOR: **MEL ANDERSON, M.D.**

BASIC INFORMATION

DEFINITION

Pulmonary tuberculosis (TB) is an infection of the lung and, occasionally, surrounding structures, caused by the bacterium *Mycobacterium tuberculosis*.

SYNONYMS

TB

ICD-9CM CODES
011.9 Pulmonary tuberculosis

EPIDEMIOLOGY & DEMOGRAPHICS

INCIDENCE (IN U.S.):
- Approximately 7 cases/100,000 persons—lowest in reported history
- >90% of new cases each year from reactivated prior infections
- 9% newly infected
- Only 10% of patients with PPD conversions (higher [8%/yr] in HIV-positive patients) will develop TB, most within 1-2 yr
- Two thirds of all new cases in racial and ethnic minorities
- Occurs most frequently in geographic areas and among populations with highest AIDS prevalence
  1. Poor, crowded urban communities
- Nearly 36% of new cases from new immigrants

PREVALENCE (IN U.S.):
- Estimated 10 million people infected
- Varies widely among population groups

PREDOMINANT SEX:
- No specific predilection
- Male predominance in AIDS, shelters, and prisons reflected in disproportionate male incidence

PREDOMINANT AGE:
- Nursing home outbreaks among elderly

PEAK INCIDENCE:
- Elderly
- HIV-positive patients, regardless of age, at highest risk

GENETICS:
- Populations with widespread low native resistance have been intensely infected when initially exposed to TB.
- Following elimination of those with least native resistance, incidence and prevalence of TB tend to decline.

PHYSICAL FINDINGS & CLINICAL PRESENTATION

- See "Etiology"
- Primary pulmonary TB infection generally asymptomatic
- Reactivation pulmonary TB
  1. Fever
  2. Night sweats
  3. Cough
  4. Hemoptysis
  5. Scanty nonpurulent sputum
  6. Weight loss
- Progressive primary pulmonary TB disease: same as reactivation pulmonary TB
- TB pleurisy
  1. Pleuritic chest pain
  2. Fever
  3. Shortness of breath
- Rare massive, suffocating, fatal hemoptysis secondary to erosion of pulmonary artery within a cavity (Rasmussen's aneurysm)
- Chest examination
  1. Not specific
  2. Usually underestimates extent of disease
  3. Rales accentuated following a cough (posttussive rales)

ETIOLOGY

- *Mycobacterium tuberculosis* (Mtb), a slow-growing, aerobic, non–spore-forming, nonmotile bacillus, with a lipid-rich cell wall
  1. Lacks pigment
  2. Produces niacin
  3. Reduces nitrate
  4. Produces heat-labile catalase
  5. Mtb staining, acid-fast, and acid-alcohol fast by Ziehl-Neelsen method, appearing as red, slightly bent, beaded rods 2-4 microns long (acid-fast bacilli [AFB]), against a blue background
  6. Polymerase chain reaction (PCR) to detect <10 organisms/ml in sputum (compared with the requisite 10,000 organisms/ml for AFB smear detection)
  7. Culture
     a. Growth on solid media (Löwenstein-Jensen; Middlebrook 7H11) in 2-6 wk
     b. Growth in liquid media (BACTEC, using a radioactive carbon source for early growth detection) often in 9-16 days
     c. Enhanced in a 5%-10% carbon dioxide atmosphere
  8. DNA fingerprinting (based on restriction fragment length polymorphism [RFLP])
     a. Facilitates immediate identification of Mtb strains in early growing cultures
     b. False-negatives possible if growth suboptimal
  9. Humans are the only reservoir for Mtb
  10. Transmission
     a. Facilitated by close exposure to high-velocity cough (unprotected by proper mask or respirators) from patient with AFB-positive sputum and cavitary lesions, producing aerosolized droplets containing AFB, which are inhaled directly into alveoli
     b. Occurs within prisons, nursing homes, and hospitals
- Pathogenesis
  1. AFB (Mtb) ingested by macrophages in alveoli, then transported to regional lymph nodes where spread is contained
  2. Some AFB may reach bloodstream and disseminate widely
  3. Primary TB (asymptomatic, minimal pneumonitis in lower or midlung fields, with hilar lymphadenopathy) essentially an intracellular infection, with multiplication of organisms continuing for 2-12 wk after primary exposure, until cell-mediated hypersensitivity (detected by positive skin test reaction to tuberculin purified protein derivative [PPD]) matures, with subsequent containment of infection
  4. Local and disseminated AFB thus contained by T-cell–mediated immune responses
     a. Recruitment of monocytes
     b. Transformation of lymphocytes with secretion of lymphokines
     c. Activation of macrophages and histiocytes
     d. Organization into granulomas, where organisms may survive within macrophages (Langhans' giant cells), but within which multiplication essentially ceases (95%) and from which spread is prohibited
  5. Progressive primary pulmonary disease
     a. May immediately follow the asymptomatic phase
     b. Necrotizing pulmonary infiltrates
     c. Tuberculous bronchopneumonia
     d. Endobronchial TB
     e. Interstitial TB
     f. Widespread miliary lung lesions
  6. Postprimary TB pleurisy with pleural effusion
     a. Develops after early primary infection, although often before conversion to positive PPD
     b. Results from pleural seeding from a peripheral lung lesion or rupture of lymph node into pleural space
     c. May produce a large (sometimes hemorrhagic) exudative effusion (with polymorphonuclear cells early, rapidly replaced by lymphocytes), frequently without pulmonary infiltrates
     d. Generally resolves without treatment
     e. Portends a high risk of subsequent clinical disease, and

therefore must be diagnosed and treated early (pleural biopsy and culture) to prevent future catastrophic TB illness
    f. May result in disseminated extrapulmonary infection
7. Reactivation pulmonary TB
    a. Occurs months to years following primary TB
    b. Preferentially involves the apical posterior segments of the upper lobes and superior segments of the lower lobes
    c. Associated with necrosis and cavitation of involved lung, hemoptysis, chronic fever, night sweats, weight loss
    d. Spread within lung occurs via cough and inhalation
8. Reinfection TB
    a. May mimic reactivation TB
    b. Ruptured caseous foci and cavities, which may produce endobronchial spread
9. Mtb in both progressive primary and reactivation pulmonary TB
    a. Intracellular (macrophage) lesions (undergoing slow multiplication)
    b. Closed caseous lesions (undergoing slow multiplication)
    c. Extracellular, open cavities (undergoing rapid multiplication)
    d. INH and rifampin are cidal in all three sites
    e. PZA especially active within acidic macrophage environment
    f. Extrapulmonary reactivation disease also possible
10. Most symptoms (fever, weight loss, anorexia) and tissue destruction (caseous necrosis) from cytokines and cell-mediated immune responses
11. Mtb has no important endotoxins or exotoxins
12. Granuloma formation related to tumor necrosis factor (TNF) secreted by activated macrophages

DIAGNOSIS

DIFFERENTIAL DIAGNOSIS

- Necrotizing pneumonia (anaerobic, gram-negative)
- Histoplasmosis
- Coccidioidomycosis
- Melioidosis
- Interstitial lung diseases (rarely)
- Cancer
- Sarcoidosis
- Silicosis
- Paragonimiasis
- Rare pneumonias
    1. *Rhodococcus equi* (cavitation)
    2. *Bacillus cereus* (50% hemoptysis)
    3. *Eikenella corrodens* (cavitation)

WORKUP

- Sputum for AFB stains
- Chest x-ray examination
- PPD
    1. Recent conversion from negative to positive within 3 mo of exposure is highly suggestive of recent infection.
    2. Single positive PPD is not helpful diagnostically.
    3. Negative PPD never rules out acute TB.
    4. Be certain that positive PPD does not reflect "booster phenomenon" (prior positive PPD may become negative after several years and return to positive only after second repeated PPD; repeat second PPD within 1 wk), which thus may mimic skin test conversion.
    5. Positive PPD reaction is determined as follows:
        a. Induration after 72 hr of intradermal injection of 0.1 ml of 5 TU-PPD
        b. 5-mm induration if HIV-positive, close contact of active TB, fibrotic chest lesions
        c. 10-mm induration if in high–medical risk groups (immunosuppressive disease or therapy, renal failure, gastrectomy, silicosis, diabetes), foreign-born high-risk group (Southeast Asia, Latin America, Africa, India), low socioeconomic groups, IV drug addict, prisoner, health care worker
        d. 15-mm induration if low risk
    6. Anergy antigen testing (using mumps, *Candida,* tetanus toxoid) may identify patients who are truly anergic to PPD and these antigens, but results are often confusing. Not recommended.
    7. Patients with TB may be selectively anergic only to PPD.
    8. Positive PPD indicates prior infection but does not itself confirm active disease.

LABORATORY TESTS

- Sputum for AFB stains and culture
    1. Induced sputum if patient not coughing productively
- Sputum from bronchoscopy if high suspicion of TB with negative expectorated induced sputum for AFB
    1. Positive AFB smear is essential before or shortly after treatment to ensure subsequent growth for definitive diagnosis and sensitivity testing
    2. Consider lung biopsy if sputum negative, especially if infiltrates are predominantly interstitial
- AFB stain-negative sputum may grow Mtb subsequently
- Gastric aspirates reliable, especially in HIV-negative patients

- CBC
    1. Variable values
        a. WBCs: low, normal, or elevated (including leukemoid reaction: >50,000)
        b. Normocytic, normochromic anemia often
    2. Rarely helpful diagnostically
- ESR usually elevated
- Thoracentesis
    1. Exudative effusion
        a. Elevated protein
        b. Decreased glucose
        c. Elevated WBCs (polymorphonuclear leukocytes early, replaced later by lymphocytes)
        d. May be hemorrhagic
    2. Pleural fluid usually AFB-negative
    3. Pleural biopsy often diagnostic—may need to be repeated for diagnosis
    4. Culture pleural biopsy tissue for AFB
- Bone marrow biopsy is often diagnostic in difficult-to-diagnose cases, especially miliary tuberculosis

IMAGING STUDIES

- Chest x-ray examination
    1. Primary infection reflected by calcified peripheral lung nodule with calcified hilar lymph node
    2. Reactivation pulmonary TB
        a. Necrosis
        b. Cavitation (especially on apical lordotic views)
        c. Fibrosis and hilar retraction
        d. Bronchopneumonia
        e. Interstitial infiltrates
        f. Miliary pattern
        g. Many of previous may also accompany progressive primary TB
    3. TB pleurisy
        a. Pleural effusion, often rapidly accumulating and massive
    4. TB activity not established by single chest x-ray examination
    5. Serial chest x-ray examinations are excellent indicators of progression or regression

TREATMENT

NONPHARMACOLOGIC THERAPY

- Bed rest during acute phase of treatment
- High-calorie, high-protein diet to reverse malnutrition and enhance immune response to TB
- Isolation in negative-pressure rooms with high-volume air replacement and circulation, with health care provider wearing proper protective 0.5- to 1-micron filter respirators, until three consecutive sputum AFB smears are negative

ACUTE GENERAL Rx

- Compliance (rigid adherence to treatment regimen) chief determinant of success
  1. Supervised directly observed therapy (DOT) recommended for all patients and mandatory for unreliable patients
- Preferred adult regimen: DOT
  1. Isoniazid (INH) 15 mg/kg (max 900 mg) + rifampin 600 mg + ethambutol (EMB) 30 mg/kg (max 2500 mg) + pyrazinamide (PZA) (2 g [<50 kg]; 2.5 g [51 to 74 kg]; 3 g [>75 kg]) thrice weekly for 6 mo
  2. Alternative, more complicated DOT regimens
- Rifapentine, a rifampin derivative with a much longer serum half-life, was shown to be as effective when administered weekly (with weekly isoniazid) as conventional regimens for drug-sensitive pulmonary tuberculosis in non-HIV-infected patients.
- Short-course daily therapy: adult
  1. HIV-negative patient: 6 mo total therapy (2 mo INH 300 mg + rifampin 600 mg + EMB 15 mg/kg [max 2500 mg]) + PZA (1.5 g [<50 kg]; 2 g [51 to 74 kg]; 2.5 g [>75 kg]) daily and until smear negative and sensitivity confirmed; then INH + rifampin daily × 4 mo
  2. HIV-positive patient: 9 mo total therapy (2 mo INH + rifampin + EMB + PZA daily until smear negative and sensitivity confirmed; then INH + rifampin qd × 7 mo)
  3. Continue treatment at least 3 mo following conversion to negative cultures
- Drug resistance (often multiple drug resistance [MDRTB]) increased by:
  1. Prior treatment
  2. Acquisition of TB in developing countries
  3. Homelessness
  4. AIDS
  5. Prisoners
  6. IV drug addicts
  7. Known contact with MDRTB
- Never add single drug to failing regimen
- Never treat TB with fewer than two to three drugs or two to three new additional drugs

---

- Monitor for clinical toxicity (especially hepatitis)
  1. Patient and physician awareness that anorexia, nausea, RUQ pain, and unexplained malaise require immediate cessation of treatment
  2. Evaluation of LFTs
     a. Minimal SGOT/SGPT elevations without symptoms generally transient and not clinically significant
- Preventive treatment for PPD conversion only (infection without disease)
  1. Must be certain that chest x-ray examination is negative and patient has no symptoms of TB
  2. INH 300 mg daily for 6-12 mo; at least 12 mo if HIV-positive
  3. Most important groups:
     a. HIV-positive
     b. Close contact of active TB
     c. Recent converter
     d. Old TB on chest x-ray examination
     e. IV drug addict
     f. Medical risk factor
     g. High-risk foreign country
     h. Homeless

CHRONIC Rx

- Generally not indicated beyond treatment described previously
- Prolonged treatment, supervised by infectious disease expert, in a few very complicated infections caused by resistant organisms

DISPOSITION

- Monthly follow-up by physician experienced in TB treatment
- Confirm sensitivity testing and alter treatment appropriately
- Frequent sputum samples until culture is negative
- Confirm chest x-ray regression at 2 to 3 mo

REFERRAL

- To infectious disease expert for:
  1. HIV-positive patient
  2. Patient with suspected drug-resistant TB
  3. Patients previously treated for TB
  4. Patients whose fever has not decreased and sputum has not converted to negative in 2-4 wk

---

  5. Patients with overwhelming pulmonary or extrapulmonary tuberculosis
- To pulmonologist for bronchoscopy or pleural biopsy

PEARLS & CONSIDERATIONS

COMMENTS

- All contacts (especially close household contacts and infants) should be properly tested for PPD conversions during 3 mo following exposure.
- Those with positive PPD should be evaluated for active TB and properly treated or given prophylaxis.

SUGGESTED READINGS

Benator D et al: Rifapentine and isoniazid once a week versus rifampicin and isoniazid twice a week for treatment of drug susceptible pulmonary tuberculosis in HIV-negative patients: a randomized clinical trial, *Lancet* 360(9332):528, 2002.

Espinal MA et al: Infectiousness of *Mycobacterium tuberculosis* in HIV-1-infected patients with tuberculosis: a prospective study, *Lancet* 355(9200):275, 2000.

Kanaya AM, Glidden DV, Chambers HF: Identifying pulmonary tuberculosis in patients with negative sputum smear results, *Chest* 120(2):349, 2001.

Karcic AA et al: An elderly woman with chronic knee pain and abnormal chest radiography, *Postgrad Med* 77(911):600, 2001.

Mulder K: Tuberculosis: a case history, *Lancet* 358(9283):776, 2001.

Salazar GE et al: Pulmonary tuberculosis in children in a developing country, *Pediatrics* 108(2):448, 2001.

Small P, Fujiwara P: Management of tuberculosis in the United States, *N Engl J Med* 345:189, 2001.

Tudo G et al: Detection of unsuspected cases of nosocomial transmission of tuberculosis by use of a molecular typing method, *Clin Infect Dis* 33(4):453, 2001.

AUTHOR: **GEORGE O. ALONSO, M.D.**

BASIC INFORMATION

DEFINITION

Urinary tract infection (UTI) is a term that encompasses a broad range of clinical entities that have in common a positive urine culture. A conventional threshold is growth of >100,000 colony-forming units per ml from a midstream-catch urine sample. In symptomatic patients, a smaller number of bacteria (between 100 and 10,000 colony-forming units per ml of midstream urine) is recognized as an infection.

SYNONYMS

UTI

ICD-9CM CODES
595.0 Acute cystitis
595.3 Trigonitis
595.2 Chronic cystitis
590.1 Acute pyelonephritis
590.0 Chronic pyelonephritis
590.8 Nonspecific pyelonephritis

CLASSIFICATION

FIRST INFECTION: The first documented UTI tends to be uncomplicated and is easily treated.

UNRESOLVED BACTERIURIA: UTI in which the urinary tract is not sterilized during therapy. Main causes are bacterial resistance, patient noncompliance with medication, resistance, mixed bacterial infection, rapid reinfection, azotemia, infected stones, Munchausen's, and papillary necrosis.

BACTERIAL PERSISTENCE: UTI in which the urine cultures become sterile during therapy, but a persistent source of infection from a site within the urinary tract that was excluded from the high urinary concentrations gives rise to reinfection by the same organism. Causes: infected stone, chronic bacterial prostatitis, atrophic infected kidney, vesicovaginal or enterovesical fistulas, obstructive uropathy, infected pyelocalyceal diverticula, infected ureteral stump following nephrectomy, infected necrotic papillae from papillary necrosis, infected urachal cysts, infected medullary sponge kidney, urethral diverticula, and foreign bodies.

REINFECTION: UTI in which a new infection occurs with new pathogens at variable intervals after a previous infection has been eradicated.

Relapse: The less common form of recurrent infection; occurs within 2 wk of treatment when the same organism reappears in the same site as the previous infection. Relapsing infections of the urinary tract most commonly occur in pyelonephritis, kidney obstruction from a stone, and prostatitis.

EPIDEMIOLOGY & DEMOGRAPHICS

INCIDENCE:
In adults, 65 yr and older, at least 10% of men and 20% of women have bacteriuria.

PATHOGENESIS:
- Four major pathways:
  1. Ascending from the urethra
  2. Lymphatic
  3. Hematogenous
  4. Direct extension from another organ system
- Other risk factors: neurologic diseases, renal failure, diabetes; anatomic abnormalities: bladder outlet obstruction, urethral stricture, vesicoureteral reflux, fistula, urinary diversion, megacystis, and infected stones; age; instrumentation, poor patient compliance, poor hygiene, infrequent voider, douches, and catheters

Catheters: All patients who require a long-term Foley catheter eventually develop significant levels of bacteriuria. Treatment is reserved for those individuals who become symptomatic (i.e., leukocytosis, fever, chills, malaise, loss of appetite, etc.). Using prophylactic antibiotics to treat patients who have chronic catheters is to be discouraged because of the risk of acquiring bacteria that are resistant to antibiotic therapy.
- Once bacteria reach the urinary tract, three factors determine whether the infection occurs (Box 1-7):
  1. Virulence of the microorganism
  2. Inoculum size
  3. Adequacy of the host defense mechanisms
- These factors also determine the anatomic level of the UTI.

Urinary Pathogens: In >95% of UTIs the infecting organism is a member of the Enterobacteriaceae, *Pseudomonas aeruginosa,* or enterococci. In contrast, the organisms that commonly colonize the distal urethra and skin of both men and women and the vagina of women are *Staphylococcus epidermidis,* diphtheroids, lactobacilli, *Gardnerella vaginalis,* and a variety of anaerobes that rarely cause UTI. Generally, the isolation of two or more bacterial species from a urine culture signifies a contaminated specimen, unless the patient is being managed with an indwelling catheter or urinary diversion or has a chronic complicated infection.

Defense Mechanisms Against Cystitis: Low pH and high osmolarity, mucopolysaccharide glycosaminoglycan protective layer, normal bladder that empties completely and has no incontinence, and the presence of estrogen

PHYSICAL FINDINGS

- UTI presentation is inconsistent and cannot be relied upon to diagnose UTI accurately or to localize the site of infection. Patients complain of:
  1. Urinary frequency, urgency
  2. Dysuria
  3. Urge incontinence
  4. Suprapubic pain
  5. Gross or microscopic hematuria
- When negative cultures are associated with significant pyuria, vaginal discharge, or hematuria, infections with *Chlamydia trachomatis, Neisseria gonorrhoeae,* and *Trichomonas vaginalis* should be considered.
- Acute pyelonephritis (PN) presents with fever, flank or abdominal pain, chills, malaise, vomiting, and diarrhea. It is these systemic symptoms that distinguish pyelonephritis from cystitis. Complications of acute pyelonephritis are renal abscess, perinephric abscess, emphysematous pyelonephritis, and pyonephrosis.

BOX 1-7 Bacterial Factors

1. The size of the inoculum
2. The virulence of the infecting organism:
   a. Virulence factors:
      i. P-fimbriae facilitate the adherence of bacteria to biologic surfaces.
      ii. K-antigens facilitate adherence and protect the organisms from the host-immune response.
      iii. O-antigens are an important source of the systemic reactions, such as fever and shock, that occur with bacterial infections.
      iv. H antigens are associated with flagella and are related to bacterial locomotion.
      v. Hemolysin may potentiate tissue damage and facilitate local bacterial growth.
      vi. Urease alkalinizes the urine and facilitates stone formation, thus potentiating infection.
   b. Biofilms harbor bacteria on prosthetic devices and may be a source of recurrent infections.
   c. The presence of sialosyl galactosyl globoside (SGG) on the surface of kidney cells. This compound is a highly powerful receptor for E. coli bacteria.
   d. Women with a deficiency in human beta-defensin-1 (HBD-1) are at greater risk for urinary tract infection.
3. Adequacy of host defense mechanisms

DIAGNOSIS

DIFFERENTIAL DIAGNOSIS

- Interstitial cystitis
- Vaginitis
- Urethritis (gonococcal, nongonococcal, *Trichomonas*)
- Frequency-urgency syndrome, prostatitis (acute and chronic)
- Obstructive uropathy
- Infected stones
- Fistulas
- Papillary necrosis
- Vesicoureteral reflux

LABORATORY TESTS

- Urinalysis with microscopic evaluation of clean-catch urine for bacteria and pyuria
- Urine C&S
- CBC with differential (shows leukocytosis)
- Antibody-coated bacteria are seen with pyelonephritis

IMAGING STUDIES

- Warranted only if renal infection or genitourinary abnormality is suspected
- KUB, VCUG, renal sonogram, IVP, CT scan, and nuclear scan
- Specialty examination: cystoscopy with occasional retrograde pyelography to rule out obstructive uropathy; stenting the obstruction possibly required

TREATMENT

NONPHARMACOLOGIC THERAPY

- Hot sitz baths, anticholinergics, urinary analgesics
- For pyelonephritis: bed rest, analgesics, antipyretics, and IV hydration

ACUTE GENERAL Rx

- Conventional therapy of 7 days; short-term therapy of 1, 3, or 5 days is not recommended for geriatric patients.
- Agents of choice: amoxicillin/clavulanate, cephalosporins, fluoroquinolones, nitrofurantoin, and trimethoprim with sulfonamide.
- For pyelonephritis: hospitalization until afebrile and stable, then at home via home care agency with IV antibiotic composed of aminoglycoside plus cephalosporin × 1 wk followed by oral agents (based on sensitivity) for 2 wk. Moderate forms of pyelonephritis have been successfully treated with fluoroquinolone therapy for 21 days, without requiring hospitalization. Most important, complicating factors such

as obstructive uropathy or infected stones must be identified and treated.
- Section III, "Urinary Tract Infection," describes an approach to the management of UTI.

PEARLS & CONSIDERATIONS

COMMENTS

- *Asymptomatic bacteriuria:* occurs in both anatomically normal and abnormal urinary tracts. Common among nursing home residents. This can clear spontaneously, persist, or lead to symptomatic kidney infection. Treatment is recommended in patients with vesicoureteral reflux, stones, obstructive uropathy, parenchymal renal disease, diabetes mellitus, and immunocompromised patients.
- Urinary incontinence and "asymptomatic" bacteriuria often coexist among nursing home patients, and antibiotics rarely correct the incontinence, especially in the absence of pyuria.
- UTI can present as delirium, particularly in patients with baseline cognitive impairments.
- *Recurrent UTI:* caused by an unresolved infection, vaginal colonization of the originally infecting organism, or reinfection with a new strain. Management of recurrent UTI includes continuous antibiotic prophylaxis, intermittent self-treatment, and postcoital prophylaxis. Prophylaxis is considered for women who experience two or more symptomatic UTIs over a 6-mo period or three or more episodes over a 12-mo period.
  1. Changes after menopause: lower levels of lactobacilli, decreased estrogen, senile atrophy of the genitalia, and loss of bladder elasticity (compliance).
  2. Biologic factors altering defense systems: the presence of sialosyl galactosyl globoside (SGG) on the surface of the kidney acts as a powerful receptor for *E. coli* and increases the risk for UTI; the presence of the blood group P1 causes increased binding of *E. coli* that is resistant to normal infection-fighting mechanisms in the body and it is believed that some individuals are deficient in a compound called *human beta-defensin-1* (HBD-1), a naturally occurring antibiotic that fights *E. coli* within the urinary tract.
  3. BPH and chronic prostatitis in men

Resistance:

- Because of the overuse of antibiotics, organisms once sensitive to a number of agents are now increasingly more resistant, making effective management of UTI and pyelonephritis more difficult and potentially more dangerous. Most important has been the increasing resistance to TMP-SMX, the current primary care provider drug of choice for acute uncomplicated UTI in women.
- Facts about bacterial resistance:
  1. Given enough antibiotic and time, resistance will develop
  2. Organisms that are resistant to one antibiotic will likely become resistant to others
  3. Resistance is progressive, moving from low to intermediate to high levels
  4. Once selected, drug resistance will not disappear
  5. When antibiotics are used by any patient, this use affects other people by changing the immediate and extended environment
  6. No counterselective steps against resistant bacteria now exist
- When choosing a treatment regimen physicians should consider such factors as:
  1. In-vitro susceptibility
  2. Adverse effects
  3. Cost effectiveness
  4. Resistance rates in the respective communities

SUGGESTED READINGS

Bent S et al: Does this woman have an acute uncomplicated urinary tract infection? *JAMA* 287:2701, 2002.

Gomolin IH et al: Efficacy and safety of ciprofloxacin oral suspension versus trimethoprim-sulfamethoxazole oral suspension for treatment of older women with acute urinary tract infection, *J Am Geriatr Soc* 49:1606, 2001.

Gupta K et al: Increasing antimicrobial resistance and the management of uncomplicated community-acquired urinary tract infections, *Ann Int Med* 135:41, 2001.

Levy SB: Multidrug resistance—a sign of the times, *N Engl J Med* 338:1376, 1998 [editorial].

McIsaac WJ et al: The impact of empirical management of acute cystitis on unnecessary antibiotic use, *Arch Int Med* 161:600, 2002.

Saint S et al: The effectiveness of a clinical practical guideline for the management of presumed uncomplicated UTI in women, *Am J Med* 106:636, 1999.

AUTHORS: **PHILIP J. ALIOTTA, M.D., M.S.H.A.,** with revisions by **TOM J. WACHTEL, M.D.**

BASIC INFORMATION

DEFINITION

Urolithiasis is the presence of calculi within the urinary tract. The five major types of urinary stones are calcium oxalate (>50%), calcium phosphate (10% to 20%), uric acid (8%), struvite (15%), and cystine (3%).

SYNONYMS

Nephrolithiasis
Renal colic

ICD-9CM CODES

592.9 Urinary calculus

EPIDEMIOLOGY & DEMOGRAPHICS

- Urinary stone disease afflicts 250,000 to 750,000 Americans/yr.
- Male:female ratio is 4:1. After the sixth decade, the ratio is 1.5:1.
- Incidence of symptomatic nephrolithiasis is greatest during the summer (resulting from increased humidity and temperatures with increased risk of dehydration and concentrated urine).
- Calcium oxalate or mixed calcium oxalate/calcium phosphate stones account for 70% of urolithiasis.

PHYSICAL FINDINGS & CLINICAL PRESENTATION

Stones may be asymptomatic or may cause the following signs and symptoms from obstruction:

- Sudden onset of flank tenderness
- Nausea and vomiting
- Patient in constant movement, attempting to lessen the pain (patients with an acute abdomen are usually still because movement exacerbates the pain)
- Pain may be referred to the testes or labium (progression of stone down the urinary ureter)
- Fever and chills accompanying the acute colic if there is superimposed infection
- Pain may radiate anteriorly over to the abdomen and result in intestinal ileus

ETIOLOGY

- Increased absorption of calcium in the small bowel: type I absorptive hypercalciuria (independent of calcium intake)
- Idiopathic hypercalciuria nephrolithiasis is the most common diagnosis for patients with calcium stones; the diagnosis is made only if there is no hypercalcemia and no known cause for hypercalciuria
- Increased vitamin D synthesis (e.g., secondary to renal phosphate loss: type III absorptive hypercalciuria)
- Renal tubular malfunction with inadequate reabsorption of calcium and resulting hypercalciuria
- Heterozygous mutations in the NPT2a gene result in hypophosphatemia and urinary phosphate loss
- Hyperparathyroidism with resulting hypercalcemia
- Elevated uric acid level (metabolic defects, dietary excess)
- Chronic diarrhea (e.g., inflammatory bowel disease) with increased oxalate absorption
- Type I (distal tubule) renal tubular acidosis (<1% of calcium stones)
- Chronic hydrochlorothiazide treatment
- Chronic infections with urease-producing organisms (e.g., *Proteus, Providencia, Pseudomonas, Klebsiella*). Struvite, or magnesium ammonium phosphate crystals, are produced when the urinary tract is colonized by bacteria, producing elevated concentrations of ammonia
- Abnormal excretion of cystine
- Chemotherapy for malignancies

DIAGNOSIS

DIFFERENTIAL DIAGNOSIS

- Urinary tract infection
- Pyelonephritis
- Diverticulitis
- PID
- Ovarian pathology
- Factitious (drug addicts)
- Appendicitis
- Small bowel obstruction
- The differential diagnosis of obstructive uropathy is described in Section II

WORKUP

- Laboratory and imaging studies. Stone analysis should be performed on recovered stones.
- A clinical algorithm for evaluation of nephrolithiasis is described in Section III.
- Box 1-8 describes past medical history significant for urolithiasis.

LABORATORY TESTS

- Urinalysis: hematuria may be present; however, its absence does not exclude urinary stones. Evaluation of urinary pH is of value in identification of type of stone (pH >7.5 is associated with struvite stones, whereas pH <5 generally is seen with uric acid or with cystine stones).
- Urine C&S should be obtained for all patients.
- Serum chemistries should include calcium, electrolytes, phosphate, and uric acid.
- Additional tests: 24-hr urine collection for calcium, uric acid, phosphate, oxalate, and citrate excretion is generally reserved for patients with recurrent stones.

BOX 1-8   Past Medical History Significant for Urolithiasis

Diseases associated with disturbances of calcium metabolism: primary hyperparathyroidism, Wilson's disease, medullary sponge kidney, osteoporosis, immobilization, sarcoidosis, osteolytic metastases, plasmacytoma, neuroendocrine tumors, Paget's disease
  Dietary history: purine gluttony, calcium excess, milk alkali, oxalate excess, sodium excess, low citrus fruit intake
  Medications: uricosurics, diuretics, analgesics, vitamins C and D, antacids (especially phosphorus-binding agents), acetazolamide, calcium channel blockers, triamterene, theophylline, protease inhibitors (indinavir), sulfonamides
Diseases associated with disturbances of oxalate metabolism: primary hyperoxaluria types I and II, Crohn's disease, ulcerative colitis, intestinal bypass surgery (especially jejunoileal bypass), ileal resection
Diseases associated with disturbances of purine metabolism
  Intrinsic metabolic disorders—anemia, neoplastic disorders (especially leukemias), intoxication, myocardial infarction, irradiation, cytotoxic chemotherapy
  Enzyme deficiency—primary gout, Lesch-Nyhan syndrome
  Altered excretion—renal insufficiency, metabolic acidosis
  Infectious history: organisms (particularly Proteus and Klebsiella), febrile upper tract involvement and dates if hospitalized.

From Nseyo UO (ed): *Urology for primary care physicians,* Philadelphia, 1999, WB Saunders.

IMAGING STUDIES

- Plain films of the abdomen can identify radioopaque stones (calcium, uric acid stones).
- Renal sonogram may be helpful.
- IVP demonstrates the size and location of the stone, as well as degree of obstruction.
- Unenhanced (noncontrast) helical CT scan does not require contrast media and can visualize the calculus (identified by the "rim sign" or "halo" representing the edematous ureteral wall around the stone). It is fast, accurate (sensitivity 15%-100%, specificity 94%-96%), and readily identifies all stone types in all locations. This modality is being used increasingly in the initial assessment of renal colic.

TREATMENT

NONPHARMACOLOGIC THERAPY

- Increase in water or other fluid intake (doubling of previous fluid intake unless patient has a history of CHF or fluid overload)
- Normal dietary calcium intake. If one does not consume enough calcium, less is available to bind to dietary oxalate; as a result, more oxalate reaches the colon, is absorbed into the bloodstream, and is excreted as calcium oxalate, setting the stage for calcium urolithiasis
- Sodium restriction (to decrease calcium excretion), decreased protein intake to 1 g/kg/day (to decrease uric acid, calcium, and oxalate excretion)
- Increase in bran (may decrease bowel transit time with increased binding of calcium and subsequent decrease in urinary calcium)

ACUTE GENERAL Rx

- Pain control (use of narcotics is generally indicated because of the severity of pain)
- Specific therapy tailored to the stone type:
  1. Uric acid calculi: control of hyperuricosuria with allopurinol 100-300 mg/day; increase urinary pH with potassium citrate, 10-mEq tablets tid
  2. Calcium stones:
     a. HCTZ 25-50 mg qd in patients with type I absorptive hypercalciuria
     b. Decrease bowel absorption of calcium with cellulose phosphate 10 g/day in patients with type I absorptive hypercalciuria
     c. Orthophosphates to inhibit vitamin B synthesis in patients with type III absorptive hypercalciuria
     d. Potassium citrate supplementation in patients with hypocitraturic calcium nephrolithiasis
     e. Purine dietary restrictions or allopurinol in patients with hyperuricosuric calcium nephrolithiasis
  3. Struvite stones:
     a. Most of the stones are large and cause obstruction and bleeding.
     b. ESWL and percutaneous nephrolithotomy are generally necessary.
     c. Prolonged use of antibiotics directed against the predominant urinary tract organism may be beneficial to prevent recurrence.
  4. Cystine stones: Hydration and alkalization of the urine to pH >6.5, penicillamine, and tiopronin can also be used to reduce the formation of cystine; captopril is also beneficial and causes fewer side effects
- Surgical treatment in patients with severe pain unresponsive to medication and patients with persistent fever or nausea or significant impediment of urine flow:
  a. Ureteroscopic stone extraction
  b. Extracorporeal shock wave lithotripsy (ESWL) for most renal stones
- In 1997 the American Urological Association issued the following guidelines for the treatment of ureteral stones:
  1. Proximal ureteral stones <1 cm in diameter: options are ESWL, percutaneous nephroureterolithotomy, and ureteroscopy
  2. Proximal ureteral stones >1 cm in diameter: options are ESWL, percutaneous nephroureterolithotomy, and ureteroscopy. Placement of a ureteral stent should be considered if the stone is causing high-grade obstruction
  3. Distal ureteral stones <1 cm in diameter: most of these pass spontaneously. ESWL and ureteroscopy are two accepted modes of therapy
  4. Distal ureteral stones >1 cm in diameter: watchful waiting, ESWL, ureteroscopy (following stone fragmentation)
- Section III describes an approach to the management of ureteral calculi.

CHRONIC Rx

Maintenance of proper hydration and dietary restrictions (see "Acute General Rx")

DISPOSITION

- >50% of patients will pass the stone within 48 hr.
- Stones will recur in approximately 50% of patients within 5 yr if no medical treatment is provided.

REFERRAL

Urology referral in complicated or recurrent urolithiasis; most patients with small uncomplicated ureteral or renal calculi can be followed as outpatient, whereas patients with persistent vomiting, suspected UTI, pain unresponsive to oral analgesics, or obstructing calculus associated with solitary kidney should be admitted to a hospital

PEARLS & CONSIDERATIONS

COMMENTS

- Early identification and aggressive treatment of urinary tract infections is indicated in all patients with struvite stones.
- Alkalinization of urine (pH >7.5 with penicillamine) is useful in patients with recurrent cystine stones.
- An algorithmic approach to the management of ureteral calculi is described in Section III.

SUGGESTED READINGS

Borghi L et al: Comparison of two diets for the prevention of recurrent stones in idiopathic hypercalciuria, *N Engl J Med* 346:77, 2002.

Prie D et al: Nephrolithiasis and osteoporosis associated with hypophosphatemia caused by mutations in the type 2a sodium-phosphate cotransporter, *N Engl J Med* 347:983, 2002.

Worster A et al: The accuracy of noncontrast helical computed tomography versus intravenous pyelography in the diagnosis of suspected acute urolithiasis: a meta-analysis, *Ann Intern Med* 40:280, 2002.

AUTHOR: **FRED F. FERRI, M.D.**

BASIC INFORMATION

DEFINITION

Urticaria is a pruritic rash involving the epidermis and the upper portions of the dermis, resulting from localized capillary vasodilation and followed by transudation of protein-rich fluid in the surrounding tissue and manifesting clinically with the presence of hives.

SYNONYMS

Hives
Wheals

ICD-9CM CODES
708.8 Other unspecified urticaria

EPIDEMIOLOGY & DEMOGRAPHICS

- At least 20% of the population will have one episode of hives during their lifetime.
- Incidence is increased in atopic patients.
- The etiology of chronic urticaria (hives lasting longer than 6 wk) is determined in only 5%-20% of cases.

PHYSICAL FINDINGS & CLINICAL PRESENTATION

- Presence of elevated, erythematous, or white nonpitting plaques that change in size and shape over time; they generally last a few hours and disappear without a trace.
- Annular configuration with central pallor (Fig. 1-51).

ETIOLOGY

- Foods (e.g., shellfish, eggs, strawberries, nuts)
- Drugs (e.g., penicillin, aspirin, sulfonamides)
- Systemic diseases (e.g., SLE, serum sickness, autoimmune thyroid disease, polycythemia vera)

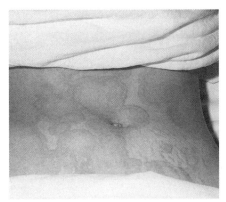

FIGURE 1-51 Wheal (urticaria). Note central cleaning, giving annular configuration. (From Noble J et al: *Textbook of primary care medicine,* ed 3, St Louis, 2001, Mosby.)

- Food additives (e.g., salicylates, benzoates, sulfites)
- Infections (viral infections, fungal infections, chronic bacterial infections)
- Physical stimuli (e.g., pressure urticaria, exercise-induced, solar urticaria, cold urticaria)
- Inhalants (e.g., mold spores, animal danders, pollens)
- Contact (nonimmunologic) urticaria (e.g., caterpillars, plants)
- Other: hereditary angioedema, urticaria pigmentosa, cold urticaria, hair bleaches, chemicals, saliva, cosmetics, perfumes, pemphigoid, emotional stress

DIAGNOSIS **Dx**

DIFFERENTIAL DIAGNOSIS

- Erythema multiforme
- Erythema marginatum
- Erythema infectiosum
- Urticarial vasculitis
- Drug eruption
- Multiple insect bites
- Bullous pemphigoid

WORKUP

- It is useful to determine whether hives are acute or chronic; a medical history focused on various etiologic factors is necessary before embarking on extensive laboratory testing.
- A diagnostic approach to chronic urticaria is described in Section III.

LABORATORY TESTS

- CBC with differential
- Stool for ova and parasites in patients with suspected parasitic infestations
- ANA, ESR, TSH, LFTs, eosinophil count are indicated only in selected patients
- Measurement of C_4 in patients who present with angioedema alone
- Skin biopsy is helpful in patients with fever, arthralgias, and elevated ESR

TREATMENT **Rx**

NONPHARMACOLOGIC THERAPY

- Remove suspected etiologic agents (e.g., stop aspirin and all nonessential drugs), restrict diet (e.g., elimination of tomatoes, nuts, eggs, shellfish).
- Elimination of yeast should be attempted in patients with chronic urticaria (*Candida albicans* sensitivity may be a factor in patients with chronic urticaria).

ACUTE GENERAL Rx

- Oral antihistamines: use of nonsedating antihistamines (e.g., loratadine [Claritin] 10 mg qd or cetirizine [Zyrtec] 10 mg qd) is preferred over first-generation antihistamines (e.g., hydroxyzine, diphenhydramine).
- Doxepin (a tricyclic antidepressant) that blocks both H_1 and H_2 receptors 25-75 mg qhs may be effective in patients with chronic urticaria.
- H_2 receptor antagonists (cimetidine, ranitidine, famotidine) can be added to H_1 antagonists in refractory cases.
- A short course of rapidly tapering oral corticosteroids may be prescribed (e.g., prednisone starting at 60 mg qd and ending at 10 mg qd over 8 days).

CHRONIC Rx

- Use of nonsedating antihistamines, doxepin, and/or oral corticosteroids (see "Acute General Rx")
- Oral corticosteroids should be reserved for refractory cases (e.g., prednisone 20 mg qd or 20 mg bid).
- Low dose of the immunosuppressant cyclosporine (2.5-3 mg/kg body weight/day) has been shown to be effective and corticosteroid sparing in chronic urticaria
- There is insufficient data to support use of leukotriene antagonists (zafirlukast, montelukast) in patients with chronic urticaria

DISPOSITION

- Most cases of urticaria resolve within 6 wk.
- Only 25% of patients with a history of chronic urticaria are completely cured after 5 yr.

PEARLS & CONSIDERATIONS **!**

COMMENTS

- Local treatment (e.g., starch baths or Aveeno baths) may be helpful in selected patients; however, local treatment is generally not rewarding.
- The management of angioedema (i.e., Dx and Rx) is the same as urticaria.

SUGGESTED READINGS

Kaplan AP: Chronic urticaria and angioedema, *N Engl J Med* 346:157, 2002.
Miller BA: Urticaria and angioedema: a practical approach, *Am Fam Physician* 69:1123, 2004.

AUTHORS: **FRED F. FERRI, M.D.,** with minor revisions by **TOM J. WACHTEL, M.D.**

BASIC INFORMATION

DEFINITION

Uterine prolapse refers to the protrusion of the uterus into or out of the vaginal canal. In a *first-degree uterine prolapse,* the cervix is visible when the perineum is depressed. In a *second-degree uterine prolapse,* the uterine cervix has prolapsed through the vaginal introitus, with the fundus remaining within the pelvis proper. In a *third-degree uterine prolapse* (i.e., *complete uterine prolapse, uterine procidentia*), the entire uterus is outside the introitus.

SYNONYMS

Genital prolapse
Uterine descensus
Pelvic organ prolapse

ICD-9CM CODES
618.8 Genital prolapse
618.1 Uterine descensus
618.8 Pelvic organ prolapse

EPIDEMIOLOGY & DEMOGRAPHICS

Most prevalent in postmenopausal multiparous women.
RISK FACTORS:
- Labor
- Vaginal childbirth
- Obesity
- Chronic coughing
- Constipation
- Pelvic tumors
- Ascites
- Strenuous physical exertion
- Caucasian race

GENETICS: Increased incidence in women with spina bifida occulta.

PHYSICAL FINDINGS & CLINICAL PRESENTATION

- Pelvic pressure
- Bearing-down sensation
- Bilateral groin pain
- Sacral backache
- Coital difficulty
- Protrusion from vagina
- Spotting
- Ulceration
- Bleeding
- Examination of patient in lithotomy, sitting, and standing positions and before, during, and after a maximum Valsalva effort
- Erosion or ulceration of the cervix possible in the most dependent area of the protrusion

ETIOLOGY

- Vaginal childbirth and chronic increases in intraabdominal pressure leading to detachments, lacerations, and denervations of the vaginal support system

- Further weakening of pelvic support system by hypoestrogenic atrophy
- Some cases from congenital or inherited weaknesses within the pelvic support system

DIAGNOSIS

DIFFERENTIAL DIAGNOSIS

- Occasionally, elongated cervix; body of the uterus remains undescended
- Diagnosis is based on history and physical examination. Currently there is only one genital tract prolapse classification system that has attained international acceptance & recognition, the Patient pelvic organ prolapse quantification (POPQ). See Boxes 1-9 and 1-10.

WORKUP

- If erosion or ulceration of the cervix is present, a Pap smear followed by a cervical biopsy should be performed if indicated.
- If urinary symptoms are significant, further urodynamic workup is indicated, looking for concurrent cystourethrocele, cystocele, enterocele, or rectocele.

LABORATORY TESTS

Urinalysis and urine culture if urinary symptoms exist

IMAGING STUDIES

Ultrasound if concurrent fibroids need further evaluation

TREATMENT

NONPHARMACOLOGIC THERAPY

- Prophylactic measures
  1. Diagnosis and treatment of chronic respiratory and metabolic disorders
  2. Correction of constipation
  3. Weight control, nutrition, and smoking cessation counseling
  4. Teaching of pelvic muscle exercises
- Supportive pessary therapy
  1. Ring-type pessary useful for first- or second-degree prolapse
  2. Gellhorn pessary preferred for more advanced prolapse
  3. Use of pessaries in conjunction with continuous hormone replacement therapy, unless contraindicated
  4. Perineorrhaphy under local anesthesia possibly needed to support the pessary if the vaginal outlet is very relaxed

ACUTE GENERAL Rx

- Patients who are only infrequently symptomatic: insertion of a tampon or diaphragm for temporary relief when prolonged standing is anticipated

---

BOX 1-9 Staging of Pelvic Organ Prolapse Based on POP-Q Examination

Stage 0	No prolapse.
Stage I	Most distal prolapse more than 1 cm above hymenal ring.
Stage II	Most distal point is 1 cm or less above hymenal ring.
Stage III	Most distal point is more than 1 cm below the hymenal ring but not further than 2 cm less the total vaginal length, i.e., > +1 cm but < + (TVL-2) cm.
Stage IV	Complete vaginal eversion.

From Pemberton J (ed): The pelvic floor, Philadelphia, 2002, WB Saunders.

BOX 1-10 Points of Reference for POP-Q

Point A Three cm above the hymen on anterior vaginal wall (Aa) or posterior vaginal wall (Ap). Point Aa roughly corresponds with the urethrovesical junction. These points can range from −3 cm (no prolapse) to +3 cm (maximal prolapse.)
Point B The lowest extent of the segment of vagina between point A and the apex of the vagina. Unlike point A they are not fixed but will be the same as A if point A is the most protruding point. In maximal prolapse it will be the same as point C.
Point C The most distal part of the cervix or vaginal vault.
Point D The posterior fornix, which is thus omitted in women with prior hysterectomy.
Genital hiatus From midline external urethral meatus to inferior hymenal ring.
Perineal body From inferior hymenal ring to middle of anal orifice.
Vaginal length This should be measured without undue stretching of the vagina.

From Pemberton J (ed): The pelvic floor, Philadelphia, 2002, WB Saunders.

CHRONIC Rx

- Hormone replacement therapy at the time of menopause helps preserve tissue strength, maintain elasticity of the vagina, and promote the durability of surgical repairs; however, the routine use of HRT is no longer recommended.
- Gold standard for therapy is vaginal hysterectomy.
- Vaginal apex should be well suspended, but a prophylactic sacrospinous ligament fixation is not routinely required.
- If occult enterocele present, McCall culdoplasty is performed.
- If vaginal approach to hysterectomy is contraindicated, abdominal hysterectomy is performed; vaginal apex likewise well supported.

- Colpocleisis is considered for the elderly patient who is sexually inactive and is a high-risk patient from a surgical point of view; can be done rapidly under local anesthesia with mild sedation if necessary.
- Other surgical options are sling operations and sacral cervicopexy.

DISPOSITION

If untreated, uterine prolapse progressively worsens.

REFERRAL

To a gynecologist/urologist if pessary fitting or surgical intervention is needed

PEARLS & CONSIDERATIONS

COMMENTS

Surgery contraindicated in mild or asymptomatic uterine prolapse because the patient will seldom benefit from the operation although exposed to its risks.

SUGGESTED READINGS

Glass RH, Curtis MG, Hopkins MP: *Glass' Office Gynecology,* ed 5, Baltimore, 1999, Lippincott Williams & Wilkins.

Thaker R: Management of uterine prolapse, *BMJ* 324:1258, 2002.

AUTHOR: **ARUNDATHI G. PRASAD, M.D.**

BASIC INFORMATION

DEFINITION

- Vision loss in the elderly incorporates the spectrum from near-normal vision to mild deficits to low vision, profound visual loss, and blindness.
- Moderate and severe vision loss can have a profound impact on the ability to perform instrumental activities of daily living such as reading, driving, check-writing, and taking medications.
- Vision loss can result in an inability to live independently and to socialize.
- Vision loss increases the risk of depression, functional impairment, and mortality.

SYNONYMS

Low vision
Blindness

ICD-9CM CODES
368.11 Sudden visual loss
368.12 Transient visual loss
369.00 Visual impairment level not further specified
369.3 Unqualified visual loss, both eyes

EPIDEMIOLOGY & DEMOGRAPHICS

- 22 million blind people worldwide are over 60 years old.
- 17% of Americans 65 to 74 years and 26% of Americans 75 years and older report vision impairment.
- 1 in 3 Americans over 75 years has signs of macular degeneration, which is the most common cause of blindness in the U.S.
- Glaucoma and cataracts are the most common causes of blindness among African Americans.
- 46% of people 75 to 85 years old have cataracts, with a higher prevalence in females.
- Patients with visual impairment have an average hospital length of stay 2.4 days longer than those without impairment.

NORMAL & ABNORMAL CHANGES IN VISION WITH AGING

Eyelids
- Thinning, dehydration, dermatochalasis (redundant skin), ectropion (eversion of the lower lid), entropion (inversion of the lid, causing corneal irritation from the lower lashes)
- Site of neoplasms, such basal cell carcinoma and squamous cell carcinoma

Tears
- Decreased production and thinning of the tear film
- Affected by rheumatoid arthritis and Sjögren's

Cornea
- Yellows with age, loses transparency, becomes more astigmatic
- Fuch's dystrophy is an autosomal dominant disease found after the fifth decade causing severe pain and loss in corneal transparency
- Affected by infections, dry eyes, and neoplasms

Pupil
- Aperture decreases by 2.5 mm between age 20 and 80, resulting in less ambient light reaching the photosensitive layer

Lens
- Yellowing of the lens with reduced amount of light reaching the retina
- Loss of accommodative amplitude (presbyopia) begins around age 40, with impairment in the fifth to sixth decades
- Cataracts

Vitreous
- Transparent but may contract, liquefy, or detach
- Vitreous hemorrhage is a complication of diabetic retinopathy that causes clouded vision

Retina
- Affected by pathologic changes in macular degeneration, diabetic retinopathy, retinal detachment, artery and vein occlusions, or hemorrhage

PHYSICAL FINDINGS & CLINICAL PRESENTATION

See Table 1-18.

ETIOLOGY

See Table 1-18.

DIAGNOSIS **Dx**

DIFFERENTIAL DIAGNOSIS

Logical approach to loss of vision: generally helpful to categorize vision loss as sudden vs. gradual, unilateral vs. bilateral, and painless vs. painful.

Sudden—Unilateral—Painless loss of vision
- Vitreous hemorrhage—may resolve spontaneously, but in people with DM, may need emergency photocoagulation
- Retinal detachment—requires urgent surgical repair
- Age-related macular degeneration/choroidal neovascular membrane—urgent angiography to detect lesions amenable to repair
- Retinal vein occlusion—urgent retinal photocoagulation
- Amaurosis fugax and central retinal artery occlusion—urgent neurovascular workup
- Anterior ischemic optic neuropathy—also requires urgent neurovascular workup, but may have nonarteritic causes

Sudden—Unilateral—Painful loss of vision
- Associated with red eye
  - Corneal ulcers and infections—emergency ophthalmologic referral for cultures and intensive antibiotic treatment
  - Corneal abrasions
  - Acute angle-closure glaucoma—emergency laser iridectomy to relieve blockage
- Associated with photophobia
  - Uveitis—may be idiopathic, but associated with sarcoid, collagen vascular disease, syphilis, and TB; refer to ophthalmology for slit lamp exam and topical steroids
- Traumatic hyphema—refer to ophthalmology and minimize intraocular pressure and risk of recurrent bleeding
- Pain and tenderness over scalp, elevated ESR—temporal arteritis
  - Requires urgent treatment with systemic corticosteroids
- Pain on eye movement—optic neuritis
  - Associated with multiple sclerosis
  - May respond to systemic corticosteroids
- Orbital cellulitis
  - Emergency referral to ophthalmologist and otorhinolaryngologist
  - Cultures, CT scanning, IV antibiotics

Sudden—Bilateral—Painless loss of vision
- Uncontrolled diabetes
- Medications, especially anticholinergics and corticosteroids

Sudden—Bilateral—Painful loss of vision
- Trauma, foreign bodies, chemical spills, exposure to UV radiation
- Corneal infections, iritis, acute glaucoma—all rarely bilateral
- Temporal arteritis

Gradual—Unilateral—Painless loss of vision
- Cataracts—require routine, nonurgent ophthalmologic follow-up
- Age-related macular degeneration—routine ophthalmologic follow-up
- Lesions in the orbit or intracranial space—visual field defects and optic atrophy with lesions compressing the optic nerve

Gradual—Unilateral—Painful loss of vision
- Inflammatory or neoplastic process of the cornea or retrobulbar space, including orbital granulomas and optic neuromas—require ophthalmologic referral and CT or MRI

Gradual—Bilateral—Painless loss of vision
- Cataracts develop with age
- Age-related macular degeneration
- Drug toxicity, such as hydroxychloroquine or ethambutol
- Compressive lesions at the optic chiasm

TABLE 1-18   Causes of Vision Loss

Disease	Symptoms	Exam Findings and Diagnostic Tests	Treatment
Amaurosis fugax	• Rapid unilateral vision loss • Curtain descending over vision • Sudden loss of a portion of visual field	• Ophthalmoscopy: retinal edema (appears whitened); milky retina with a cherry red fovea • Evaluate for ischemic disease, including neuroimaging, carotid Doppler ultrasonography, or echocardiogram • May need to evaluate for hypercoagulable state	• Treat hypertensive crisis • Treat ischemic disease • Treat hypercoagulable state
Anterior ischemic optic neuropathy (AION)	• Sudden unilateral vision loss • May become progressive	• Ophthalmoscopy: optic disc swollen; nerve fiber layer splinter hemorrhages • Check ESR and CRP (association with temporal arteritis)	• High-dose glucocorticoids • May need temporal artery biopsy
Retinal detachment	• Floaters • Flashing lights • Peripheral scotoma • Afferent pupil defect and decreased acuity if fovea involved	• Ophthalmoscopy: elevated, folded retinal tissue • Decreased visual acuity	• Laser surgery
Retinal vein occlusion	• Similar to amaurosis fugax, but more prolonged	• Ophthalmoscopy: engorged, phlebitic veins; retinal hemorrhages • May need to evaluate for hypercoagulable state	• Treat underlying hypertension and diabetes • Treat hypercoagulable state • Aspirin
Toxic optic neuropathy	• Acute bilateral vision loss • Central scotoma	• Optic disc swelling • History of drug exposure: carbon monoxide, ethylene glycol, methanol, amiodarone, ciprofloxacin, digitalis, thallium, isoniazid, and others • Ophthalmoscopy	• Discontinue offending agent
Age-related macular degeneration	• Blurring of central vision (peripheral intact) • Central scotoma • Glare sensitivity • Decreased color perception • Hallucinations	• Ophthalmoscopy: drusen; degeneration of the retinal pigmented epithelium • Fluorescein angiography showing choroidal neovascular lesions	• Vitamin and mineral supplements may reduce risk • Laser photocoagulation • Photodynamic therapy
Glaucoma	• Early = asymptomatic • Headache or blurred vision after exercise • Haloes or cloudy vision in low illumination • Blurred vision • Loss of peripheral vision or tunnel vision	• Ophthalmoscopy: optic nerve cupping (increased cup to disk ratio); nasalization of retinal vessels • Loss of visual fields • Visual field testing showing loss of fields • Tonometry showing increased intraocular pressure	• Eyedrops, including beta blockers, cholinergic agonists, prostaglandin analogs, carbonic anhydrase inhibitors • Surgery, including iridotomy or filtration surgery
Presbyopia	• Loss of ability to focus on close objects	• Visual acuity testing showing loss of accommodative amplitude	• Prescriptive lenses • Bifocal contact lenses • Corrective corneal surgery • Lens implantation
Cataract	• Blurred vision • Light sensitivity • Small local opacity • Double vision • Worsening myopia • Reduced contrast sensitivity	• Reduced visual acuity • Loss of red reflex • Focal or diffuse opacity of lens	• Absorptive lenses that filter glare • Lens prescription adjustment • Intraocular lens implantation surgery
Diabetic retinopathy	• May be asymptomatic, especially nonproliferative type • Floaters • Blurred vision • Decreased color perception • Decreased night vision • Symptoms worse in the morning	• Ophthalmoscopy: retinal changes, including hemorrhages and exudates; macular edema; vitreous hemorrhage; vascular changes including looping	• Control blood sugar • Treat hypertension and hypercholesterolemia • Focal laser photocoagulation • Scatter laser photocoagulation • Vitrectomy

Gradual—Bilateral—Painful loss of vision
- Chronic inflammatory process, associated with collagen vascular disease or sarcoidosis

TREATMENT

WORKUP, LABORATORY TESTS, IMAGING STUDIES

See Table 1-18.

NONPHARMACOLOGIC THERAPY

See individual topics for condition-specific treatment.
- Vision rehabilitation
  - Useful for patients with macular degeneration, cataracts, glaucoma, diabetic retinopathy, or visual field loss.
  - Patients with low visual acuity (<20/50), central or peripheral vision loss, reduced contrast sensitivity, glare, and light/dark adaptation difficulties may benefit.
  - Assessment of need for low-vision devices, reading ability, impairment in activities of daily living, ability to travel.
- Low-vision devices
  - Magnifiers and telescopic systems for macular degeneration and visual field losses
  - Absorptive and tinted lenses for glare
  - Visual field expansion devices, including mirrors and prisms
  - Illumination control for light/dark adaptation
  - Use of increased bright color or color contrast

REFERRAL

See individual topics for condition-specific referral.
- Ophthalmologist—emergent visit with acute symptoms
- Otolaryngologist—for neoplastic or infectious concerns

- Low-vision evaluation
  - For patients with vision not corrected by glasses, lenses, medical treatments, or surgery
  - Specialized tests of function, including contrast sensitivity, Amsler grid (for macular degeneration), visual field testing, color vision testing, and photostress tests
- Lighthouse for the Blind: local chapters providing support, services, products, referrals, and rehabilitation services for visually impaired persons
- Local Department on Aging chapters: information about senior centers that provide services and rehabilitation for vision loss

PEARLS & CONSIDERATIONS

Don't forget the impact of vision loss on the elderly, including increased depression, loss of functional status, and increased mortality.

PREVENTION

- Antioxidants for macular degeneration
  - Lutein alone or with antioxidants was helpful in the Veterans' Lutein Antioxidant Supplement Trial.
  - The Age-Related Eye Diseases Study showed benefit of antioxidants in patients with advanced macular degeneration, but other studies have not shown benefit of antioxidants for primary prevention.
- Diabetic retinopathy
  - Better glycemic control: Most of the preventive benefit is achieved by reducing a high HbA1c to 9%, and little is achieved by reducing from 9% to 7%.
  - Control hypertension
  - Control hyperlipidemia
- Smoking cessation to reduce the risk of macular degeneration, cataracts, and diabetic retinopathy
- Avoid ultraviolet light damage

PATIENT/FAMILY EDUCATION

- General vision and information and referral for vision disorders: http://www.visionchannel.net
- Lighthouse for the Blind: http://www.lighthouse.org
- American Council for the Blind: http://www.acb.org
- Macular degeneration: www.mdsupport.org
- Glaucoma Service Foundation To Prevent Blindness: http://www.wills-glaucoma.org/index.htm

CROSS REFERENCES

Please refer to the following topics for more information about specific diseases causing vision loss:
Cataracts
Glaucoma, Chronic Open-Angle
Glaucoma, Primary Closed-Angle
Macular Degeneration
Red Eye, Acute (algorithm)

SUGGESTED READINGS

Harvey PT: Common eye diseases of elderly people: identifying and treating causes of vision loss, *Gerontology* 49:1-11, 2003.
Quillen DA: Common causes of vision loss in elderly patients, *Amer Fam Phys* 60:99-108, 1999.
Reuben DB et al: The prognostic value of sensory impairment in older persons, *J Am Geriatr Soc* 47:930-935, 1999.
Rosenthal BP: Screening and treatment of age-related and pathologic vision changes, *Geriatrics* 58:27-31, 2001.
Shingleton BJ, O'Donoghue MW: Blurred vision, *N Engl J Med* 343:556-562, 2000.

AUTHORS: **HOLLY M. HOLMES, M.D.,** and **JOSEPH W. SHEGA, M.D.**

BASIC INFORMATION

DEFINITION

Vulvar cancer is an abnormal cell proliferation arising on the vulva and exhibiting malignant potential. The majority are of squamous cell origin; however, other types include adenocarcinoma, basal cell carcinoma, sarcoma, and melanoma (Fig. 1-52).

SYNONYMS

Squamous cell carcinoma of the vulva (90%)
Basal cell carcinoma of the vulva
Adenocarcinoma of the vulva
Melanoma of the vulva
Bartholin gland carcinoma
Verrucous carcinoma of the vulva
Vulvar sarcoma

ICD-9CM CODES
184.4 Vulvar neoplasm

EPIDEMIOLOGY & DEMOGRAPHICS

PREVALENCE: Vulvar cancer is uncommon. It comprises 4% of malignancies of the female genital tract. It is the fourth most common gynecologic malignancy.
INCIDENCE: 1.8 cases/100,000 persons

MEAN AGE AT DIAGNOSIS: Predominantly a disease of menopause. Mean age at diagnosis is 65 yr.

PHYSICAL FINDINGS & CLINICAL PRESENTATION

- Vulvar pruritus or pain is present.
- May produce a malodor or discharge or present as bleeding.
- Raised lesion, may have fleshy, ulcerated, leukoplakic, or warty appearance; may have multifocal lesions.
- Lesions are usually located on labia majora, but may be seen on labia minora, clitoris, and perineum.
- The lymph nodes of groin may be palpable.

ETIOLOGY

- The exact etiology is unknown.
- Vulvar intraepithelial neoplasia has been reported in 20%-30% of invasive squamous cell carcinoma of the vulva, but the malignant potential is unknown.
- Human papillomavirus is found in 30%-50% of vulvar carcinoma, but its exact role is unclear.
- Chronic pruritus, wetness, industrial wastes, arsenicals, hygienic agents, and vulvar dystrophies have been implicated as causative agents.

DIAGNOSIS

DIFFERENTIAL DIAGNOSIS

- Lymphogranuloma inguinale
- Tuberculosis
- Vulvar dystrophies
- Vulvar atrophy
- Paget's disease

WORKUP

- Diagnosis is made histologically by biopsy
- Thorough examination of the lesion and assessment of spread
- Possible colposcopy of adjacent areas
- Cytologic smear of vagina and cervix
- Cystoscopy and proctosigmoidoscopy may be necessary

IMAGING STUDIES

- Chest radiography
- CT scan and MRI for assessing local tumor spread

TREATMENT

NONPHARMACOLOGIC THERAPY

- Treatment is individualized depending on the stage of the tumor.
- Stage I tumors with <1 mm stromal invasion are treated with complete local excision without groin node dissection.
- Stage I tumors with >1 mm stromal invasion are treated with complete local excision with groin node dissection.
- Stage II tumors require radical vulvectomy with bilateral groin node dissection.
- Advanced-stage disease may require the addition of radiation and chemotherapy to the surgical regimen.
- Section III describes a treatment algorithm for management of vulvar cancer.

DISPOSITION

Five-year survival ranges from 90% for stage I to 15% for stage IV.

REFERRAL

Vulvar cancer should be managed by a gynecologic oncologist and radiation oncologist.

SUGGESTED READINGS

Canavan TP, Cohen D: Vulvar cancer, *Am Fam Physician* 66(7):1269, 2002.
Coleman RL, Santoso JT: Vulvar carcinoma, *Curr Treat Opt Oncol* 1(2):177, 2000.
Grandys EC Jr, Aroris JV: Innovations in the management of vulvar carcinoma, *Curr Opin Obstet Gynecol* 12(1):15, 2000.

AUTHOR: **GIL FARKASH, M.D.**

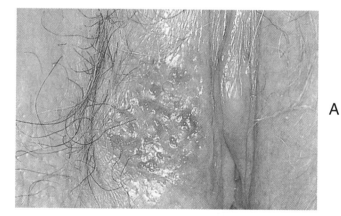
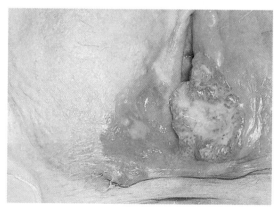

FIGURE 1-52   A, Basal cell carcinoma of the vulva. **B,** Ulcerative squamous cell carcinoma of the vulva. (From Symonds EM, Macpherson MBA: *Color atlas of obstetrics and gynecology,* St Louis, 1994, Mosby.)

BASIC INFORMATION

DEFINITION

Estrogen-deficient vulvovaginitis is the irritation and/or inflammation of the vulva and vagina because of progressive thinning and atrophic changes secondary to estrogen deficiency (Fig. 1-53).

SYNONYMS

Atrophic vaginitis

ICD-9CM CODES
616.10 Vulvovaginitis

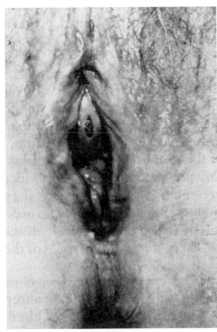

FIGURE 1-53 Advanced postmenopausal atrophy of the vulva in a 72-year-old woman. (From Symonds EM, Macpherson MBA: *Color atlas of obstetrics and gynecology,* St Louis, 1994, Mosby.)

EPIDEMIOLOGY & DEMOGRAPHICS

- Seen most often in postmenopausal women

PHYSICAL FINDINGS & CLINICAL PRESENTATION

- Thinning of pubic hair, labia minora and majora
- Decreased secretions from the vestibular glands, with vaginal dryness
- Regression of subcutaneous fat
- Vulvar and vaginal itching
- Dyspareunia
- Dysuria and urinary frequency
- Vaginal spotting

ETIOLOGY

Estrogen deficiency

DIAGNOSIS **Dx**

DIFFERENTIAL DIAGNOSIS

- Infectious vulvovaginitis
- Squamous cell hyperplasia
- Lichen sclerosus
- Vulva malignancy
- Vaginal malignancy
- Cervical and endometrial malignancy

WORKUP

- Pelvic examination
- Speculum examination
- Pap smear
- Possible endometrial biopsy if bleeding

TREATMENT **Rx**

ACUTE GENERAL Rx

- Premarin 0.625 mg PO qd
- Estraderm patch 0.05 mg × 2 per week

- If uterus present:
  1. Estrogen + 2.5 mg PO Provera qd *or*
  2. Estrogen + 10 mg PO Provera × 10 days each mo
- Systemic use of HRT or ERT is controversial at this time.
- Conjugated estrogen vaginal cream intravaginally. Estradiol vaginal cream 0.01%
  2 to 4 g/day × 2 wk then
  1 to 2 g/day × 2 wk then
  1 to 2 g × 3 days/wk
- Vagifen (estradial vaginal tablets) 25 mg inserted intravaginally daily for 2 wk then twice weekly. May take up to 12 wk to feel the full benefits of the medication.
- Conjugated estrogen vaginal cream: 2-4 g qd (3 wk on, 1 wk off) for 3-5 mo.

CHRONIC Rx

See "Acute General Rx." May discontinue vaginal estrogen cream once symptoms alleviate.

DISPOSITION

The symptoms should be improved with the therapy. Caution for vaginal bleeding if uterus present

REFERRAL

To obstetrician/gynecologist if vaginal bleeding

SUGGESTED READING

Bornstein J et al: The classic approach to diagnosis of vulvovaginitis: a critical analysis, *Infect Dis Obstet Gynecol* 9(2):105, 2001.

AUTHOR: **JULIE ANNE SZUMIGALA, M.D.**

BASIC INFORMATION

DEFINITION

Pressure ulcers: localized areas of tissue necrosis that develop when soft tissue is compressed between a bony prominence and an external surface for a prolonged period.

Arterial ulcers: areas of arteriosclerosis that lead to insufficient oxygenation of the skin and underlying tissues.

Diabetic ulcers: a chronic ulcer in a diabetic patient due to extrinsic factors (e.g., trauma, injury) or intrinsic factors (e.g., neuropathy, microvascular disease).

Venous ulcers: a discontinuity of the epidermis occurring as a result of venous hypertension and venous insufficiency.

SYNONYMS

Decubitus ulcers
Bedsores
Pressure sores
Dermal ulcers

ICD-9CM CODES
707.0 Decubitus ulcers
440.23 Arterial peripheral vascular
disease with ulceration
459.81 Venous insufficiency
707.10-707.9 codes specify ulcer sites

EPIDEMIOLOGY & DEMOGRAPHICS

- The incidence of pressure ulcers in acute care facilities has ranged from 2.7% to 29.5%. Prevalence has varied from 3.5% to 29.5%. High-risk populations include quadriplegic patients (60% prevalence), elderly patients admitted for femoral fracture (66% incidence), and critical care patients (33% incidence).
- Risk factors for pressure ulcers:
  - Altered sensation or response to discomfort
  - Altered mobility
  - Significant changes in weight
  - Bowel or bladder incontinence
- Risk factors for arterial ulcers:
  - Arterial insufficiency
  - Tobacco abuse
- Risk factors for diabetic ulcers:
  - Diabetic neuropathy
  - Structural foot deformity
  - Peripheral arterial occlusive disease
- Risk factors for venous ulcers:
  - Venous insufficiency
  - History of leg injury, obesity, phlebitis, varicose vein surgery
  - History of prolonged sitting or standing

PHYSICAL FINDINGS & CLINICAL PRESENTATION

Pressure ulcers usually occur over bony prominences and are graded or staged to classify the degree of tissue damage observed.

Stage I: nonblanchable erythema of intact skin

Stage II: partial-thickness skin loss involving the epidermis, dermis, or both

Stage III: full-thickness skin loss involving damage or necrosis of subcutaneous tissue that may extend down to, but not through, underlying fascia or muscle

Stage IV: full-thickness skin loss with extensive destruction and tissue damage to muscle, bone, or supporting structures

ETIOLOGY

- Prolonged unrelieved pressure often associated with impaired or restricted mobility
- Friction or shearing forces on skin
- See Definition
- See Risk Factors

DIAGNOSIS

DIFFERENTIAL DIAGNOSIS

Diabetic ulcers (DU)
Venous stasis ulcers (VU)
Arterial ulcers (AU)
See Table 1-19.

WORKUP

Many pressure ulcers are preventable, with a comprehensive risk assessment in place.

Risk assessment:

- Consider all bed- or chair-bound persons, or those whose ability to reposition is impaired, to be at risk for pressure ulcers.
- Select and use a method of risk assessment, such as the Norton Scale or Braden Scale, that ensures systematic evaluation of individual risk factors.

- Assess all at-risk patients at the time of admission to health care facilities and at regular intervals thereafter.
- Identify all individual risk factors (decreased mental status, moisture, incontinence, nutritional deficits) to direct specific preventive treatments. Modify care according to the individual factors.
- All ulcers should have a description of the ulcer (i.e., stage, location, size); the wound bed (i.e., epithelialization, granulation tissue, necrotic tissue, eschar); the presence of any exudates, which includes type and amount; the wound edges (i.e., undermining, sinus tracts, tunneling, fistulas); signs of infection; and pain.

LABORATORY TESTS

- CBC with differential
- Sed rate
- Albumin

IMAGING STUDIES

X-ray

TREATMENT

NONPHARMACOLOGIC THERAPY

Special mattresses/beds (e.g., low air loss mattress) may help reduce skin pressure. They can be used preventively or as part of a treatment program.

CHRONIC Rx

Pressure ulcers:

- Managing tissue loads. Reduce skin pressure through repositioning and pressure-reducing devices. Positioning devices should be used to raise the ulcer off the support surface. Prevent shear injury by maintaining the head of the bed at the lowest level of elevation and for the shortest period that is consistent with medical conditions and other restrictions.

TABLE 1-19 **Differential Diagnosis of Ulcers**

	Location	Cause	Appearance
PU—pressure ulcers	Bony prominences	Pressure	Crater
DU—diabetic ulcers	Pressure points (callus)	Repetitive trauma; neuropathy	Well-marked borders
VU—venous statis ulcers	Gaiter area	Venous stasis	Irregular
AU—arterial ulcers	Distal points	Vascular insufficiency	Gangrene

From Thomas D: Wound care: prevention, management, and nursing care, American Medical Director's Association Annual Symposium, Phoenix, Arizona, 2004. Copyright 2004.

- Ulcer care. Any necrotic tissue observed during initial or subsequent assessments should be debrided. The clinician should select the debridement method (sharp, mechanical, enzymatic, or autolytic) most appropriate to the patient's condition and goals. Ulcer wounds should be cleansed (preferably with normal saline) at each dressing change, using a minimum amount of mechanical force. Select a dressing that will keep the ulcer bed continuously moist while allowing the surrounding intact skin to remain dry. Consider whirlpool therapy for cleansing pressure ulcers that contain thick exudates, slough, or necrotic tissue.
- Managing bacterial colonization and infection. All Stage II, III, and IV pressure ulcers are colonized with bacteria. Effective cleansing and debridement will minimize colonization. More frequent cleansing and debridement may be needed if purulence or a foul odor develops. A topical antibiotic should be considered if a clean ulcer continues to have exudates despite optimal care for 2 to 4 weeks. Topical antiseptics should not be used. Swab cultures have no diagnostic value; however, if the ulcer does not respond to topical antibiotic therapy, quantitative bacterial cultures, preferably by means of tissue biopsy, should be obtained to evaluate for osteomyelitis. Systemic antibiotics should be given to patients with bacteremia, sepsis, advancing cellulitis, or osteomyelitis.
- Operative repair. Operative procedures should be considered for clean Stage III or IV ulcers that do not respond to optimal care and include direct closure, skin grafting, skin flaps, musculocutaneous flaps, and free flaps. Quality of life, patient preferences, treatment goals, risk of recurrence, and anticipated rehabilitative outcomes should be considered.
- Education and quality improvement. Institutions and health care agencies are responsible for developing and implementing pressure ulcer prevention and treatment programs for patients, families, and caregivers. In addition, a quality improvement program should be established.

Arterial ulcers:
- Restore adequate vascular supply whenever possible.
- Consider aspirin 325 mg qd, cilostazol (Pletal) 100 mg bid, or pentoxifylline (Trental) 400 mg tid.
- Manage underlying medical issues, e.g., hypertension, diabetes.
- Maintain moderate level of exercise.
- Smoking cessation.
- Avoid caffeine, cold temperatures, and constrictive garments.
- Keep wounds clean.
- Use nonocclusive moist wound dressings.
- Manage local infection.
- Treatment failure may lead to amputation.

Diabetic ulcers:
- Offload mechanical stress.
- Sharp wound debridement.
- Revascularization.
- Moist wound dressing.
- Manage local infection.
- Treatment failure may lead to amputation.

Venous ulcers:
- Use a compression bandage system.
- Manage local infection.
- Moist wound dressing.
- Use bioengineered skin appropriately.

COMPLEMENTARY & ALTERNATIVE MEDICINE

- Nutritional and vitamin supplementation have a strength of evidence C, per ACHPR.
- Encourage dietary intake and supplementation if an individual with a pressure ulcer is malnourished.
- A daily high-potency vitamin/mineral is recommended for all patients suspected of having deficiencies.

DISPOSITION

When systematic risk assessments are done and preventive measures are followed, many pressure ulcers can be prevented. Most ulcers heal when appropriate management strategies are followed.

REFERRAL

Surgical referral when clean Stage III or IV pressure ulcers do not respond to optimal patient care.

SUGGESTED READINGS

National Pressure Ulcer Advisory Panel: Statement on pressure ulcer prevention: http://www.npuap.org/positn1.html

Thomas D: Wound care: prevention, management, and nursing care, American Medical Director's Association Annual Symposium, Phoenix, Arizona, 2004.

Treatment of pressure ulcers, Clinical Practice Guidelines Number 15, AHCPR Publication No. 95-0652, Rockville, Md, 1994, US Department of Health and Human Services, Public Health Service, Agency for Health Care Policy and Research.

AUTHOR: **LAURA TRICE, M.D.**

Differential Diagnosis

ABDOMINAL DISTENTION
ICD-9CM # 787.3

NONMECHANICAL OBSTRUCTION

Excessive intraluminal gas.
Intraabdominal infection.
Trauma.
Retroperitoneal irritation (renal colic, neoplasms, infections, hemorrhage).
Vascular insufficiency (thrombosis, embolism).
Mechanical ventilation.
Extraabdominal infection (sepsis, pneumonia, empyema, osteomyelitis of spine).
Metabolic/toxic abnormalities (hypokalemia, uremia, lead poisoning).
Chemical irritation (perforated ulcer, bile, pancreatitis).
Peritoneal inflammation.
Severe pain, pain medications.

MECHANICAL OBSTRUCTION

Neoplasm (intraluminal, extraluminal).
Adhesions, endometriosis.
Infection (intraabdominal abscess, diverticulitis).
Gallstones.
Foreign body, bezoars.
Hernias.
Volvulus.
Stenosis at surgical anastomosis, radiation stenosis.
Fecaliths.
Inflammatory bowel disease.
Gastric outlet obstruction.
Hematoma.
Other: parasites, superior mesenteric artery (SMA) syndrome, pneumatosis intestinalis, annular pancreas, Hirschsprung's disease, intussusception, meconium.

ABDOMINAL PAIN, DIFFUSE
ICD-9CM # 789.67

Early appendicitis.
Aortic aneurysm.
Gastroenteritis.
Intestinal obstruction.
Diverticulitis.
Peritonitis.
Mesenteric insufficiency or infarction.
Pancreatitis.
Inflammatory bowel disease.
Irritable bowel.
Mesenteric adenitis.
Metabolic: toxins, lead poisoning, uremia, drug overdose, diabetic ketoacidosis (DKA), heavy metal poisoning.
Sickle cell crisis.
Pneumonia (rare).
Trauma.
Urinary tract infection.
Other: acute intermittent porphyria, tabes dorsalis, periarteritis nodosa, Henoch-Schönlein purpura, adrenal insufficiency.

ABDOMINAL PAIN, EPIGASTRIC
ICD-9CM # 789.66

Gastric: peptic ulcer disease (PUD), gastric outlet obstruction, gastric ulcer.
Duodenal: PUD, duodenitis.
Biliary: cholecystitis, cholangitis.

Hepatic: hepatitis.
Pancreatic: pancreatitis.
Intestinal: high small bowel obstruction, early appendicitis.
Cardiac: angina, MI, pericarditis.
Pulmonary: pneumonia, pleurisy, pneumothorax.
Subphrenic abscess.
Vascular: dissecting aneurysm, mesenteric ischemia.

ABDOMINAL PAIN, LEFT LOWER QUADRANT
ICD-9CM # 789.64

Intestinal: diverticulitis, intestinal obstruction, perforated ulcer, inflammatory bowel disease, perforated descending colon, inguinal hernia, neoplasm, appendicitis.
Reproductive: ovarian cyst, torsion of ovarian cyst, tuboovarian abscess.
Renal: renal or ureteral calculi, pyelonephritis, neoplasm.
Vascular: leaking aortic aneurysm.
Psoas abscess.
Trauma.

ABDOMINAL PAIN, LEFT UPPER QUADRANT
ICD-9CM # 789.32

Gastric: PUD, gastritis, pyloric stenosis, hiatal hernia.
Pancreatic: pancreatitis, neoplasm, stone in pancreatic duct or ampulla.
Cardiac: MI, angina pectoris.
Splenic: splenomegaly, ruptured spleen, splenic abscess, splenic infarction.
Renal: calculi, pyelonephritis, neoplasm.
Pulmonary: pneumonia, empyema, pulmonary infarction.
Vascular: ruptured aortic aneurysm.
Cutaneous: herpes zoster.
Trauma.
Intestinal: high fecal impaction, perforated colon, diverticulitis.

ABDOMINAL PAIN, PERIUMBILICAL
ICD-9CM # 789.65

Intestinal: small bowel obstruction or gangrene, early appendicitis.
Vascular: mesenteric thrombosis, dissecting aortic aneurysm.
Pancreatic: pancreatitis.
Metabolic: uremia, DKA.
Trauma.

ABDOMINAL PAIN, RIGHT LOWER QUADRANT
ICD-9CM # 789.63

Intestinal: acute appendicitis, regional enteritis, incarcerated hernia, cecal diverticulitis, intestinal obstruction, perforated ulcer, perforated cecum, Meckel's diverticulitis.
Reproductive: ovarian cyst, torsion of ovarian cyst.
Renal: renal and ureteral calculi, neoplasms, pyelonephritis.
Vascular: leaking aortic aneurysm.
Psoas abscess.
Trauma.
Cholecystitis.

ABDOMINAL PAIN, RIGHT UPPER QUADRANT
ICD-9CM # 789.61

Biliary: calculi, infection, inflammation, neoplasm.
Hepatic: hepatitis, abscess, hepatic congestion, neoplasm, trauma.

Gastric: PUD, pyloric stenosis, neoplasm, alcoholic gastritis, hiatal hernia.

Pancreatic: pancreatitis, neoplasm, stone in pancreatic duct or ampulla.

Renal: calculi, infection, inflammation, neoplasm, rupture of kidney.

Pulmonary: pneumonia, pulmonary infarction, right-sided pleurisy.

Intestinal: retrocecal appendicitis, intestinal obstruction, high fecal impaction, diverticulitis.

Cardiac: myocardial ischemia (particularly involving the inferior wall), pericarditis.

Cutaneous: herpes zoster.

Trauma.

Fitz-Hugh-Curtis syndrome (perihepatitis).

ABDOMINAL PAIN, SUPRAPUBIC

ICD-9CM # 789.85

Intestinal: colon obstruction or gangrene, diverticulitis, appendicitis.

Reproductive system: torsion of ovarian cyst.

Cystitis, rupture of urinary bladder.

ACHES AND PAINS, DIFFUSE[13]

ICD-9CM # 719.49

Postviral arthralgias/myalgias.

Bilateral soft tissue rheumatism.

Overuse syndromes.

Fibrositis.

Hypothyroidism.

Metabolic bone disease.

Paraneoplastic syndrome.

Myopathy (polymyositis, dermatomyositis).

RA.

Sjögren's syndrome.

Polymyalgia rheumatica.

Hypermobility.

Benign arthralgias/myalgias.

Chronic fatigue syndrome.

Hypophosphatemia.

ACIDOSIS, METABOLIC

ICD-9CM # 276.2

METABOLIC ACIDOSIS WITH INCREASED AG (AG ACIDOSIS)

Lactic acidosis.

Ketoacidosis (diabetes mellitus, alcoholic ketoacidosis).

Uremia (chronic renal failure).

Ingestion of toxins (paraldehyde, methanol, salicylate, ethylene glycol).

High-fat diet (mild acidosis).

METABOLIC ACIDOSIS WITH NORMAL AG (HYPERCHLOREMIC ACIDOSIS)

Renal tubular acidosis (including acidosis of aldosterone deficiency).

Intestinal loss of HCO_3^- (diarrhea, pancreatic fistula).

Carbonic anhydrase inhibitors (e.g., acetazolamide).

Dilutional acidosis (as a result of rapid infusion of bicarbonate-free isotonic saline).

Ingestion of exogenous acids (ammonium chloride, methionine, cystine, calcium chloride).

Ileostomy.

Ureterosigmoidostomy.

Drugs: amiloride, triamterene, spironolactone, β-blockers.

ACIDOSIS RESPIRATORY

ICD-9CM # 276.2

Pulmonary disease (COPD, severe pneumonia, pulmonary edema, interstitial fibrosis).

Airway obstruction (foreign body, severe bronchospasm, laryngospasm).

Thoracic cage disorders (pneumothorax, flail chest, kyphoscoliosis).

Defects in muscles of respiration (myasthenia gravis, hypokalemia, muscular dystrophy).

Defects in peripheral nervous system (amyotrophic lateral sclerosis, poliomyelitis, Guillain-Barré syndrome, botulism, tetanus, organophosphate poisoning, spinal cord injury).

Depression of respiratory center (anesthesia, narcotics, sedatives, vertebral artery embolism or thrombosis, increased intracranial pressure).

Failure of mechanical ventilator.

ACUTE SCROTUM

ICD-9CM # 608.9

Testicular torsion.

Epididymitis.

Testicular neoplasm.

Orchitis.

ADNEXAL MASS[14]

ICD-9CM # VARIES WITH SPECIFIC DISORDER

Ovary (neoplasm, endometriosis, functional cyst).

Fallopian tube (neoplasm, tuboovarian abscess, hydrosalpinx, paratubal cyst).

Uterus (fibroid, neoplasm).

Retroperitoneum (neoplasm, abdominal wall hematoma or abscess).

Urinary tract (pelvic kidney, distended bladder, urachal cyst).

Inflammatory bowel disease.

GI tract neoplasm.

Diverticular disease.

Appendicitis.

Bowel loop with feces.

ADRENAL MASSES[22]

ICD-9CM # 194.0 ADRENOCORTICAL CARCINOMA
255.8 ADRENAL HYPERPLASIA

UNILATERAL ADRENAL MASSES

Functional lesions

Adrenal adenoma.

Adrenal carcinoma.

Pheochromocytoma.

Primary aldosteronism, adenomatous type.

Nonfunctional lesions

Incidentaloma of adrenal.

Ganglioneuroma.

Myelolipoma.

Hematoma.

Adenolipoma.

Metastasis.

BILATERAL ADRENAL MASSES

Functional lesions

ACTH-dependent Cushing's syndrome.

Congenital adrenal hyperplasia.

Pheochromocytoma.

Conn's syndrome, hyperplastic variety.

Micronodular adrenal disease.
Idiopathic bilateral adrenal hypertrophy.
Nonfunctional lesions
Infection (tuberculosis, fungi).
Infiltration (leukemia, lymphoma).
Replacement (amyloidosis).
Hemorrhage.
Bilateral metastases.

ADYNAMIC ILEUS[14]

ICD-9CM # 560.1

Abdominal trauma.
Infection (retroperitoneal, pelvic, intrathoracic).
Laparotomy.
Metabolic disease (hypokalemia).
Renal colic.
Skeletal injury (rib fracture, vertebral fracture).
Medications (e.g., narcotics).

ALKALOSIS, METABOLIC

ICD-9CM # 276.3

CHLORIDE-RESPONSIVE

Vomiting.
Nasogastric (NG) suction.
Diuretics.
Posthypercapnic alkalosis.
Stool losses (laxative abuse, cystic fibrosis, villous adenoma).
Massive blood transfusion.
Exogenous alkali administration.

CHLORIDE-RESISTANT

Hyperadrenocorticoid states (Cushing's syndrome, primary hyperaldosteronism, secondary mineralocorticoidism [licorice, chewing tobacco]).
Hypomagnesemia.
Hypokalemia.
Bartter's syndrome.

ALKALOSIS, RESPIRATORY

ICD-9CM # 276.3

Hypoxemia (pneumonia, pulmonary embolism, atelectasis, high-altitude living).
Drugs (salicylates, xanthenes, progesterone, epinephrine, thyroxine, nicotine).
Central nervous system (CNS) disorders (tumor, cerebrovascular accident [CVA], trauma, infections).
Psychogenic hyperventilation (anxiety, hysteria).
Hepatic encephalopathy.
Gram-negative sepsis.
Hyponatremia.
Sudden recovery from metabolic acidosis.
Assisted ventilation.

ALVEOLAR CONSOLIDATION

ICD-9CM # 514

Infection.
Neoplasm (bronchoalveolar carcinoma, lymphoma).
Aspiration.
Trauma.
Hemorrhage (Wegener's Goodpasture, bleeding diathesis).
ARDS.
CHF.

Renal failure.
Eosinophilic pneumonia.
Bronchiolitis obliterans.
Pulmonary alveolar proteinosis.

AMNESIA

ICD-9CM # 292.83 DRUG INDUCED
300.12 HYSTERICAL
780.9 RETROGRADE
437.7 TRANSIENT GLOBAL

Degenerative diseases (e.g., Alzheimer's, Huntington's disease).
CVA (especially when involving thalamus, basal forebrain, and hippocampus).
Head trauma.
Postsurgical (e.g., mammillary body surgery, bilateral temporal lobectomy).
Infections (herpes simplex encephalitis, meningitis).
Wernicke-Korsakoff syndrome.
Cerebral hypoxia.
Hypoglycemia.
CNS neoplasms.
Creutzfeldt-Jakob disease.
Medications (e.g., midazolam and other benzodiazepines).
Psychosis.
Malingering.

ANAL INCONTINENCE[14]

ICD-9CM # 787.6

TRAUMATIC

Nerve injured in surgery.
Spinal cord injury.
Obstetric trauma.
Sphincter injury.

NEUROLOGIC

Spinal cord lesions.
Dementia.
Autonomic neuropathy (e.g., diabetes mellitus).
Gynecologic: pudendal nerve stretched during surgery.
Hirschsprung's disease.

MASS EFFECT

Carcinoma of anal canal.
Carcinoma of rectum.
Foreign body.
Fecal impaction.
Hemorrhoids.

MEDICAL

Inflammatory disease.
Diarrhea.
Laxative abuse.

ANAPHYLAXIS[11]

ICD-9CM # 995.0

PULMONARY

Laryngeal edema.
Epiglottitis.
Foreign body aspiration.
Pulmonary embolus.
Asphyxiation.
Hyperventilation.

CARDIOVASCULAR

Myocardial infarction.
Arrhythmia.
Hypovolemic shock.
Cardiac arrest.

CNS

Vasovagal reaction.
CVA.
Seizure disorder.
Drug overdose.

ENDOCRINE

Hypoglycemia.
Pheochromocytoma.
Carcinoid syndrome.

PSYCHIATRIC

Vocal cord dysfunction syndrome.
Munchausen's disease.
Panic attack/globus hystericus.

OTHER

Hereditary angioedema.
Cord urticaria.
Idiopathic urticaria.
Mastocytosis.
Serum sickness.
Idiopathic capillary leak syndrome.
Sulfite exposure.
Scombroid poisoning (tuna, blue fish, mackerel).

ANEMIA, DRUG-INDUCED[10]

ICD-9CM # 283.0

DRUGS THAT MAY INTERFERE WITH RED CELL PRODUCTION BY INDUCING MARROW SUPPRESSION OR APLASIA

Alcohol.
Antineoplastic drugs.
Antithyroid drugs.
Antibiotics.
Oral hypoglycemic agents.
Phenylbutazone.
Azidothymidine (AZT).

DRUGS THAT INTERFERE WITH VITAMIN B$_{12}$, FOLATE, OR IRON ABSORPTION OR UTILIZATION

Nitrous oxide.
Anticonvulsant drugs.
Antineoplastic drugs.
Isoniazid, cycloserine A.

DRUGS CAPABLE OF PROMOTING HEMOLYSIS

Immune mediated
Penicillins.
Quinine.
Alpha-methyldopa.
Procainamide.
Mitomycin C.
Oxidative stress
Antimalarials.
Sulfonamide drugs.
Nalidixic acid.

DRUGS THAT MAY PRODUCE OR PROMOTE BLOOD LOSS

Aspirin.
Alcohol.
Nonsteroidal antiinflammatory agents.
Corticosteroids.
Anticoagulants.

ANEMIA, LOW RETICULOCYTE COUNT[1]

ICD-9CM # 285.9

MICROCYTIC ANEMIA (MCV <80)

Iron deficiency.
Thalassemia minor.
Sideroblastic anemia.
Lead poisoning.

MACROCYTIC ANEMIA (MCV >100)

Megaloblastic anemias.
Folate deficiency.
Vitamin B$_{12}$ deficiency.
Drug-induced megaloblastic anemia.
Nonmegaloblastic macrocytosis.
Liver disease.
Hypothyroidism.

NORMOCYTIC ANEMIA (MCV 80-100)

Early iron deficiency.
Aplastic anemia.
Myelophthisic disorders.
Endocrinopathies.
Anemia of chronic disease.
Uremia.
Mixed nutritional deficiency.

ANEMIA, MEGALOBLASTIC[22]

ICD-9CM # 281.0 PERNICIOUS ANEMIA
       281.1 B$_{12}$ DEFICIENCY
       281.2 FOLATE DEFICIENCY
       281.3 B$_{12}$ WITH FOLATE DEFICIENCY
       281.4 PROTEIN OR AMINO ACID DEFICIENCY
       281.8 NUTRITIONAL
       281.9 NOS

COBALAMIN (CBL) DEFICIENCY

Nutritional Cbl deficiency (insufficient Cbl intake): vegetarians, vegans, breast-fed infants of mothers with pernicious anemia.

Abnormal intragastric events (inadequate proteolysis of food Cbl): atrophic gastritis, partial gastrectomy with hypochlorhydria.

Loss/atrophy of gastric oxyntic mucosa (deficient IF molecules): total or partial gastrectomy, pernicious anemia (PA), caustic destruction (lye).

Abnormal events in small bowel lumen:
Inadequate pancreatic protease (R-Cbl not degraded, Cbl not transferred to IF).
- Insufficiency of pancreatic protease—pancreatic insufficiency.
- Inactivation of pancreatic protease—Zollinger-Ellison syndrome.

Usurping of luminal Cbl (inadequate Cbl binding to IF).
- By bacteria—stasis syndromes (blind loops, pouches of diverticulosis, strictures, fistulas, anastomoses); impaired

bowel motility (scleroderma, pseudoobstruction), hypogammaglobulinemia.
- By *Diphyllobothrium latum.*

Disorders of ileal mucosa/IF receptors (IF-Cbl not bound to IF receptors):

Diminished or absent IF receptors—ileal bypass/resection/fistula.

Abnormal mucosal architecture/function—tropical/nontropical sprue, Crohn's disease, TB ileitis, infiltration by lymphomas, amyloidosis.

IF-/post IF-receptor defects—Imerslund-Graesbeck syndrome, TC II deficiency.

Drug-induced effects (slow K, biguanides, cholestyramine, colchicine, neomycin, PAS).

DISORDERS OF PLASMA CBL TRANSPORT (TC II-CBL NOT DELIVERED TO TC II RECEPTORS)

Congenital TC II deficiency, defective binding of TC II-Cbl to TC II receptors (rare).

METABOLIC DISORDERS (CBL NOT UTILIZED BY CELL)

Inborn enzyme errors (rare).

Acquired disorders: (Cbl oxidized to cob[III]alamin)—N_2O inhalation.

FOLATE DEFICIENCY

Nutritional causes

Decreased dietary intake—poverty and famine (associated with kwashiorkor, marasmus), institutionalized individuals (psychiatric/nursing homes), chronic debilitating disease/goats' milk (low in folate), special diets (slimming), cultural/ethnic cooking techniques (food folate destroyed) or habits (folate-rich foods not consumed).

Decreased diet and increased requirements:
- Pathologic: intrinsic hematologic disease (autoimmune hemolytic disease), drugs, malaria; hemoglobinopathies (SS, thalassemia), RBC membrane defects (hereditary spherocytosis, paroxysmal nocturnal hemoglobinopathy); abnormal hematopoiesis (leukemia/lymphoma, myelodysplastic syndrome, agnogenic myeloid metaplasia with myelofibrosis); infiltration with malignant disease; dermatologic (psoriasis).

Folate malabsorption

With normal intestinal mucosa:
- Some drugs (controversial).
- Congenital folate malabsorption (rare).

With mucosal abnormalities—tropical and nontropical sprue, regional enteritis.

Defective cellular folate uptake—familial aplastic anemia (rare)

Inadequate cellular utilization

Folate antagonists (methotrexate).

Hereditary enzyme deficiencies involving folate.

Drugs (multiple effects on folate metabolism)

Alcohol, sulfasalazine, triamterine, pyrimethamine, trimethoprim-sulfamethoxazole, diphenylhydantoin, barbiturates.

MISCELLANEOUS MEGALOBLASTIC ANEMIAS (NOT CAUSED BY CBL OR FOLATE DEFICIENCY)

Congenital disorders of DNA synthesis (rare)

Orotic aciduria, Lesch-Nyhan syndrome, congenital dyserythropoietic anemia.

Acquired disorders of DNA synthesis

Thiamine-responsive megaloblastosis (rare).

Malignancy—erythroleukemia—refractory sideroblastic anemias—all antineoplastic drugs that inhibit DNA synthesis.

Toxic—alcohol.

ANEURYSMS, THORACIC AORTA

ICD-9CM # 441.2

Trauma.

Infection.

Inflammatory (syphilis, Takayasu's disease).

Collagen vascular disease (rheumatoid arthritis, ankylosing spondylitis).

Annuloaortic ectasia (Marfan's syndrome, Ehlers-Danlos syndrome).

Congenital.

Coarctation.

Cystic medial necrosis.

ARTERIAL OCCLUSION[7]

ICD-9CM # 444.22 ARTERIAL OCCLUSION, LOWER EXTREMITIES
444.21 ARTERIAL OCCLUSION, UPPER EXTREMITIES

Thromboembolism (post-MI, mitral stenosis, rheumatic valve disease, atrial fibrillation, atrial myxoma, marantic endocarditis, bacterial endocarditis, Libman-Sacks endocarditis).

Atheroembolism (microemboli composed of cholesterol, calcium, and platelets from proximal atherosclerotic plaques).

Arterial thrombosis (endothelial injury, altered arterial blood flow, trauma, severe atherosclerosis, acute vasculitis).

Vasospasm.

Trauma.

Hypercoagulable states.

Miscellaneous (irradiation, drugs, infections, necrotizing).

ARTHRITIS, MONOARTICULAR AND OLIGOARTICULAR[2]

ICD-9CM # 715.3 OSTEOARTHRITIS, LOCALIZED
711.9 INFECTIOUS ARTHRITIS
716.6 MONOARTICULAR ARTHRITIS
5TH DIGIT TO BE ADDED TO THE ABOVE DEPENDING ON SITE OF ARTHRITIS

0. SITE UNSPECIFIED
1. SHOULDER REGION
2. UPPER ARM
3. FOREARM
4. HAND
5. PELVIC REGION AND THIGH
6. LOWER LEG
7. ANKLE AND/OR FOOT
8. OTHER SPECIFIED EXCEPT SPINE

Septic arthritis (*S. aureus, Neisseria gonorrhea, Meningococci, Streptococci, S. pneumoniae, enteric gram-neg bacilli*).

Crystalline-induced arthritis (gout, pseudogout, calcium oxalate, hydroxyapatite and other basic calcium/phosphate crystals).

Traumatic joint injury.

Hemarthrosis.

Monoarticular or oligoarticular flare of an inflammatory polyarticular rheumatic disease (RA, psoriatic arthritis, Reiter's syndrome, SLE).

ARTHRITIS, POLYARTICULAR

ICD-9CM # 715.09 GENERALIZED OSTEOARTHRITIS, MULTIPLE SITES
716.89 ARTHRITIS, MULTIPLE SITES

RA.

SLE, other connective tissue diseases, erythema nodosum, palindromic rheumatism, relapsing polychondritis.

Psoriatic arthritis, ankylosing spondylitis.
Sarcoidosis.
Lyme arthritis, bacterial endocarditis, *Neisseria gonorrhoeae* infection, rheumatic fever, Reiter's disease.
Crystal deposition disease.
Hypersensitivity to serum or drugs.
Hepatitis B, HIV, rubella, mumps.
Other: serum sickness, leukemias, lymphomas, enteropathic arthropathy, Whipple's disease, Behçet's syndrome, Henoch-Schönlein purpura, familial Mediterranean fever, hypertrophic pulmonary osteoarthropathy.

ASCITES

ICD-9CM # 789.5 ASCITES NOS
197.6 ASCITES, CANCEROUS (MALIGNANT)
457.8 ASCITES, CHYLOUS

Hypoalbuminemia: nephrotic syndrome, protein-losing gastroenteropathy, starvation.
Cirrhosis.
Hepatic congestion: CHF, constrictive pericarditis, tricuspid insufficiency, hepatic vein obstruction (Budd-Chiari syndrome), inferior vena cava or portal vein obstruction.
Peritoneal infections: TB and other bacterial infections, fungal diseases, parasites.
Neoplasms: primary hepatic neoplasms, metastases to liver or peritoneum, lymphomas, leukemias, myeloid metaplasia.
Lymphatic obstruction: mediastinal tumors, trauma to the thoracic duct, filariasis.
Ovarian disease: Meigs' syndrome, struma ovarii.
Chronic pancreatitis or pseudocyst: pancreatic ascites.
Leakage of bile: bile ascites.
Urinary obstruction or trauma: urine ascites.
Myxedema.
Chylous ascites.

ATAXIA

ICD-9CM # 781.3 ATAXIA NOS
303.0 ALCOHOLIC, ACUTE
303.9 ALCOHOLIC, CHRONIC
334.3 CEREBELLAR
331.89 CEREBRAL
334.0 FRIEDREICH'S
300.11 HYSTERICAL

Vertebral-basilar artery ischemia.
Diabetic neuropathy.
Tabes dorsalis.
Vitamin B_{12} deficiency.
Multiple sclerosis and other demyelinating diseases.
Meningomyelopathy.
Cerebellar neoplasms, hemorrhage, abscess, infarct.
Nutritional (Wernicke's encephalopathy).
Paraneoplastic syndromes.
Parainfectious: Guillain-Barré syndrome.
Toxins: phenytoin, alcohol, sedatives, organophosphates.
Wilson's disease (hepatolenticular degeneration).
Hypothyroidism.
Myopathy.
Cerebellar and spinocerebellar degeneration: ataxia/telangiectasia, Friedreich's ataxia.
Frontal lobe lesions: tumors, thrombosis of anterior cerebral artery, hydrocephalus.
Labyrinthine destruction: neoplasm, injury, inflammation, compression.
Hysteria.
AIDS.

BACK PAIN

ICD-9CM # 724.5 BACK PAIN (POSTURAL)
724.2 LOW BACK PAIN
307.89 BACK PAIN PSYCHOGENIC
724.8 STIFF BACK
847.9 BACK STRAIN
724.6 BACKACHE, SACROILIAC

Trauma: injury to bone, joint, or ligament.
Mechanical: obesity, fatigue, scoliosis.
Degenerative: osteoarthritis.
Infections: osteomyelitis, subarachnoid or spinal abscess, TB, meningitis, basilar pneumonia.
Metabolic: osteoporosis, osteomalacia, vertebral compression.
Vascular: leaking aortic aneurysm, subarachnoid or spinal hemorrhage/infarction.
Neoplastic: myeloma, Hodgkin's disease, carcinoma of pancreas, metastatic neoplasm from breast, prostate, lung.
GI: penetrating ulcer, pancreatitis, cholelithiasis, inflammatory bowel disease.
Renal: hydronephrosis, calculus, neoplasm, renal infarction, pyelonephritis.
Hematologic: sickle cell crisis, acute hemolysis.
Gynecologic: neoplasm of uterus or ovary, dysmenorrhea, salpingitis, uterine prolapse.
Inflammatory: ankylosing spondylitis, psoriatic arthritis, Reiter's syndrome.
Lumbosacral strain.
Psychogenic: malingering, hysteria, anxiety.
Endocrine: adrenal hemorrhage or infarction.

BLEEDING, LOWER GI

ICD-9CM # 578.9

(ORIGINATING BELOW THE LIGAMENT OF TREITZ)

Small intestine
Ischemic bowel disease (mesenteric thrombosis, embolism, vasculitis, trauma).
Small bowel neoplasm: leiomyomas, carcinoids.
Hereditary hemorrhagic telangiectasia (Rendu-Osler-Weber syndrome).
Meckel's diverticulum and other small intestine diverticula.
Aortoenteric fistula.
Intestinal hemangiomas: blue rubber bleb nevi, intestinal hemangiomas, cutaneous vascular nevi.
Hamartomatous polyps: Peutz-Jeghers syndrome (intestinal polyps, mucocutaneous pigmentation).
Infections of small bowel: tuberculous enteritis, enteritis necroticans.
Volvulus.
Intussusception.
Lymphoma of small bowel, sarcoma, Kaposi's sarcoma.
Irradiation ileitis.
AV malformation of small intestine.
Inflammatory bowel disease.
Polyarteritis nodosa.
Other: pancreatoenteric fistulas, Henoch-Schönlein purpura, Ehlers-Danlos syndrome, systemic lupus erythematosus, amyloidosis, metastatic melanoma.
Colon
Carcinoma (particularly left colon).
Diverticular disease.
Inflammatory bowel disease.
Ischemic colitis.
Colonic polyps.

Vascular abnormalities: angiodysplasia, vascular ectasia.
Radiation colitis.
Infectious colitis.
Uremic colitis.
Aortoenteric fistula.
Lymphoma of large bowel.
Hemorrhoids.
Anal fissure.
Trauma, foreign body.
Solitary rectal/cecal ulcers.
Long-distance running.

BLEEDING, UPPER GI

ICD-9CM # 578.9

(ORIGINATING ABOVE THE LIGAMENT OF TREITZ)

Oral or pharyngeal lesions: swallowed blood from nose or oropharynx.

Swallowed hemoptysis

Esophageal: varices, ulceration, esophagitis, Mallory-Weiss tear, carcinoma, trauma.

Gastric: peptic ulcer (including Cushing and Curling's ulcers), gastritis, angiodysplasia, gastric neoplasms, hiatal hernia, gastric diverticulum, pseudoxanthoma elasticum, Rendu-Osler-Weber syndrome.

Duodenal. peptic ulcer, duodenitis, angiodysplasia, aortoduodenal fistula, duodenal diverticulum, duodenal tumors, carcinoma of ampulla of Vater, parasites (e.g., hookworm), Crohn's disease.

Biliary: hematobilia (e.g., penetrating injury to liver, hepatobiliary malignancy, endoscopic papillotomy).

BLINDNESS

ICD-9CM # 369.4

Cataracts.
Glaucoma.
Diabetic retinopathy.
Macular degeneration.
Trauma.
CVA.
Corneal scarring.
Temporal arteritis.

BONE LESIONS, PREFERENTIAL SITE OF ORIGIN[21]

ICD-9CM # 170.0 SKULL AND FACE
     170.1 MANDIBLE
     170.2 VERTEBRAL COLUMN
     170.3 RIBS, STERNUM, CLAVICLE
     170.4 SCAPULA, LONG BONES UPPER LIMB
     170.5 SHORT BONES AND UPPER LIMB
     170.6 PELVIC BONES, SACRUM COCCYX
     170.7 LONG BONES LOWER LIMB
     170.8 SHORT BONES LOWER LIMB
     170.9 BONE CANCER NOS
     198.5 BONE CANCER, METASTATIC

EPIPHYSIS

Chondroblastoma.
Giant-cell tumor—after fusion of growth plate.
Langerhans' cell histiocytosis.
Clear cell chondrosarcoma.
Osteosarcoma.

METAPHYSIS

Parosteal sarcoma.
Chondrosarcoma.
Fibrosarcoma.
Nonossifying fibroma.
Giant cell tumor—before fusion of growth plate.
Unicameral bone cyst.
Aneurysmal bone cyst.

DIAPHYSIS

Myeloma.
Ewing's tumor.
Reticulum cell sarcoma.

METADIAPHYSEAL

Fibrosarcoma.
Fibrous dysplasia.
Enchondroma.
Osteoid osteoma.
Chondromyofibroma.

BRADYCARDIA, SINUS[7]

ICD-9CM # 427.89

Idiopathic.
Degenerative processes (e.g., Lev's disease, Lenegre's disease).

Medications

Beta blockers.
Some calcium channel blockers (diltiazem, verapamil).
Digoxin (when vagal tone is high).
Class I antiarrhythmic agents (e.g., procainamide).
Class III antiarrhythmic agents (amiodarone, sotalol).
Clonidine.
Lithium carbonate.

Acute myocardial ischemia and infarction

Right or left circumflex coronary artery occlusion or spasm.
High vagal tone (e.g., athletes).

BREAST MASS

ICD-9CM # 611.72

Fibrocystic breasts.
Benign tumors (fibroadenoma, papilloma).
Mastitis (acute bacterial mastitis, chronic mastitis).
Malignant neoplasm.
Fat necrosis.
Hematoma.
Duct ectasia.
Mammary adenosis.

BREATH ODOR[20]

ICD-9CM # 784.9 HALITOSIS

Sweet, fruity: DKA, starvation ketosis.
Fishy, stale: uremia (trimethylamines).
Ammonia-like: uremia (ammonia).
Musty fish, clover: fetor hepaticus (hepatic failure).
Foul, feculent: intestinal obstruction/diverticulum.
Foul, putrid: nasal/sinus pathology (infection, foreign body, cancer), respiratory infections (empyema, lung abscess, bronchiectasis).
Halitosis: tonsillitis, gingivitis, respiratory infections, Vincent's angina, gastroesophageal reflux, achalasia.
Cinnamon: pulmonary TB.

BULLOUS DISEASES

ICD-9CM # 694.9 BULLOUS DERMATOSES
          694.5 BULLOUS PEMPHIGOID
          694.4 PEMPHIGUS VULGARIS
          694.4 PEMPHIGUS FOLIACEUS

Bullous pemphigoid.
Pemphigus vulgaris.
Pemphigus foliaceus.
Paraneoplastic pemphigus.
Cicatricial pemphigoid.
Erythema multiforme.
Dermatitis herpetiformis.
Herpes.
Impetigo.
Erosive lichen planus.
Linear IgA bullous dermatosis.
Epidermolysis bullosa acquisita.

CALCIFICATION ON CHEST X-RAY

ICD-9CM # 722.92

Lung neoplasm (primary or metastatic).
Silicosis.
Idiopathic pulmonary fibrosis.
Tuberculosis.
Histoplasmosis.
Disseminated varicella infection.
Mitral stenosis (end-stage).
Secondary hyperparathyroidism.

CARDIAC ARREST, NONTRAUMATIC[14]

ICD-9CM # 427.5 CARDIAC ARREST NOS

Cardiac (coronary artery disease, cardiomyopathies, structural abnormalities, valve dysfunction, arrhythmias).
Respiratory (upper airway obstruction, hypoventilation, pulmonary embolism, asthma, COPD exacerbation, pulmonary edema).
Circulatory (tension pneumothorax, pericardial tamponade, PE, hemorrhage, sepsis).
Electrolyte abnormalities (hypokalemia or hyperkalemia, hypomagnesemia or hypermagnesemia, hypocalcemia).
Medications (tricyclic antidepressants, digoxin, theophylline, calcium channel blockers).
Drug abuse (cocaine, heroin, amphetamines).
Toxins (carbon monoxide, cyanide).
Environmental (drowning/near-drowning, electrocution, lightning, hypothermia or hyperthermia, venomous snakes).

CARDIAC ENLARGEMENT[7]

ICD-9CM # 429.3 CARDIOMEGALY, IDIOPATHIC
          746.89 CARDIOMEGALY, CONGENITAL
          402.0 CARDIOMEGALY, MALIGNANT
          402.1 CARDIOMEGALY, BENIGN

CARDIAC CHAMBER ENLARGEMENT

Chronic volume overload
Mitral or aortic regurgitation.
Left-to-right shunt (PDA, VSD, AV fistula).
Cardiomyopathy
Ischemic.
Nonischemic.
Decompensated pressure overload
Aortic stenosis.
Hypertension.

High-output states
Severe anemia.
Thyrotoxicosis.
Bradycardia
Severe sinus bradycardia.
Complete heart block.

LEFT ATRIUM

LV failure of any cause.
Mitral valve disease.
Myxoma.

RIGHT VENTRICLE

Chronic volume overload.
Tricuspid or pulmonic regurgitation.
Left-to-right shunt (ASD).
Decompensated pressure overload:
    Pulmonic stenosis.
    Pulmonary artery hypertension:
        Primary.
        Secondary (PE, COPD).
Pulmonary venoocclusive disease.

RIGHT ATRIUM

RV failure of any cause.
Tricuspid valve disease.
Myxoma.
Ebstein's anomaly.

MULTICHAMBER ENLARGEMENT

Hypertrophic cardiomyopathy.
Acromegaly.
Severe obesity.

PERICARDIAL DISEASE

Pericardial effusion with or without tamponade.
Effusive constrictive disease.
Pericardial cyst, loculated effusion.

PSEUDOCARDIOMEGALY

Epicardial fat.
Chest wall deformity (pectus excavatum, straight back syndrome).
Low lung volumes.
AP chest x-ray.
Mediastinal tumor, cyst.

CARDIAC MURMURS

ICD-9CM # CODE VARIES WITH SPECIFIC DISORDER

SYSTOLIC

Mitral regurgitation (MR).
Tricuspid regurgitation (TR).
Ventricular septal defect (VSD).
Aortic stenosis (AS).
Idiopathic hypertrophic subaortic stenosis (IHSS).
Pulmonic stenosis (PS).
Innocent murmur of childhood.
Coarctation of aorta.
Mitral valve prolapse (MVP).

DIASTOLIC

Aortic regurgitation (AR).
Atrial myxoma.
Mitral stenosis (MS).
Pulmonary artery branch stenosis.
Tricuspid stenosis (TS).

Graham Steell murmur (diastolic decrescendo murmur heard in severe pulmonary hypertension).
Pulmonic regurgitation (PR).
Severe mitral regurgitation (MR).
Austin Flint murmur (diastolic rumble heard in severe AR).
Severe VSD and patent ductus arteriosus.

CONTINUOUS

Patent ductus arteriosus.
Pulmonary AV fistula.

CAVITARY LESION ON CHEST X-RAY[9]

ICD-9CM # 793.1 CHEST X-RAY LUNG SHADOW

NECROTIZING INFECTIONS

Bacteria: anaerobes, *Staphylococcus aureus,* enteric gram-negative bacteria, *Pseudomonas aeruginosa, Legionella* species, *Haemophilus influenzae, Streptococcus pyogenes, Streptococcus pneumoniae* (?), *Rhodococcus, Actinomyces.*
Mycobacteria: *Mycobacterium tuberculosis, Mycobacterium kansasii,* MAI.
Bacteria-like: *Nocardia* species.
Fungi: *Coccidioides immitis, Histoplasma capsulatum, Blastomyces hominis, Aspergillus* species, *Mucor* species.
Parasitic: *Entamoeba histolytica, Echinococcus, Paragonimus westermani.*

CAVITARY INFARCTION

Bland infarction (with or without superimposed infection).
Lung contusion.

SEPTIC EMBOLISM

S. aureus, anaerobes, others.

VASCULITIS

Wegener's granulomatosis, periarteritis.

NEOPLASMS

Bronchogenic carcinoma, metastatic carcinoma, lymphoma.

MISCELLANEOUS LESIONS

Cysts, blebs, bullae, or pneumatocele with or without fluid collections.
Sequestration.
Empyema with air-fluid level.
Bronchiectasis.

CEREBROVASCULAR DISEASE, ISCHEMIC[23]

ICD-9CM # 437.9

VASCULAR DISORDERS

Large-vessel atherothrombotic disease.
Lacunar disease.
Arterial-to-arterial embolization.
Carotid or vertebral artery dissection.
Fibromuscular dysplasia.
Migraine.
Venous thrombosis.
Radiation.
Complications of arteriography.
Multiple, progressive intracranial arterial occlusions.

INFLAMMATORY DISORDERS

Giant cell arteritis.
Polyarteritis nodosa.
Systemic lupus erythematosus.

Granulomatous angiitis.
Takayasu's disease.
Arteritis associated with amphetamine, cocaine, or phenylpropanolamine.
Syphilis, mucormycosis.
Sjögren's syndrome.
Behçet's syndrome.

CARDIAC DISORDERS

Rheumatic heart disease.
Mural thrombus.
Arrhythmias.
Mitral valve prolapse.
Prosthetic heart valve.
Endocarditis.
Myxoma.
Paradoxical embolus.

HEMATOLOGIC DISORDERS

Thrombotic thrombocytopenic purpura.
Sickle cell disease.
Hypercoagulable states.
Polycythemia.
Thrombocytosis.
Leukocytosis.
Lupus anticoagulant.

CHEST PAIN (NONPLEURITIC)[4]

ICD-9CM # 786.50 CHEST PAIN NOS
786.59 CHEST DISCOMFORT

Cardiac: myocardial ischemia/infarction, myocarditis.
Esophageal: spasm, esophagitis, ulceration, neoplasm, achalasia, diverticula, foreign body.
Referred pain from subdiaphragmatic GI structures.
Gastric and duodenal: hiatal hernia, neoplasm, PUD.
Gallbladder and biliary: cholecystitis, cholelithiasis, impacted stone, neoplasm.
Pancreatic: pancreatitis, neoplasm.
Dissecting aortic aneurysm.
Pain originating from skin, breasts, and musculoskeletal structures: herpes zoster, mastitis, cervical spondylosis.
Mediastinal tumors: lymphoma, thymoma.
Pulmonary: neoplasm, pneumonia, pulmonary embolism/infarction.
Psychoneurosis.
Chest pain associated with mitral valve prolapse.

CHEST PAIN (PLEURITIC)

ICD-9CM # 786.52 CHEST PAIN, PLEURITIC

Cardiac: pericarditis, postpericardiotomy/Dressler's syndrome.
Pulmonary: pneumothorax, hemothorax, embolism/infarction, pneumonia, empyema, neoplasm, bronchiectasis, pneumomediastinum, TB, carcinomatous effusion.
GI: liver abscess, pancreatitis, esophageal rupture, Whipple's disease with associated pericarditis or pleuritis.
Subdiaphragmatic abscess.
Pain originating from skin and musculoskeletal tissues: costochondritis, chest wall trauma, fractured rib, interstitial fibrositis, myositis, strain of pectoralis muscle, herpes zoster, soft tissue and bone tumors.
Collagen vascular diseases with pleuritis.
Psychoneurosis.
Familial Mediterranean fever.

CHOLESTASIS[7]

ICD-9CM # 574.71

EXTRAHEPATIC

Choledocholithiasis.
Bile duct stricture.
Cholangiocarcinoma.
Pancreatic carcinoma.
Chronic pancreatitis.
Papillary stenosis.
Ampullary cancer.
Primary sclerosing cholangitis.
Choledochal cysts.
Parasites (e.g., ascaris, clonorchis).
AIDS.
Cholangiography.
Biliary atresia.
Portal lymphadenopathy.
Mirizzi's syndrome.

INTRAHEPATIC

Viral hepatitis.
Alcoholic hepatitis.
Drug induced.
Ductopenia syndromes.
Primary biliary cirrhosis.
Benign recurrent intrahepatic cholestasis.
Byler's disease.
Primary sclerosing cholangitis.
Alagille's syndrome.
Sarcoid.
Lymphoma.
Postoperative.
Total parenteral nutrition.
Alpha-1-antitrypsin deficiency.

CLUBBING

ICD-9CM # 781.5 CLUBBING FINGER

Pulmonary neoplasm (lung, pleura).
Other neoplasm (GI, liver, Hodgkin's, thymus, osteogenic sarcoma).
Pulmonary infectious process (empyema, abscess, bronchiectasis, TB, chronic pneumonitis).
Extrapulmonary infectious process (subacute bacterial endocarditis, intestinal TB, bacterial or amebic dysentery, arterial graft sepsis).
Pneumoconiosis.
Sarcoidosis.
Cyanotic congenital heart disease.
Endocrine (Graves' disease, hyperparathyroidism).
Inflammatory bowel disease.
Celiac disease.
Chronic liver disease, cirrhosis.
Pulmonary AV malformations.
Idiopathic.
Thyroid acropachy.
Hereditary (pachydermoperiostosis).
Chronic trauma (jackhammer operators, machine workers).

CONSTIPATION

ICD-9CM # 564.0

Intestinal obstruction.
Fecal impaction.
Diverticular disease.
GI neoplasm.
Strangulated femoral hernia.
Gallstone ileus.
Tuberculous stricture.
Adhesions.
Ameboma.
Volvulus.
Intussusception.
Inflammatory bowel disease.
Hematoma of bowel wall, secondary to trauma or anticoagulants.
Poor dietary habits: insufficient bulk in diet, inadequate fluid intake.
Change from daily routine: travel, hospital admission, physical inactivity.
Acute abdominal conditions: renal colic, biliary colic, appendicitis, ischemia.
Hypercalcemia or hypokalemia, uremia.
Irritable bowel syndrome, anorexia nervosa, depression.
Painful anal conditions: hemorrhoids, fissure, stricture.
Decreased intestinal peristalsis: old age, spinal cord injuries, myxedema, diabetes, multiple sclerosis, parkinsonism and other neurologic diseases.
Drugs: codeine, morphine, antacids with aluminum, verapamil, anticonvulsants, anticholinergics, disopyramide, cholestyramine, alosetron, iron supplements.
Hirschsprung's disease.

COUGH

ICD-9CM # 786.2

Infectious process (viral, bacterial).
Postinfectious.
"Smoker's cough."
Rhinitis (allergic, vasomotor, postinfectious).
Asthma.
Exposure to irritants (noxious fumes, smoke, cold air).
Drug-induced (especially ACE inhibitors, β-blockers).
GERD.
Interstitial lung disease.
Lung neoplasms.
Lymphomas, mediastinal neoplasms.
Bronchiectasis.
Cardiac (CHF, pulmonary edema, mitral stenosis, pericardial inflammation).
Recurrent aspiration.
Inflammation of larynx, pleura, diaphragm, mediastinum.
Cystic fibrosis.
Anxiety.
Other: pulmonary embolism, foreign body inhalation, aortic aneurysm, Zenker's diverticulum, osteophytes, substernal thyroid, thyroiditis, PMR.

CYANOSIS

ICD-9CM # 782.5 CYANOSIS NOS

Congenital heart disease with right-to-left shunt.
Pulmonary embolism.
Hypoxia.
Pulmonary edema.
Pulmonary disease (oxygen diffusion and alveolar ventilation abnormalities).
Hemoglobinopathies.
Decreased cardiac output.
Vasospasm.
Arterial obstruction.
Pulmonary AV fistulas.
Elevated hemidiaphragm.

Neoplasm (bronchogenic carcinoma, mediastinal neoplasm, intrahepatic lesion).
Substernal thyroid.
Infectious process (pneumonia, empyema, TB, subphrenic abscess, hepatic abscess).
Atelectasis.
Idiopathic.
Eventration.
Phrenic nerve dysfunction (myelitis, myotonia, herpes zoster).
Trauma to phrenic nerve or diaphragm (e.g., surgery).
Aortic aneurysm.
Intraabdominal mass.
Pulmonary infarction.
Pleurisy.
Radiation therapy.
Rib fracture.
Superior vena cava syndrome.

DELIRIUM[14]

ICD-9CM # 780.09 DELIRIUM NOS
293.0 ACUTE DELIRIUM

PHARMACOLOGIC AGENTS

Anxiolytics (benzodiazepines).
Antidepressants (e.g., amitriptyline, doxepin, imipramine).
Cardiovascular agents (e.g., methyldopa, digitalis, reserpine, propranolol, procainamide, captopril, disopyramide).
Antihistamine.
Cimetidine.
Corticosteroids.
Antineoplastics.
Drugs of abuse (alcohol, cannabis, amphetamines, cocaine, hallucinogens, opioids, sedative-hypnotics, phencyclidine).

METABOLIC DISORDERS

Hypercalcemia.
Hypercarbia.
Hypoglycemia.
Hyponatremia.
Hypoxia.

INFLAMMATORY DISORDERS

Sarcoidosis.
SLE.
Giant cell arteritis.

ORGAN FAILURE

Hepatic encephalopathy.
Uremia.

NEUROLOGIC DISORDERS

Alzheimer's disease.
CVA.
Encephalitis (including HIV).
Encephalopathies.
Epilepsy.
Huntington's disease.
Multiple sclerosis.
Neoplasms.
Normal pressure hydrocephalus.
Parkinson's disease.
Pick's disease.
Wilson's disease.

ENDOCRINE DISORDERS

Addison's disease.
Cushing's disease.
Panhypopituitarism.

Parathyroid disease.
Recurrent menstrual psychosis.
Sydenham's chorea.
Thyroid disease.

DEFICIENCY STATES

Niacin.
Thiamine, vitamin B_{12}, and folate.

DIPLOPIA, BINOCULAR

ICD-9CM # 368.2

Cranial nerve palsy (3rd, 4th, 6th).
Thyroid eye disease.
Myasthenia gravis.
Decompensated strabismus.
Orbital trauma with blow-out fracture.
Orbital pseudotumor.
Cavernous sinus thrombosis.

DYSPAREUNIA[5]

ICD-9CM # 625.0 DYSPAREUNIA
608.89 DYSPAREUNIA, MALE
302.76 DYSPAREUNIA, PSYCHOGENIC

INTROITAL

Vaginismus.
Intact or rigid hymen.
Clitoral problems.
Vulvovaginitis.
Vaginal atrophy: hypoestrogen.
Vulvar dystrophy.
Bartholin or Skene gland infection.
Inadequate lubrication.
Operative scarring.

MIDVAGINAL

Urethritis.
Trigonitis.
Cystitis.
Short vagina.
Operative scarring.
Inadequate lubrication.

DEEP

Pelvic infection.
Uterine retroversion.
Ovarian pathology.
Gastrointestinal.
Orthopedic.
Abnormal penile size or shape.

DYSPHAGIA

ICD-9CM # 787.2

Esophageal obstruction: neoplasm, foreign body, achalasia, stricture, spasm, esophageal web, diverticulum, Schatzki's ring.
Peptic esophagitis with stricture, Barrett's stricture.
External esophageal compression: neoplasms (thyroid neoplasm, lymphoma, mediastinal tumors), thyroid enlargement, aortic aneurysm, vertebral spurs, aberrant right subclavian artery (dysphagia lusoria).
Hiatal hernia, GERD.
Oropharyngeal lesions: pharyngitis, glossitis, stomatitis, neoplasms.
Hysteria: globus hystericus.

Neurologic and/or neuromuscular disturbances: bulbar paralysis, myasthenia gravis, ALS, multiple sclerosis, parkinsonism, CVA, diabetic neuropathy.
Toxins: poisoning, botulism, tetanus, postdiphtheritic dysphagia.
Systemic diseases: scleroderma, amyloidosis, dermatomyositis.
Candida and herpes esophagitis.
Presbyesophagus.

DYSPNEA
ICD-9CM # 786.00

Upper airway obstruction: trauma, neoplasm, epiglottitis, laryngeal edema, tongue retraction, laryngospasm, abductor paralysis of vocal cords, aspiration of foreign body.
Lower airway obstruction: neoplasm, COPD, asthma, aspiration of foreign body.
Pulmonary infection: pneumonia, abscess, empyema, TB, bronchiectasis.
Pulmonary hypertension.
Pulmonary embolism/infarction.
Parenchymal lung disease.
Pulmonary vascular congestion.
Cardiac disease: ASHD, valvular lesions, cardiac dysrhythmias, cardiomyopathy, pericardial effusion, cardiac shunts.
Space-occupying lesions: neoplasm, large hiatal hernia, pleural effusions.
Disease of chest wall: severe kyphoscoliosis, fractured ribs, sternal compression, morbid obesity.
Neurologic dysfunction: Guillain-Barré syndrome, botulism, polio, spinal cord injury.
Interstitial pulmonary disease: sarcoidosis, collagen vascular diseases, DIP, Hamman-Rich pneumonitis, etc.
Pneumoconioses: silicosis, berylliosis, etc.
Mesothelioma.
Pneumothorax, hemothorax, pleural effusion.
Inhalation of toxins.
Cholinergic drug intoxication.
Carcinoid syndrome.
Hematologic: anemia, polycythemia, hemoglobinopathies.
Thyrotoxicosis, myxedema.
Diaphragmatic compression caused by abdominal distention, subphrenic abscess, ascites.
Lung resection.
Metabolic abnormalities: uremia, hepatic coma, DKA.
Sepsis.
Atelectasis.
Psychoneurosis.
Diaphragmatic paralysis.

DYSURIA
ICD-9CM # 788.1 DYSURIA
306.53 DYSURIA, PSYCHOGENIC

Urinary tract infection.
Estrogen deficiency (in postmenopausal female).
Vaginitis.
Genital infection (e.g., herpes, condyloma).
Interstitial cystitis.
Chemical irritation (e.g., deodorant aerosols, douches).
Meatal stenosis or stricture.
Reiter's syndrome.
Bladder neoplasm.
GI etiology (diverticulitis, Crohn's disease).
Impaired bladder or sphincter action.
Urethral carbuncle.

Chronic fibrosis posttrauma.
Radiation therapy.
Prostatitis.
Urethritis (gonococcal, *Chlamydiae*).
Behçet's syndrome.
Stevens-Johnson syndrome.

EDEMA, GENERALIZED
ICD-9CM # 782.3 EDEMA NOS

Congestive heart failure (CHF).
Cirrhosis.
Nephrotic syndrome.
Idiopathic.
Acute nephritic syndrome.
Myxedema.
Medications (NSAIDs, estrogens, vasodilators).

EDEMA, LEG, UNILATERAL[14]
ICD-9CM # 782.3

WITH PAIN
DVT.
Postphlebitic syndrome.
Popliteal cyst rupture.
Gastrocnemius rupture.
Cellulitis.
Psoas or other abscess.

WITHOUT PAIN
DVT.
Postphlebitic syndrome.
Other venous insufficiency (after saphenous vein harvest, varicosities).
Lymphatic obstruction/lymphedema (carcinoma, lymphoma, sarcoidosis, filariasis, retroperitoneal fibrosis).

EDEMA OF LOWER EXTREMITIES
ICD-9CM # 782.3

CHF (right-sided).
Hepatic cirrhosis.
Nephrosis.
Myxedema.
Lymphedema.
Abdominal mass: neoplasm, cyst.
Venous compression from abdominal aneurysm.
Varicose veins.
Bilateral cellulitis.
Bilateral thrombophlebitis.
Vena cava thrombosis, venous thrombosis.
Retroperitoneal fibrosis.

EPILEPSY
ICD-9CM # 345.9 EPILEPSY NOS

Psychogenic spells.
Transient ischemic attack.
Hypoglycemia.
Syncope.
Narcolepsy.
Migraine.
Paroxysmal vertigo.
Arrhythmias.
Drug reaction.

EPISTAXIS
ICD-9CM # 784.7

Trauma.
Medications (nasal sprays, NSAIDs, anticoagulants, antiplatelets).
Nasal polyps.
Cocaine use.
Coagulopathy (hemophilia, liver disease, DIC, thrombocytopenia).
Systemic disorders (hypertension, uremia).
Infections.
Anatomic malformations.
Rhinitis.
Nasal polyps.
Local neoplasms (benign and malignant).
Desiccation.
Foreign body.

ERECTILE DYSFUNCTION, ORGANIC[18]
ICD-9CM # 607.84

Neurogenic abnormalities: somatic nerve neuropathy, central nervous system abnormalities.
Psychogenic causes: depression, performance anxiety, marital conflict.
Endocrine causes: hyperprolactinemia, hypogonadotropic hypogonadism, testicular failure, estrogen excess.
Trauma: pelvic fracture, prostate surgery, penile fracture.
Systemic disease: diabetes mellitus, renal failure, hepatic cirrhosis.
Medications: diuretics, antidepressants, H2 blockers, exogenous hormones, alcohol, antihypertensives, nicotine abuse, finasteride, etc.
Structural abnormalities: Peyronie's disease.

EYE PAIN
ICD-9CM # 379.91

Foreign body.
Herpes zoster.
Trauma.
Conjunctivitis.
Iritis.
Iridocyclitis.
Uveitis.
Blepharitis.
Ingrown lashes.
Orbital or periorbital cellulitis/abscess.
Sinusitis.
Headache.
Glaucoma.
Inflammation of lacrimal gland.
Tic douloureux.
Cerebral aneurysm.
Cerebral neoplasm.
Entropion.
Retrobulbar neuritis.
UV light.
Dry eyes.
Irritation or inflammation from eyedrops, dust, cosmetics, etc.

FACIAL PAIN
ICD-9CM # 784.0

Infection, abscess.
Postherpetic neuralgia.
Trauma, posttraumatic neuralgia.

Tic douloureux.
Cluster headache, "lower-half headache."
Geniculate neuralgia.
Anxiety, somatization syndrome.
Glossopharyngeal neuralgia.
Carotidynia.

FACIAL PARALYSIS[16]
ICD-9CM # 351.0 FACIAL (7TH NERVE) PALSY

INFECTION
Bacterial: otitis media, mastoiditis, meningitis, Lyme disease.
Viral: herpes zoster, mononucleosis, varicella, rubella, mumps, Bell's palsy.
Mycobacterial: TB, meningitis, leprosy.
Miscellaneous: syphilis, malaria.

TRAUMA
Temporal bone fracture, facial laceration.
Surgery.

NEOPLASM
Malignant: squamous cell carcinoma, basal cell and adenocystic tumors, leukemia, parotid neoplasms, metastic tumors.
Benign: facial nerve neuroma, vestibular schwannoma, cholesteatoma.

IMMUNOLOGIC
Guillain-Barré syndrome, periarteritis nodosa.
Reaction to tetanus antiserum.

METABOLIC
Hypothyroidism.
DM.

FAILURE TO THRIVE
ICD-9CM # 783.4

MALABSORPTION
Pancreatic insufficiency (chronic pancreatitis).
Short bowel syndrome.
Celiac disease.
Other intestinal mucosal abnormalities.

INSUFFICIENT CALORIC INTAKE
Food shortage (poverty).
Depression.
Dementia.
Functional (inability to shop or prepare food).

GASTROINTESTINAL IMPEDIMENTS TO TRANSIT
Oropharyngeal dysphagia (SP stroke).
Esophageal dysphagia (cancer, stricture).
Gastric cancer.
Pyloric stenosis.
Bowel obstruction.

INCREASED NEEDS
Addison's Disease.
Hyperthyroidism.
CHF.
Malignancy.
Renal or hepatic disease.
COPD.
Diabetes mellitus.

CHRONIC INFECTIONS

Tuberculosis.
HIV.

FATIGUE

ICD-9CM # 780.7 FATIGUE NOS
       300.5 FATIGUE PSYCHOGENIC
       780.7 CHRONIC FATIGUE SYNDROME

Depression.
Anxiety, emotional stress.
Inadequate sleep.
Prolonged physical activity.
Anemia.
Hypothyroidism.
Medications (β-blockers, anxiolytics, antidepressants, sedating antihistamines, clonidine, methyldopa).
Viral or bacterial infections.
Sleep apnea syndrome.
Dieting.
Renal failure, CHF, COPD, liver disease.

FATTY LIVER

ICD-9CM # 571.8

Obesity.
Alcohol abuse.
Diabetes mellitus.
Medications (tetracycline, valproic acid, glucocorticoids, amiodarone, estrogen, methotrexate).
Reye's syndrome.
Wilson's disease.
Nonalcoholic steatosis and steatohepatitis.

FLATULENCE AND BLOATING[19]

ICD-9CM # 787.3

Ingestion of nonabsorbable carbohydrates.
Ingestion of carbonated beverages.
Malabsorption: pancreatic insufficiency, biliary disease, celiac disease, bacterial overgrowth in small intestine.
Lactase deficiency.
Irritable bowel syndrome.
Anxiety disorders.
Food poisoning, giardiasis.

GAIT ABNORMALITY

ICD-9CM # 781.2 GAIT ABNORMALITY

Parkinsonism.
Degenerative joint disease (hips, back, knees).
Multiple sclerosis.
Trauma, foot pain.
CVA.
Cerebellar lesions.
Infections (tabes, encephalitis, meningitis).
Sensory ataxia.
Dystonia, cerebral palsy, neuromuscular disorders.
Metabolic abnormalities.

GOITER

ICD-9CM # 240.9 GOITER, UNSPECIFIED
       241.9 GOITER, ADENOMATOUS
       246.1 GOITER, CONGENITAL
       240.9 GOITER, NONTOXIC DIFFUSE
       241.1 GOITER, NONTOXIC MULTINODULAR
       240.0 SIMPLE GOITER
       242.1 THYROTOXIC GOITER

Thyroiditis.
Toxic multinodular goiter.
Graves' disease.
Medications (PTU, methimazole, sulfonamides, sulfonylureas, ethionamide, amiodarone, lithium, etc.).
Iodine deficiency.
Sarcoidosis, amyloidosis.
Defective thyroid hormone synthesis.
Resistance to thyroid hormone.

GYNECOMASTIA

ICD-9CM # 611.1 GYNECOMASTIA, NONPUERPERAL

Physiologic (aging).
Drugs (estrogen and estrogen precursors, digitalis, testosterone and exogenous androgens, cimetidine, spironolactone, ketoconazole, amiodarone, ACE inhibitors, isoniazid, phenytoin, methyldopa, metoclopramide, phenothiazine).
Increased prolactin level (prolactinoma).
Liver disease.
Adrenal disease.
Thyrotoxicosis.
Increased estrogen production (hCG-producing tumor, testicular tumor, bronchogenic carcinoma).
Secondary hypogonadism.
Primary gonadal failure (trauma, castration, viral orchitis, granulomatous disease).
Defects in androgen synthesis.
Testosterone deficiency.
Klinefelter's syndrome.

HALITOSIS

ICD-9CM # 784.9

Tobacco use.
Alcohol use.
Dry mouth (mouth breathing, inadequate fluid intake).
Foods (onion, garlic, meats, nuts).
Disease of mouth or nose (infections, cancer, inflammation).
Medications (antihistamines, antidepressants).
Systemic disorders (diabetes, uremia).
GI disorders (esophageal diverticula, hiatal hernia, GERD, achalasia).
Sinusitis.
Pulmonary disorders (bronchiectasis, pneumonia, neoplasms, TB).

HEADACHE[6]

ICD-9CM # 784.0 HEADACHE NOS
       307.81 HEADACHE, TENSION
       346.2 HEADACHE, CLUSTER
       346.9 HEADACHE, MIGRAINE
       784.0 HEADACHE, VASCULAR

Vascular: migraine, cluster headaches, temporal arteritis, hypertension, cavernous sinus thrombosis.
Musculoskeletal: neck and shoulder muscle contraction, strain of extraocular and/or intraocular muscles, cervical spondylosis, temporomandibular arthritis.

Infections: meningitis, encephalitis, brain abscess, sepsis, sinusitis, osteomyelitis, parotitis, mastoiditis.
Cerebral neoplasm.
Subdural hematoma.
Cerebral hemorrhage/infarct.
Normal pressure hydrocephalus (NPH).
Postlumbar puncture.
Cerebral aneurysm, arteriovenous malformations.
Posttrauma.
Dental problems: abscess, periodontitis, poorly fitting dentures.
Trigeminal neuralgia, glossopharyngeal neuralgia.
Otitis and other ear diseases.
Glaucoma and other eye diseases.
Metabolic: uremia, carbon monoxide inhalation, hypoxia.
Pheochromocytoma, hypoglycemia, hypothyroidism.
Effort induced: benign exertional headache, cough, headache, coital cephalalgia.
Drugs: alcohol, nitrates, histamine antagonists.
Paget's disease of the skull.
Emotional, psychiatric.

HEARING LOSS, ACUTE[14]

ICD-9CM # 388.2

Infectious: mumps, measles, influenza, herpes simplex, herpes zoster, CMV, mononucleosis, syphilis.
Vascular: macroglobulinemia, sickle cell disease, Berger's disease, leukemia, polycythemia, fat emboli, hypercoagulable states.
Metabolic: diabetes, hyperlipoproteinemia.
Conductive: cerumen impaction, foreign bodies, otitis media, otitis externa, barotrauma, trauma.
Medications: aminoglycosides, loop diuretics, antineoplastics, salicylates, vancomycin.
Neoplasm: acoustic neuroma, metastatic neoplasm.

HEARTBURN AND INDIGESTION[19]

ICD-9CM # 787.1 HEARTBURN
536.8 INDIGESTION

Reflux esophagitis.
Gastritis.
Nonulcer dyspepsia.
Functional GI disorder (anxiety disorder, social/environmental stresses).
Excessive intestinal gas (ingestion of flatulogenic foods, GI stasis, constipation).
Gas entrapment (hepatitis or splenic flexure syndrome).
Neoplasm (adenocarcinoma of stomach or esophagus, lymphoma).
Gallbladder disease.

HEEL PAIN, PLANTAR[13]

ICD-9CM # 729.5

SKIN

Keratoses.
Verruca.
Ulcer.
Fissure.

CONNECTIVE TISSUE

Fat
Atrophy.
Panniculitis.
Dense connective tissue
Inflammatory fasciitis.
Fibromatosis.

Enthesopathy.
Bursitis.
Bone (calcaneus)
Stress fracture.
Paget's disease.
Benign bone cyst/tumor.
Malignant bone tumor.
Metabolic bone disease (osteopenia).
Nerve
Tarsal tunnel.
Plantar nerve entrapment.
S1 nerve root radiculopathy.
Painful peripheral neuropathy.

INFECTION

Dermatomycoses.
Acute osteomyelitis.
Plantar abscess.

MISCELLANEOUS

Foreign body.
Nonunion calcaneus fracture.
Psychogenic.
Idiopathic.

HEMATURIA

ICD-9CM # 599.7 HEMATURIA, BENIGN (ESSENTIAL)

Use the mnemonic TICS:
T (trauma): blow to kidney, insertion of Foley catheter or foreign body in urethra, prolonged and severe exercise, very rapid emptying of overdistended bladder.
(tumor): hypernephroma, papillary carcinoma of the bladder, prostatic and urethral neoplasms.
(toxins): turpentine, phenols, sulfonamides and other antibiotics, cyclophosphamide, NSAIDs.
I (infections): glomerulonephritis, TB, cystitis, prostatitis, urethritis, Schistosoma haematobium, yellow fever, blackwater fever.
(inflammatory processes): Goodpasture's syndrome, periarteritis, postirradiation.
C (calculi): renal, ureteral, bladder, urethra.
(cysts): simple cysts, polycystic disease.
(congenital anomalies): hemangiomas, aneurysms, AVM.
S (surgery): invasive procedures, prostatic resection, cystoscopy.
(sickle cell disease and other hematologic disturbances): hemophilia, thrombocytopenia, anticoagulants.
(somewhere else): bleeding genitals, factitious (drug addicts).

HEMATURIA, CAUSED BY AGE AND SEX

ICD-9CM # 599.7 HEMATURIA BENIGN (ESSENTIAL)
OTHER CODES FOR HEMATURIA VARY
WITH CAUSE OF HEMATURIA

60 YR AND OLDER (WOMEN)
Acute urinary tract infection.
Bladder cancer.
Vaginal trauma or irritation.
Urolithiasis.

60 YR AND OLDER (MEN)
Acute urinary tract infection.
Benign prostatic hyperplasia.
Bladder cancer.
Urolithiasis.
Trauma.

HEMIPARESIS/HEMIPLEGIA

ICD-9CM # 436.0 ACQUIRED DUE TO ACUTE CVA, FLACCID
436.1 ACQUIRED DUE TO CVA, ACUTE, SPASTIC

CVA.
Transient ischemic attack.
Cerebral neoplasm.
Multiple sclerosis or other demyelinating disorder.
CNS infection.
Migraine.
Hypoglycemia.
Subdural hematoma.
Vasculitis.
Todd's paralysis.
Epidural hematoma.
Metabolic (hyperosmolar state, electrolyte imbalance).
Psychiatric disorders.
Congenital disorders.
Leukodystrophies.

HEMOPTYSIS

ICD-9CM # 786.3

CARDIOVASCULAR

Pulmonary embolism/infarction.
Left ventricular failure.
Mitral stenosis.
AV fistula.
Severe hypertension.
Erosion of aortic aneurysm.

PULMONARY

Neoplasm (primary or metastatic).
Infection.
Pneumonia: *Streptococcus pneumoniae*, *Klebsiella pneumoniae*, *Staphylococcus aureus*, *Legionella pneumophila*.
Bronchiectasis.
Abscess.
TB.
Bronchitis.
Fungal infections (aspergillosis, coccidioidomycosis).
Parasitic infections (amebiasis, ascariasis, paragonimiasis).
Vasculitis: Wegener's granulomatosis, Churg-Strauss syndrome, Henoch-Schönlein purpura.
Goodpasture's syndrome.
Trauma (needle biopsy, foreign body, right-sided heart catheterization, prolonged and severe cough).
Bullous emphysema.
Pulmonary sequestration.
Pulmonary AV fistula.
SLE.
Idiopathic pulmonary hemosiderosis.
Drugs: aspirin, anticoagulants, penicillamine.
Pulmonary hypertension.
Mediastinal fibrosis.

OTHER

Epistaxis, trauma.
Laryngeal bleeding (laryngitis, laryngeal neoplasm).
Hematologic disorders (clotting abnormalities, DIC, thrombocytopenia).

HICCUPS[11]

ICD-9CM # 786.8

TRANSIENT HICCUPS

Sudden excitement, emotion.
Gastric distention.
Esophageal obstruction.
Alcohol ingestion.
Sudden change in temperature.

PERSISTENT OR CHRONIC HICCUPS

Toxic/metabolic: uremia, DM, hyperventilation, hypocalcemia, hypokalemia, hyponatremia, gout, fever.
Drugs: benzodiazepines, steroids, α-methyldopa, barbiturates.
Surgery/general anesthesia.
Thoracic/diaphragmatic disorders: pneumonia, lung cancer, asthma, pleuritis, pericarditis, myocardial infarction, aortic aneurysm, esophagitis, esophageal obstruction, diaphragmatic hernia or irritation.
Abdominal disorders: gastric ulcer or cancer, hepatobiliary or pancreatic disease, IBD, bowel obstruction, intraabdominal or subphrenic abscess, prostatic infection or cancer.
Central nervous system disorders: traumatic, infectious, vascular, structural.
Ear, nose, and throat disorders: pharyngitis, laryngitis, tumor, irritation of auditory canal.
Psychogenic disorders.
Idiopathic disorders.

HOARSENESS

ICD-9CM # 784.49

Allergic rhinitis.
Infections (laryngitis, epiglottitis, tracheitis, croup).
Vocal cord polyps.
Voice strain.
Irritants (tobacco smoke).
Vocal cord trauma (intubation, surgery).
Neoplastic involvement of vocal cord (primary or metastatic).
Neurologic abnormalities (multiple sclerosis, ALS, parkinsonism).
Endocrine abnormalities (puberty, menopause, hypothyroidism).
Other (laryngeal webs or cysts, psychogenic, muscle tension abnormalities).

HYPERCALCEMIA

ICD-9CM # 275.42 HYPERCALCEMIA DISORDER

Malignancy: increased bone resorption via osteoclast-activating factors, secretion of PTH-like substances, prostaglandin E2, direct erosion by tumor cells, transforming growth factors, colony-stimulating activity. Hypercalcemia is common in the following neoplasms:
Solid tumors: breast, lung, pancreas, kidneys, ovary.
Hematologic cancers: myeloma, lymphosarcoma, adult.
T-cell lymphoma, Burkitt's lymphoma.
Hyperparathyroidism: increased bone resorption, GI absorption, and renal absorption; etiology:
Parathyroid hyperplasia, adenoma.
Hyperparathyroidism or renal failure with secondary hyperparathyroidism.
Granulomatous disorders: increased GI absorption (e.g., sarcoidosis).

Paget's disease: increased bone resorption, seen only during periods of immobilization.

Vitamin D intoxication, milk-alkali syndrome; increased GI absorption.

Thiazides: increased renal absorption.

Other causes: familial hypocalciuric hypercalcemia, thyrotoxicosis, adrenal insufficiency, prolonged immobilization, vitamin A intoxication, recovery from acute renal failure, lithium administration, pheochromocytoma, disseminated SLE.

HYPERHIDROSIS[3]

ICD-9CM # 780.8 HYPERHIDROSIS

CORTICAL

Emotional.
Familial dysautonomia.
Congenital ichthyosiform erythroderma.
Epidermolysis bullosa.
Nail-patella syndrome.
Jadassohn-Lewandowsky syndrome.
Pachyonychia congenita.
Palmoplantar keratoderma.

HYPOTHALAMIC

Drugs
Antipyretics.
Emetics.
Insulin.
Meperidine.
Exercise
Infection
Defervescence.
Chronic illness.
Metabolic
Debility.
Diabetes mellitus.
Hyperpituitarism.
Hyperthyroidism.
Hypoglycemia.
Obesity.
Porphyria.
Cardiovascular
Heart failure.
Shock.
Vasomotor
Cold injury.
Raynaud's phenomenon.
Rheumatoid arthritis.
Neurologic
Abscess.
Familial dysautonomia.
Postencephalitic.
Tumor.
Miscellaneous
Chédiak-Higashi syndrome.
Compensatory.
Phenylketonuria.
Pheochromocytoma.
Vitiligo.
Medullary
Physiologic gustatory sweating.
Encephalitis.
Granulosis rubra nasi.
Syringomyelia.
Thoracic sympathetic trunk injury.

Spinal
Cord transection.
Syringomyelia.
Changes in blood flow
Mallucci syndrome.
Arteriovenous fistula.
Klippel-Trenaunay syndrome.
Glomus tumor.
Blue rubber bleb nevus syndrome.

HYPERKALEMIA

ICD-9CM # 276.7

Pseudohyperkalemia.
   Hemolyzed specimen.
   Severe thrombocytosis (platelet count >1 million/ml).
   Severe leukocytosis (white blood cell count >100,000/ml).
   Fist clenching during phlebotomy.
Excessive potassium intake (often in setting of impaired excretion).
   Potassium replacement therapy.
   High-potassium diet.
   Salt substitutes with potassium.
   Potassium salts of antibiotics.
Decreased renal excretion.
   Potassium-sparing diuretics (e.g., spironolactone, triamterene, amiloride).
   Renal insufficiency.
   Mineralocorticoid deficiency.
   Hyporeninemic hypoaldosteronism (DM).
   Tubular unresponsiveness to aldosterone (e.g., SLE, multiple myeloma, sickle cell disease).
   Type 4 RTA.
   ACE inhibitors.
   Heparin administration.
   NSAIDs.
   Trimethoprim-sulfamethoxazole.
   β-Blockers.
   Pentamidine.
Redistribution (excessive cellular release).
   Acidemia (each 0.1 decrease in pH increases the serum potassium by 0.4 to 0.6 mEq/L). Lactic acidosis and ketoacidosis cause minimal redistribution.
   Insulin deficiency.
   Drugs (e.g., succinylcholine, markedly increased digitalis level, arginine, β-adrenergic blockers).
   Hypertonicity.
   Hemolysis.
   Tissue necrosis, rhabdomyolysis, burns.
   Hyperkalemic periodic paralysis.

HYPOCALCEMIA

ICD-9CM # 275.41

Renal insufficiency: hypocalcemia caused by:
   Increased calcium deposits in bone and soft tissue secondary to increased serum $PO_4$23 level.
   Decreased production of 1,25-dihydroxyvitamin D.
   Excessive loss of 25-OHD (nephrotic syndrome).
Hypoalbuminemia: each decrease in serum albumin (g/L) will decrease serum calcium by 0.8 mg/dl but will not change free (ionized) calcium.
Vitamin D deficiency:
   Malabsorption (most common cause).
   Inadequate intake.
   Low sun exposure.

Section II

DIFFERENTIAL DIAGNOSIS

Decreased production of 1,25-dihydroxyvitamin D (vitamin D-dependent rickets, renal failure).

Decreased production of 25-OHD (parenchymal liver disease).

Accelerated 25-OHD catabolism (phenytoin, phenobarbital).

End-organ resistance to 1,25-dihydroxyvitamin D.

Hypomagnesemia: hypocalcemia caused by:

Decreased PTH secretion.

Inhibition of PTH effect on bone.

Pancreatitis, hyperphosphatemia, osteoblastic metastases: hypocalcemia is secondary to increased calcium deposits (bone, abdomen).

Pseudohypoparathyroidism (PHP): autosomal recessive disorder characterized by short stature, shortening of metacarpal bones, obesity, and mental retardation; the hypocalcemia is secondary to congenital end-organ resistance to PTH.

Idiopathic hypoparathyroidism, surgical removal of parathyroids (e.g., neck surgery).

"Hungry bones syndrome": rapid transfer of calcium from plasma into bones after removal of a parathyroid tumor.

Sepsis.

Massive blood transfusion (as a result of EDTA in blood).

HYPOCAPNIA

ICD-9CM # 786.01

Hyperventilation.

Pneumonia, pneumonitis.

Fever, sepsis.

Medications (salicylates, β-adrenergic agonists, progesterone, methylxanthines).

Pulmonary disease (asthma, interstitial fibrosis).

Pulmonary embolism.

Hepatic failure.

Metabolic acidosis.

High altitude.

CHF.

Pain.

CNS lesions.

HYPOKALEMIA

ICD-9CM # 276.8

Cellular shift (redistribution) and undetermined mechanisms.

Alkalosis (each 0.1 increase in pH decreases serum potassium by 0.4 to 0.6 mEq/L).

Insulin administration.

Vitamin B_{12} therapy for megaloblastic anemias, acute leukemias.

Hypokalemic periodic paralysis: rare familial disorder manifested by recurrent attacks of flaccid paralysis and hypokalemia.

β-Adrenergic agonists (e.g., terbutaline), decongestants, bronchodilators, theophylline, caffeine.

Barium poisoning, toluene intoxication, verapamil intoxication, chloroquine intoxication.

Correction of digoxin intoxication with digoxin antibody fragments (Digibind).

Increased renal excretion.

Drugs:

Diuretics, including carbonic anhydrase inhibitors (e.g., acetazolamide).

Amphotericin B.

High-dose sodium penicillin, nafcillin, ampicillin, or carbenicillin.

Cisplatin.

Aminoglycosides.

Corticosteroids, mineralocorticoids.

Foscarnet sodium.

RTA: distal (type 1) or proximal (type 2).

Diabetic ketoacidosis (DKA), ureteroenterostomy.

Magnesium deficiency.

Postobstruction diuresis, diuretic phase of ATN.

Osmotic diuresis (e.g., mannitol).

Bartter's syndrome: hyperplasia of juxtaglomerular cells leading to increased renin and aldosterone, metabolic alkalosis, hypokalemia, muscle weakness, and tetany.

Increased mineralocorticoid activity (primary or secondary aldosteronism), Cushing's syndrome.

Chronic metabolic alkalosis from loss of gastric fluid (increased renal potassium secretion).

GI loss.

Vomiting, nasogastric suction.

Diarrhea.

Laxative abuse.

Villous adenoma.

Fistulas.

Inadequate dietary intake (e.g., anorexia nervosa).

Cutaneous loss (excessive sweating).

High dietary sodium intake, excessive use of licorice.

HYPOMAGNESEMIA

ICD-9CM # 275.2

GI and nutritional

Defective GI absorption (malabsorption).

Inadequate dietary intake (e.g., alcoholics).

Parenteral therapy without magnesium.

Chronic diarrhea, villous adenoma, prolonged nasogastric suction, fistulas (small bowel, biliary).

Excessive renal losses

Diuretics.

RTA.

Diuretic phase of ATN.

Endocrine disturbances (DKA, hyperaldosteronism, hyperthyroidism, hyperparathyroidism), SIADH, Bartter's syndrome, hypercalciuria, hypokalemia.

Cisplatin, alcohol, cyclosporine, digoxin, pentamidine, mannitol, amphotericin B, foscarnet, methotrexate.

Antibiotics (gentamicin, ticarcillin, carbenicillin).

Redistribution: hypoalbuminemia, cirrhosis, administration of insulin and glucose, theophylline, epinephrine, acute pancreatitis, cardiopulmonary bypass.

Miscellaneous: sweating, burns, prolonged exercise, lactation, "hungry-bones" syndrome.

HYPOTENSION, POSTURAL

ICD-9CM # 458.0

Antihypertensive medications (especially α-blockers, diuretics, ACE inhibitors).

Volume depletion (hemorrhage, dehydration).

Impaired cardiac output (constrictive pericarditis, aortic stenosis).

Peripheral autonomic dysfunction (DM, Guillain-Barré).

Idiopathic orthostatic hypotension.

Central autonomic dysfunction (Shy-Drager syndrome).

Peripheral venous disease.

Adrenal insufficiency.

IMPOTENCE[15]

ICD-9CM # 302.72 PSYCHOSEXUAL
607.84 ORGANIC
997.99 ORGANIC POSTPROSTATECTOMY

Psychogenic.
Endocrine: hyperprolactinemia, DM, Cushing's syndrome, hypothyroidism or hyperthyroidism, abnormality of hypothalamic-pituitary-testicular axis.
Vascular: arterial insufficiency, venous leakage, AV malformation, local trauma.
Medications.
Neurogenic: autonomic or sensory neuropathy, spinal cord trauma or tumor, CVA, multiple sclerosis, temporal lobe epilepsy.
Systemic illness: renal failure, COPD, cirrhosis of liver, myotonic dystrophy.
Peyronie's disease.
Prostatectomy.

INSOMNIA[19]

ICD-9CM # 780.52 INSOMNIA NOS
307.42 INSOMNIA, CHRONIC ASSOCIATED
WITH ANXIETY OR DEPRESSION
780.51 INSOMNIA WITH SLEEP APNEA

Anxiety disorder, psychophysiologic insomnia.
Depression.
Drugs (e.g., caffeine, amphetamines, cocaine), hypnotic-dependent sleep disorder.
Pain, fibromyalgia.
Inadequate sleep hygiene.
Restless leg syndrome.
Obstructive sleep apnea.
Sleep bruxism.
Medical illness (e.g., GERD, sleep-related asthma, parkinsonism and movement disorders).
Narcolepsy.
Other: periodic leg movement of sleep, central sleep apnea, REM behavioral disorder.

INTESTINAL PSEUDOOBSTRUCTION[22]

ICD-9CM # 560.1 ADYNAMIC INTESTINAL OBSTRUCTION
564.9 INTESTINAL DISORDER, FUNCTIONAL

"PRIMARY" (IDIOPATHIC INTESTINAL PSEUDOOBSTRUCTION)

Hollow visceral myopathy:
  Familial.
  Sporadic.
Neuropathic:
  Abnormal myenteric plexus.
  Normal myenteric plexus.

SECONDARY

Scleroderma.
Myxedema.
Amyloidosis.
Muscular dystrophy.
Hypokalemia.
Chronic renal failure.
Diabetes mellitus.
Drug toxicity caused by:
  Anticholinergics.
  Opiate narcotics.
Ogilvie's syndrome.

ISCHEMIC COLITIS, NONOCCLUSIVE[11]

ICD-9CM # 557.1

ACUTE DIMINUTION OF COLONIC INTRAMURAL BLOOD FLOW

Small vessel obstruction
Collagen-vascular disease.
Vasculitis, diabetes.
Nonocclusive hypoperfusion
Hemorrhage.
CHF, MI, arrhythmias.
Sepsis.
Vasoconstricting agents: vasopressin, ergot.
Increased viscosity: polycythemia, sickle cell disease, thrombocytosis.

INCREASED DEMAND ON MARGINAL BLOOD FLOW

Increased motility
Mass lesion, stricture.
Constipation.
Increased intraluminal pressure
Bowel obstruction.
Colonoscopy.
Barium enema.

JOINT PAIN, ANTERIOR HIP, MEDIAL THIGH, KNEE[16]

ICD-9CM # 719.4 ADD 5TH DIGIT
0 SITE NOS
1 SHOULDER REGION
2 UPPER ARM (ELBOW, HUMERUS)
3 FOREARM (RADIUS, WRIST, ULNA)
4 HAND
5 PELVIC REGION AND THIGH
6 LOWER LEG (FIBULA, PATELLA, TIBIA)
7 ANKLE AND/OR FOOT

ACUTE

Acute rheumatic fever.
Adductor muscle strain.
Avascular necrosis.
Crystal arthritis.
Femoral artery (pseudo) aneurysm.
Fracture (femoral neck or intertrochanteric).
Hemarthrosis.
Hernia.
Herpes zoster.
Iliopectineal bursitis.
Iliopsoas tendinitis.
Inguinal lymphadenitis.
Osteomalacia.
Painful transient osteoporosis of hip.
Septic arthritis.

SUBACUTE AND CHRONIC

Adductory muscle strain.
Amyloidosis.
Acute rheumatic fever.
Femoral artery aneurysm.
Hernia (inguinal or femoral).
Iliopectineal bursitis.
Iliopsoas tendinitis.
Inguinal lymphadenopathy.
Osteochondromatosis.
Osteomyelitis.
Osteitis deformans (Paget's disease).
Osteomalacia (pseudofracture).

Postherpetic neuralgia.
Sterile synovitis (e.g., rheumatoid arthritis, psoriatic, systemic lupus erythematosus).

JOINT PAIN, HIP, LATERAL THIGH[16]

ICD-9CM # 959.6 HIP INJURY
719.95 HIP JOINT DISORDER
843.9 HIP STRAIN

ACUTE

Herpes zoster.
Iliotibial tendinitis.
Impacted fracture of femoral neck.
Lateral femoral cutaneous neuropathy (meralgia paresthetica).
Radiculopathy: L4-5.
Trochanteric avulsion fracture (greater trochanter).
Trochanteric bursitis.
Trochanteric fracture.

SUBACUTE AND CHRONIC

Lateral femoral cutaneous neuropathy (meralgia paresthetica).
Osteomyelitis.
Postherpetic neuralgia.
Radiculopathy: L4-5.
Tumors.

JOINT PAIN, POSTERIOR HIPS, THIGH, BUTTOCKS[16]

ICD-9CM # 719.4 ADD 5TH DIGIT
0 SITE NOS
1 SHOULDER REGION
2 UPPER ARM (ELBOW, HUMERUS)
3 FOREARM (RADIUS, WRIST, ULNA)
4 HAND
5 PELVIC REGION AND THIGH
6 LOWER LEG (FIBULA, PATELLA, TIBIA)
7 ANKLE AND/OR FOOT

ACUTE

Gluteal muscle strain.
Herpes zoster.
Ischial bursitis.
Ischial or sacral fracture.
Osteomalacia (pseudofracture).
Sciatic neuropathy.
Radiculopathy: L5-S1.

SUBACUTE AND CHRONIC

Gluteal muscle strain.
Ischial bursitis.
Lumbar spinal stenosis.
Osteoarthritis of hip.
Osteitis deformans (Paget's disease).
Osteomyelitis.
Osteochondromatosis.
Osteomalacia (pseudofracture).
Postherpetic neuralgia.
Radiculopathy: L5-S1.
Tumors.

JOINT SWELLING

ICD-9CM # 719.0 ADD 5TH DIGIT
0 SITE NOS
1 SHOULDER REGION
2 UPPER ARM (ELBOW, HUMERUS)
3 FOREARM (RADIUS, WRIST, ULNA)
4 HAND
5 PELVIC REGION AND THIGH
6 LOWER LEG (FIBULA, PATELLA, TIBIA)
7 ANKLE AND/OR FOOT

Trauma.
Osteoarthritis.
Gout.
Pyogenic arthritis.
Pseudogout.
Rheumatoid arthritis.
Viral syndrome.

KNEE PAIN[16]

ICD-9CM # 844.1 COLLATERAL LIGAMENT SPRAIN,
MEDIAL
844.2 CRUCIATE LIGAMENT SPRAIN
716.96 KNEE INFLAMMATION
959.7 KNEE INJURY
718.86 KNEE INSTABILITY
836.1 LATERAL MENISCUS TEAR
836.0 MEDIAL MENISCUS TEAR
844.8 PATELLAR SPRAIN
719.56 KNEE STIFFNESS
719.06 KNEE SWELLING

DIFFUSE

Articular.
Anterior.
Prepatellar bursitis.
Patellar tendon enthesopathy.
Chondromalacia patellae.
Patellofemoral osteoarthritis.
Cruciate ligament injury.
Medial plica syndrome.

MEDIAL

Anserine bursitis.
Spontaneous osteonecrosis.
Osteoarthritis.
Medial meniscal tear.
Medial collateral ligament bursitis.
Referred pain from hip and L3.
Fibromyalgia.

LATERAL

Iliotibial band syndrome.
Meniscal cyst.
Lateral meniscal tear.
Collateral ligament.
Peroneal tenosynovitis.

POSTERIOR

Popliteal cyst (Baker's cyst).
Tendinitis.
Aneurysms, ganglions, sarcoma.

LEG CRAMPS, NOCTURNAL
ICD-9CM # 729.82 MUSCLE CRAMPS

Diabetic neuropathy.
Medications.
Electrolyte abnormalities (hypokalemia, hyponatremia, hypocalcemia, hyperkalemia, hypophosphatemia).
Respiratory alkalosis.
Uremia.
Hemodialysis.
Peripheral nerve injury.
ALS.
Alcohol use.
Heat cramps.
Vitamin B_{12} deficiency.
Hyperthyroidism.
Contractures.
DVT.
Hypoglycemia.
Peripheral vascular insufficiency.
Baker cyst.

LEG PAIN WITH EXERCISE
ICD-9CM # 729.82 MUSCLE CRAMPS

Shin splints.
Arteriosclerosis obliterans.
Neurogenic (spinal cord compression or ischemia).
Venous claudication.
Popliteal cyst.
DVT.
Thromboangiitis obliterans.
Adventitial cysts.
Popliteal artery entrapment syndrome.
McArdle's syndrome.

LEG ULCERS[16]
ICD-9CM # 440.23 LOWER LIMB, ARTERIOSCLEROTIC
707.1 LOWER LIMB, CHRONIC
707.1 LOWER LIMB, NEUROGENIC
250.70 LOWER LIMB, CHRONIC DIABETES
MELLITUS TYPE II
250.71 LOWER LIMB, CHRONIC, DIABETES
MELLITUS TYPE I

VASCULAR

Arterial: arteriosclerosis, thromboangiitis obliterans, AV malformation, cholesterol emboli.
Venous: superficial varicosities, incompetent perforators, DVT, lymphatic abnormalities.

VASCULITIS HEMATOLOGIC

Sickle cell anemia, thalassemia, polycythemia vera, leukemia, cold agglutinin disease.
Macroglobulinemia, protein C and protein S deficiency, cryoglobulinemia, lupus anticoagulant, antiphospholipid syndrome.

INFECTIOUS

Fungus: blastomycosis, coccidioidomycosis, histoplasmosis, sporotrichosis.
Bacterial: furuncle, ecthyma, septic emboli.
Protozoal: leishmaniasis.

METABOLIC

Necrobiosis lipoidica diabeticorum.
Localized bullous pemphigoid.
Gout, calcinosis cutis, Gaucher's disease.

TUMORS

Basal cell carcinoma, squamous cell carcinoma, melanoma.
Mycosis fungoides, Kaposi's sarcoma, metastatic neoplasms.

TRAUMA

Pressure ulcer.
Burns, cold injury, radiation dermatitis.
Insect bites.
Factitial, excessive pressure.

NEUROPATHIC

Diabetic trophic ulcers.
Tabes dorsalis, syringomyelia.

DRUGS

Warfarin, IV colchicine extravasation, methotrexate, halogens, ergotism, hydroxyurea.

PANNICULITIS

Weber-Christian disease.
Pancreatic fat necrosis, alpha-antitrypsinase deficiency.

LYMPHADENOPATHY[7]
ICD-9CM # 785.6

GENERALIZED

AIDS.
Lymphoma: Hodgkin's disease, non-Hodgkin's lymphoma.
Leukemias, reticuloendotheliosis.
Viral infections (infectious mononucleosis, CMV).
Diffuse skin infection: generalized furunculosis, multiple tick bites.
Parasitic infections: toxoplasmosis, filariasis, leishmaniasis, Chagas' disease.
Serum sickness.
Collagen vascular diseases (RA, SLE).
Dengue (arbovirus infection).
Sarcoidosis and other granulomatous diseases.
Drugs: INH, hydantoin derivatives, antithyroid and antileprosy drugs.
Secondary syphilis.
Hyperthyroidism, lipid-storage diseases.

LOCALIZED

Cervical nodes
Infections of the head, neck, ears, sinuses, scalp, pharynx.
Lymphoma.
TB.
Malignancy of head and neck.
Scalene/supraclavicular nodes
Lymphoma.
Lung neoplasm.
Bacterial or fungal infection of thorax or retroperitoneum.
GI malignancy.
Axillary nodes
Infections of hands and arms.
Cat-scratch disease.
Neoplasm (lymphoma, melanoma, breast carcinoma).
Brucellosis.
Epitrochlear nodes
Infections of the hand.
Lymphoma.
Tularemia.
Sarcoidosis, secondary syphilis (usually bilateral).
Inguinal nodes
Infections of leg or foot, folliculitis (pubic hair).
LGV, syphilis.

Lymphoma.
Pelvic malignancy.
Pasteurella pestis.
Hilar nodes
Sarcoidosis.
TB.
Lung carcinoma.
Fungal infections, systemic.
Mediastinal nodes
Sarcoidosis.
Lymphoma.
Lung neoplasm.
TB.
Mononucleosis.
Histoplasmosis.
Abdominal/retroperitoneal nodes
Lymphoma.
TB.
Neoplasm (ovary, testes, prostate, and other malignancies).

MEDIASTINAL MASSES OR WIDENING ON CHEST X-RAY

ICD-9CM # 785.6 ADENOPATHY
519.3 DISEASE NEC
793.2 SHIFT (CXR)

Lymphoma: Hodgkin's disease and non-Hodgkin's lymphoma.
Sarcoidosis.
Vascular: aortic aneurysm, ectasia or tortuosity of aorta or bronchocephalic vessels.
Carcinoma: lungs, esophagus.
Esophageal diverticula.
Hiatal hernia.
Achalasia.
Prominent pulmonary outflow tract: pulmonary hypertension, pulmonary embolism, right-to-left shunts.
Trauma: mediastinal hemorrhage.
Pneumomediastinum.
Lymphadenopathy caused by silicosis and other pneumoconioses.
Leukemias.
Infections: TB, viral (rare), *Mycoplasma* (rare), fungal, tularemia.
Substernal thyroid.
Thymoma.
Teratoma.
Bronchogenic cyst.
Pericardial cyst.
Neurofibroma, neurosarcoma, ganglioneuroma.

MESENTERIC ISCHEMIA, NONOCCLUSIVE[14]

ICD-9CM # 557.0 MESENTERIC ARTERY EMBOLISM OR INFARCTION
557.1 MESENTERIC ARTERY INSUFFICIENCY, CHRONIC
902.39 MESENTERIC VEIN INJURY

Cardiovascular disease resulting in low-flow states (CHF, cardiogenic shock, post cardiopulmonary bypass, dysrhythmias).
Septic shock.
Drug induced (cocaine, vasopressors, ergot alkaloid poisoning).

METASTATIC NEOPLASMS

ICD-9CM # 198.5 BONE AND BONE MARROW
198.3 BRAIN AND SPINAL CORD
197.7 LIVER
197.0 LUNG

To: Bone	To: Brain	To: Liver	To: Lung
Breast	Lung	Colon	Breast
Lung	Breast	Stomach	Colon
Prostate	Melanoma	Pancreas	Kidney
Thyroid	GU tract	Breast	Testis
Kidney	Colon	Lymphomas	Stomach
Bladder	Sinuses	Bronchus	Thyroid
Endometrium	Sarcoma	Lung	Melanoma
Cervix	Skin	Sarcoma	
Melanoma	Thyroid	Kidney	

MONONEUROPATHY

ICD-9CM # 355.9

Herpes zoster.
Herpes simplex.
Vasculitis.
Trauma, compression.
Diabetes.
Postinfectious or inflammatory.

MUSCLE WEAKNESS

ICD-9CM # 728.9

Physical deconditioning.
Impaired cardiac output (e.g., mitral stenosis, mitral regurgitation).
Uremia, liver failure.
Electrolyte abnormalities (hypokalemia, hyperkalemia, hypophosphatemia, hypercalcemia), hypoglycemia.
Drug-induced (e.g., statin myopathy).
Muscular dystrophies.
Steroid myopathy.
Alcoholic myopathy.
Myasthenia gravis, Lambert-Eaton syndrome.
Infections (polio, botulism, HIV, hepatitis, diphtheria, tick paralysis, neurosyphilis, brucellosis, TB, trichinosis).
Pernicious anemia, other anemias, beriberi.
Psychiatric illness (depression, somatization syndrome).
Organophosphate or arsenic poisoning.
Inflammatory myopathies (e.g., collagen vascular disease, RA, sarcoidosis).
Endocrinopathies (e.g., adrenal insufficiency, hypothyroidism), diabetic neuropathy.
Other: motor neuron disease, mitochondrial myopathy, rhabdomyolysis.

MUSCLE WEAKNESS, LOWER MOTOR NEURON VERSUS UPPER MOTOR NEURON[23]

ICD-9CM # 728.9

LOWER MOTOR NEURON

Weakness, usually severe.
Marked muscle atrophy.
Fasciculations.
Decreased muscle stretch reflexes.
Clonus not present.
Flaccidity.
No Babinski's sign.

Asymmetric and may involve one limb only in the beginning to become generalized as the disease progresses.

UPPER MOTOR NEURON

Weakness, usually less severe.
Minimal disuse muscle atrophy.
No fasciculations.
Increased muscle stretch reflexes.
Clonus may be present.
Spasticity.
Babinski's sign.
Often initial impairment of only skilled movements.
In the limbs the following muscles may be the only ones weak or weaker than the others: triceps; wrist and finger extensors; interossei; iliopsoas; hamstrings; and foot dorsiflexors, inverters and extroverters.

MYOCARDIAL ISCHEMIA[22]

ICD-9CM # 414.8 ISCHEMIA (CHRONIC)
411.89 ISCHEMIA, ACUTE WITHOUT MI

Atherosclerotic obstructive coronary artery disease.
Nonatherosclerotic coronary artery disease:
  Coronary artery spasm.
  Congenital coronary artery anomalies:
    -Anomalous origin of coronary artery from pulmonary artery.
    -Aberrant origin of coronary artery from aorta or another coronary artery.
    -Coronary arteriovenous fistula.
    -Coronary artery aneurysm.
Acquired disorders of coronary arteries:
  Coronary artery embolism.
  Dissection:
    -Surgical.
    -During percutaneous coronary angioplasty.
    -Aortic dissection.
    -Spontaneous.
  Extrinsic compression:
    -Tumors.
    -Granulomas.
    -Amyloidosis.
  Collagen-vascular disease:
    -Polyarteritis nodosa.
    -Temporal arteritis.
    -Rheumatoid arthritis.
    -Systemic lupus erythematosus.
    -Scleroderma.
  Miscellaneous disorders:
    -Irradiation.
    -Trauma.
    -Kawasaki's disease.
  Syphilis.
Hereditary disorders:
  Pseudoxanthoma elasticum.
  Gargoylism.
  Progeria.
  Homocystinuria.
  Primary oxaluria.
"Functional" causes of myocardial ischemia in absence of anatomic coronary artery disease:
  Syndrome X.
  Hypertrophic cardiomyopathy.
  Dilated cardiomyopathy.
  Muscle bridge.
  Hypertensive heart disease.
  Pulmonary hypertension.
  Valvular heart disease, aortic stenosis, aortic regurgitation.

NAUSEA AND VOMITING

ICD-9CM # 787.01

Infections (viral, bacterial).
Intestinal obstruction.
Metabolic (uremia, electrolyte abnormalities, DKA, acidosis, etc.).
Severe pain.
Anxiety, fear.
Psychiatric disorders (bulimia, anorexia nervosa).
Medications (NSAIDs, erythromycin, morphine, codeine, aminophylline, chemotherapeutic agents, etc.).
Withdrawal from substance abuse (drugs, alcohol).
Head trauma.
Vestibular or middle ear disease.
Migraine headache.
CNS neoplasms.
Radiation sickness.
PUD.
Carcinoma of GI tract.
Reye's syndrome.
Eye disorders.
Abdominal trauma.

NECK MASS[16]

ICD-9CM # 784.2

CONGENITAL ANOMALIES

Thyroglossal duct cyst.
Bronchial apparatus anomalies.
Teratomas.
Ranula.
Dermoid cysts.
Hemangioma.
Laryngoceles.
Cystic hygroma.

NONNEOPLASTIC INFLAMMATORY ETIOLOGIES

Folliculitis.
Adenopathy secondary to peritonsillar abscess.
Retropharyngeal or parapharyngeal abscess.
Salivary gland infections.
Viral infections (mononucleosis, HIV, CMV).
TB.
Cat-scratch disease.
Toxoplasmosis.
Actinomyces.
Atypical mycobacterium.
Jugular vein thrombus.

NEOPLASM (PRIMARY OR METASTATIC)

Lipoma.

NECK PAIN[16]

ICD-9CM # 723.1 NECK PAIN
(NONDISCO-
GENIC)
959.09 NECK INJURY

INFLAMMATORY DISEASES

Rheumatoid arthritis (RA).
Spondyloarthropathies.

NONINFLAMMATORY DISEASE

Cervical osteoarthritis.
Diskogenic neck pain.

Diffuse idiopathic skeletal hyperostosis.
Fibromyalgia or myofascial pain.

INFECTIOUS CAUSES

Meningitis.
Osteomyelitis.
Infectious diskitis.

NEOPLASMS

Primary.
Metastatic.

REFERRED PAIN

Temporomandibular joint pain.
Cardiac pain.
Diaphragmatic irritation.
Gastrointestinal sources (gastric ulcer, gallbladder, pancreas).

NEUROGENIC BLADDER[17]

ICD-9CM # 396.54

SUPRATENTORIAL

CVA.
Parkinson's disease.
Alzheimer's disease.
Cerebral palsy.

SPINAL CORD

Spinal cord injury.
Spinal stenosis.
Central cord syndrome.
ALS.
Multiple sclerosis.
Myelodysplasia.

PERIPHERAL NEUROPATHY

Diabetes.
Alcohol.
Shingles.
Syphilis.

NEUROLOGIC DEFICIT, FOCAL[14]

ICD-9CM # 436 CVA
435.9 TIA

TRAUMATIC: INTRACRANIAL, INTRASPINAL

Subdural hematoma.
Intraparenchymal hemorrhage.
Epidural hematoma.
Traumatic hemorrhagic necrosis.

INFECTIOUS

Brain abscess.
Epidural and subdural abscesses.
Meningitis.

NEOPLASTIC

Primary central nervous system tumors.
Metastatic tumors.
Syringomyelia.
Vascular.
Thrombosis.
Embolism.
Spontaneous hemorrhage: arteriovenous malformation, aneurysm, hypertensive.

METABOLIC

Hypoglycemia.
B_{12} deficiency.
Postseizure.
Hyperosmolar nonketotic.

OTHER

Migraine.
Bell's palsy.
Psychogenic.

NEUROLOGIC DEFICIT, MULTIFOCAL[14]

ICD-9CM # 436 CVA
435.9 TIA

Acute disseminated encephalomyelitis: postviral or postimmunization.
Infectious encephalomyelitis: poliovirus, enteroviruses, arbovirus, herpes zoster, Epstein-Barr virus.
Granulomatous encephalomyelitis: sarcoid.
Autoimmune: systemic lupus erythematosus.
Other: familial spinocerebellar degenerations.

NEUROPATHIES, PAINFUL[23]

ICD-9CM # 355.9 NEUROPATHY NOS
357.5 ALCOHOLIC
357.8 CHRONIC PROGRESSIVE OR RELAPSING
356.2 CONGENITAL SENSORY
356.0 DEJERINE-SOTTAS
356.60 DIABETIC POLYNEUROPATHY, TYPE II
356.61 DIABETIC POLYNEUROPATHY, TYPE I

MONONEUROPATHIES

Compressive neuropathy (carpal tunnel, meralgia paresthetica).
Trigeminal neuralgia.
Ischemic neuropathy.
Polyarteritis nodosa.
Diabetic mononeuropathy.
Herpes zoster.
Idiopathic and familial brachial plexopathy.

POLYNEUROPATHIES

Diabetes mellitus.
Paraneoplastic sensory neuropathy.
Nutritional neuropathy.
Multiple myeloma.
Amyloid.
Dominantly inherited sensory neuropathy.
Toxic (arsenic, thallium, metronidazole).
AIDS-associated neuropathy.
Tangier's disease.
Fabry's disease.

NYSTAGMUS

ICD-9CM # 379.50 NYSTAGMUS NOS
386.11 BENIGN POSITIONAL
386.2 CENTRAL POSITIONAL
379.59 CONGENITAL

Medications (meperidine, barbiturates, phenytoin, phenothiazines, etc.).
Multiple sclerosis.
Congenital.
Neoplasm (cerebellar, brainstem, cerebral).
Labyrinthine or vestibular lesions.

CNS infections.
Optic atrophy.
Other: Arnold-Chiari malformation, syringobulbia, chorioretinitis, meningeal cysts.

OPHTHALMOPLEGIA[1]

ICD-9CM # 378.9 OPHTHALMOPLEGIA NOS
378.52 CEREBELLAR ATAXIA SYNDROME
376.22 EXOPHTHALMIC

BILATERAL

Botulism.
Myasthenia gravis.
Wernicke's encephalopathy.
Acute cranial polyneuropathy.
Brainstem stroke.

UNILATERAL

Carotid-posterior (3rd cranial nerve, pupil involved communicating aneurysm).
Diabetic-idiopathic (3rd or 6th cranial nerve, pupil spared).
Myasthenia gravis.
Brainstem stroke.

PALPITATIONS[19]

ICD-9CM # 785.1 PALPITATIONS

Anxiety.
Electrolyte abnormalities (hypokalemia, hypomagnesemia).
Exercise.
Hyperthyroidism.
Ischemic heart disease.
Ingestion of stimulant drugs (cocaine, amphetamines, caffeine).
Medications (digoxin, β-blockers, calcium channel antagonists, hydralazines, diuretics, minoxidil).
Hypoglycemia in type 1 DM.
Mitral valve prolapse.
Wolff-Parkinson-White (WPW) syndrome.
Sick sinus syndrome.

PANCYTOPENIA[22]

ICD-9CM # 284.8

PANCYTOPENIA WITH HYPOCELLULAR BONE MARROW

Acquired aplastic anemia.
Constitutional aplastic anemia.
Exposure to chemical or physical agents, including ionizing irradiation and chemotherapeutic agents.
Some hematologic malignancies, including myelodysplasia and aleukemic leukemia.

PANCYTOPENIA WITH NORMAL OR INCREASED CELLULARITY OF HEMATOPOIETIC ORIGIN

Some hematologic malignancies, including myelodysplasia, and some leukemias, lymphomas, and myelomas.
Paroxysmal nocturnal hemoglobinuria.
Hypersplenism.
Vitamin B_{12}, folate deficiencies.
Overwhelming infection.

PANCYTOPENIA WITH BONE MARROW REPLACEMENT

Tumor metastatic to marrow.
Metabolic storage diseases.
Osteopetrosis.
Myelofibrosis.

PARESTHESIAS

ICD-9CM # 782.0

Multiple sclerosis.
Nutritional deficiencies (thiamin, vitamin B_{12}, folic acid).
Compression of spinal cord or peripheral nerves.
Medications (e.g., INH, lithium, nitrofurantoin, gold, cisplatin, hydralazine, amitriptyline, sulfonamides, amiodarone, metronidazole, dapsone, disulfiram, chloramphenicol).
Toxic chemicals (e.g., lead, arsenic, cyanide, mercury, organophosphates).
DM.
Myxedema.
Alcohol.
Sarcoidosis.
Neoplasms.
Infections (HIV, Lyme disease, herpes zoster, leprosy, diphtheria).
Charcot-Marie-Tooth syndrome and other hereditary neuropathies.
Guillain-Barré neuropathy.

PELVIC MASS

ICD-9CM # 789.39

Hemorrhagic ovarian cyst.
Simple ovarian cyst (follicle or corpus luteum).
Ovarian carcinoma, carcinoma of fallopian tube, colorectal carcinoma, metastatic carcinoma, prostate carcinoma, bladder carcinoma, lymphoma, Hodgkin's disease.
Cystadenoma, teratoma.
Leiomyoma.
Leiomyosarcoma.
Diverticulitis, diverticular abscess.
Appendiceal abscess, tuboovarian abscess.
Paraovarian cyst.
Hydrosalpinx.

PERICARDIAL EFFUSION

ICD-9CM # 420.90

Pericarditis.
Uremia.
Myxedema.
Neoplasm (leukemia, lymphoma, metastatic).
Hemorrhage (trauma, leakage of thoracic aneurysm).
SLE, rheumatoid disease.
Myocardial infarction.

PLEURAL EFFUSIONS

ICD-9CM # 511.9 PLEURAL EFFUSION, UNSPECIFIED

EXUDATIVE

Neoplasm: bronchogenic carcinoma, breast carcinoma, mesothelioma, lymphoma, ovarian carcinoma, multiple myeloma, leukemia, Meigs' syndrome.
Infections: viral pneumonia, bacterial pneumonia, *Mycoplasma,* TB, fungal and parasitic diseases, extension from subphrenic abscess.
Trauma.
Collagen vascular diseases: SLE, RA, scleroderma, polyarteritis, Wegener's granulomatosis.
Pulmonary infarction.
Pancreatitis.
Postcardiotomy/Dressler's syndrome.
Drug-induced lupus erythematosus (hydralazine, procainamide).
Postabdominal surgery.

Ruptured esophagus.
Chronic effusion secondary to congestive failure.

TRANSUDATIVE

CHF.
Hepatic cirrhosis.
Nephrotic syndrome.
Hypoproteinemia from any cause.
Meigs' syndrome.

POLYNEUROPATHY[23]

ICD-9CM # 357.9

PREDOMINANTLY MOTOR

Guillain-Barré syndrome.
Porphyria.
Diphtheria.
Lead.
Hereditary sensorimotor neuropathy, types I and II.
Paraneoplastic neuropathy.

PREDOMINANTLY SENSORY

Diabetes.
Amyloidosis.
Leprosy.
Lyme disease.
Paraneoplastic neuropathy.
Vitamin B_{12} deficiency.
Hereditary sensory neuropathy, types I-IV.

PREDOMINANTLY AUTONOMIC

Diabetes.
Amyloidosis.
Alcoholic neuropathy.
Familial dysautonomias.

MIXED SENSORIMOTOR

Systemic diseases: renal failure, hypothyroidism, acromegaly, rheumatoid arthritis, periarteritis nodosa, systemic lupus erythematosus, multiple myeloma, macroglobulinemia, remote effect of malignancy.
Medications: isoniazid, nitrofurantoin, ethambutol, chloramphenicol, chloroquine, vincristine, vinblastine, dapsone, disulfiram, diphenylhydantoin, cisplatin, L-tryptophan.
Environmental toxins: N-hexane, methyl N-butyl ketone, acrylamide, carbon disulfide, carbon monoxide, hexachlorophene, organophosphates.
Deficiency disorders: malabsorption, alcoholism, vitamin B_1 deficiency, Refsum's disease, metachromatic leukodystrophy.

POLYNEUROPATHY, DRUG-INDUCED[23]

ICD-9CM # 357.6

DRUGS IN ONCOLOGY

Vincristine.
Procarbazine.
Cisplatin.
Misonidazole.
Metronidazole (Flagyl).
Taxol.

DRUGS IN INFECTIOUS DISEASES

Isoniazid.
Nitrofurantoin.
Dapsone.
ddC (dideoxycytidine).
ddI (dideoxyinosine).

DRUGS IN CARDIOLOGY

Hydralazine.
Perhexiline maleate.
Procainamide.
Disopyramide.

DRUGS IN RHEUMATOLOGY

Gold salts.
Chloroquine.

DRUGS IN NEUROLOGY AND PSYCHIATRY

Diphenylhydantoin.
Glutethimide.
Methaqualone.

MISCELLANEOUS

Disulfiram (Antabuse).
Vitamin: pyridoxine (megadoses).

POLYNEUROPATHY, SYMMETRIC[23]

ICD-9CM # 357.9

ACQUIRED NEUROPATHIES

Toxic:
  Drugs.
  Industrial toxins.
  Heavy metals.
  Abused substances.
Metabolic/endocrine:
  Diabetes.
  Chronic renal failure.
  Hypothyroidism.
  Polyneuropathy of critical illness.
Nutritional deficiency:
  Vitamin B12 deficiency.
  Alcoholism.
  Vitamin E deficiency.
Paraneoplastic:
  Carcinoma.
  Lymphoma.
Plasma cell dyscrasia:
  Myeloma, typical, atypical, and solitary forms.
  Primary systemic amyloidosis.
Idiopathic chronic inflammatory demyelinating polyneuropathies.
Polyneuropathies associated with peripheral nerve autoantibodies.
Acquired immunodeficiency syndrome.

INHERITED NEUROPATHIES

Neuropathies with biochemical markers
Refsum's disease.
Bassen-Kornzweig disease.
Tangier's disease.
Metachromatic leukodystrophy.
Krabbe's disease.
Adrenomyeloneuropathy.
Fabry's disease.
Neuropathies without biochemical markers or systemic involvement
Hereditary motor neuropathy.
Hereditary sensory neuropathy.
Hereditary sensorimotor neuropathy.

POLYURIA

ICD-9CM # 788.42

DM.
Diabetes insipidus.
Primary polydipsia (compulsive water drinking).
Hypercalcemia.
Hypokalemia.
Postobstructive uropathy.
Diuretic phase of renal failure.
Drugs: diuretics, caffeine, alcohol, lithium.
Sickle cell trait or disease, chronic pyelonephritis (failure to concentrate urine).
Anxiety, cold weather.

PORTAL HYPERTENSION[1]

ICD-9CM # 572.3

INCREASED RESISTANCE TO FLOW

Presinusoidal
Portal or splenic vein occlusion (thrombosis, tumor).
Schistosomiasis.
Sarcoidosis.
Sinusoidal
Cirrhosis (all causes).
Alcoholic hepatitis.
Postsinusoidal
Venoocclusive disease.
Budd-Chiari syndrome.
Constrictive pericarditis.

INCREASED PORTAL BLOOD FLOW

Splenomegaly not caused by liver disease.
Arterioportal fistula.

POSTMENOPAUSAL VAGINAL BLEEDING

ICD-9CM # 627.1

Hormone replacement therapy.
Neoplasm (uterine, ovarian, cervical, vaginal, vulvar).
Atrophic vaginitis.
Vaginal infection.
Polyp.
Extragenital (GI, urinary).
Tamoxifen.
Trauma.

PRURITUS

ICD-9CM # 698.9 PRURITUS NOS
         697.0 PRURITUS ANI
         698.1 PRURITUS, GENITAL ORGANS

Dry skin.
Drug-induced eruption, fiberglass exposure.
Scabies.
Skin diseases.
Myeloproliferative disorders: mycosis fungoides, Hodgkin's lymphoma, multiple myeloma, polycythemia vera.
Cholestatic liver disease.
Endocrine disorders: DM, thyroid disease, carcinoid.
Carcinoma: breast, lung, gastric.
Chronic renal failure.
Iron deficiency.
AIDS.
Neurosis.
Sjögren's syndrome.

PULMONARY LESIONS

ICD-9CM # 518.3 PULMONARY INFILTRATE
         518.89 PULMONARY NODULE
         508.9 PULMONARY DISORDER DUE TO
                UNSPECIFIED EXTERNAL AGENT
         861.20 PULMONARY INJURY NOS

TB.
Legionella pneumophila.
Mycoplasma pneumoniae.
Viral pneumonia.
Pneumocystis carinii.
Hypersensitivity pneumonitis.
Aspiration pneumonia.
Fungal disease (aspergillosis, histoplasmosis).
ARDS associated with pneumonia.
Psittacosis.
Sarcoidosis.
Septic emboli.
Metastatic cancer.
Multiple pulmonary emboli.
Rheumatoid nodules.

PULMONARY NODULE, SOLITARY

ICD-9CM # 518.89

Bronchogenic carcinoma.
Granuloma from histoplasmosis.
TB granuloma.
Granuloma from coccidioidomycosis.
Metastatic carcinoma.
Bronchial adenoma.
Bronchogenic cyst.
Hamartoma.
AV malformation.
Other: fibroma, intrapulmonary lymph node, sclerosing hemangioma, bronchopulmonary sequestration.

PURPURA

ICD-9CM # 287.2 PURPURA NOS
         287.0 AUTOIMMUNE
         287.0 HENOCH-SCHÖNLEIN
         287.3 IDIOPATHIC THROMBOCYTOPENIC
         446.6 THROMBOCYTOPENIC

THROMBOTIC

Trauma.
Septic emboli, atheromatous emboli.
DIC.
Thrombocytopenia.
Meningococcemia.
Rocky Mountain spotted fever.
Hemolytic-uremic syndrome.
Viral infection: echo, coxsackie.
Scurvy.
Other: left atrial myxoma, cryoglobulinemia, vasculitis, hyperglobulinemic purpura.

QT INTERVAL PROLONGATION[12]

ICD-9CM # 794.31

Drugs:
   Class I antiarrhythmics (e.g., disopyramide, procainamide, quinidine).
   Class III antiarrhythmics.
   Tricyclic antidepressants.
   Phenothiazines.

Astemizole.
Terfenadine.
Adenosine.
Antibiotics (e.g., erythromycin and other macrolides).
Antifungal agents.
Pentamidine, chloroquine.
Ischemic heart disease.
Cerebrovascular disease.
Rheumatic fever.
Myocarditis.
Mitral valve prolapse.
Electrolyte abnormalities.
Hypocalcemia.
Hypothyroidism.
Liquid protein diets.
Organophosphate insecticides.
Congenital prolonged QT syndrome.

RECTAL PAIN

ICD-9CM # 569.42

Anal fissure.
Thrombosed hemorrhoid.
Anorectal abscess.
Foreign bodies.
Fecal impaction.
Neoplasms (primary or metastatic).
Pelvic inflammatory disease.
Inflammation of sacral nerves.
Compression of sacral nerves.
Prostatitis.
Other: proctalgia fugax, uterine abnormalities, myopathies, coccygodynia.

RED EYE

ICD-9CM # 379.93

Infectious conjunctivitis (bacterial, viral).
Allergic conjunctivitis.
Acute glaucoma.
Keratitis (bacterial, viral).
Iritis.
Trauma.

RENAL FAILURE, INTRINSIC OR PARENCHYMAL CAUSES[22]

ICD-9CM # 584. ACUTE, USE 4TH DIGIT
    .5 WITH ACUTE TUBULAR NECROSIS
    .6 WITH CORTICAL NECROSIS
    .7 WITH MEDULLARY NECROSIS
    .8 WITH OTHER UNSPECIFIED PATHOLOGIC
       CONDITION IN KIDNEY
    .9 RENAL FAILURE UNSPECIFIED
    585 RENAL FAILURE, CHRONIC

ABNORMALITIES OF THE VASCULATURE

Renal arteries: atherosclerosis, thromboembolism, arteritis.
Renal veins: thrombosis.
Microvasculature: vasculitis, thrombotic microangiopathy.

ABNORMALITIES OF GLOMERULI (ACUTE GLOMERULONEPHRITIS)

Antiglomerular membrane disease (Goodpasture's syndrome).
Immune complex glomerulonephritis: SLE, postinfectious, idiopathic, membranoproliferative.

ABNORMALITIES OF INTERSTITIUM (ACUTE INTERSTITIAL NEPHRITIS)

Drugs (e.g., antibiotics, NSAIDs, diuretics, anticonvulsants, allopurinol).
Infectious pyelonephritis.
Infiltrative: lymphoma, leukemia, sarcoidosis.

ABNORMALITIES OF TUBULES

Physical obstruction (uric acid, oxalate, light chains).
Acute tubular necrosis:
    Ischemic.
    Toxic (antibiotics, chemotherapy, immunosuppressives, radiocontrast dyes, heavy metals, myoglobin, hemolysed RBCs).

RENAL FAILURE, POSTRENAL CAUSES[22]

ICD-9CM # 584. ACUTE, USE 4TH DIGIT
    .5 WITH ACUTE TUBULAR NECROSIS
    .6 WITH CORTICAL NECROSIS
    .7 WITH MEDULLARY NECROSIS
    .8 WITH OTHER UNSPECIFIED PATHOLOGIC
       CONDITION IN KIDNEY
    .9 RENAL FAILURE UNSPECIFIED
    585 RENAL FAILURE, CHRONIC

RENAL FAILURE, PRERENAL CAUSES[22]

ICD-9CM # 584. ACUTE, USE 4TH DIGIT
    .5 WITH ACUTE TUBULAR NECROSIS
    .6 WITH CORTICAL NECROSIS
    .7 WITH MEDULLARY NECROSIS
    .8 WITH OTHER UNSPECIFIED PATHOLOGIC
       CONDITION IN KIDNEY
    .9 RENAL FAILURE UNSPECIFIED
    585 RENAL FAILURE, CHRONIC

DECREASED CARDIAC OUTPUT

CHF.
Arrhythmias.
Pericardial constriction or tamponade.
Pulmonary embolism.

HYPOVOLEMIA

GI tract loss (vomiting, diarrhea, nasogastric suction).
Blood losses (trauma, GI tract surgery).
Renal losses (diuretics, mineralocorticoid deficiency, postobstructive diuresis).
Skin losses (burns).

VOLUME REDISTRIBUTION (DECREASE IN EFFECTIVE BLOOD VOLUME)

Hypoalbuminemic states (cirrhosis, nephrosis).
Sequestration of fluid in "third" space (ischemic bowel, peritonitis, pancreatitis).
Peripheral vasodilation (sepsis, vasodilators, anaphylaxis).

ALTERED RENAL VASCULAR RESISTANCE

Increase in afferent vascular resistance (NSAIDs, liver disease, sepsis, hypercalcemia, cyclosporine).
Decrease in efferent arteriolar tone (ACE inhibitors).

RESPIRATORY FAILURE, HYPOVENTILATORY[16]

ICD-9CM # 518.81 RESPIRATORY FAILURE

ABNORMAL RESPIRATORY CAPACITY (NORMAL RESPIRATORY WORKLOADS)

Acute depression of central nervous system:
    Various causes.

Chronic central hypoventilation syndromes:
    Obesity-hypoventilation syndrome.
    Sleep apnea syndrome.
    Hypothyroidism.
    Shy-Drager syndrome (multisystem atrophy syndrome).
Acute toxic paralysis syndromes:
    Botulism.
    Tetanus.
    Toxic ingestion or bites.
    Organophosphate poisoning.
Neuromuscular disorders (acute and chronic):
    Myasthenia gravis.
    Guillain-Barré syndrome.
    Drugs.
    Amyotrophic lateral sclerosis.
    Muscular dystrophies.
    Polymyositis.
    Spinal cord injury.
    Traumatic phrenic nerve paralysis.

ABNORMAL PULMONARY WORKLOADS

Chronic obstructive pulmonary disease:
    Chronic bronchitis.
    Asthmatic bronchitis.
    Emphysema.
Asthma and acute bronchial hyperreactivity syndromes.
Upper airway obstruction.
Interstitial lung diseases.

ABNORMAL EXTRAPULMONARY WORKLOADS

Chronic thoracic cage disorders:
    Severe kyphoscoliosis.
    After thoracoplasty.
    After thoracic cage injury.
Acute thoracic cage trauma and burns.
Pneumothorax.
Pleural fibrosis and effusions.
Abdominal processes.

SCROTAL PAIN[16]

ICD-9CM # 878.2 SCROTAL INJURY, TRAUMATIC
**   608.9 SCROTAL DISORDER NOS**
**   608.4 SCROTAL CELLULITIS**
**   608.83 SCROTAL HEMORRHAGE,**
**   NONTRAUMATIC**
**   608.4 SCROTAL NODULE, INFLAMMATORY**

Torsion:
    Appendages.
    Spermatic cord.
Infection:
    Orchitis.
    Abscess.
    Epididymitis.
Neoplasia:
    Benign.
    Malignant.
Incarcerated hernia.
Trauma.
Hydrocele.
Spermatocele.
Varicocele.

SCROTAL SWELLING

ICD-9CM # 608.86

Hydrocele.
Varicocele.

Neoplasm.
Acute epididymitis.
Orchitis.
Trauma.
Hernia.
Torsion of spermatic cord.
Torsion of epididymis.
Torsion of testis.
Insect bite.
Folliculitis.
Sebaceous cyst.
Thrombosis of spermatic vein.
Other: lymphedema, dermatitis, fat necrosis, Henoch-Schönlein
    purpura, idiopathic scrotal edema.

SEIZURE

ICD-9CM # 780.39

Syncope.
Alcohol abuse/withdrawal.
TIA.
Hemiparetic migraine.
Psychiatric disorders.
Carotid sinus hypersensitivity.
Hyperventilation, prolonged breath holding.
Hypoglycemia.
Narcolepsy.
Movement disorders (tics, hemiballismus).
Hyponatremia.
Brain tumor (primary or metastatic).
Tetanus.
Strychnine, phencyclidine poisoning.

SEXUALLY TRANSMITTED DISEASES, ANORECTAL REGION[14]

ICD-9CM # 569.49 INFECTION AND REGION

ULCERATIVE

Lymphogranuloma venereum.
Herpes simplex virus.
Early (primary) syphilis.
Chancroid (Haemophilus ducreyi).
Cytomegalovirus.
Idiopathic (usually HIV positive).

NONULCERATIVE

Condyloma acuminatum.
Gonorrhea.
Chlamydia (Chlamydia trachomatis).
Syphilis.

SHOULDER PAIN

ICD-9CM # 952.2 SHOULDER INJURY
**   718.81 SHOULDER INSTABILITY**
**   726.19 SHOULDER LIGAMENT OR MUSCLE**
**   INSTABILITY**
**   840.9 SHOULDER STRAIN, SITE UNSPECIFIED**

WITH LOCAL FINDINGS IN SHOULDER

Trauma: contusion, fracture, muscle strain, trauma to spinal
    cord.
Arthrosis, arthritis, RA, ankylosing spondylitis.
Bursitis, synovitis, tendinitis, tenosynovitis.
Aseptic (avascular) necrosis.
Local infection: septic arthritis, osteomyelitis, abscess, herpes
    zoster, TB.

Section II   DIFFERENTIAL DIAGNOSIS

WITHOUT LOCAL FINDINGS IN SHOULDER

Cardiovascular disorders: ischemic heart disease, pericarditis, aortic aneurysm.
Subdiaphragmatic abscess, liver abscess.
Cholelithiasis, cholecystitis.
Pulmonary lesions: apical bronchial carcinoma, pleurisy, pneumothorax, pneumonia.
GI lesions: PUD, gastric neoplasm, peptic esophagitis.
Pancreatic lesions: carcinoma, calculi, pancreatitis.
CNS abnormalities: neoplasm, vascular abnormalities.
Multiple sclerosis.
Syringomyelia.
Polymyositis/dermatomyositis.
Psychogenic.
Polymyalgia rheumatica.

SHOULDER PAIN BY LOCATION

ICD-9CM # 952.2 SHOULDER INJURY
726.19 SHOULDER LIGAMENT OR MUSCLE INSTABILITY
840.8 SHOULDER SEPARATION

TOP OF SHOULDER (C4)

Cervical source.
Acromioclavicular.
Sternoclavicular.
Diaphragmatic.

SUPEROLATERAL (C5)

Rotator cuff tendinitis.
Impingement.
Adhesive capsulitis.
Glenohumeral arthritis.

ANTERIOR

Bicipital tendinitis and rupture.
Glenoid labral tear.
Adhesive capsulitis.
Glenohumeral arthritis.
Osteonecrosis.

AXILLARY

Neoplasm (Pancoast's, mediastinal).
Herpes zoster.

SMALL BOWEL OBSTRUCTION[14]

ICD-9CM # 751.1 SMALL INTESTINE OBSTRUCTION, CONGENITAL
560.81 SMALL INTESTINE OBSTRUCTION DUE TO ADHESION

INTRINSIC

Inflammatory (Crohn's, radiation enteritis).
Neoplasms (metastatic or primary).
Intussusception.
Traumatic (hematoma).

EXTRINSIC

Hernias (internal and external).
Adhesions.
Volvulus.
Compressing masses (tumors, abscesses, hematomas).

INTRALUMINAL

Foreign body.
Gallstones.
Bezoars.
Barium.
Ascaris infestation.

SPLENOMEGALY

ICD-9CM # 789.2 SPLENOMEGALY UNSPECIFIED
789.51 CHRONIC CONGESTIVE
789.2 UNKNOWN ORIGIN

Hepatic cirrhosis.
Neoplastic involvement: CML, CLL, lymphoma, multiple myeloma.
Bacterial infections: TB, infectious endocarditis, typhoid fever, splenic abscess.
Viral infections: infectious mononucleosis, viral hepatitis, HIV.
Gaucher's disease and other lipid storage diseases.
Sarcoidosis.
Parasitic infections (malaria, kala-azar, histoplasmosis).
Hereditary and acquired hemolytic anemias.
Idiopathic thrombocytopenic purpura (ITP).
Collagen vascular disorders: SLE, RA (Felty's syndrome), polyarteritis nodosa.
Serum sickness, drug hypersensitivity reaction.
Splenic cysts and benign tumors: hemangioma, lymphangioma.
Thrombosis of splenic or portal vein.
Polycythemia vera, myeloid metaplasia.

STEATOHEPATITIS

ICD-9CM # 571.8

Alcohol abuse.
Obesity.
Diabetes mellitus.
Parenteral nutrition.
Medications (high-dose estrogen, amiodarone, corticosteroids, methotrexate, nifedipine).
Jejunoileal bypass.
Abetalipoproteinemia.
Wilson's disease.

STROKE[22]

ICD-9CM # 436 ACUTE STROKE

Hypoglycemia.
Drug overdose or intoxication.
Hysterical conversion reaction.
Hyperventilation.
Metabolic encephalopathy.
Migraine.
Syncope.
Transient global amnesia.
Seizures.
Vestibular vertigo.

TARDIVE DYSKINESIA[16]

ICD-9CM # 781.3 DYSKINESIA
300.11 HYSTERICAL DYSKINESIA
333.82 OROFACIAL DYSKINESIA
307.9 PSYCHOGENIC DYSKINESIA

DIFFERENTIAL DIAGNOSIS

Medications (antidepressants, anticholinergics, amphetamines, antipsychotics, lithium, L-dopa, phenytoin).
Brain neoplasms.
Ill-fitting dentures.

Huntington's disease.
Idiopathic dystonias (tics, blepharospasm, aging).
Wilson's disease.
Extrapyramidal syndrome (postanoxic or postencephalitic).
Torsion dystonia.

TASTE AND SMELL LOSS[1]

ICD-9CM # 781.1 SMELL AND TASTE DISTURBANCE OF SENSATION

TASTE

Local: radiation therapy.
Systemic: cancer, renal failure, hepatic failure, nutritional deficiency (vitamin B_{12}, zinc), Cushing's syndrome, hypothyroidism, DM, infection (influenza), drugs (antirheumatic and antiproliferative).
Neurologic: Bell's palsy, familial dysautonomia, multiple sclerosis.

SMELL

Local: allergic rhinitis, sinusitis, nasal polyposis, bronchial asthma.
Systemic: renal failure, hepatic failure, nutritional deficiency (vitamin B_{12}), Cushing's syndrome, hypothyroidism, DM, infection (viral hepatitis, influenza), drugs (nasal sprays, antibiotics).
Neurologic: head trauma, multiple sclerosis, Parkinson's disease, frontal brain tumor.

TENDINOPATHY[14]

ICD-9CM # 727.9

INTRINSIC FACTORS

Anatomic factors
Malalignment.
Muscle weakness or imbalance.
Muscle inflexibility.
Decreased vascularity.
Systemic factors
Inflammatory conditions (e.g., SLE).
Quinolone-induced tendinopathy.
Age-related factors
Tendon degeneration.
Increased tendon stiffness.
Tendon calcification.
Decreased vascularity.

EXTRINSIC FACTORS

Repetitive mechanical load
Excessive duration.
Excessive frequency.
Excessive intensity.
Poor technique.
Workplace factors.
Equipment problems
Footwear.
Athletic field surface.
Equipment factors (e.g., racquet size).
Protective gear.

THROMBOCYTOPENIA

ICD-9CM # 287.3 CONGENITAL OR PRIMARY
287.4 SECONDARY
287.5 THROMBOCYTOPENIA NOS

INCREASED DESTRUCTION

Immunologic
Drugs: quinine, quinidine, digitalis, procainamide, thiazide diuretics, sulfonamides, phenytoin, aspirin, penicillin, heparin, gold, meprobamate, sulfa drugs, phenylbutazone, nonsteroidal antiinflammatory drugs (NSAIDs), methyldopa, cimetidine, furosemide, INH, cephalosporins, chlorpropamide, organic arsenicals, chloroquine, platelet glycoprotein IIb/IIIa receptor inhibitors, ranitidine, indomethacin, carboplatin, ticlopidine, clopidogrel.
Idiopathic thrombocytopenic purpura (ITP).
Transfusion reaction: transfusion of platelets with plasminogen activator (PLA) in recipients without PLA-1.
Collagen vascular diseases (e.g., systemic lupus erythematosus [SLE]).
Autoimmune hemolytic anemia.
Lymphoreticular disorders (e.g., CLL).
Nonimmunologic
Prosthetic heart valves.
Thrombotic thrombocytopenic purpura (TTP).
Sepsis.
DIC.
Hemolytic-uremic syndrome (HUS).
Giant cavernous hemangioma.

DECREASED PRODUCTION

Abnormal marrow.
Marrow infiltration (e.g., leukemia, lymphoma, fibrosis).
Marrow suppression (e.g., chemotherapy, alcohol, radiation).
Hereditary disorders.
Wiskott-Aldrich syndrome: X-linked disorder characterized by thrombocytopenia, eczema, and repeated infections.
May-Hegglin anomaly: increased megakaryocytes but ineffective thrombopoiesis.
Vitamin deficiencies (e.g., vitamin B_{12}, folic acid).

SPLENIC SEQUESTRATION, HYPERSPLENISM

DILUTIONAL, AS A RESULT OF MASSIVE TRANSFUSION

THROMBOCYTOSIS

ICD-9CM # 289.9 THROMBOCYTOSIS, ESSENTIAL

Iron deficiency.
Posthemorrhage.
Neoplasms (GI tract).
CML.
Polycythemia vera.
Myelofibrosis with myeloid metaplasia.
Infections.
After splenectomy.
Hemophilia.
Pancreatitis.
Cirrhosis.
Idiopathic.

TREMOR

ICD-9CM # 781.0 TREMOR NOS
         333.1 BENIGN ESSENTIAL TREMOR
         333.1 FAMILIAL TREMOR

TREMOR PRESENT AT REST

Parkinsonism.
CNS neoplasms.
Tardive dyskinesia.

POSTURAL TREMOR (PRESENT DURING MAINTENANCE OF A POSTURE)

Essential senile tremor.

ACTION TREMOR (PRESENT WITH MOVEMENT)

Anxiety.
Medications (bronchodilators, caffeine, corticosteroids, lithium, etc.).
Endocrine disorders (hyperthyroidism, pheochromocytoma, carcinoid).
Withdrawal from substance abuse.

URINARY RETENTION, ACUTE

ICD-9CM # 788.20

Mechanical obstruction: urethral stone, foreign body, urethral stricture, BPH, prostate carcinoma, prostatitis, trauma with hematoma formation).
Neurogenic bladder.
Neurologic disease (MS, parkinsonism, tabes dorsalis, CVA).
Spinal cord injury.
CNS neoplasm (primary or metastatic).
Spinal anesthesia.
Lower urinary tract instrumentation.
Medications (antihistamines, antidepressants, narcotics, anticholinergics).
Abdominal or pelvic surgery.
Alcohol toxicity.
Anxiety.
Encephalitis.
Postoperative pain.
Encephalitis.
Spina bifida occulta.

URINE, RED[17]

ICD-9CM # CODE VARIES WITH SPECIFIC DIAGNOSIS

WITH A POSITIVE DIPSTICK

Hematuria.
Hemoglobinuria: negative urinalysis.
Myoglobinuria: negative urinalysis.

WITH A NEGATIVE DIPSTICK

Drugs
Aminosalicylic acid.
Deferoxamine mesylate.
Ibuprofen.
Phenacetin.
Phenolphthalein.
Phensuximide.
Rifampin.
Anthraquinone laxatives.
Doxorubicin.
Methyldopa.
Phenazopyridine.
Phenothiazine.
Phenytoin.
Dyes
Azo dyes.
Eosin.
Foods
Beets, berries, maize.
Rhodamine B.
Metabolic
Porphyrins.
Serratia marcescens (red diaper syndrome).
Urate crystalluria.

UROPATHY, OBSTRUCTIVE[22]

ICD-9CM # 599.6

INTRINSIC CAUSES

Intraluminal
Intratubular deposition of crystals (uric acid, sulfas).
Stones.
Papillary tissue.
Blood clots.
Intramural
Functional.
Ureter (ureteropelvic or ureterovesical dysfunction).
Bladder (neurogenic): spinal cord defect or trauma, diabetes, multiple sclerosis, Parkinson's disease, cerebrovascular accidents.
Bladder neck dysfunction.
Anatomic
Tumors.
Infection, granuloma.
Strictures.

EXTRINSIC CAUSES

Originating in the reproductive system
Prostate: benign hypertrophy or cancer.
Uterus: tumors, prolapse.
Ovary: abscess, tumor, cysts.
Originating in the vascular system
Aneurysms (aorta, iliac vessels).
Aberrant arteries (ureteropelvic junction).
Venous (ovarian veins, retrocaval ureter).
Originating in the gastrointestinal tract: Crohn's disease, pancreatitis, appendicitis, tumors
Originating in the retroperitoneal space
Inflammations.
Fibrosis.
Tumor, hematomas.

VERTIGO

ICD-9CM # 780.4 VERTIGO NOS
         386.11 BENIGN PAROXYSMAL POSITIONAL
         386.2 CENTRAL ORIGIN
         386.10 PERIPHERAL
         386.12 VESTIBULAR (NEURONITIS)

PERIPHERAL

Otitis media.
Acute labyrinthitis.
Vestibular neuronitis.
Benign positional vertigo.
Meniere's disease.
Ototoxic drugs: streptomycin, gentamicin.
Lesions of the eighth nerve: acoustic neuroma, meningioma, mononeuropathy, metastatic carcinoma.
Mastoiditis.

CNS OR SYSTEMIC

Vertebrobasilar artery insufficiency.
Posterior fossa tumor or other brain tumors.
Infarction/hemorrhage of cerebral cortex, cerebellum, or brainstem.
Basilar migraine.
Metabolic: drugs, hypoxia, anemia, fever.
Hypotension/severe hypertension.
Multiple sclerosis.
CNS infections: viral, bacterial.
Temporal lobe epilepsy.
Arnold-Chiari malformation, syringobulbia.
Psychogenic: ventilation, hysteria.

VISION LOSS, ACUTE, PAINFUL

ICD-9CM # 368.11 VISION LOSS, SUDDEN

Acute angle-closure glaucoma.
Corneal ulcer.
Uveitis.
Endophthalmitis.
Factitious.
Somatization syndrome.
Trauma.

VISION LOSS, ACUTE, PAINLESS

ICD-9CM # 368.11 VISION LOSS, SUDDEN

Retinal artery occlusion.
Optic neuritis.
Retinal vein occlusion.
Vitreous hemorrhage.
Retinal detachment.
Exudative macular degeneration.
CVA.
Ischemic optic neuropathy.
Factitious.
Somatization syndrome, anxiety reaction.

VISION LOSS, CHRONIC, PROGRESSIVE

ICD-9CM # 369.9 VISION LOSS NOS

Cataract.
Macular degeneration.
Cerebral neoplasm.
Refractive error.
Open-angle glaucoma.

VISION LOSS, MONOCULAR, TRANSIENT

ICD-9CM # 369.9

Thromboembolism.
Vasculitis.
Migraine (vasospasm).
Anxiety reaction.
CNS tumor.
Temporal arteritis.
Multiple sclerosis.

VOLUME DEPLETION[1]

ICD-9CM # 276.5

Gastrointestinal losses:
    Upper: bleeding, nasogastric suction, vomiting.
    Lower: bleeding, diarrhea, enteric or pancreatic fistula, tube drainage.

Renal losses:
    Salt and water: diuretics, osmotic diuresis, postobstructive diuresis, acute tubular necrosis (recovery phase), salt-losing nephropathy, adrenal insufficiency, renal tubular acidosis.
Water loss: diabetes insipidus.
Skin and respiratory losses:
    Sweat, burns, insensible losses.
Sequestration without external fluid loss:
    Intestinal obstruction, peritonitis, pancreatitis, rhabdomyolysis, internal bleeding.

VOLUME EXCESS[1]

ICD-9CM # CODE VARIES WITH SPECIFIC DIAGNOSIS

PRIMARY RENAL SODIUM RETENTION (INCREASED EFFECTIVE CIRCULATING VOLUME)

Renal failure, nephritic syndrome, acute glomerulonephritis.
Primary hyperaldosteronism.
Cushing syndrome.
Liver disease.

SECONDARY RENAL SODIUM RETENTION (DECREASED EFFECTIVE CIRCULATING VOLUME)

Heart failure.
Liver disease.
Nephrotic syndrome (minimal change disease).

VOMITING

ICD-9CM # 787.03

GI disturbances:
Obstruction: esophageal, pyloric, intestinal.
Infections: viral or bacterial enteritis, viral hepatitis, food poisoning, gastroenteritis.
Pancreatitis.
Appendicitis.
Biliary colic.
Peritonitis.
Perforated bowel.
Diabetic gastroparesis.
Other: gastritis, PUD, IBD, GI tract neoplasms.
Drugs: morphine, digitalis, cytotoxic agents, bromocriptine.
Severe pain: MI, renal colic.
Metabolic disorders: uremia, acidosis/alkalosis, hyperglycemia, DKA, thyrotoxicosis.
Trauma: blows to the testicles, epigastrium.
Vertigo.
Reye's syndrome.
Increased intracranial pressure.
CNS disturbances: trauma, hemorrhage, infarction, neoplasm, infection, hypertensive encephalopathy, migraine.
Radiation sickness.
Motion sickness.
Bulimia, anorexia nervosa.
Psychogenic: emotional disturbances, offensive sights or smells.
Severe coughing.
Pyelonephritis.
Boerhaave's syndrome.
Carbon monoxide poisoning.

VULVAR LESIONS[5]

ICD-9CM # 625.8 VULVAR MASS
098.0 VULVAR ULCER, GONOCOCCAL
091.0 VULVAR ULCER, SYPHILITIC
616.51 BEHÇET'S
624.0 LEUKOPLAKIA
624.8 DYSPLASIA
233.3 CARCINOMA
616.9 INFLAMMATORY LESION
624.4 VULVAR SCAR (OLD)
624.1 VULVAR ATROPHY

RED LESION

Infection/infestation
Fungal infection:
    Candida.
    Tinea cruris.
    Intertrigo.
    Pityriasis versicolor.
Sarcoptes scabiei.
Erythrasma: *Corynebacterium minutissimum.*
Granuloma inguinale: *Calymmatobacterium granulomatis.*
Folliculitis: *Staphylococcus aureus.*
Hidradenitis suppurativa.
Behçet's syndrome.
Inflammation
Reactive vulvitis.
Chemical irritation:
    Detergent.
    Dyes.
    Perfume.
    Spermicide.
    Lubricants.
    Hygiene sprays.
    Podophyllum.
    Topical 5-FU.
    Saliva.
    Gentian violet.
    Semen.
Mechanical trauma: scratching.
Vestibular adenitis.
Essential vulvodynia.
Psoriasis.
Seborrheic dermatitis.
Neoplasm
Vulvar intraepithelial neoplasia (VIN):
    Mild dysplasia.
    Moderate dysplasia.
    Severe dysplasia.
    Carcinoma-in-situ.
Vulvar dystrophy.
Bowen's disease.
Invasive cancer:
    Squamous cell carcinoma.
    Malignant melanoma.
    Sarcoma.
    Basal cell carcinoma.
    Adenocarcinoma.
    Paget's disease.
    Undifferentiated.

WHITE LESION

Vulvar dystrophy:
    Lichen sclerosus.
    Vulvar dystrophy.
    Vulvar hyperplasia.
    Mixed dystrophy.
VIN.

Vitiligo.
Partial albinism.
Intertrigo.
Radiation treatment.

DARK LESION

Lentigo.
Nevi (mole).
Neoplasm (see Neoplasm, Vulvar, below).
Reactive hyperpigmentation.
Seborrheic keratosis.
Pubic lice.

ULCERATIVE LESION

Infection
Herpes simplex.
Vaccinia.
Treponema pallidum.
Granuloma inguinale.
Pyoderma.
Tuberculosis.
Noninfection
Behçet's disease.
Crohn's disease.
Pemphigus.
Pemphigoid.
Hidradenitis suppurativa (see Neoplasm, Vulvar, below).
Neoplasm
Basal cell carcinoma.
Squamous cell carcinoma.
Vulvar tumor <1 cm:
    Condyloma acuminatum.
    Molluscum contagiosum.
    Epidermal inclusion.
    Vestibular cyst.
    Mesenephric duct.
    VIN.
    Hemangioma.
    Hidradenoma.
    Neurofibroma.
    Syringoma.
    Accessory breast tissue.
    Acrochordon.
    Endometriosis.
    Fox-Fordyce disease.
    Pilonidal sinus.
Vulvar tumor >1 cm:
    Bartholin cyst or abscess.
    Lymphogranuloma venereum.
    Fibroma.
    Lipoma.
    Verrucous carcinoma.
    Squamous cell carcinoma.
    Hernia.
    Edema.
    Hematoma.
    Acrochordon.
    Epidermal cysts.
    Neurofibromatosis.
    Accessory breast tissue.

WEIGHT GAIN

ICD-9CM # 783.1 ABNORMAL WEIGHT GAIN
278.00 OBESITY

Sedentary lifestyle.
Fluid overload.
Discontinuation of tobacco abuse.

Endocrine disorders (hypothyroidism, hyperinsulinism associated with maturity-onset DM, Cushing's syndrome, hypogonadism, insulinoma, hyperprolactinemia, acromegaly).

Medications (nutritional supplements, antidepressants, glucocorticoids, etc.).

Anxiety disorders with compulsive eating.

Laurence-Moon-Biedl syndrome, Prader-Willi syndrome, other congenital diseases.

Hypothalamic injury (rare; <100 cases reported in medical literature).

WEIGHT LOSS

ICD-9CM # 783.2 ABNORMAL WEIGHT LOSS

Malignancy.

Psychiatric disorders (depression, anorexia nervosa).

New-onset DM.

Malabsorption.

COPD.

AIDS.

Uremia, liver disease.

Thyrotoxicosis, pheochromocytoma, carcinoid syndrome.

Addison's disease.

Intestinal parasites.

Peptic ulcer disease.

Inflammatory bowel disease.

Food faddism.

Postgastrectomy syndrome.

WHEEZING

ICD-9CM # 786.09

Asthma.

COPD.

Interstitial lung disease.

Infections (pneumonia, bronchitis, bronchiolitis, epiglottitis).

Cardiac asthma.

GERD with aspiration.

Foreign body aspiration.

Pulmonary embolism.

Anaphylaxis.

Obstruction airway (neoplasm, goiter, edema or hemorrhage from trauma, aneurysm, strictures, spasm).

Carcinoid syndrome.

XEROSTOMIA[16]

ICD-9CM # 527.7

Medications

Tricyclic antidepressants: amitriptyline (Elavil), doxepin (Sinequan).

Antihistamines: diphenhydramine (Benadryl), chlorpheniramine (Chlor-Trimeton), promethazine (Phenergan), and many cold and decongestant preparations.

Anticholinergic agents: antiemetics such as scopolamine, antispasmodic agents such as oxybutynin chloride (Ditropan).

Dehydration

Debility.

Fever.

Polyuria

Alcohol intake.

Arrhythmia.

Diabetes.

Previous head and neck irradiation

Systemic diseases

Sjögren's syndrome.

Sarcoidosis.

Amyloidosis.

REFERENCES

1. Andreoli TE, editor: *Cecil essentials of medicine,* ed 5, Philadelphia, 2001, WB Saunders.
2. Barkin RM, Rosen P: *Emergency pediatrics: a guide to ambulatory care,* ed 5, St Louis, 1998, Mosby.
3. Behrman RE: *Nelson textbook of pediatrics,* ed 16, Philadelphia, 2000, WB Saunders.
4. Conn R: *Current diagnosis,* ed 9, Philadelphia, 1997, WB Saunders.
5. Danakas G, editor: *Practical guide to the care of the gynecologic/obstetric patient,* St Louis, 1997, Mosby.
6. Goldberg RJ: *The care of the psychiatric patient,* ed 22, St Louis, 1998, Mosby.
7. Goldman L, Ausiello D: *Cecil textbook of medicine,* ed 21, Philadelphia, 2004, WB Saunders.
8. Goldman L, Braunwauld E, editors: *Primary cardiology,* Philadelphia, 1998, WB Saunders.
9. Gorbach SL: *Infectious diseases,* ed 2, Philadelphia, 1998, WB Saunders.
10. Harrington J: *Consultation in internal medicine,* ed 2, St Louis, 1997, Mosby.
11. Kassirer J, editor: *Current therapy in adult medicine,* ed 4, St Louis, 1998, Mosby.
12. Khan MG: *Rapid ECG interpretation,* Philadelphia, 2003, WB Saunders.
13. Klippel J, editor: *Practical rheumatology,* London, 1995, Mosby.
14. Marx J, editor: *Rosen's emergency medicine: concepts and clinical practice,* ed 5, St Louis, 2002, Mosby.
15. Moore WT, Eastman RC: *Diagnostic endocrinology,* ed 2, St Louis, 1996, Mosby.
16. Noble J, editor: *Primary care medicine,* ed 3, St Louis, 2001, Mosby.
17. Nseyo UO: *Urology for primary care physicians,* Philadelphia, 1999, WB Saunders.
18. Rakel RE: *Principles of family practice,* ed 6, Philadelphia, 2002, WB Saunders.
19. Seller RH: *Differential diagnosis of common complaints,* ed 4, Philadelphia, 2000, WB Saunders.
20. Siedel HM, editor: *Mosby's guide to physical examination,* ed 4, St Louis, 1999, Mosby.
21. Specht N: *Practical guide to diagnostic imaging,* St Louis, 1998, Mosby.
22. Stein JH, editor: *Internal medicine,* ed 5, St Louis, 1998, Mosby.
23. Wiederholt WC: *Neurology for non-neurologists,* ed 4, Philadelphia, 2000, WB Saunders.

Section III

Clinical Algorithms

PLEASE NOTE: These algorithms are designed to assist clinicians in the evaluation and treatment of patients. They may not apply to all patients with a particular condition and are not intended to replace a clinician's individual judgment.

ICD-9CM # 995.81

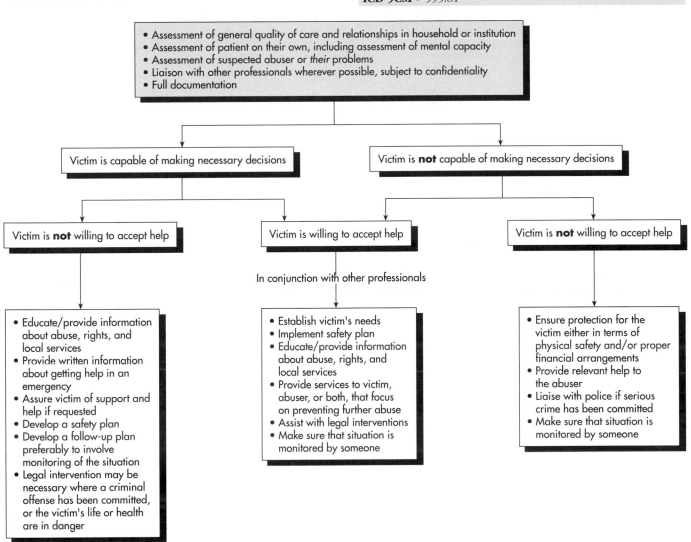

- Assessment of general quality of care and relationships in household or institution
- Assessment of patient on their own, including assessment of mental capacity
- Assessment of suspected abuser or *their* problems
- Liaison with other professionals wherever possible, subject to confidentiality
- Full documentation

Victim is capable of making necessary decisions

Victim is **not** capable of making necessary decisions

Victim is **not** willing to accept help

Victim is willing to accept help

Victim is **not** willing to accept help

In conjunction with other professionals

- Educate/provide information about abuse, rights, and local services
- Provide written information about getting help in an emergency
- Assure victim of support and help if requested
- Develop a safety plan
- Develop a follow-up plan preferably to involve monitoring of the situation
- Legal intervention may be necessary where a criminal offense has been committed, or the victim's life or health are in danger

- Establish victim's needs
- Implement safety plan
- Educate/provide information about abuse, rights, and local services
- Provide services to victim, abuser, or both, that focus on preventing further abuse
- Assist with legal interventions
- Make sure that situation is monitored by someone

- Ensure protection for the victim either in terms of physical safety and/or proper financial arrangements
- Provide relevant help to the abuser
- Liaise with police if serious crime has been committed
- Make sure that situation is monitored by someone

FIGURE 3-1 Management of geriatric abuse. (From Tallis RC, Fillit HM [eds]: *Brocklehurst's text-book of geriatric medicine and gerontology,* ed 6, London, 2003, Churchill Livingstone.)

Section III

CLINICAL ALGORITHMS

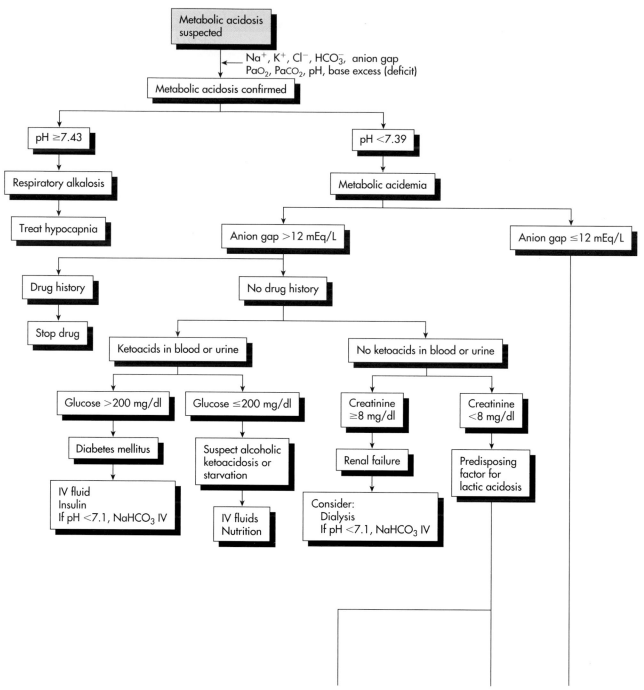

FIGURE 3-2 Suspected metabolic acidosis. (From Greene HL, Johnson WP, Lemke D [eds]: *Decision making in medicine,* ed 2, St Louis, 1998, Mosby.)

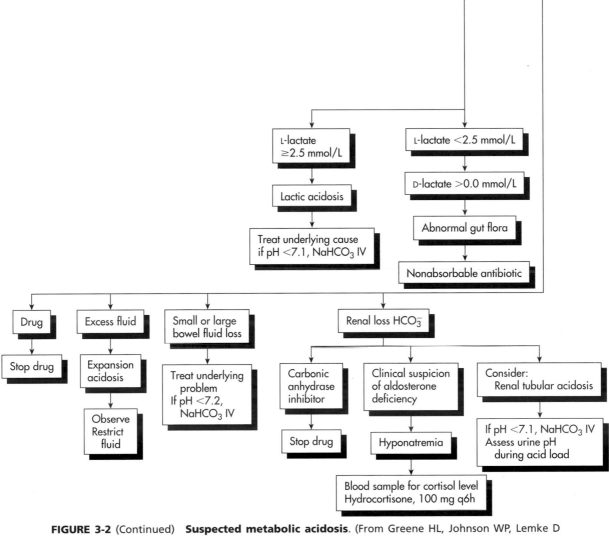

FIGURE 3-2 (Continued)   **Suspected metabolic acidosis**. (From Greene HL, Johnson WP, Lemke D [eds]: *Decision making in medicine*, ed 2, St Louis, 1998, Mosby.)

Step I: Ask about alcohol use
  Consumption
    Per week
    Per occasion
  CAGE questions (1 point for each yes answer):
    Have you ever felt that you should **C**ut down on your
      drinking?
    Have people **A**nnoyed you by criticizing your drinking?
    Have you ever felt bad or **G**uilty about your drinking?
    Have you ever had a drink first thing in the morning
      to steady your nerves or to get rid of a hangover
      (**E**ye opener)?

Men: >14 drinks/week or >4 per occasion
Women: >7 drinks/week or >3 per occasion
or
CAGE score ≥1

Step II: Assess for alcohol-related problems
At risk: **May be alcohol-dependent:**
  Drinking above recommended   CAGE score ≥3 or ≥1 of the
    levels or in high-risk situations   following:
  Personal or family history of   Preoccupied with drinking
    alcohol-related problems   Unable to stop once started
Current alcohol-related problems: Drinking to avoid
  CAGE score 1-2 (in past year)   withdrawal symptoms
  Evidence of alcohol-related   Tolerance
    medical or behavioral
    problems

Step III: Advise appropriate action
State medical concerns about drinking
Agree on plan of action:
  At risk or current problems: **Alcohol-dependent:**
    Advise to cut down   Advise to abstain
    Set specific drinking goal   Refer to specialist

Step IV: Monitor patient progress
  All patients: **Patients referred for**
    Consider scheduling   **alcohol treatment:**
      separate follow-up   Review updates from
      visit or phone call   treatment specialist
    Review progress and   Monitor for depression
      reinforce efforts at   and anxiety
      each follow-up visit

FIGURE 3-3   Screening and brief intervention for alcohol problems in clinical practice. (From Goldman L, Ausiello D [eds]: *Cecil textbook of medicine*, ed 22, Philadelphia, 2004, WB Saunders.)

ICD-9CM # 273.6

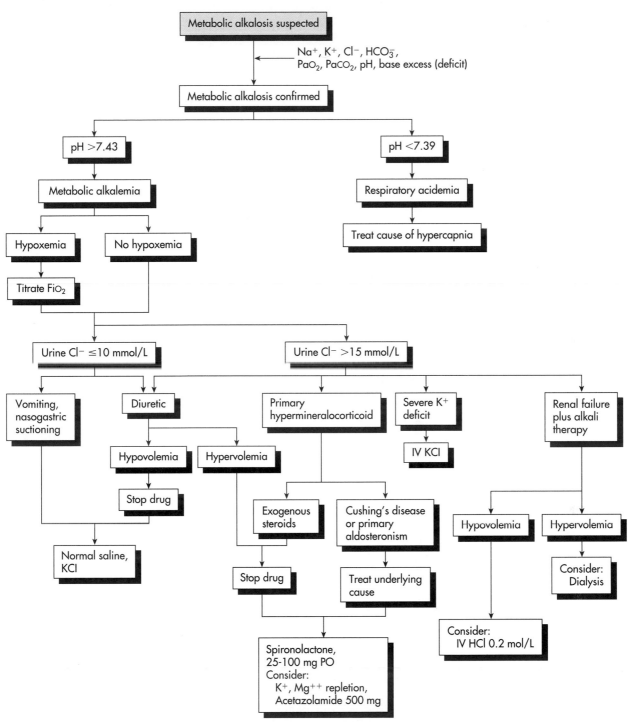

FIGURE 3-4   Suspected metabolic alkalosis. (From Greene HL, Johnson WP, Lemke D [eds]: *Decision making in medicine,* ed 2, St Louis, 1998, Mosby.)

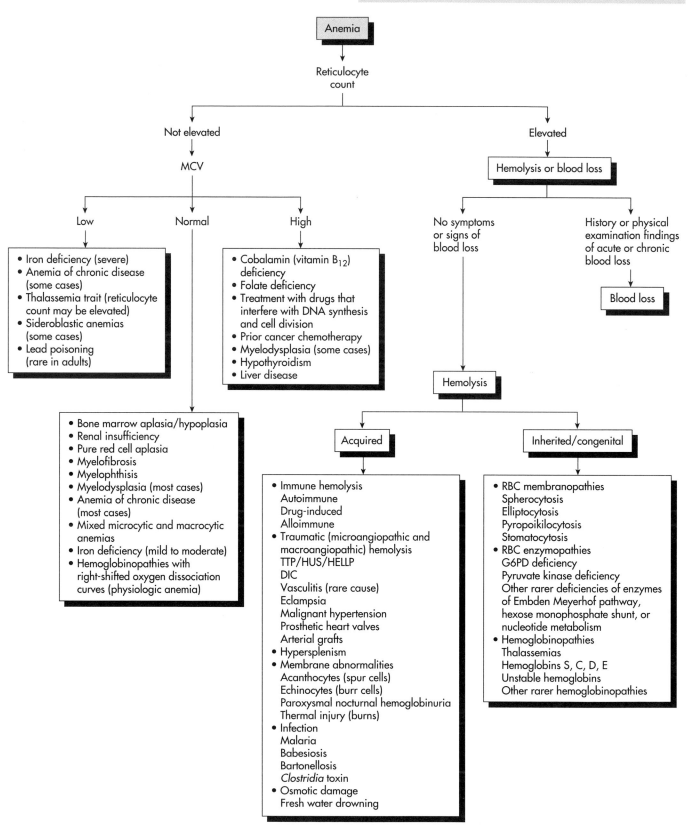

FIGURE 3-5 Algorithm for diagnosis of anemias. *DIC,* Disseminated intravascular coagulation; *HELLP,* hepatomegaly-elevated *l*iver (function tests)-*l*ow platelets; *HUS,* hemolytic-uremic syndrome; *MCV,* mean corpuscular volume; *RBC,* red blood cell; *TTP,* thrombotic thrombocytopenic purpura. (From Goldman L, Ausiello D [eds]: *Cecil textbook of medicine,* ed 22, Philadelphia, 2004, WB Saunders.)

ANEMIA, MACROCYTIC

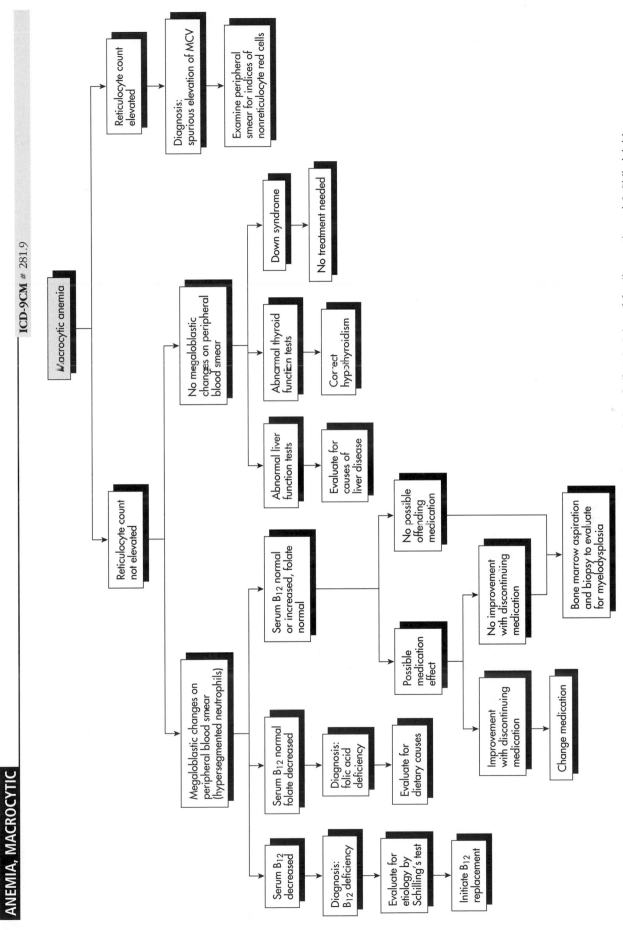

FIGURE 3-6   Differential diagnosis of macrocytic anemia. (From Rakel RE [ed]: *Principles of family practice*, ed 6, Philadelphia, 2002, WB Saunders.)

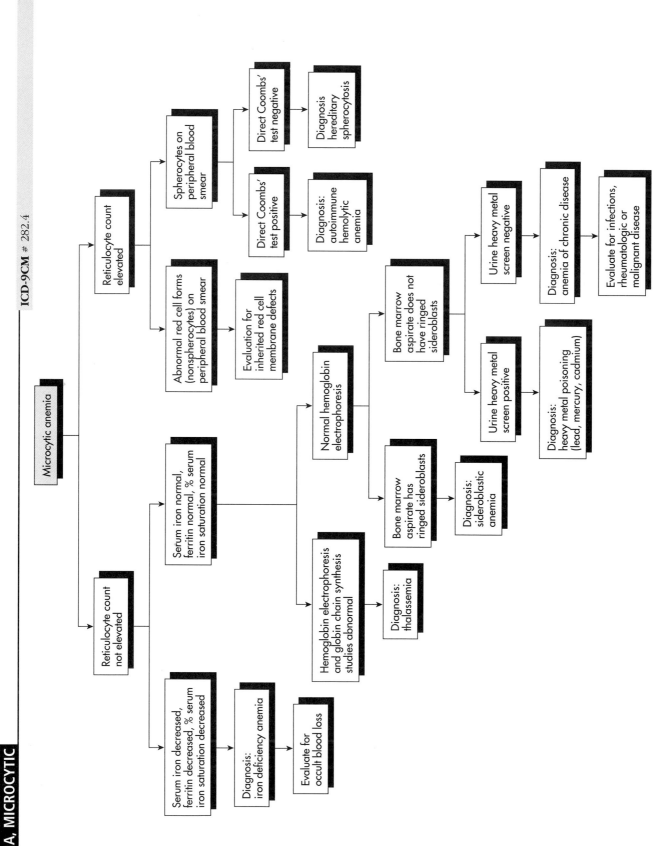

FIGURE 3-7   Differential diagnosis of microcytic anemia. (From Rakel RE [ed]: *Principles of family practice*, ed 6, Philadelphia, 2002, WB Saunders.)

ANEMIA, WITH RETICULOCYTOSIS

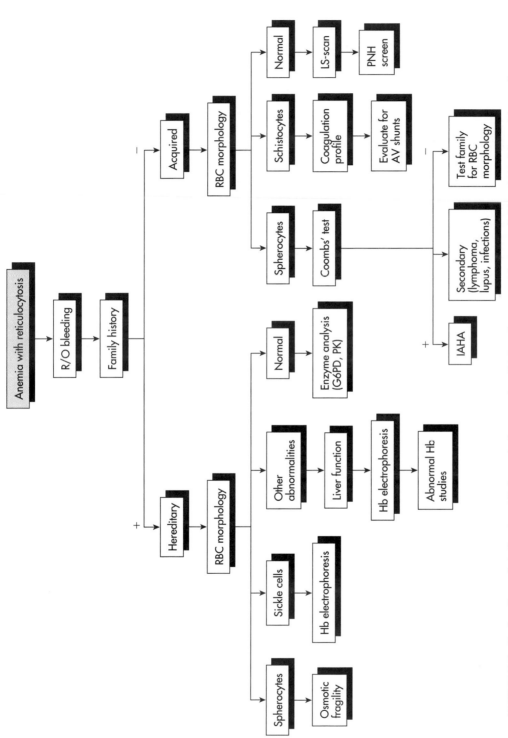

FIGURE 3-8   Evaluation of patients with hemolytic anemia. *AV,* Arteriovenous; *Hb,* hemoglobin; *IAHA,* idiopathic autoimmune hemolytic anemia; *LS,* liver spleen; *PK,* pyruvate kinase; *PNH,* paroxysmal nocturnal hemoglobinuria; *RBC,* red blood cell. (From Stein JH: *Internal medicine,* ed 5, St Louis, 1997, Mosby.)

ICD-9CM # 783.0

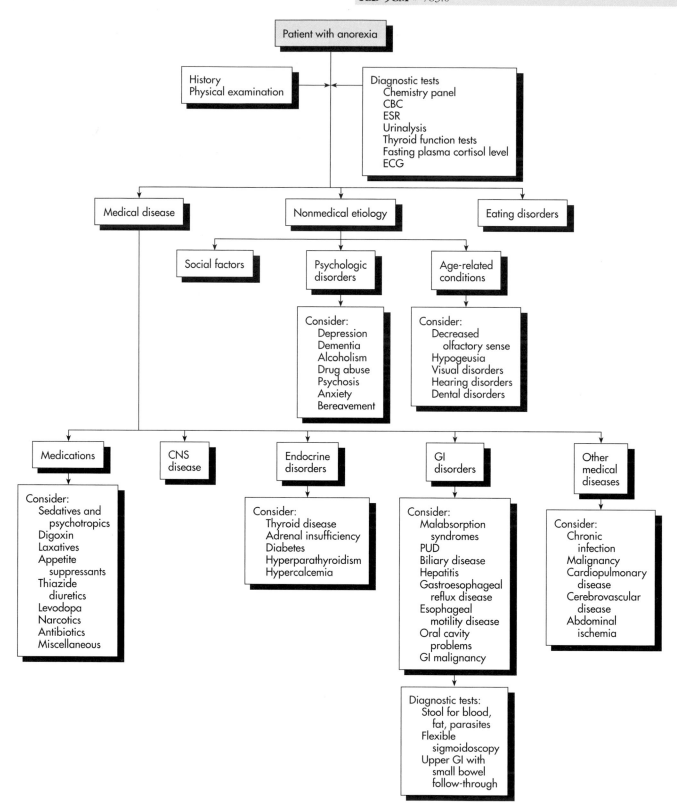

FIGURE 3-9   Evaluation of anorexia. *CBC,* Complete blood count; *CNS,* central nervous system; *ECG,* electrocardiogram; *ESR,* erythrocyte sedimentation rate; *GI,* gastrointestinal; *PUD,* peptic ulcer disease. (From Greene HL, Johnson WP, Lemcke D [eds]: *Decision making in medicine,* ed 2, St Louis, 1998, Mosby.)

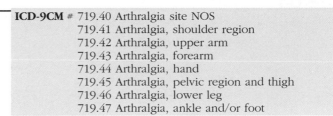

ICD-9CM # 719.40 Arthralgia site NOS
719.41 Arthralgia, shoulder region
719.42 Arthralgia, upper arm
719.43 Arthralgia, forearm
719.44 Arthralgia, hand
719.45 Arthralgia, pelvic region and thigh
719.46 Arthralgia, lower leg
719.47 Arthralgia, ankle and/or foot

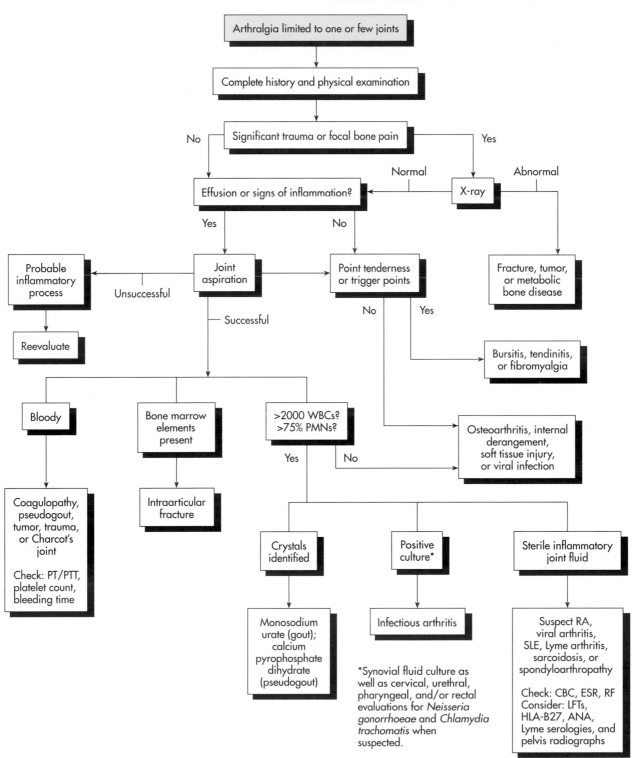

FIGURE 3-10 A diagnostic approach to arthralgia in a few joints. *ANA,* Antinuclear antibodies; *CBC,* complete blood count; *ESR,* erythrocyte sedimentation rate; *LFTs,* liver function tests; *PMNs,* polymorphonuclear neutrophils; *PT,* prothrombin time; *PTT,* partial thromboplastin time; *RA,* rheumatoid arthritis; *RF,* rheumatoid factor; *SLE,* systemic lupus erythematosus; *WBCs,* white blood cells. (Modified from American College of Rheumatology Ad Hoc Committee on Clinical Guidelines: *Arthritis Rheum* 39:1, 1996.)

Section III

CLINICAL ALGORITHMS

ICD-9CM # 789.5 Ascites NOS
197.6 Ascites, cancerous
(malignant) M8000/6
457.8 Chylous
014.0 Tuberculous

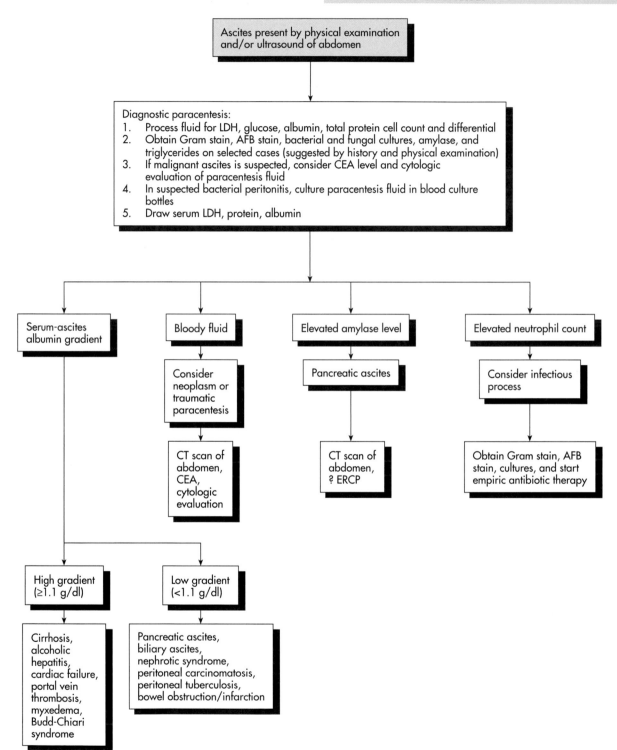

FIGURE 3-11 Evaluation of ascites. *AFB,* Acid-fast bacillus; *CEA,* carcinoembryonic antigen; *CT,* computed tomography; *ERCP,* endoscopic retrograde cholangiopancreatography; *LDH,* lactate dehydrogenase.

ICD-9CM # 493.9 Asthma, unspecified
493.1 Intrinsic asthma
493.0 Extrinsic asthma

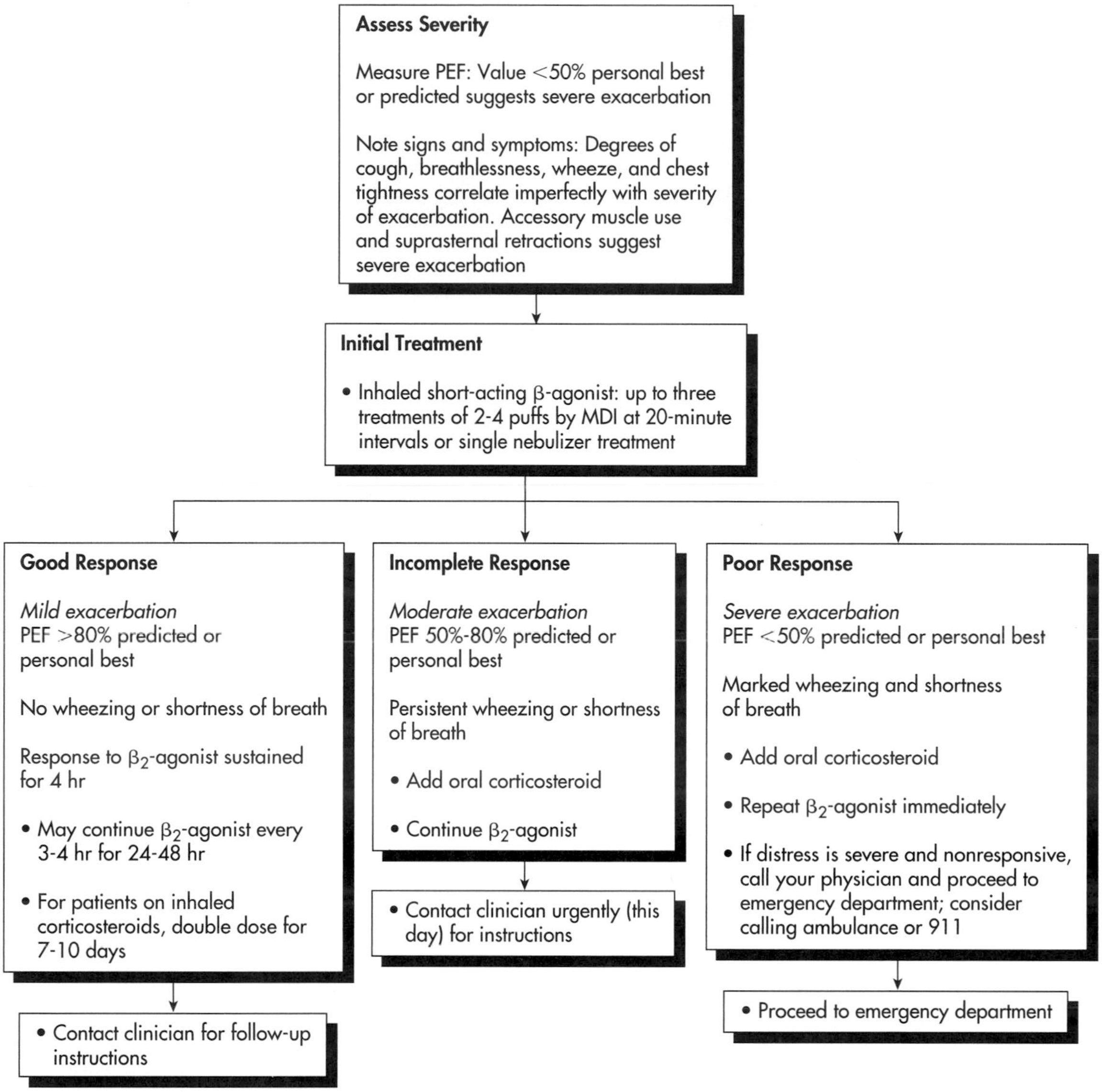

Assess Severity

Measure PEF: Value <50% personal best or predicted suggests severe exacerbation

Note signs and symptoms: Degrees of cough, breathlessness, wheeze, and chest tightness correlate imperfectly with severity of exacerbation. Accessory muscle use and suprasternal retractions suggest severe exacerbation

Initial Treatment

• Inhaled short-acting β-agonist: up to three treatments of 2-4 puffs by MDI at 20-minute intervals or single nebulizer treatment

Good Response

Mild exacerbation
PEF >80% predicted or personal best

No wheezing or shortness of breath

Response to β$_2$-agonist sustained for 4 hr

• May continue β$_2$-agonist every 3-4 hr for 24-48 hr

• For patients on inhaled corticosteroids, double dose for 7-10 days

• Contact clinician for follow-up instructions

Incomplete Response

Moderate exacerbation
PEF 50%-80% predicted or personal best

Persistent wheezing or shortness of breath

• Add oral corticosteroid

• Continue β$_2$-agonist

• Contact clinician urgently (this day) for instructions

Poor Response

Severe exacerbation
PEF <50% predicted or personal best

Marked wheezing and shortness of breath

• Add oral corticosteroid

• Repeat β$_2$-agonist immediately

• If distress is severe and nonresponsive, call your physician and proceed to emergency department; consider calling ambulance or 911

• Proceed to emergency department

FIGURE 3-12   Home management of acute asthma. *MDI,* Metered-dose inhaler; *PEF,* peak expiratory flow rate. (Modified from National Asthma Education and Prevention Program, National Heart, Lung, and Blood Institute, Expert Panel Report 2: *Guidelines for the diagnosis and management of asthma,* NIH Pub No 97-4051, July 1997.)

ICD-9CM # 847.9

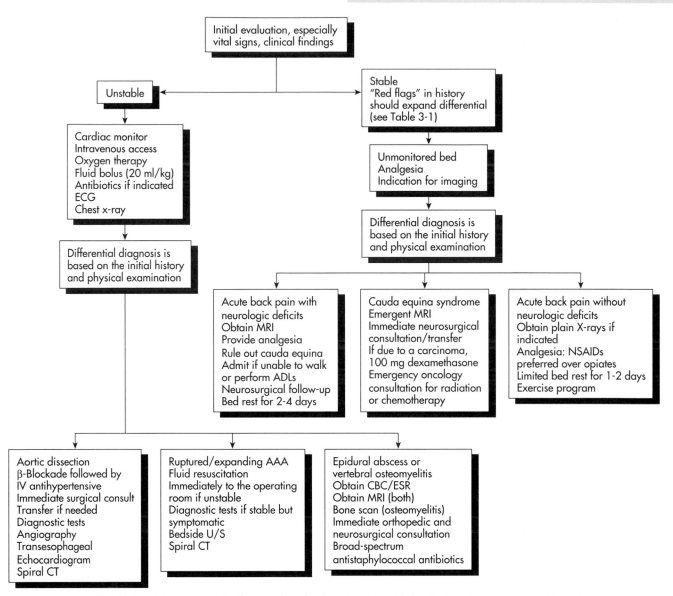

FIGURE 3-13 Management of acute low back pain. *AAA,* Abdominal aortic aneurysm; *ADL,* activities of daily living; *CBC,* complete blood count; *CT,* computed tomography; *ECG,* electrocardiogram; *ESR,* erythrocyte sedimentation rate; *IV,* intravenous; *NSAIDs,* nonsteroidal antiinflammatory drugs. (From Marx JA [ed]: *Rosen's emergency medicine,* ed 5, St Louis 2002, Mosby.)

TABLE 3-1 Red Flags for Potentially Serious Conditions

Possible Fracture	Possible Tumor or Infection	Possible Cauda Equina Syndrome
From Medical History		
Major trauma, such as vehicle accident or fall from height	Age over 50 or under 20 yr	Saddle anesthesia
Minor trauma or even strenuous lifting (in older or potentially osteoporotic patient)	History of cancer	Recent onset of bladder dysfunction, such as urinary retention, increased frequency, or overflow incontinence
	Constitutional symptoms, such as recent fever or chills or unexplained weight loss	Severe or progressive neurologic deficit in the lower extremity
	Risk factors for spinal infection: recent bacterial infection (e.g., urinary tract infection); intravenous drug abuse; or immune suppression (from steroids, transplant, or human immunodeficiency virus)	
	Pain that worsens when supine; severe nighttime pain	

ICD-9CM # 578.9

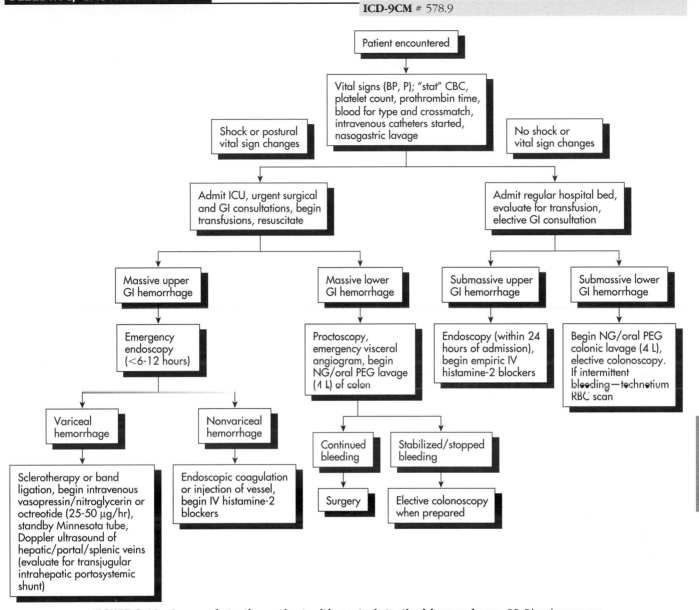

FIGURE 3-14 Approach to the patient with gastrointestinal hemorrhage. *BP,* Blood pressure; *CBC,* complete blood count; *GI,* gastrointestinal; *ICU,* intensive care unit; *IV,* intravenous; *NG,* nasogastric; *P,* weight; *PEG,* percutaneous endoscopic gastrostomy; *RBC,* red blood cell. (From Goldman L, Ausiello D [eds]: *Cecil textbook of medicine,* ed 22, Philadelphia, 2004, WB Saunders.)

ICD-9CM # 427.89 Unspecified bradycardia
427.81 Chronic bradycardia
770.8 Newborn bradycardia
427.89 Postoperative bradycardia
337 Reflex bradycardia
427.89 Sinus bradycardia

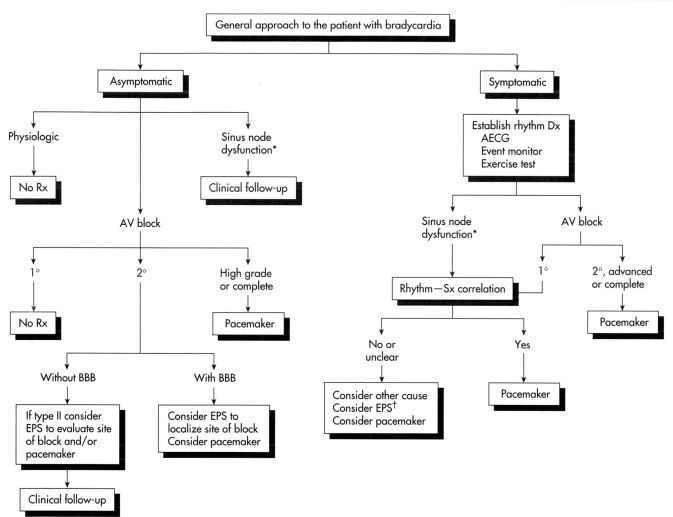

*Includes bradycardia-tachycardia syndrome.
†EPS includes sinus node function and ventricular arrhythmia induction studies.

FIGURE 3-15 General approach to the patient with bradycardia. *AECG,* Ambulatory electrocardiography; *AV,* atrioventricular; *BBB,* bundle branch block; *Dx,* diagnostic; *EPS,* electrophysiologic study; *Rx,* treatment; *Sx,* symptoms; 1°, first-degree; 2°, second-degree. (From Goldman L, Braunwald E [eds]: *Primary cardiology,* Philadelphia, 1998, WB Saunders.)

ICD-9CM # V76.10

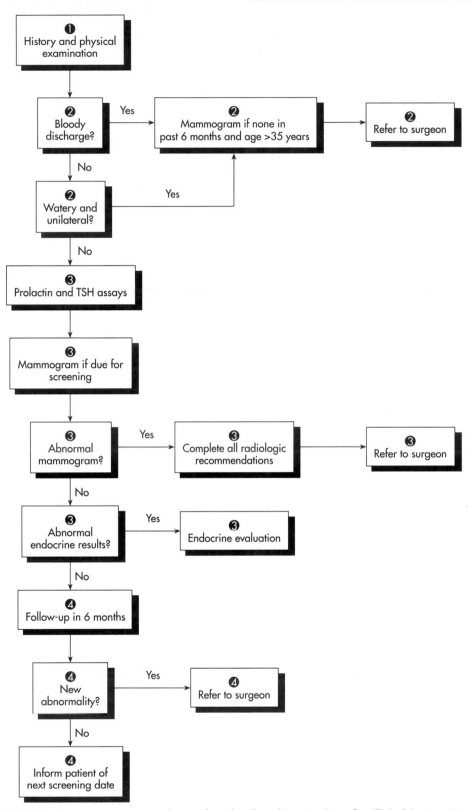

FIGURE 3-16   Breast cancer screening and evaluation. (From Institute for Clinical Systems Integration, Minneapolis: *Postgrad Med* 100:182-187, 1996.)

Continued on following page

FIGURE 3-16 (Continued)

1. **Screening mammogram.*** Patients are most commonly referred to a radiologist for screening mammography. Occasionally, however, patients are referred for diagnostic mammography based on symptoms or findings on breast exam. In the event of an abnormal finding on the mammogram, complete evaluation under the direction of a radiologist is recommended. It is the responsibility of the radiologist to complete the radiologic assessment so that the best possible characterization of the abnormality can be provided in an expeditious fashion to the primary care physician who ordered the original study. Any recommendations for referral to a surgeon for possible biopsy should be made directly to the primary care physician. The ultimate responsibility to make the referral will rest with the primary care physician.

2. **Abnormal mammogram. Sorting abnormalities. Suspicious for cancer?** On obtaining an abnormal finding on a mammogram, the radiologist determines whether further mammographic images are required for completion of the evaluation process. This may include a repeated image of the involved breast at 6 months to document stability of a low-risk, probably benign lesion. Alternatively, spot compression, magnification, or both may be necessary to obtain further characterization of indeterminate breast lesions. These additional studies should be done with the radiologist present to reduce the risk of patient recall for further studies necessary to evaluate the same lesion.

   On completion of these views, each and every abnormality uncovered for each independent lesion of the breast studied should be sorted according to the nature of the abnormality. The radiologist should classify the lesion as representing either suspicious microcalcifications, architectural distortion, or a soft-tissue mass. For any lesions identified as demonstrating microcalcifications that suggest cancer, biopsy will be recommended. It is up to the primary care physician to make the referral to a surgeon for biopsy. If a soft-tissue mass is identified on the mammogram, it should be studied further to determine its relative risk for malignancy. Any suspect lesions identified as having associated microcalcifications, architectural distortion, or interval growth when compared with the previous mammogram should likewise be referred to a surgeon for possible biopsy.

3. **Ultrasound results.** When the mass is not immediately suggestive of cancer, an ultrasound should be performed to determine whether the lesion is solid. A solid mass should be further characterized for its level of benignity according to three criteria:

   - Size less than 15 mm
   - Three or fewer lobulations
   - More than 50% of the margin of the lesion appearing well circumscribed in any view

   Patients who have lesions that fit all three criteria may be observed and then evaluated with a 6-month follow-up study. Any lesion that does not fit all three criteria for benignity should be characterized as indeterminate, and biopsy should be considered. Likewise, any solid mass that is palpable should be referred to a surgeon for possible open biopsy. Finally, any lesion that appears to be new since the last screening mammogram should be considered for biopsy.

4. **Aspiration and results.** If the ultrasound of the soft-tissue mass demonstrates that it is a cystic lesion, the cyst should be further categorized by the criteria listed in the algorithm: irregular wall, as seen on ultrasonography; internal echoes; complex, septated appearance; and palpability within the region of the ultrasound-proven cyst. A positive finding for any of these criteria would be an indication for ultrasound-directed aspiration of the cyst. Aspiration should also be offered if the patient requests it.

   After cyst aspiration, a single-view mammogram should be obtained to demonstrate complete resolution of the lesion. If the lesion is sufficiently complex, a cyst pneumogram may be performed. Should any residual mass be present or if the cyst pneumogram findings are abnormal, biopsy should be recommended. If, on the other hand, the mass is a simple cyst that does not fit any of the previously listed criteria, the patient should be returned to the screening process, and completion of this evaluation should be reported to the ordering health care provider.

---

*ICSI healthcare guidelines are designed to assist clinicians by providing an analytic framework for the evaluation and treatment of patients. They are not intended either to replace a clinician's judgment or to establish a protocol for all patients with a particular condition. A guideline will rarely establish the only approach to a problem. In addition, guidelines are "living documents" that are expected to be imperfect and are subject to annual review and revision.

ICSI is a nonprofit organization that provides healthcare quality improvement services to 20 medical groups affiliated with HealthPartners in central and southern Minnesota and western Wisconsin. The guidelines are developed through a process that involves physicians, nurses, and other healthcare professionals from beginning to end, and healthcare purchasers are included in decision making. To order any of the more than 40 guidelines ICSI has developed, contact the ICSI Publications Fulfillment Center, in care of the ARDEL Group, 6518 Walker St., Suite 150, Minneapolis, MN 55426; 612-927-6707.

BREAST, ROUTINE SCREEN OR PALPABLE MASS EVALUATION

ICD-9CM # 611.72 Breast mass or lump, nonpuerperal

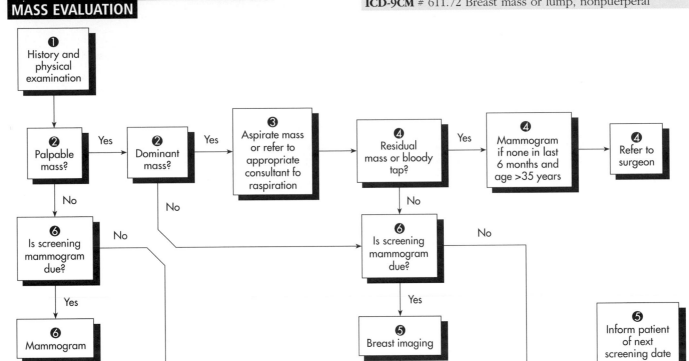

FIGURE 3-17   Breast cancer screening and evaluation. (From Institute for Clinical Systems Integration, Minneapolis: *Postgrad Med* 100:182, 1996.)

1. **History and physical examination.*** Primary care evaluation is initiated with history taking aimed at uncovering and characterizing any breast-related symptom. A risk assessment should also be undertaken for identified risk factors, including patient age over 50 years, any past personal history of breast cancer, history of hyperplasia on previous breast biopsies, and family history of breast cancer in first-degree relatives (mother, sister, daughter). Physical examination should include inspection of the breast for any evidence of ulceration or contour changes and inspection of the nipple for Paget's disease. Palpation should be performed with the patient in both the upright and supine positions to determine the presence of any palpable mass.

2. **Palpable mass? Dominant mass?** A dominant mass is a palpable finding that is discrete and clearly different from the surrounding parenchyma. If a palpable mass is identified, it should be determined whether it represents a dominant (i.e., discrete) mass, which requires immediate evaluation. The primary care physician or appropriate consultant should attempt to aspirate any dominant mass because a simple cyst may be uncovered, in which case aspiration completes the evaluation process.

3. **Aspirate mass or refer for aspiration.** Aspiration of a dominant palpable mass should be performed by the primary care physician or by the appropriate consultant. The breast skin is prepped with alcohol. Then, with the lesion immobilized by the nonoperating hand, an 18- to 25-gauge needle mounted on a 10-ml syringe is directed to the central portion of the mass for a single attempt at aspiration. Successful aspiration of a simple cyst would yield a nonbloody fluid with complete resolution of the dominant mass. Typical watery fluid may be discarded. However, cyst fluid that is bloody or unusually tenacious should be examined cytologically.

Continued on following page

FIGURE 3-17 (Continued)

4. **Residual mass or bloody tap? Mammogram if none in past 6 months. Refer to surgeon.** Should the mass remain after the attempt at aspiration or should frank blood be aspirated during the process, the presence of a malignant process cannot be ruled out. Patients with a residual mass or bloody tap should be referred to a surgeon for possible biopsy. Before the referral, a mammogram should be obtained for any patient over age 35 years who has not had a mammogram within the preceding 6 months. In patients 35 years and under, obtaining any other breast-imaging studies should be left to the discretion of the surgeon or radiologist.

5. **Is screening mammogram due? Breast imaging. Follow-up clinical breast examination. Refer to surgeon.** Should physical examination demonstrate a palpable mass that is not clearly a discrete and dominant mass, its size, location, and character should be documented in anticipation of a follow-up examination. A screening mammogram should be obtained if one has not been done within the recommended interval. If no mammogram is required or if a required mammogram demonstrates no abnormality, a follow-up examination in 1 month is indicated. Should any residual mass be identified, the patient should be referred to a surgeon for possible biopsy. Patients with a persisting non-dominant palpable mass that does not resolve within 1 month and those with any recurring cystic mass should be referred for surgical evaluation. If no mass is apparent at the time of the follow-up examination, the patient should then be informed of the appropriate date for her next screening examination, according to the recommended intervals.

6. **Screening mammogram and results.** After completion of the physical examination, the appropriateness of a routine screening mammogram should be determined. If a mammogram is done, the radiologist should provide the results to the primary care physician for reporting to the patient. Should any abnormalities be uncovered, it will be the responsibility of the radiologist to complete any additional imaging studies required for the complete radiographic characterization of the lesion. The radiologist should make certain that all recommended additional views, follow-up studies, and ultrasound examinations have been completed before referral to a surgeon. However, it is important that the primary care physician who ordered the mammogram review the results of these studies to understand fully the opinion of the radiologist and to ensure that all recommendations of the radiologist have been completed. Should the radiologist recommend that surgical consultation is warranted, it will be the responsibility of the primary care physician to establish this referral.

NOTE: *The importance of communication between the surgical consultant and the primary care physician cannot be overstated. Biopsy results should be reported both to the surgeon and to the primary care physician. More important, patients who do not require biopsy after surgical consultation should be returned to the routine screening process. This process is under the supervision of the primary care physician. Therefore it is absolutely necessary for the primary care physician to know when the patient reenters the routine screening population. In the event that new symptoms arise during the screening interval, the patient should be evaluated by the primary care physician using the primary care evaluation process of this guideline.*

---

*ICSI healthcare guidelines are designed to assist clinicians by providing an analytic framework for the evaluation and treatment of patients. They are not intended either to replace a clinician's judgment or to establish a protocol for all patients with a particular condition. A guideline will rarely establish the only approach to a problem. In addition, guidelines are "living documents" that are expected to be imperfect and are subject to annual review and revision.

ICSI is a nonprofit organization that provides healthcare quality improvement services to 20 medical groups affiliated with HealthPartners in central and southern Minnesota and western Wisconsin. The guidelines are developed through a process that involves physicians, nurses, and other healthcare professionals from beginning to end, and healthcare purchasers are included in decision making. To order any of the more than 40 guidelines ICSI has developed, contact the ICSI Publications Fulfillment Center, in care of the ARDEL Group, 6518 Walker St., Suite 150, Minneapolis, MN 55426; 612-927-6707.

CARDIOMEGALY ON CHEST X-RAY

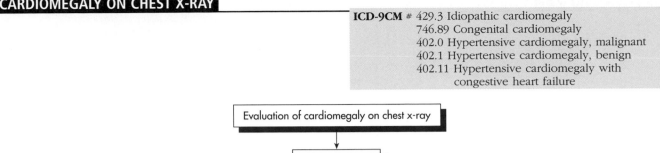

ICD-9CM # 429.3 Idiopathic cardiomegaly
746.89 Congenital cardiomegaly
402.0 Hypertensive cardiomegaly, malignant
402.1 Hypertensive cardiomegaly, benign
402.11 Hypertensive cardiomegaly with
congenital heart failure

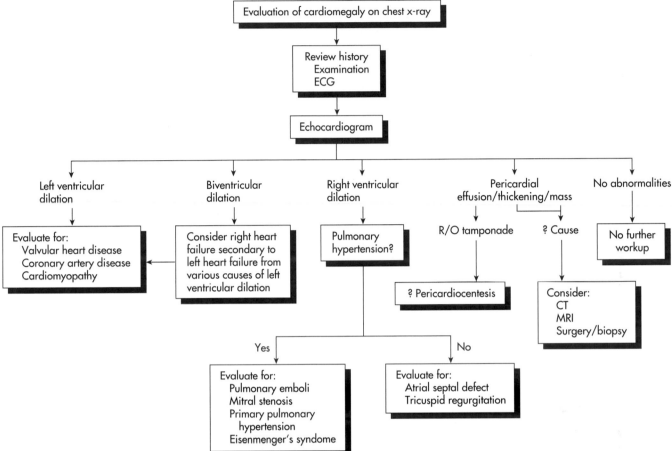

FIGURE 3-18 Approach to the patient with cardiomegaly. When cardiomegaly is found on the chest radiograph, the history and physical examination should be reviewed and an electrocardiogram (ECG) performed before obtaining a two-dimensional Doppler echocardiographic study. Cardiomegaly may be explained by left ventricular dilation, biventricular dilation, right ventricular dilation, or pericardial abnormalities, or it may be found to be spurious on the echocardiogram. Rarely, isolated abnormalities of the atrium, particularly the left atrium, may cause abnormalities on the chest radiograph but will not cause true cardiomegaly. Depending on the echocardiographic findings, further tests can help elucidate the cause of echocardiographically confirmed cardiomegaly. *CT*, Computer tomography; *MRI*, magnetic resonance imaging; *R/O*, rule out. (From Goldman L, Branwald E [eds]: *Primary cardiology,* Philadelphia, 1998, WB Saunders.)

ICD-9CM # 437.1 Cerebral ischemia (chronic)
435.9 Cerebral ischemia intermittent (transient)

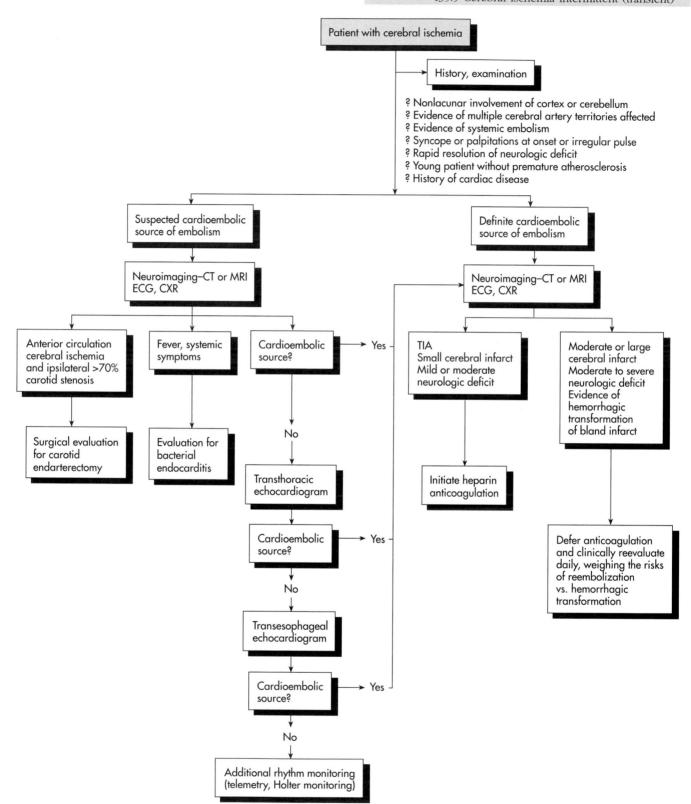

FIGURE 3-19   Evaluation of patients with cerebral ischemia for a cardioembolic source. *CT,* computed tomography; *CXR,* chest radiograph; *ECG,* electrocardiogram; *MRI,* magnetic resonance imaging; *TIA,* transient ischemic attack. (From Johnson R [ed]: *Current therapy in neurologic disease,* ed 5, St Louis, 1997, Mosby.)

CHRONIC OBSTRUCTIVE PULMONARY DISEASE

ICD-9CM # 496 COPD
492.8 Emphysema

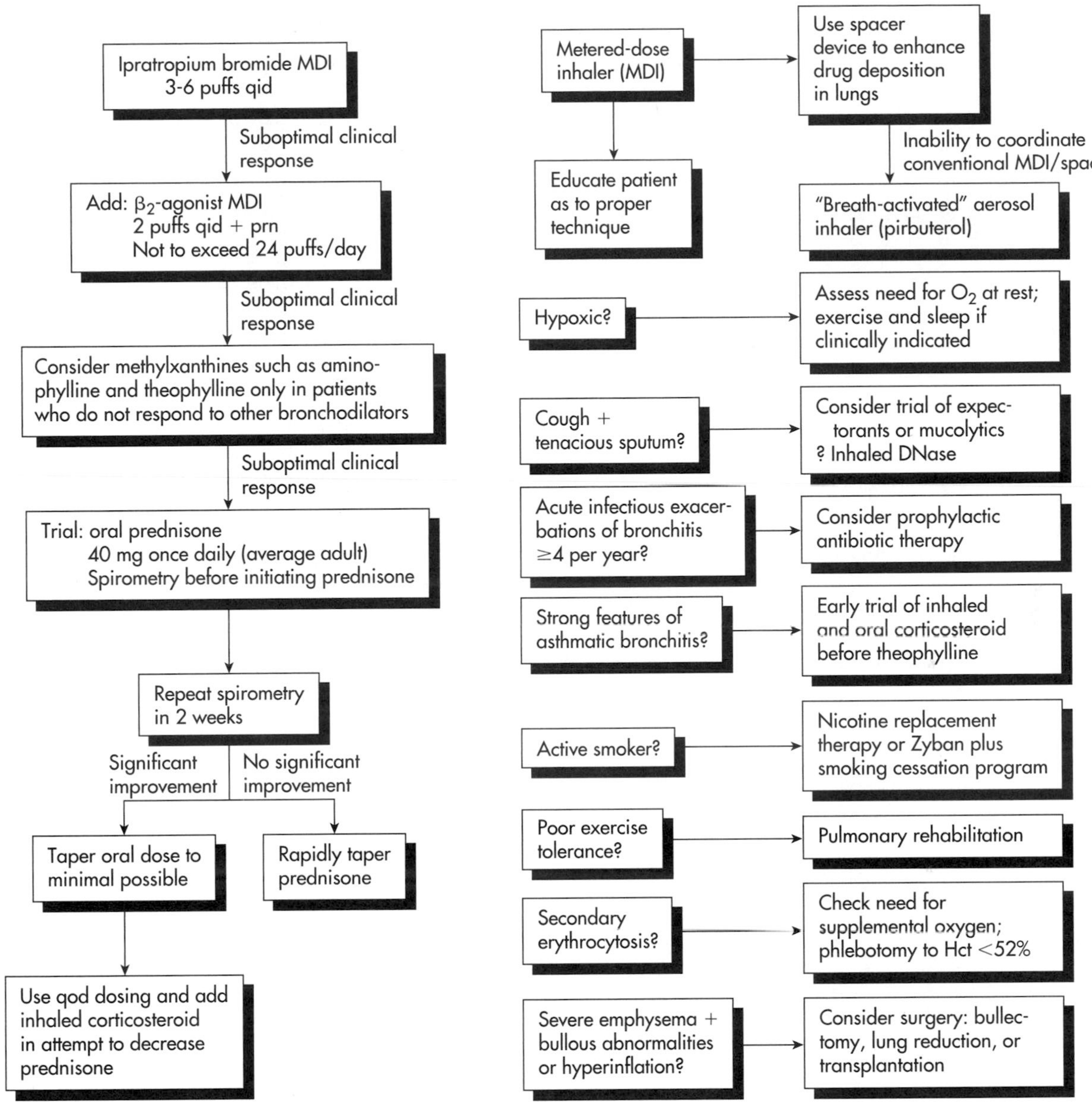

FIGURE 3-20 Managed care guide: pharmacotherapy and general management approaches for chronic obstructive pulmonary disease (COPD). *DNase,* Deoxyribonuclease; *Hct,* hematocrit; *prn,* as needed; *qid,* four times a day; *qod,* every other day. (Modified from Noble J: *Primary care medicine,* ed 3, St Louis, 2001, Mosby.)

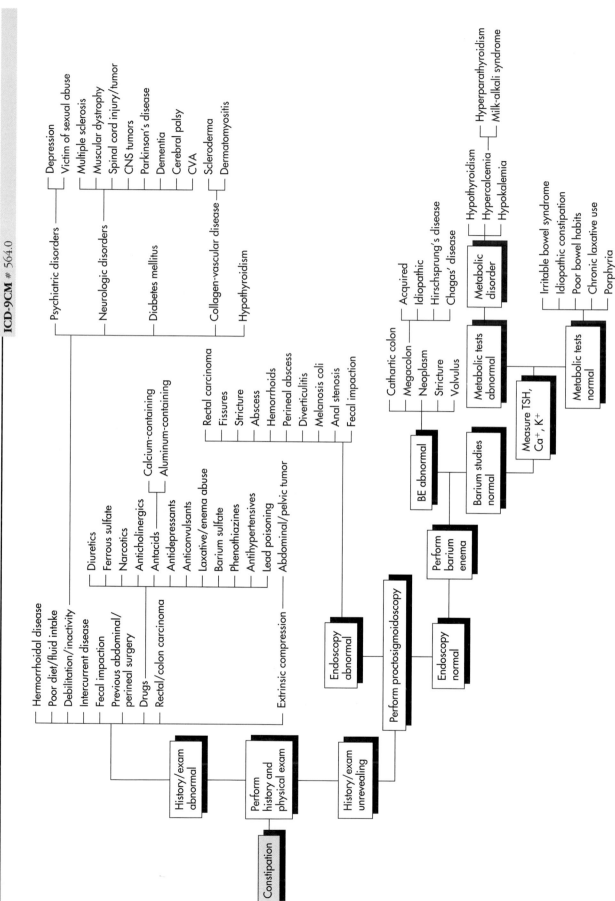

FIGURE 3-21   Constipation. *BE,* Barium enema; *CNS,* central nervous system; *CVA,* cerebral vascular accident; *TSH,* thyroid-stimulating hormone. (From Healey PM: *Common medical diagnosis: an algorithmic approach,* ed 3, Philadelphia, 2000, WB Saunders.)

ICD-9CM # 786.2

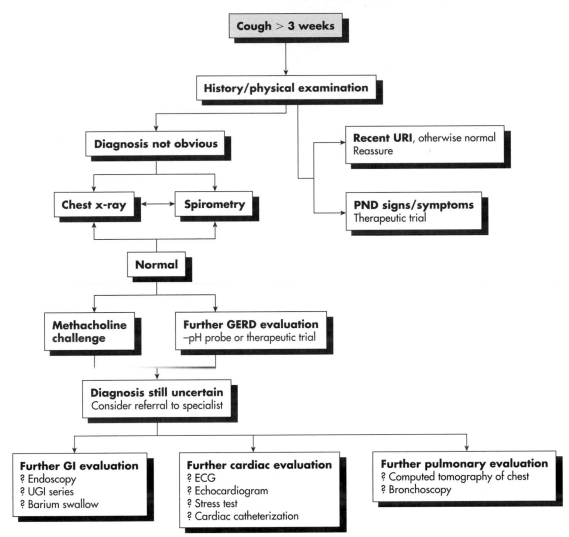

FIGURE 3-22 Diagnostic approach to chronic cough. *ECG,* Electrocardiogram; *GERD,* gastro-esophageal reflux disease; *PND,* paroxysmal nocturnal dyspnea; *UGI,* upper gastrointestinal tract; *URI,* upper respiratory infection. (From Carlson KJ et al: *Primary care of women,* ed 2, St Louis, 2002, Mosby.)

ICD-9CM # 782.5 Cyanosis NOS

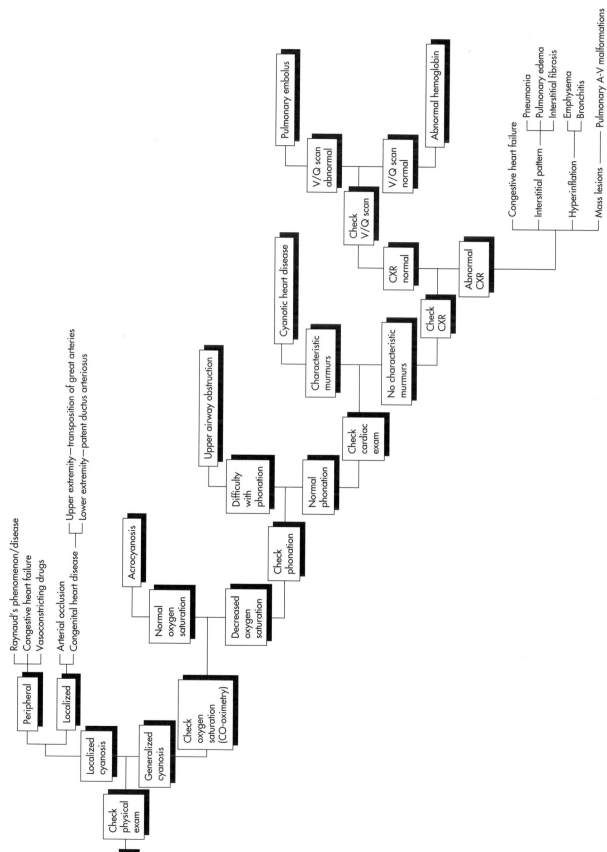

FIGURE 3-23　Cyanosis. *A-V,* Arteriovenous; *CXR,* chest x-ray; *V/Q,* ventilation-perfusion. (From Healey PM: *Common medical diagnosis: an algorithmic approach,* ed 3, Philadelphia, 2000, WB Saunders.)

DELIRIUM, GERIATRIC PATIENT

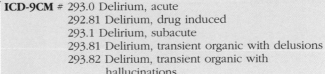

ICD-9CM # 293.0 Delirium, acute
292.81 Delirium, drug induced
293.1 Delirium, subacute
293.81 Delirium, transient organic with delusions
293.82 Delirium, transient organic with hallucinations

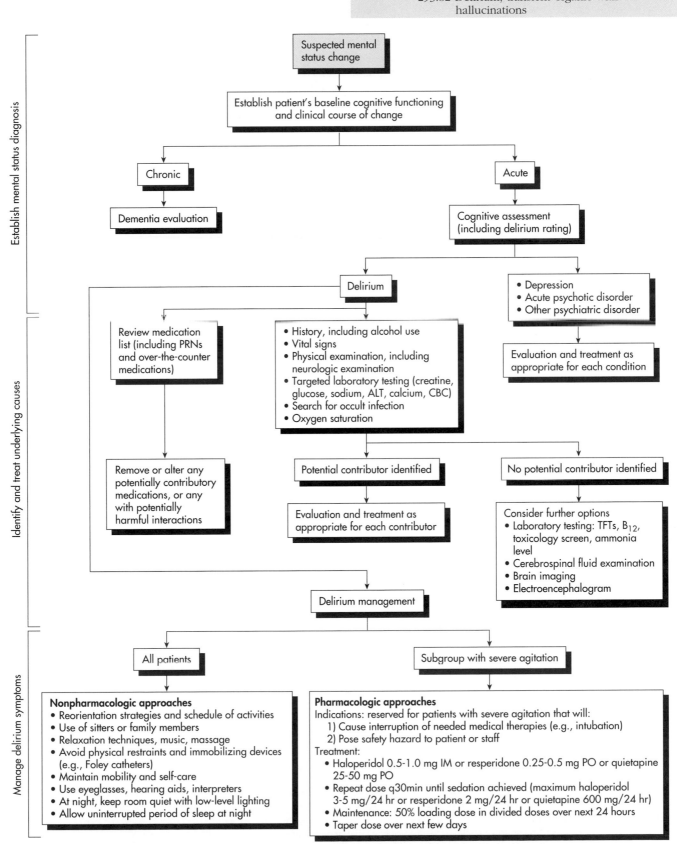

Section III

CLINICAL ALGORITHMS

FIGURE 3-24 Algorithm for evaluation of suspected mental status change in an older patient.
ALT, Alanine aminotransferase; *CBC,* complete blood count; *IM,* intramuscular; *NG,* nasogastric; *PO,* by mouth; *PRNs,* as needed; *TFTs,* thyroid function tests. (Adapted from Goldman L, Ausiello D [eds]: *Cecil textbook of medicine,* ed 22, Philadelphia, 2004, WB Saunders.)

ICD-9CM # 290.10 Dementia, presenile
290.0 Dementia, senile
437.0 Dementia, arteriosclerotic

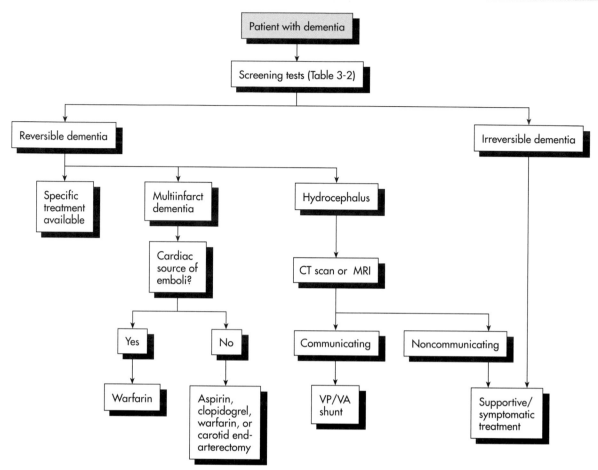

FIGURE 3-25 Management of dementia. *VA,* ventriculoatrial; *VP,* ventriculoperitoneal.

TABLE 3-2 **Screening Tests for Diagnosis of Dementia**

Test	Rationale	Remarks
Blood Test		
Complete blood count	Assess general nutritional status	
Creatine, ALT	Exclude renal or hystic disease	
Serum B_{12} level	Exclude vitamin B_{12} deficiency	Consider antiparietal cell antibody or Schilling's test if B_{12} level is low
TSH + free T4 *or* TSH + FTI	Exclude primary and secondary hypothyroidism	
HIV serology	Exclude HIV infection	Perform only if indicated; consent from patient required
Calcium	Exclude hypercalcemia or hypocalcemia	
Cerebrospinal Fluid		
Cell count/protein level	Exclude chronic meningitis	Perform only if indicated
Cytology	Exclude carcinomatous meningitis	Perform only if indicated
VDRL	Exclude neurosyphilis	Perform only if indicated; check serum TPHA and HIV serology if CSF VDRL is positive
CT Scan/MRI of the Brain	Identify infarcts and white matter changes; exclude presence of neoplasm, demyelinating disease, and hydrocephalus; location of atrophy may suggest the diagnosis (e.g., parahippocampal atrophy in Alzheimer's disease, frontotemporal atrophy in Pick's disease)	
Electroencephalogram	Exclude metabolic encephalopathies; useful if Creutzfeldt-Jakob disease or status epilepticus is suspected	Perform only if indicated
Neuropsychologic Evaluation	Help to characterize pattern of cognitive impairment, which may aid in the classification of dementia; rule out pseudodementia from depression	

From Johnson RT, Griffin JW: *Current therapy in neurologic disease,* ed 5, St Louis, 1997, Mosby.
ALT, Alanine aminotransferase; *CSF,* cerebrospinal fluid; *CT,* computed tomography; *FTI,* free thyroxine index; *HIV,* human immunodeficiency virus; *MRI,* magnetic resonance imaging; *T₄,* thyroxine; *TPHA, Treponema pallidum* hemagglutination assay; *TSH,* thyroid-stimulating hormone; *VDRL,* Venereal Disease Research Laboratory test.

DEPRESSION

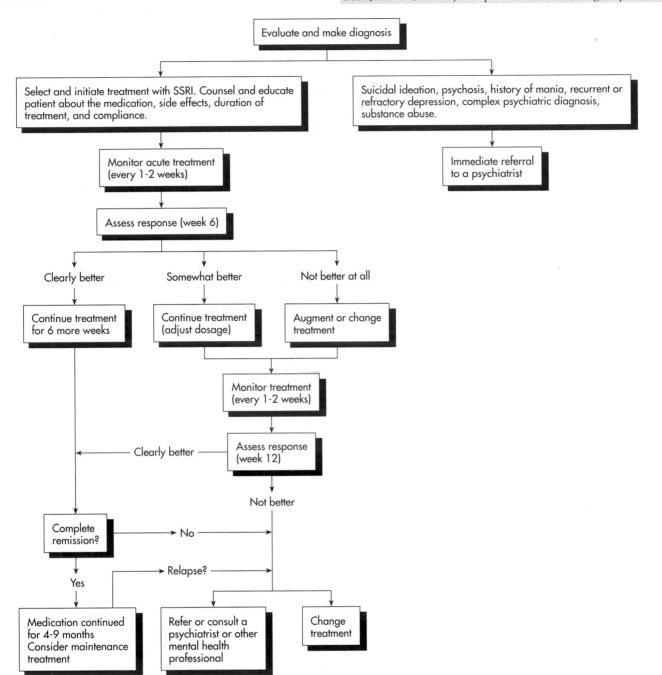

FIGURE 3-26 Guidelines for the treatment of depression in the primary care setting. *SSRI,* Selective serotonin reuptake inhibitor. NOTE: Time of assessment (weeks 6 and 12) rests on very modest data. It may be necessary to revise the treatment plan earlier for patients who fail to respond. (From AHCPR Quick Reference Guide of Clinicians, No. 5: *Depression in primary care: Detection, diagnosis and treatment,* 1993; and American Psychiatric Association: *Diagnostic and statistical manual of mental disorders,* ed 4, Washington, DC, 1994, American Psychiatric Association.)

Section III

CLINICAL ALGORITHMS

ICD-9CM # 787.91

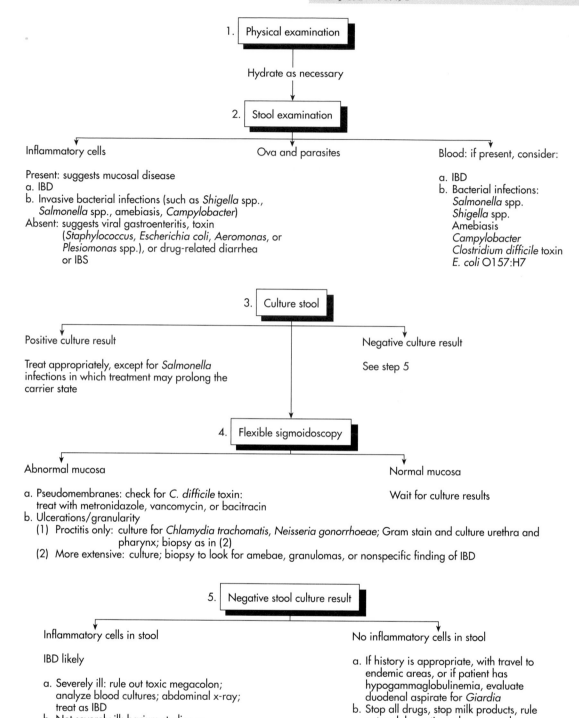

FIGURE 3-27 **Diagnostic steps in the assessment of acute diarrhea.** *IBD,* Inflammatory bowel disease; *IBS,* irritable bowel syndrome. (From Stein JH [ed]: *Internal medicine,* ed 5, St Louis, 1998, Mosby.)

1. Diagnostic steps 1 to 4 as in Fig. 3-27

   a. Results diagnostic for infectious diarrhea (uncommon in chronic diarrhea except for *Clostridium difficile* after antibiotics), inflammatory bowel disease, or overt drug-induced diarrhea

   b. Results nondiagnostic; usually without inflammatory cells in stool

2. Stool volume

   a. Small volume: usually seen in infectious diarrhea or inflammatory bowel disease (consider colonoscopy), but can also be seen in malabsorption syndromes and irritable bowel syndrome

   b. Large volume: suggests malabsorption syndromes, secretory diarrhea, or laxative abuse

3. Stool Sudan stain

Positive

Suggests malabsorption syndrome, pancreatic insufficiency, bile salt insufficiency, or mucosal disease

Negative

See step 4

4. Oral intake stopped

Diarrhea continues

   a. Secretory diarrhea: stool osmolality = stool $(Na^+ + K^+) \times 2$

   b. Nasogastric suction

     (1) Diarrhea stops

       (a) Zollinger-Ellison syndrome: gastric analysis, gastrin, secretin stimulation

       (b) Laxative abuse: see step 5

     (2) Diarrhea continues

       (a) Secretory diarrhea: plasma VIP, calcitonin, urinary 5-HIAA abdominal ultrasound, computed tomography, and/or selective mesenteric angiogram to identify tumor

       (b) Laxative abuse: see step 5

Diarrhea stops

   a. Malabsorption syndromes: stool osmolality > plasma osmolality

   b. Laxative ingestion: see step 5

   c. Congenital chloridorrhea

     (1) Stool electrolytes: chloride concentration greater than the sum of sodium and potassium concentrations in stool water

     (2) No fecal osmotic gap

5. Laxative abuse detection

   a. Screening tests

     (1) Detailed history

     (2) Sigmoidoscopy and biopsy for melanosis coli

     (3) Barium enema: dilated, hypomotile "cathartic colon"

   b. Specific tests

     (1) Urine screening test for senna

     (2) Chromatographic test for bisacodyl

     (3) Stool test for fecal sulfate and phosphate

     (4) Magnesium concentration in fecal water (atomic absorption spectrophotometry)

6. Radiologic studies

Perform barium studies only after stool examination, culture, and studies requiring quantitative measurements of the stool have been completed.

FIGURE 3-28 Diagnostic approach to the patient with chronic diarrhea. *5-HIAA*, 5-Hydroxyindoleacetic acid; *VIP*, vasoactive intestinal polypeptide. (Modified from Stein JH [ed]: *Internal medicine*, ed 5, St Louis, 1998, Mosby.)

ICD-9CM # 563.3 Dyspepsia atonic
536.8 Dyspepsia disorders other unspecified function of stomach
306.4 Dyspepsia, psychogenic

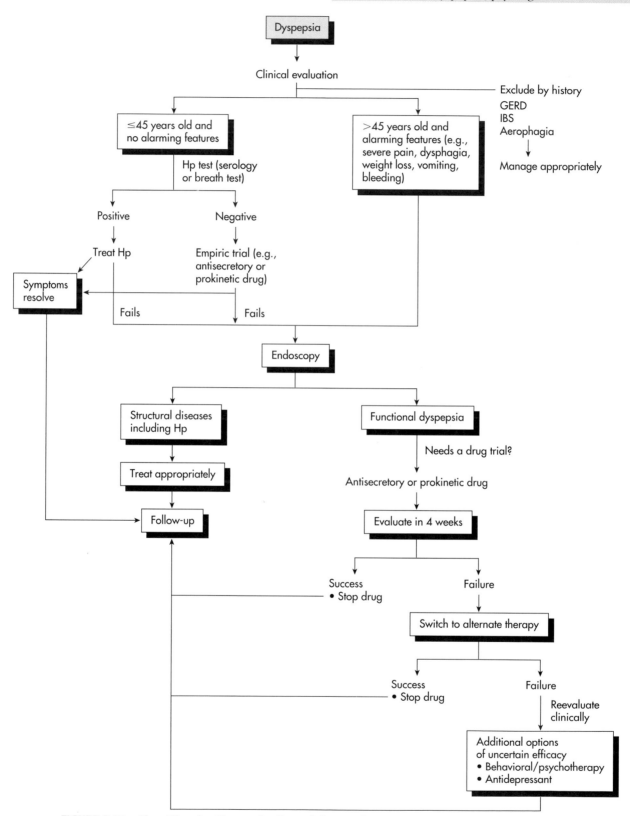

FIGURE 3-29 Algorithm for the evaluation of dyspepsia. *GERD,* Symptomatic gastroesophageal reflux disease; *Hp, Helicobacter pylori; IBS,* irritable bowel syndrome. (From Goldman L, Ausiello D [eds]: *Cecil textbook of medicine,* ed 22, Philadelphia, 2004, WB Saunders.)

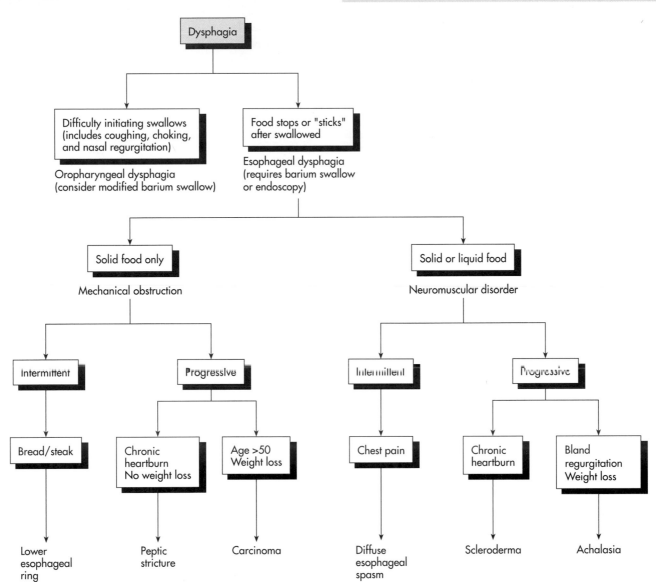

FIGURE 3-30 Differential diagnosis of dysphagia. (Adapted from Andreoli TE [ed]: *Cecil essentials of medicine,* ed 5, Philadelphia, 2001, WB Saunders.)

ICD-9CM # 786.00

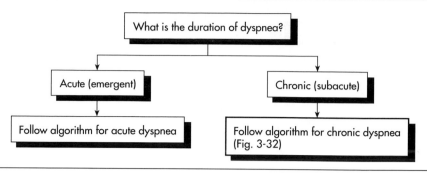

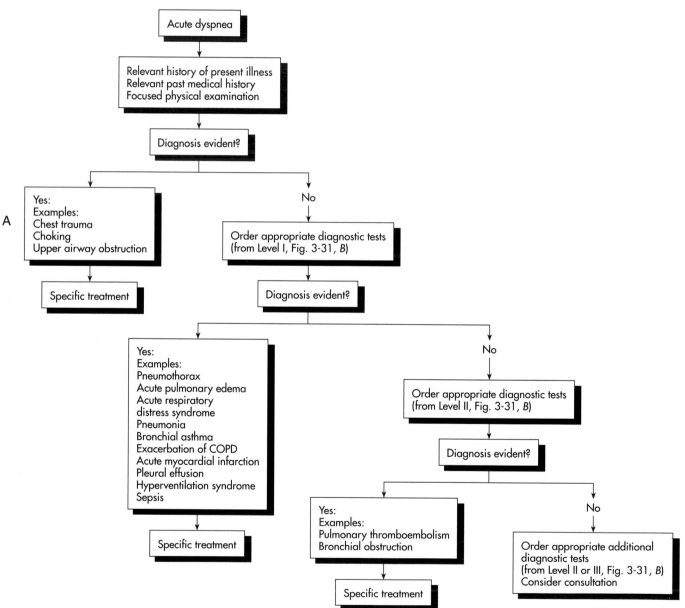

FIGURE 3-31   A, Evaluation of the patient with dyspnea. *COPD,* Chronic obstructive pulmonary disease. (From Stein J [ed]: *Internal medicine,* ed 5, St Louis, 1998, Mosby.)

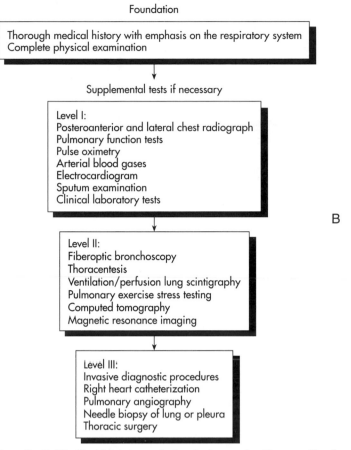

Foundation

Thorough medical history with emphasis on the respiratory system
Complete physical examination

Supplemental tests if necessary

Level I:
Posteroanterior and lateral chest radiograph
Pulmonary function tests
Pulse oximetry
Arterial blood gases
Electrocardiogram
Sputum examination
Clinical laboratory tests

Level II:
Fiberoptic bronchoscopy
Thoracentesis
Ventilation/perfusion lung scintigraphy
Pulmonary exercise stress testing
Computed tomography
Magnetic resonance imaging

Level III:
Invasive diagnostic procedures
Right heart catheterization
Pulmonary angiography
Needle biopsy of lung or pleura
Thoracic surgery

B

FIGURE 3-31 (Continued)   **B, Medical history and physical examination are the foundation for the diagnosis of respiratory system disease.** Diagnostic tests of increasing levels of complexity and invasiveness are performed if necessary to supplement the initial history and physical examination. (From Stein J [ed]: *Internal medicine,* ed 5, St Louis, 1998, Mosby.)

ICD-9CM # 786.00

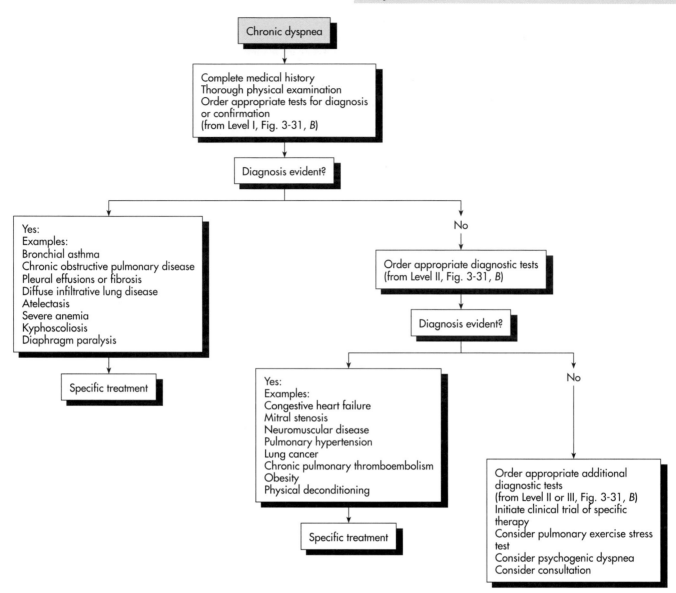

FIGURE 3-32 Chronic dyspnea. (From Stein J [ed]: *Internal medicine,* ed 5, St Louis, 1998, Mosby.)

EDEMA, GENERALIZED

ICD-9CM # 782.3 Edema NOS
782.3 Edema, lower extremities

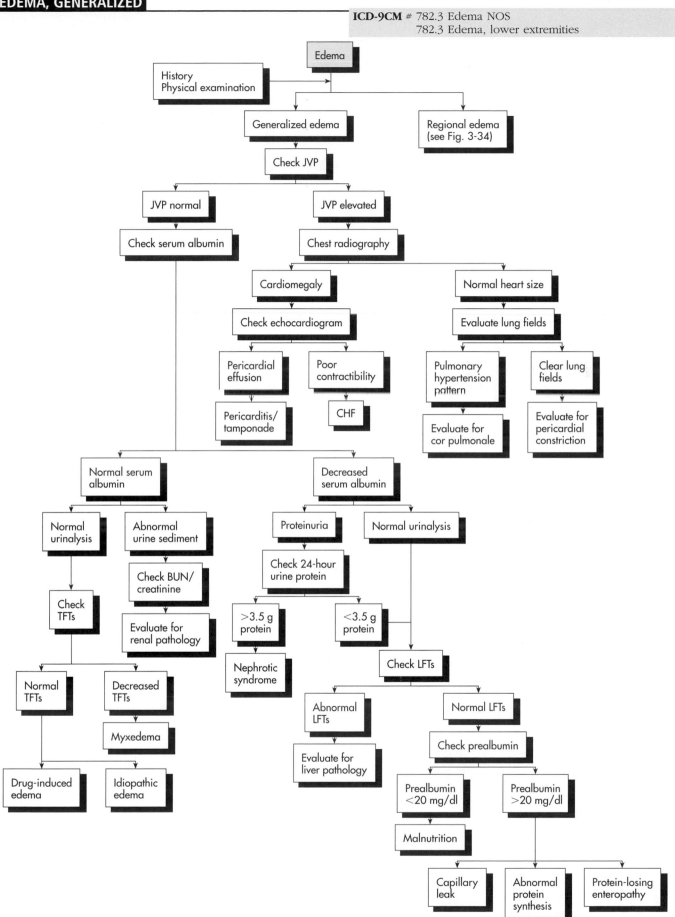

FIGURE 3-33 Evaluation of generalized edema. *BUN,* Blood urea nitrogen; *CHF,* congestive heart failure; *JVP,* jugular venous pressure; *LFT,* liver function tests; *TFT,* thyroid function tests. (From Greene HL, Johnson WP, Lemcke D [eds]: *Decision making in medicine,* ed 2, St Louis, 1998, Mosby.)

ICD-9CM # 250.6

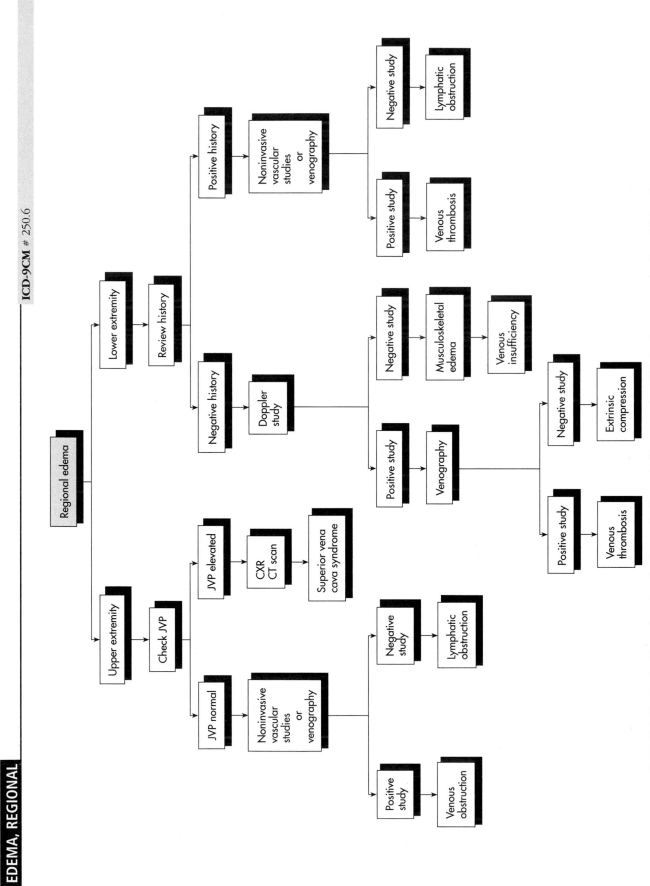

FIGURE 3-34 Evaluation of regional edema. *CT,* Computed tomography; *CXR,* chest x-ray examination; *JVP,* jugular venous pressure. (From Greene HL, Johnson WP, Lemcke D [eds]: *Decision making in medicine,* ed 2, St Louis, 1998, Mosby.)

FATIGUE

ICD-9CM # 780.7 Fatigue, general

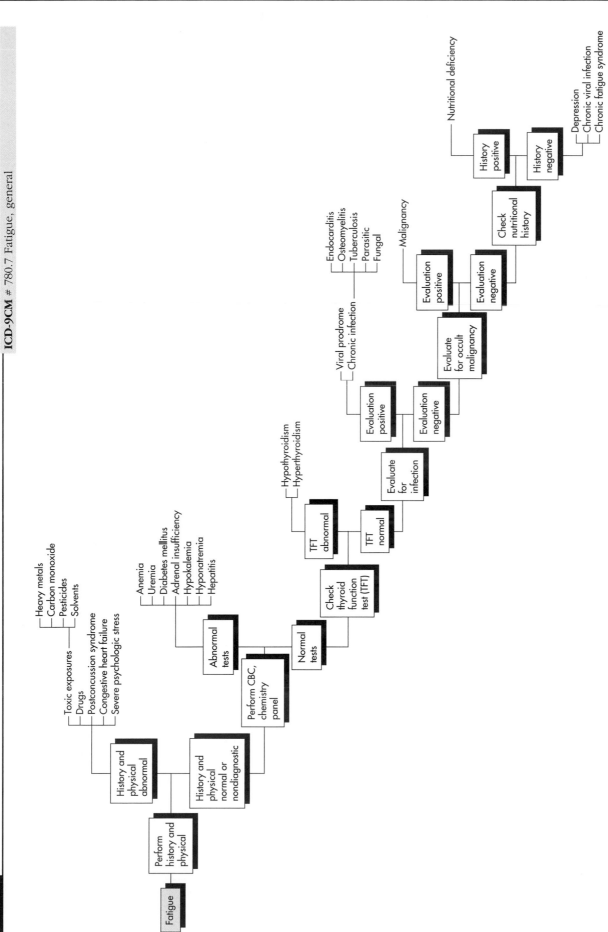

FIGURE 3-35 Evaluation of fatigue. *CBC,* Complete blood count. (From Healey PM: *Common medical diagnosis: an algorithmic approach,* ed 3, Philadelphia, 2000, WB Saunders.)

ICD-9CM # 787.6

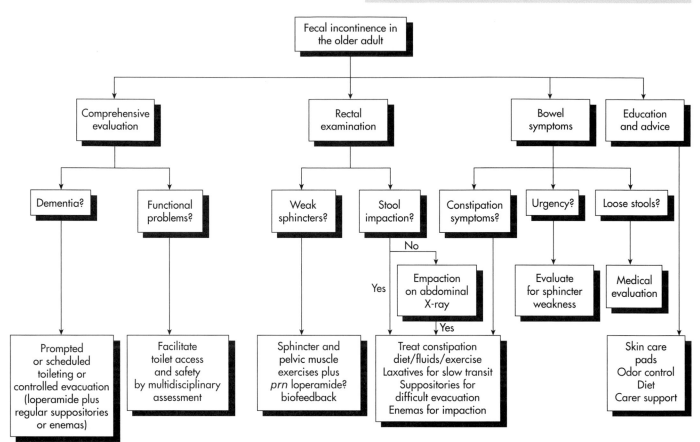

FIGURE 3-36   Evaluation of fecal incontinence. (From Tallis RC, Fillit HM [eds]: *Brocklehurst's text-book of geriatric medicine and gerontology,* ed 6, London, 2003, Churchill Livingstone.)

BOX 3-1   Clinical Assessment of Fecal Incontinence in Older People

Emphasis in older people is on a *structured clinical approach* to identify all contributing factors for fecal incontinence

History
- Duration of fecal incontinence
- Frequency of episodes
- Type (constant soiling, small amounts, complete bowel movement)
- Stool consistency (diarrhea, hard stool)
- Unconscious leakage or symptoms of urgency
- Constipation symptoms/current laxative use
- Systemic illness (confusion, depression, weight loss, anemia)
- Antibiotic use

General examination
- Cognitive and mood assessment
- Neurological profile (stroke, autonomic neuropathy, Parkinson's disease)

Toilet access
- Evaluate ability to use toilet based on muscle strength, coordination, vision, limb function, and cognition
- Place in context of current living environment

Specific examination
Abdominal inspection for distension and tenderness
- Perineal inspection for skin breakdown, dermatitis, surgical scars
- Perianal sensation/cutaneous anal reflex
- Observe for excessive downward motion of the pelvic floor when asking patient to bear down in the lateral lying position
- Digital examination for stool impaction
- Digital examination for evaluation of impaired sphincter tone
  - Anal gaping, and/or easy insertion of finger (internal sphincter)
  - Reduced squeeze pressure (external sphincter)
- Ask patient to strain while sitting on commode and observe for rectal prolapse

From Tallis RC, Fillit HM (eds): *Brocklehurst's textbook of geriatric medicine and gerontology,* ed 6, London, 2003, Churchill Livingstone.

FEVER OF UNDETERMINED ORIGIN

ICD-9CM # 780.6 Pyrexia of undetermined origin

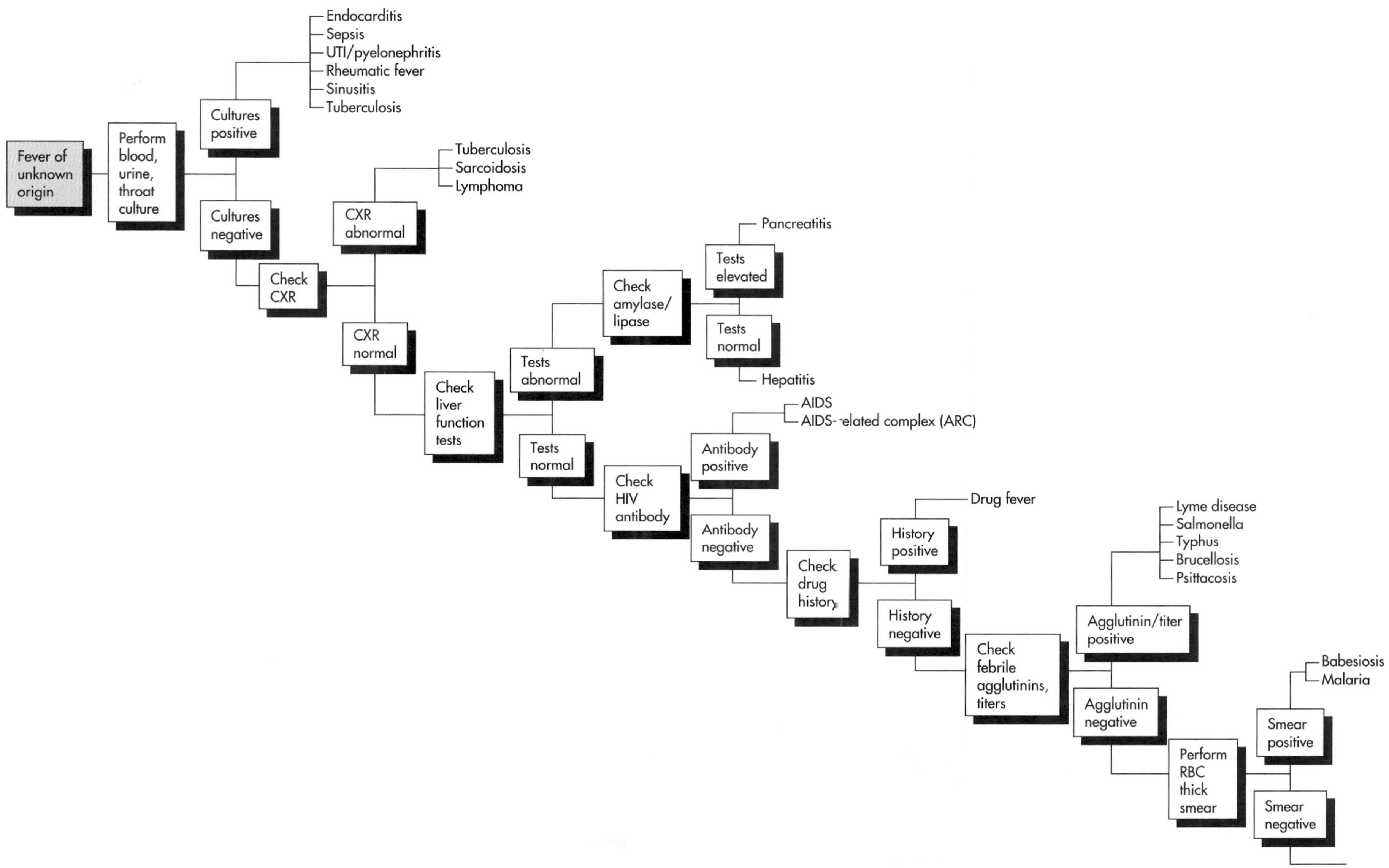

FIGURE 3-37 Approach to the patient with fever of undetermined origin. *AIDS,* Acquired immunodeficiency syndrome; *ANA,* antinuclear antibody; *CT,* computed tomography; *CSR,* chest x-ray; *ESR,* erythrocyte sedimentation rate; *GI,* gastrointestinal; *HIV,* human immunodeficiency virus; *RBC,* red blood cell; *UTI,* urinary tract infection. (From Healey PM: *Common medical diagnosis: an algorithmic approach,* ed 3, Philadelphia, 2000, WB Saunders.)

Continued on following page

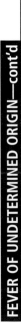

FEVER OF UNDETERMINED ORIGIN—cont'd

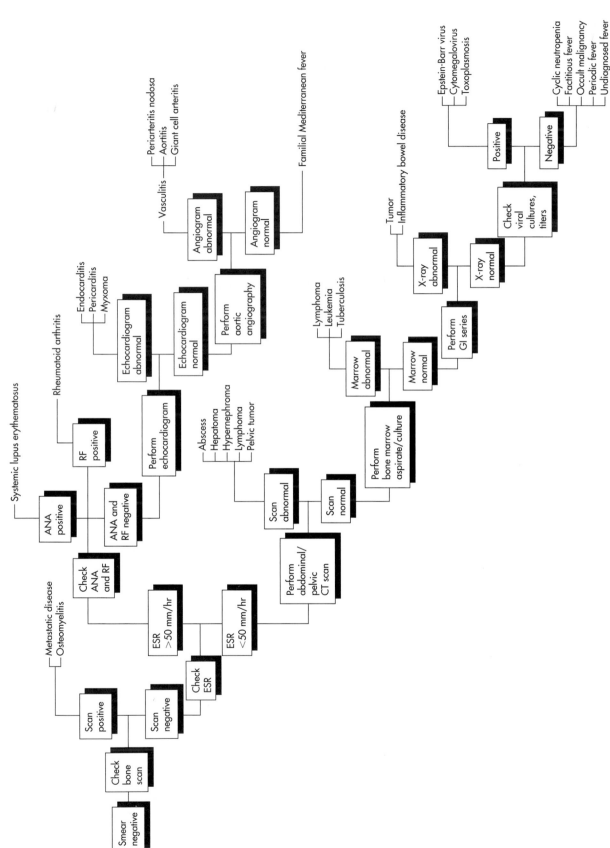

FIGURE 3-37 (Continued) *AIDS,* Acquired immunodeficiency syndrome; *ANA,* antinuclear antibody; *CT,* computed tomography; *CSR,* chest x-ray; *ESR,* erythrocyte sedimentation rate; *GI,* gastrointestinal; *HIV,* human immunodeficiency virus; *RBC,* red blood cell; *RF,* rheumatoid factor; *UTI,* urinary tract infection. (From Healey PM: *Common medical diagnosis: an algorithmic approach,* ed 3, Philadelphia, 2000, WB Saunders.)

FRACTURE, BONE

ICD-9CM # 829.0 Fracture bone(s) NOS closed
829.1 Fracture bone(s) NOS open

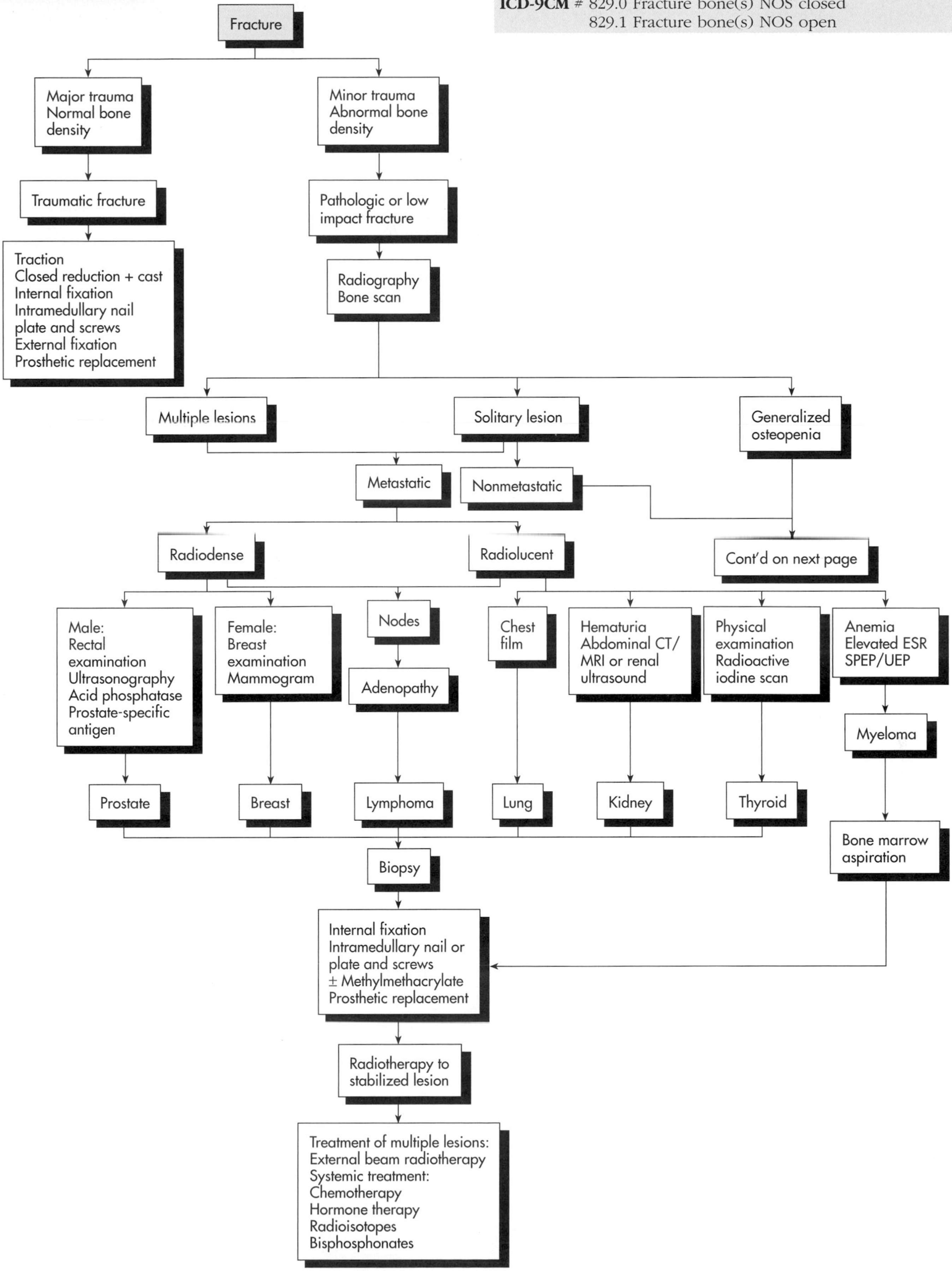

FIGURE 3-38 Bone fracture. *CT,* Computed tomography; *ESR,* erythrocyte sedimentation rate; *MRI,* magnetic resonance imaging; *SPEP,* serum protein electrophoresis; *UEP,* urine electrophoresis. (From Greene HL, Johnson WP, Lemcke D [eds]: *Decision making in medicine,* ed 2, St Louis, 1998, Mosby.)

Continued on following page

Section III

CLINICAL ALGORITHMS

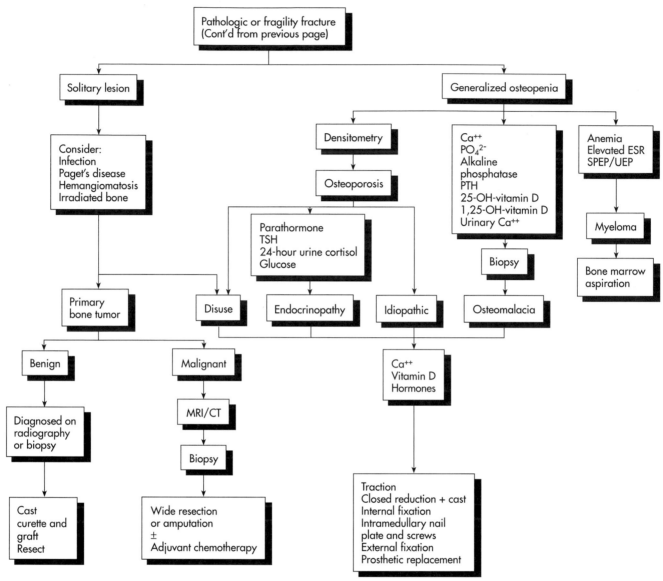

FIGURE 3-38 (Continued)

GOITER EVALUATION AND MANAGEMENT

ICD-9CM # 240.9 Goiter, unspecified
240.0 Goiter, simple
241.9 Goiter, adenomatous
246.1 Goiter, congenital
242.1 Goiter, uninodular with thyrotoxicosis
242.2 Goiter, multinodular with thyrotoxicosis

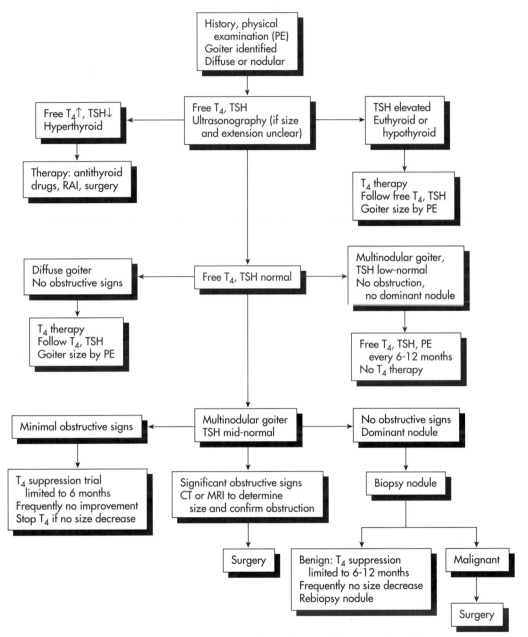

FIGURE 3-39 Evaluation and management of patients with nontoxic diffuse and nodular goiter and undetermined thyroid status. *CT,* Computed tomography; *MRI,* magnetic resonance imaging; *RAI,* radioactive iodine; *TSH,* thyroid-stimulating hormone. (From Goldman L, Ausiello D [eds]: *Cecil textbook of medicine,* ed 22, Philadelphia, 2004, WB Saunders.)

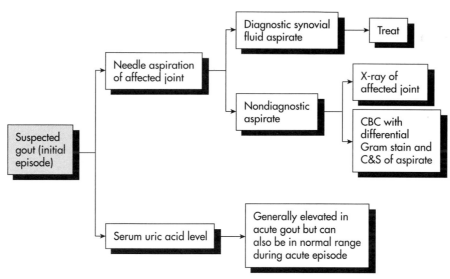

FIGURE 3-40 Evaluation of suspected gout. *CBC,* Complete blood count; *C&S,* culture and sensitivity. (From Ferri FF: *Ferri's best test: a practical guide to clinical laboratory medicine and diagnostic imaging,* Philadelphia, 2004, Elsevier Mosby.)

BOX 3-2   **Gout**

Diagnostic imaging
Best test
None
Ancillary tests
Plain radiograph of affected joint when diagnosis is unclear

Lab evaluation
Best test
Examination of synovial fluid aspirate from affected joint for presence of urate crystals (needle-shaped and birefringent)
Ancillary tests
Serum uric acid level
CBC with differential, ESR if infectious process is suspected
Gram stain and C&S of synovial fluid aspirate

From Ferri FF: *Ferri's best test: a practical guide to clinical laboratory medicine and diagnostic imaging,* Philadelphia, 2004, Elsevier Mosby.
  CBC, Complete blood count; *C&S,* culture and sensitivity; *ESR,* erythrocyte sedimentation rate.

ICD-9CM # 611.1 Gynecomastia nonpuerperal

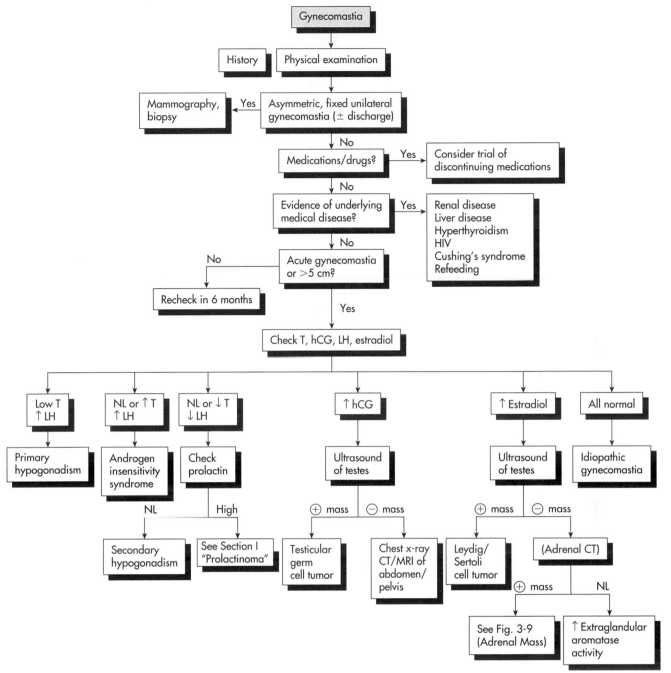

FIGURE 3-41 Evaluation of gynecomastia. *CT,* Computed tomography; *hCG,* human chorionic gonadotropin; *HIV,* human immunodeficiency syndrome; *LH,* luteinizing hormone; *MRI,* magnetic resonance imaging; *NL,* normal limits; *T,* testosterone. (From Noble J: *Primary care medicine,* ed 3, St Louis, 2001, Mosby.)

ICD-9CM # 389.00 Hearing loss, conductive
389.10 Hearing loss, sensorineural

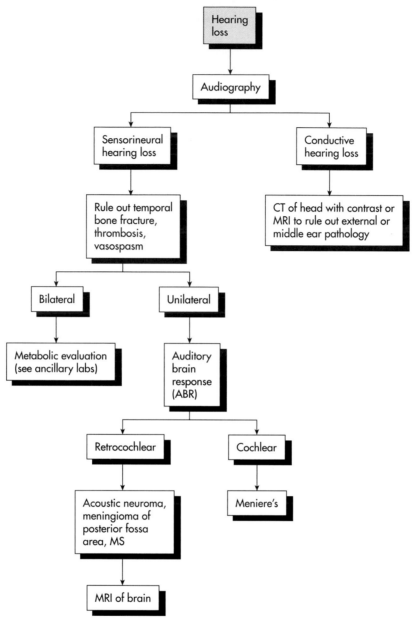

FIGURE 3-42 Evaluation of hearing loss. *CT,* Computed tomography; *MRI,* magnetic resonance imaging. (From Ferri FF: *Ferri's best test: a practical guide to clinical laboratory medicine and diagnostic imaging,* Philadelphia, 2004, Elsevier Mosby.)

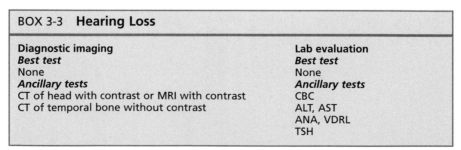

BOX 3-3   **Hearing Loss**

Diagnostic imaging	**Lab evaluation**
Best test	***Best test***
None	None
Ancillary tests	***Ancillary tests***
CT of head with contrast or MRI with contrast	CBC
CT of temporal bone without contrast	ALT, AST
	ANA, VDRL
	TSH

From Ferri FF: *Ferri's best test: a practical guide to clinical laboratory medicine and diagnostic imaging.* *ALT,* Alanine aminotransferase; *ANA,* antibody to nuclear antigens; *AST,* angiotension sensitivity test; *CBC,* complete blood count; *CT,* computed tomography; *TSH,* thyroid-stimulating hormone; *VDRL,* Venereal Disease Research Laboratory test.

ICD-9CM # 787.1

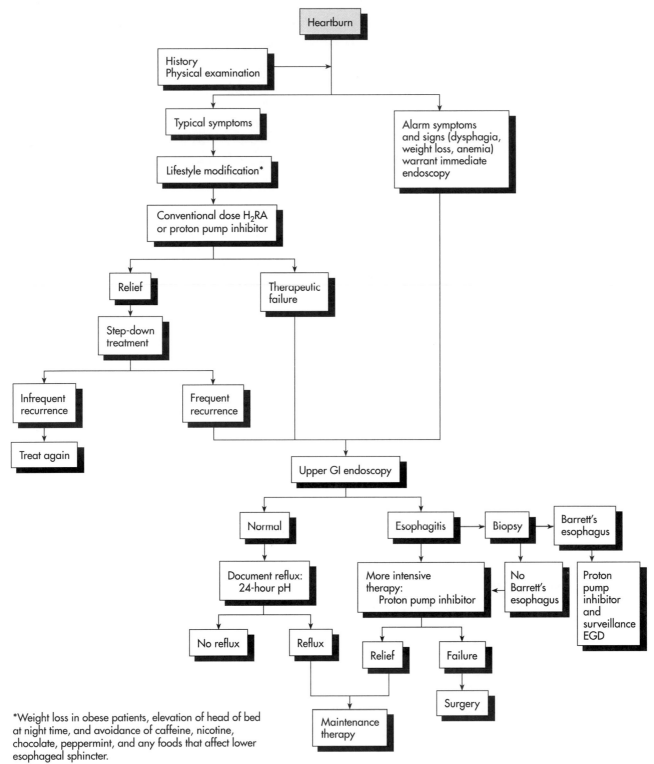

*Weight loss in obese patients, elevation of head of bed at night time, and avoidance of caffeine, nicotine, chocolate, peppermint, and any foods that affect lower esophageal sphincter.

FIGURE 3-43 Treatment of a patient with heartburn. *EGD,* Esophagogastroduodenoscopy; *GI,* gastrointestinal; *H₂RA,* H₂ receptor antagonist. (Adapted from Sampliner RE: Heartburn. In Greene HL, Johnson WP, Lemcke D [eds]: *Decision making in medicine,* ed 2, St Louis, 1998, Mosby.)

ICD-9CM # 599.7

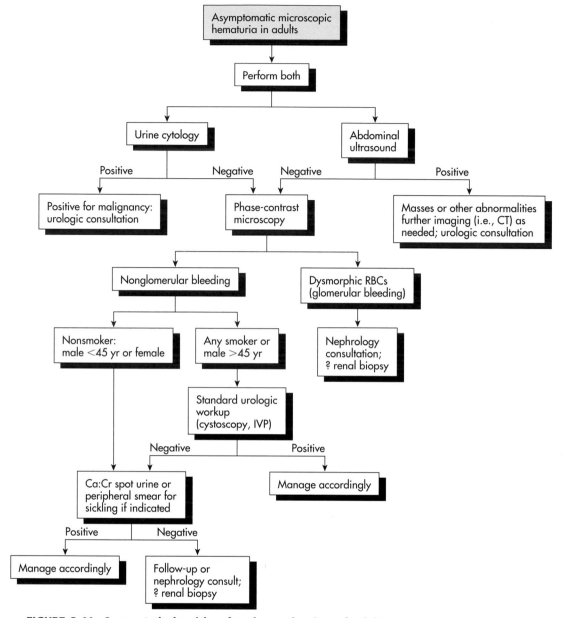

FIGURE 3-44 Suggested algorithm for the evaluation of adult asymptomatic microscopic hematuria. These patients must have no symptoms referable to the hematuria and a negative urinalysis except for red blood cells (RBCs). Adults with gross hematuria require a full urologic evaluation. *Ca:Cr,* Calcium:creatinine ratio; *IVP,* intravenous pyelogram. (From Nseyo UO [ed]: *Urology for primary care physicians,* Philadelphia, 1999, WB Saunders.)

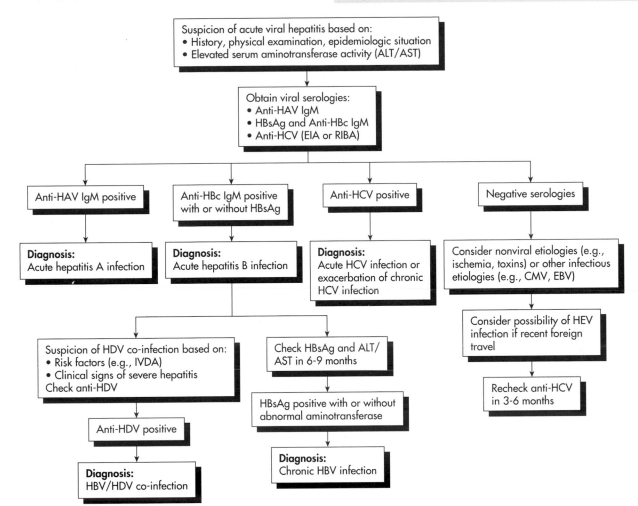

FIGURE 3-45 **A flow diagram showing the use of specific serologic tests for the diagnosis of acute viral hepatitis in relation to the clinical and epidemiologic setting. Co-infections and superinfections of chronic hepatitis B or C patients should always be considered in cases that do not fit well with the clinical or serologic picture.** *CMV,* Cytomegalovirus; *EBV,* Epstein-Barr virus; *EIA,* enzyme immunoassay; *HBV,* hepatitis B virus; *HCV,* hepatitis C virus; *HDV,* hepatitis D virus; *HEV,* hepatoencephalomyelitis virus; *IVDA,* intravenous drug abuse; *RIBA,* recombinant immunoblot assay. (From Mandell GL: *Mandell, Douglas, and Bennett's principles and practice of infectious diseases,* ed 5, New York, 2000, Churchill Livingstone.)

ICD-9CM # 789.1

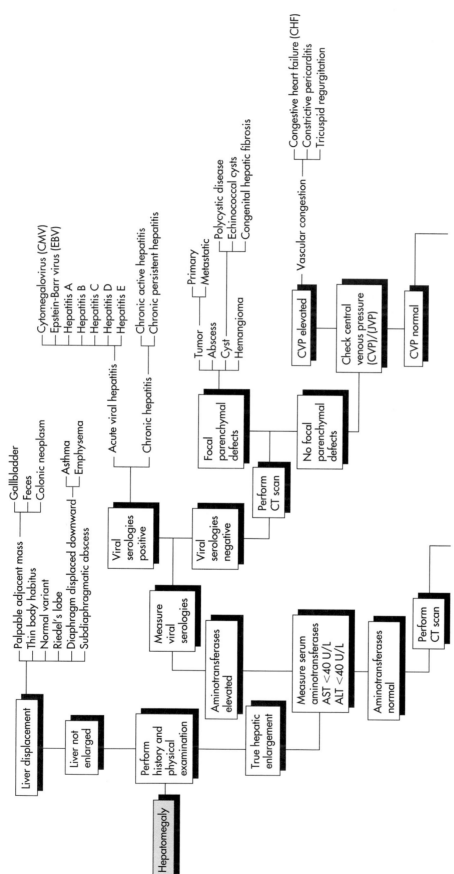

FIGURE 3-46 Hepatomegaly. *ALT,* Alanine aminotransferase; *AST,* aspartate aminotransferase; *CT,* computed tomography; *JVP,* jugular venous pressure. (From Healey PM: *Common medical diagnosis: an algorithmic approach,* ed 3, Philadelphia, 2000, WB Saunders.)

HEPATOMEGALY—cont'd

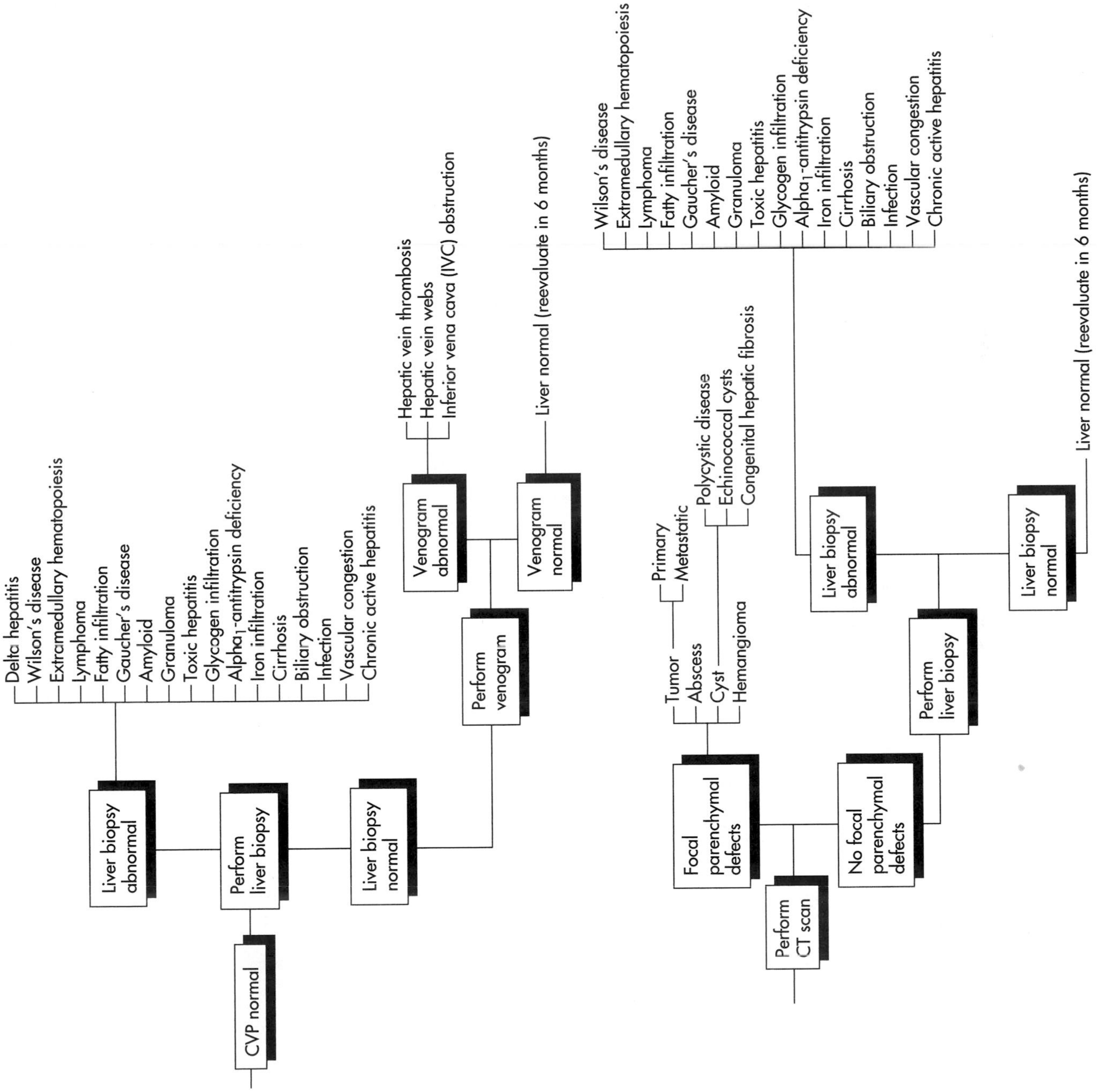

Perform liver biopsy

Liver biopsy abnormal
- Delta hepatitis
- Wilson's disease
- Extramedullary hematopoiesis
- Lymphoma
- Fatty infiltration
- Gaucher's disease
- Amyloid
- Granuloma
- Toxic hepatitis
- Glycogen infiltration
- Alpha₁-antitrypsin deficiency
- Iron infiltration
- Cirrhosis
- Biliary obstruction
- Infection
- Vascular congestion
- Chronic active hepatitis

CVP normal

Liver biopsy normal

Perform venogram

Venogram abnormal
- Hepatic vein thrombosis
- Hepatic vein webs
- Inferior vena cava (IVC) obstruction

Venogram normal
- Liver normal (reevaluate in 6 months)

Perform CT scan

Focal parenchymal defects
- Tumor
  - Primary
  - Metastatic
- Abscess
- Cyst
  - Polycystic disease
  - Echinococcal cysts
  - Congenital hepatic fibrosis
- Hemangioma

No focal parenchymal defects

Perform liver biopsy

Liver biopsy abnormal
- Wilson's disease
- Extramedullary hematopoiesis
- Lymphoma
- Fatty infiltration
- Gaucher's disease
- Amyloid
- Granuloma
- Toxic hepatitis
- Glycogen infiltration
- Alpha₁-antitrypsin deficiency
- Iron infiltration
- Cirrhosis
- Biliary obstruction
- Infection
- Vascular congestion
- Chronic active hepatitis

Liver biopsy normal
- Liver normal (reevaluate in 6 months)

FIGURE 3-46 (Continued)

ICD-9CM # 053.9

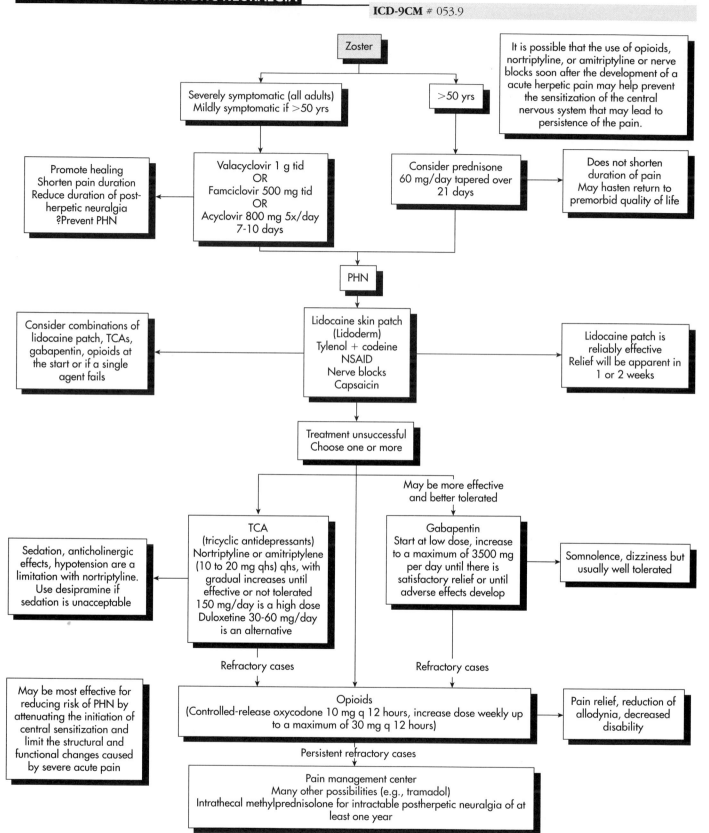

FIGURE 3-47   Treatment of herpes zoster and postherpetic neuralgia. *PHN*, postherpetic neuralgia; *TCA*, tricyclic antidepressant; *NSAID*, nonsteroidal antiinflammatory drug. (Adapted from Habif TA:
Clinical dermatology, ed 4, St Louis, 2004, Mosby.)

ICD-9CM # 275.24

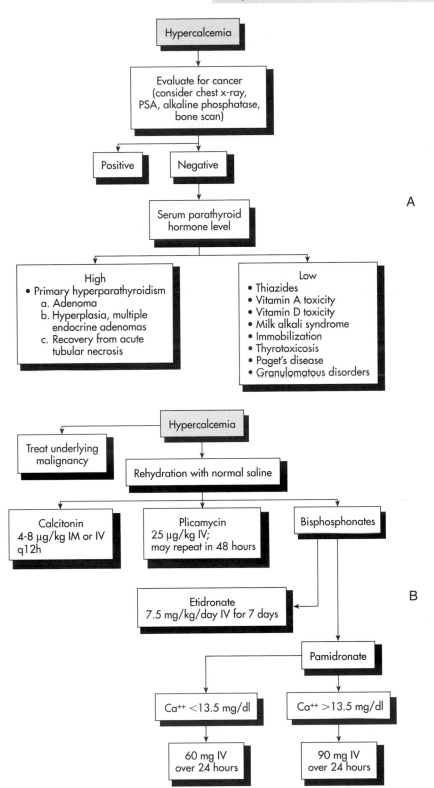

FIGURE 3-48 A, Evaluation of hypercalcemia. *PSA,* Prostate-specific antigen. **B, Therapy for hypercalcemia.** *IM,* Intramuscularly; *IV,* intravenously. (From Noble J [ed]: *Primary care medicine,* ed 3, St Louis, 2001, Mosby.) (From Wachtel TJ, Stein MD: *Practical guide to the care of the ambulatory patient,* ed 2, St Louis, 2000, Mosby.)

ICD-9CM # 276.7

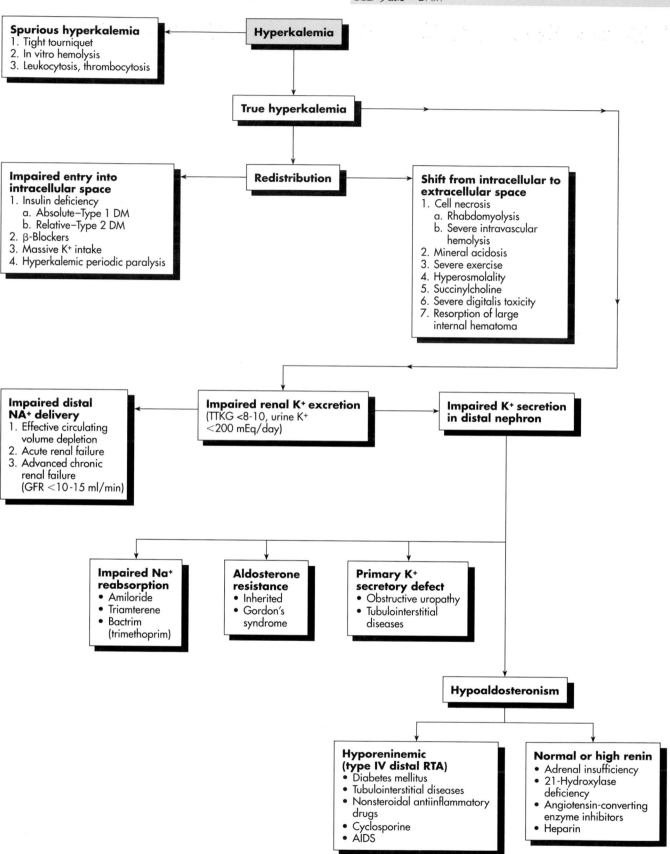

FIGURE 3-49 **Diagnostic approach to hyperkalemia.** *AIDS,* Acquired immunodeficiency syndrome; *DM,* diabetes mellitus; *GFR,* glomerular filtration rate; *RTA,* renal tubular acidosis; *TTKG,* transtubular potassium gradient. (From Andreoli TE [ed]: *Cecil essentials of medicine,* ed 4, Philadelphia, 1997, WB Saunders.)

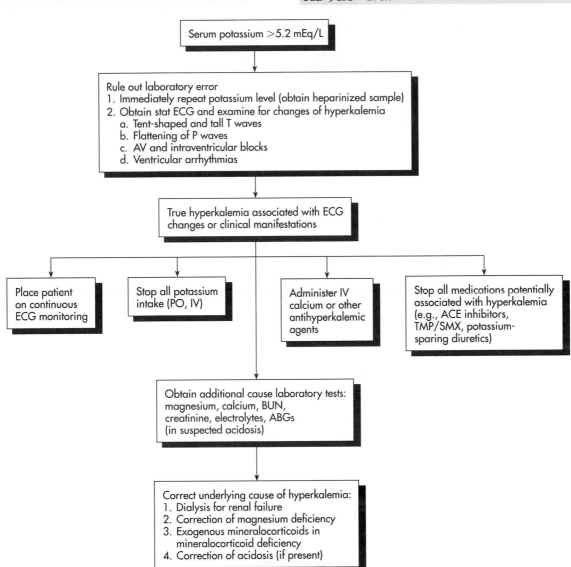

FIGURE 3-50 Evaluation and treatment of hyperkalemia. *ABGs,* Arterial blood gases; *ACE,* angiotensin-converting enzyme; *AV,* atrioventricular; *BUN,* blood urea nitrogen; *ECG,* electrocardiogram; *IV,* intravenous; *PO,* oral; *TMP/SMX,* trimethoprim-sulfamethoxazole. (From Ferri F: *Practical guide to the care of the medical patient,* ed 6, St Louis, 2004, Mosby.)

HYPERNATREMIA

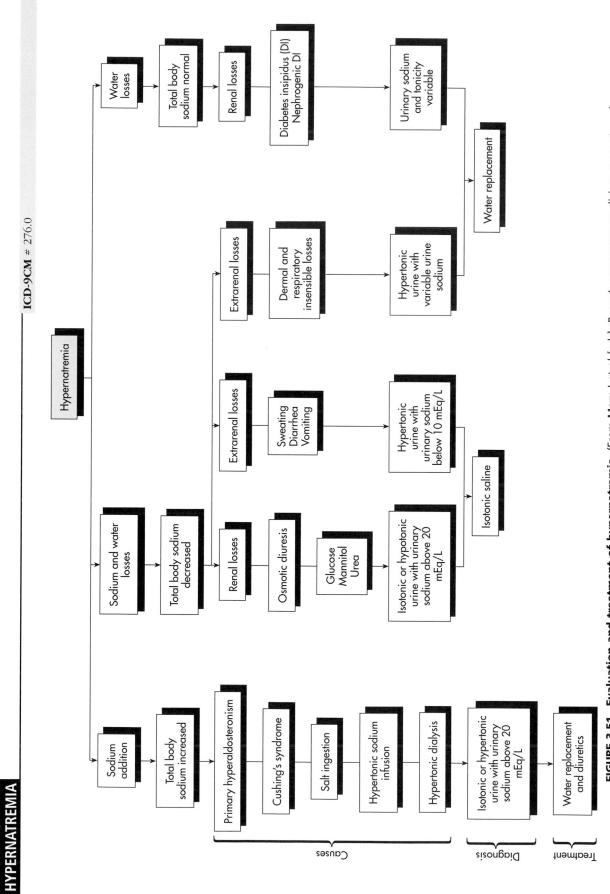

FIGURE 3-51 **Evaluation and treatment of hypernatremia.** (From Marx J et al [eds]: *Rosen's emergency medicine: concepts and clinical practice*, ed 6, St Louis, 2004, Mosby.)

HYPERTENSION, SECONDARY CAUSES

ICD-9CM # 401.1 Essential hypertension
401.0 Malignant hypertension due to renal artery stenosis
405.01 Malignant hypertension secondary to renal artery stenosis
437.2 Hypertensive encephalopathy

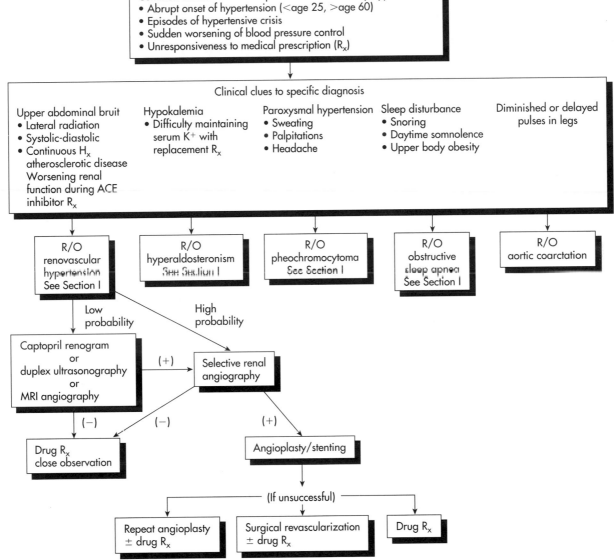

FIGURE 3-52 **Algorithm for identifying patients for evaluation of secondary causes of hypertension.** *ACE,* Angiotension-converting enzyme; *Hx,* history; *K+,* potassium; *R/O,* rule out. (From Goldman L, Ausiello D [eds]: *Cecil textbook of medicine,* ed 22, Philadelphia, 2004, WB Saunders.)

Section III

CLINICAL ALGORITHMS

ICD-9CM # 242.9

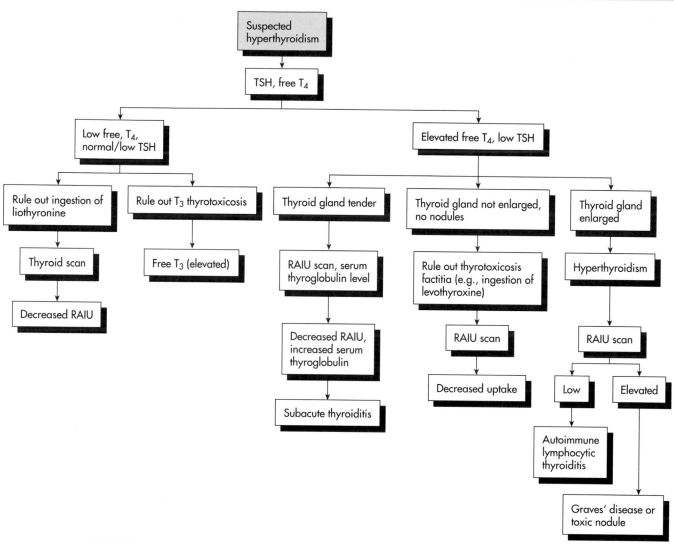

FIGURE 3-53   Hyperthyroidism. *RAIU,* Radioactive iodine uptake; *TSH,* thyroid-stimulating hormone.

ICD-9CM # 275.41

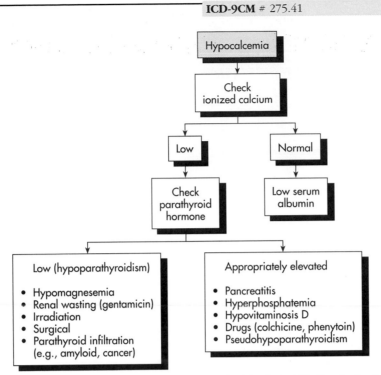

FIGURE 3-54 Evaluation of hypocalcemia. (From Wachtel TJ, Stein MD: *Practical guide to the care of the ambulatory patient,* ed 2, St Louis, 2000, Mosby.)

ICD-9CM # 256.3 Hypogonadism, female
257.2 Hypogonadism, male

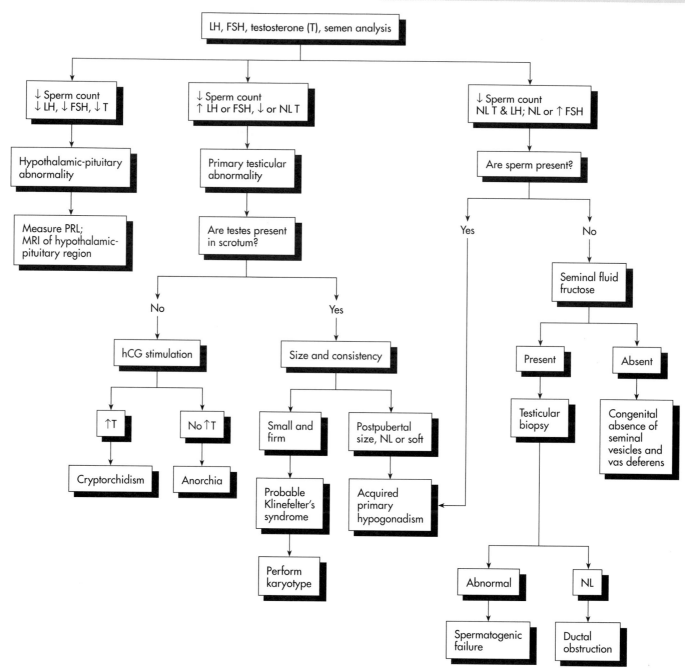

FIGURE 3-55 Laboratory evaluation of hypogonadism. *FSH,* Follicle-stimulating hormone; *hCG,* human chorionic gonadotropin; *LH,* luteinizing hormone; *MRI,* magnetic resonance imaging; *NL,* normal; *PRL,* prolactin; ↑, elevated; ↓, decreased or low. (From Andreoli TE [ed]: *Cecil essentials of medicine,* ed 5, Philadelphia, 2001, WB Saunders.)

ICD-9CM # 276.8

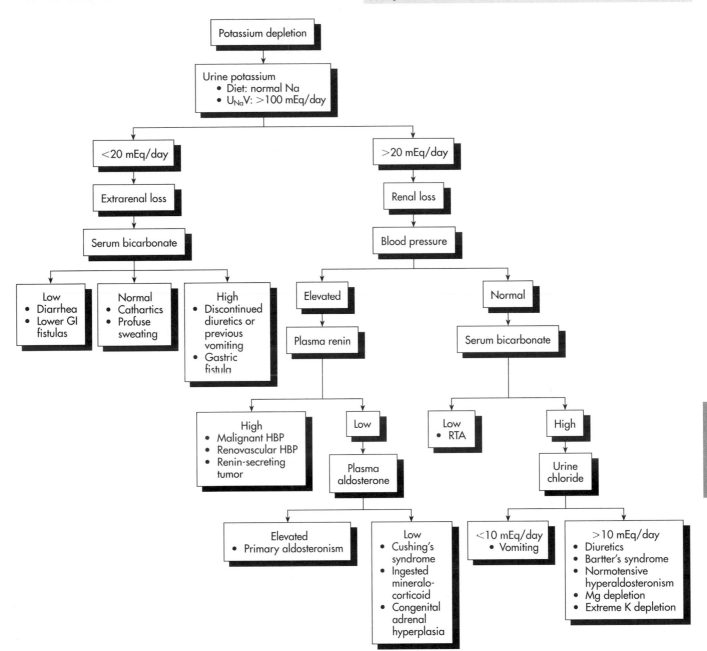

FIGURE 3-56 Diagnostic approach to hypokalemia. Because renal potassium wasting may improve during sodium restriction, diminished potassium excretion is indicative of extrarenal loss only when the diet (and therefore the urine) is rich in sodium. *GI*, Gastrointestinal; *HBP*, high blood pressure; *RTA*, renal tubular acidosis; $U_{Na}V$, urinary sodium volume. (From Stein JH [ed]: *Internal medicine,* ed 5, St Louis, 1998, Mosby.)

ICD-9CM # 276.1

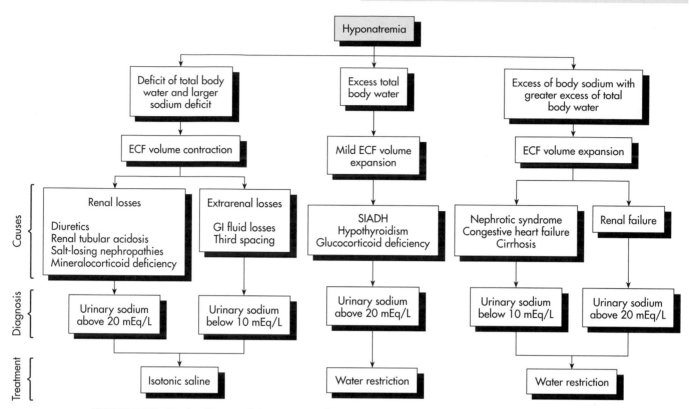

FIGURE 3-57 **Evaluation and treatment of asymptomatic, mild hyponatremia.** *ECF,* Extracellular fluid; *GI,* gastrointestinal; *SIADH,* syndrome of inappropriate secretion of antidiuretic hormone. (From Marx J et al [eds]: *Rosen's emergency medicine: concepts and clinical practice,* ed 5, St Louis, 2002, Mosby.)

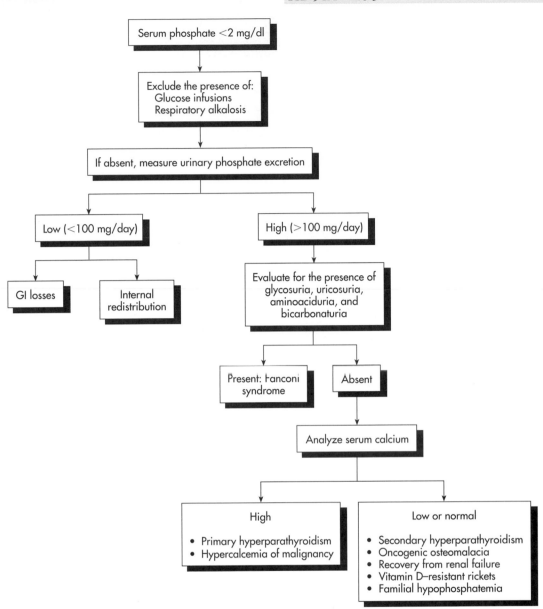

FIGURE 3-58 Diagnostic workup of hypophosphatemia. *GI*, Gastrointestinal. (From Stein JH [ed]: *Internal medicine,* ed 5, St Louis, 1998, Mosby.)

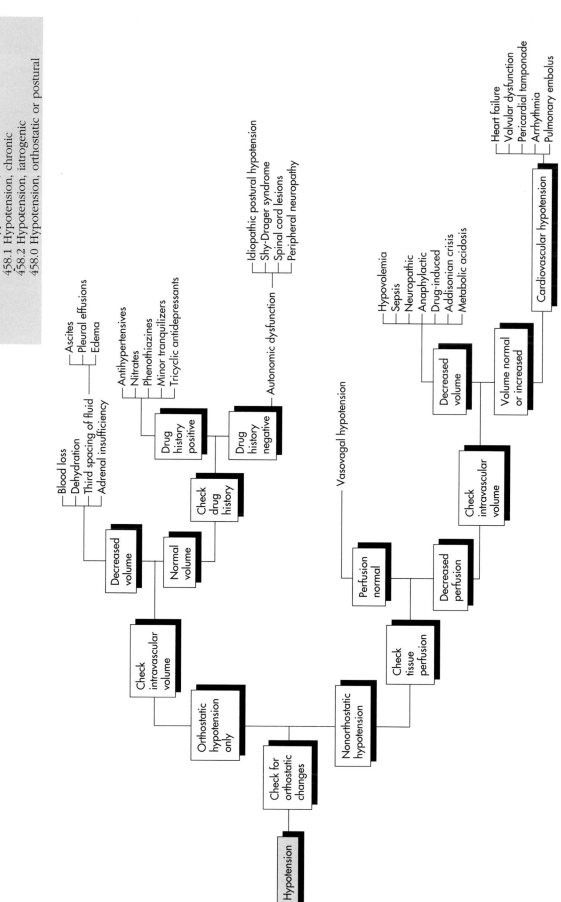

ICD-9CM # 458.9 Hypotension, NOS
458.1 Hypotension, chronic
458.2 Hypotension, iatrogenic
458.0 Hypotension, orthostatic or postural

FIGURE 3-59 Hypotension. (From Healey PM: *Common medical diagnosis: an algorithmic approach*, ed 3, Philadelphia, 2000, WB Saunders.)

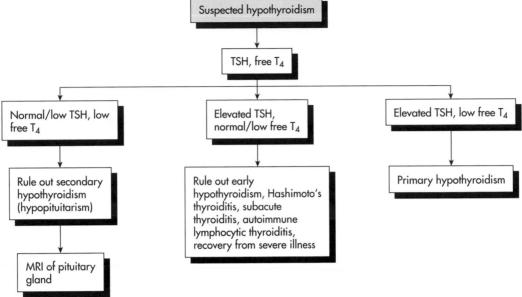

FIGURE 3-60 **Hypothyroidism.** *MRI,* Magnetic resonance imaging; *TSH,* thyroid-stimulating hormone.

JAUNDICE AND HEPATOBILIARY DISEASE

ICD-9CM # 782.4 Jaundice NOS
277.4 Bilirubin excretion disorders
576.8 Jaundice, obstructive

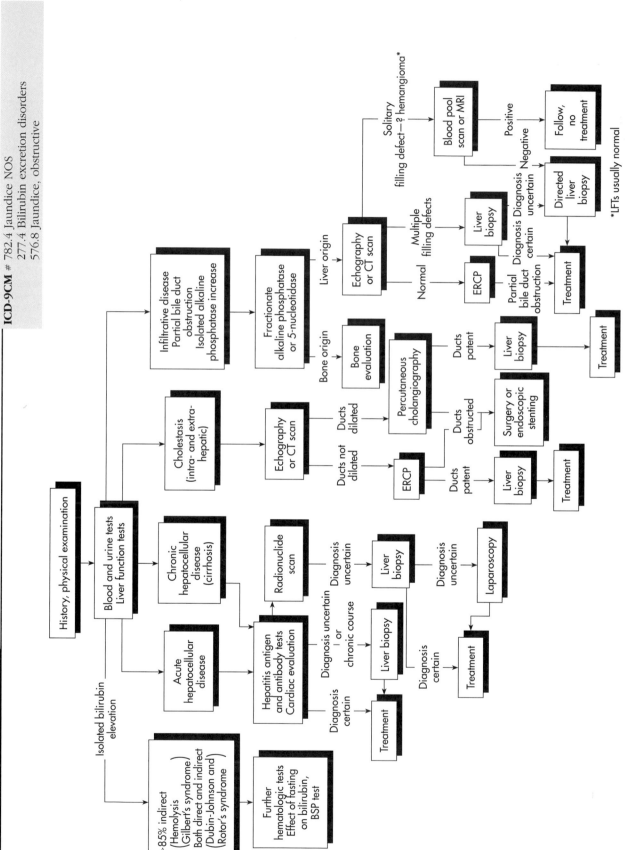

FIGURE 3-61 Evaluation of jaundice and hepatobiliary disease. *BSP,* Bromsulphalein; *CT,* computed tomography; *ERCP,* endoscopic retrograde cholangiopancreatography; *LFTs,* liver function tests; *MRI,* magnetic resonance imaging. (From Stein JH [ed]: *Internal medicine,* ed 5, St Louis, 1998, Mosby.)

ICD-9CM # 719.0

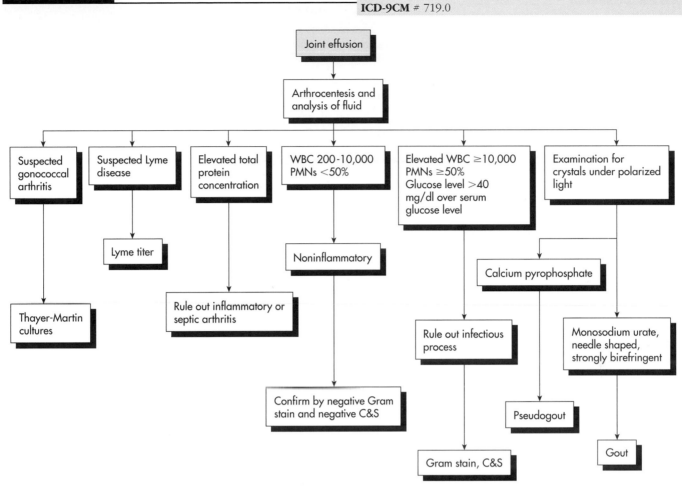

FIGURE 3-62   Joint effusion. *C&S,* Culture and sensitivity; *WBC,* white blood cell count.

ICD-9CM # 719.00

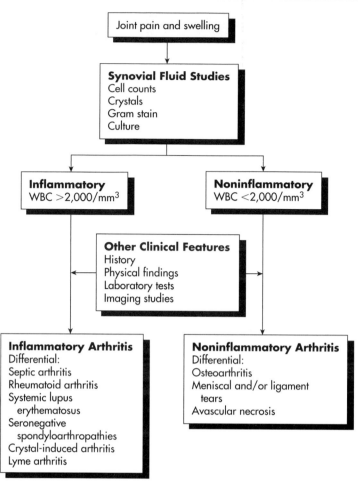

FIGURE 3-63 **Diagnostic approach for swollen joints.** *WBC,* White blood cell count. (From Goldman L, Ausiello D [eds]: *Cecil textbook of medicine,* ed 22, Philadelphia, 2004, WB Saunders.)

ICD-9CM # 440.23 Ulcer, lower limb, arteriosclerotic
707.1 Ulcer, lower limb, chronic
707.1 Ulcer, lower limb, neurogenic
707.9 Ulcer, non-healing
707.0 Pressure ulcer

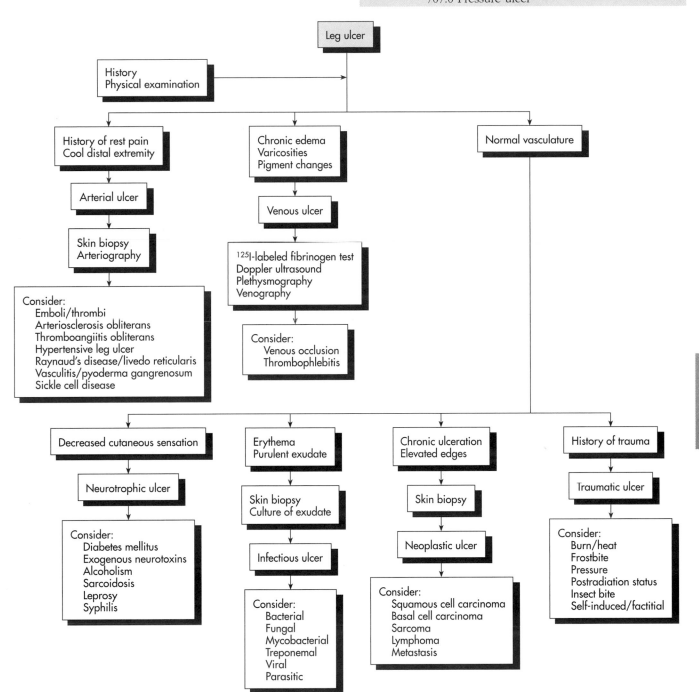

FIGURE 3-64   Leg ulcer. (From Greene HL, Johnson WP, Lemcke D [eds]: *Decision making in medicine,* ed 2, St Louis, 1998, Mosby.)

ICD-9CM # 573.9

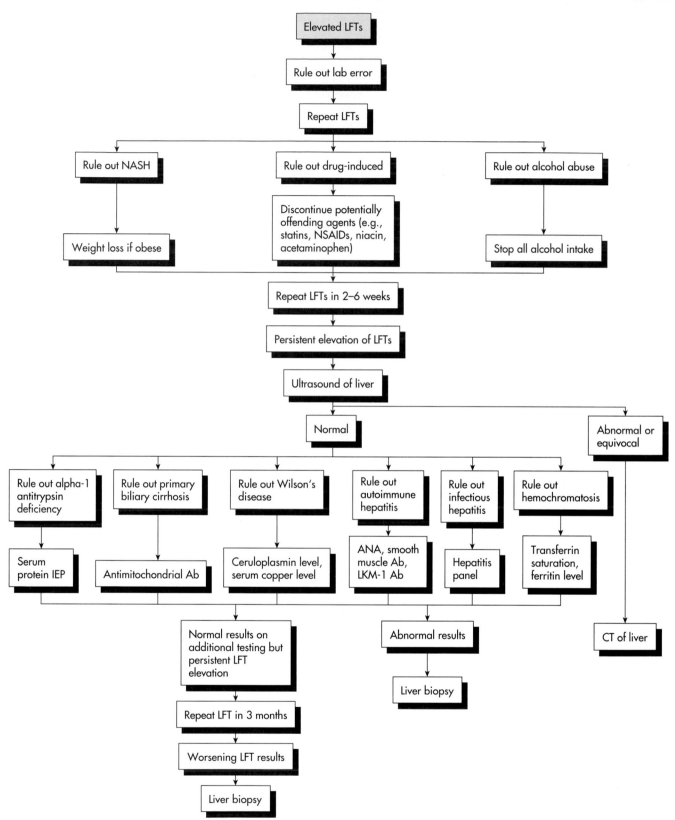

FIGURE 3-65 Liver function test elevations. *Ab,* Antibody; *ANA,* antibody to nuclear antigens; *CT,* computed tomography; *IEP,* immuno-electrophoresis; *LFT,* liver function test; *LKM,* liver-kidney microsome; *NSAIDs,* nonsteroidal antiinflammatory drugs.

LYMPHADENOPATHY, AXILLARY

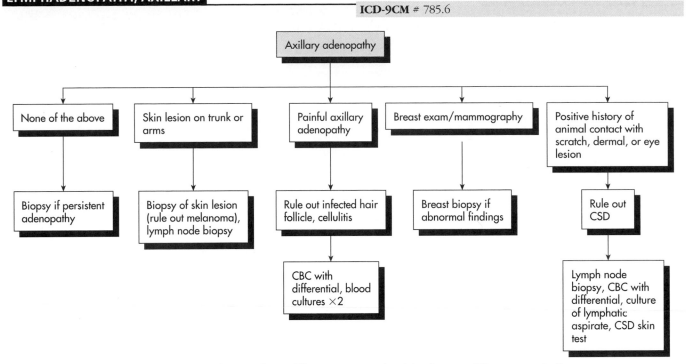

FIGURE 3-66 Lymphadenopathy, axillary. *CBC,* Complete blood count; *CSD,* cat-scratch disease.

ICD-9CM # 785.6

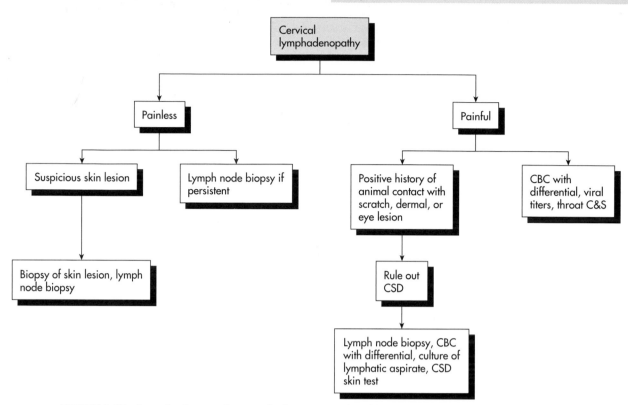

FIGURE 3-67 Lymphadenopathy, cervical. *CBC,* Complete blood count; *C&S,* culture and sensitivity; *CSD,* cat-scratch disease.

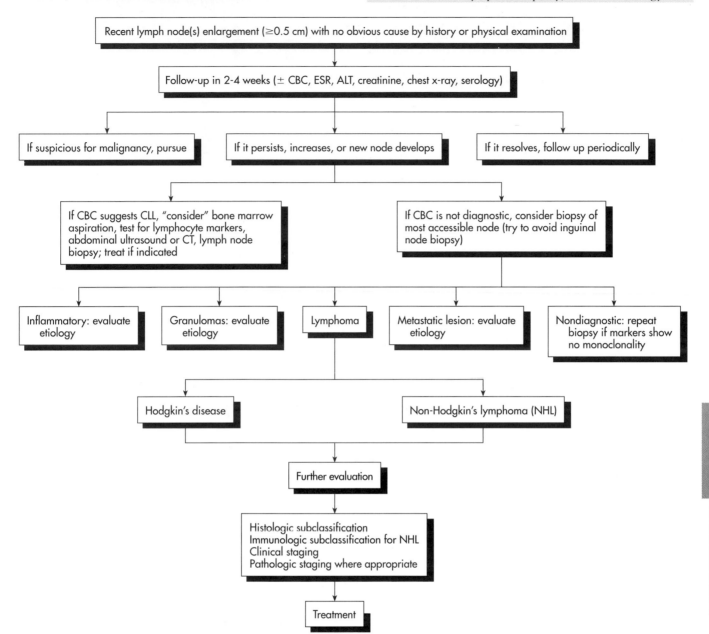

FIGURE 3-68 Workup of lymphadenopathy. *ALT,* Alanine aminotransferase; *CBC,* complete blood count; *CLL,* chronic lymphocytic leukemia; *CT,* computed tomography; *ESR,* erythrocyte sedimentation rate. (Modified from Noble J [ed]: *Primary care medicine,* ed 3, St Louis, 2001, Mosby.)

ICD-9CM # 579.9

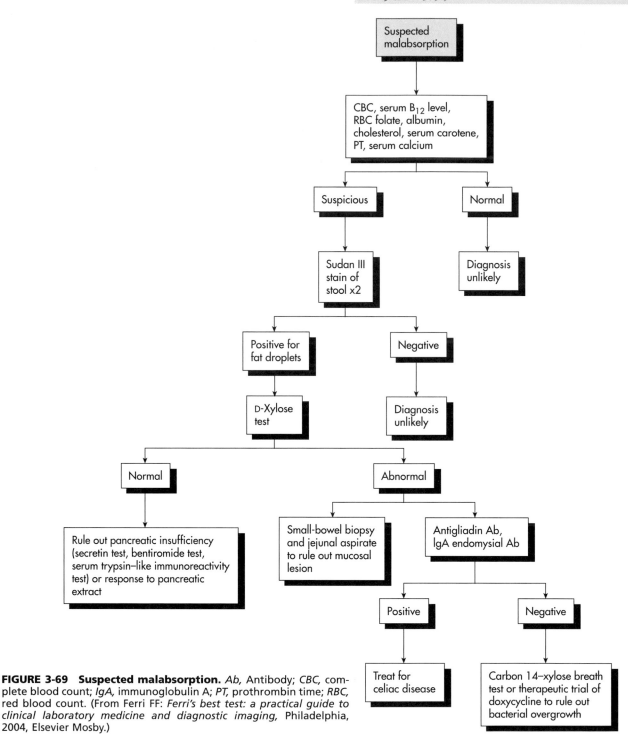

FIGURE 3-69 Suspected malabsorption. *Ab,* Antibody; *CBC,* complete blood count; *IgA,* immunoglobulin A; *PT,* prothrombin time; *RBC,* red blood count. (From Ferri FF: *Ferri's best test: a practical guide to clinical laboratory medicine and diagnostic imaging,* Philadelphia, 2004, Elsevier Mosby.)

BOX 3-4 **Malabsorption, Suspected**	
Diagnostic imaging	**Ancillary tests**
Best test	Albumin, total protein
Small-bowel series	ALT, AST, PT
Ancillary test	Serum lytes, BUN, creatinine
CT of pancreas with IV contrast	Sudan III stain of stool for fecal leukocytes
Lab evaluation	CBC, RBC folate, serum iron, serum carotene, cholesterol, serum calcium
Best test	Hydrogen 14-C xylose breath test
Biopsy of small bowel	D-Xylose test, secretin test
	Quantitative fecal test
	Antigliadin antibody, IgA endomysial antibody

From Ferri FF: *Ferri's best test: a practical guide to clinical laboratory medicine and diagnostic imaging,* Philadelphia, 2004, Elsevier Mosby.
ALT, Alanine aminotransferase; *AST,* aspartate aminotransferase; *BUN,* blood urea nitrogen; *CBC,* complete blood count; *CT,* computed tomography; *IgA,* immunoglobulin A; *IV,* intravenous; *PT,* prothrombin time; *RBC,* red blood count.

ICD-9CM # 203.0

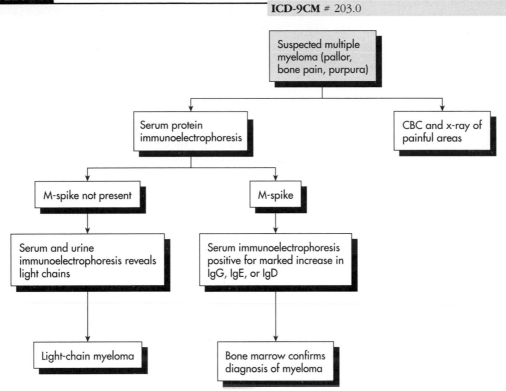

FIGURE 3-70 **Multiple myeloma.** *CBC,* Complete blood count; *Ig,* immunoglobulin.

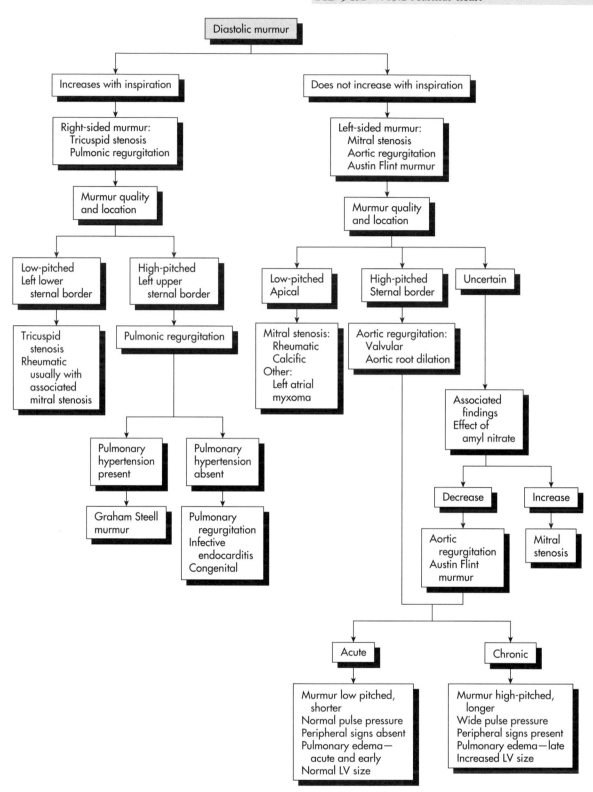

FIGURE 3-71 Diastolic murmur. *LV,* Left ventricle. (From Greene HL, Johnson WP, Lemke D [eds]: *Decision making in medicine,* ed 2, St Louis, 1998, Mosby.)

ICD-9CM # 785.2 Murmur heart

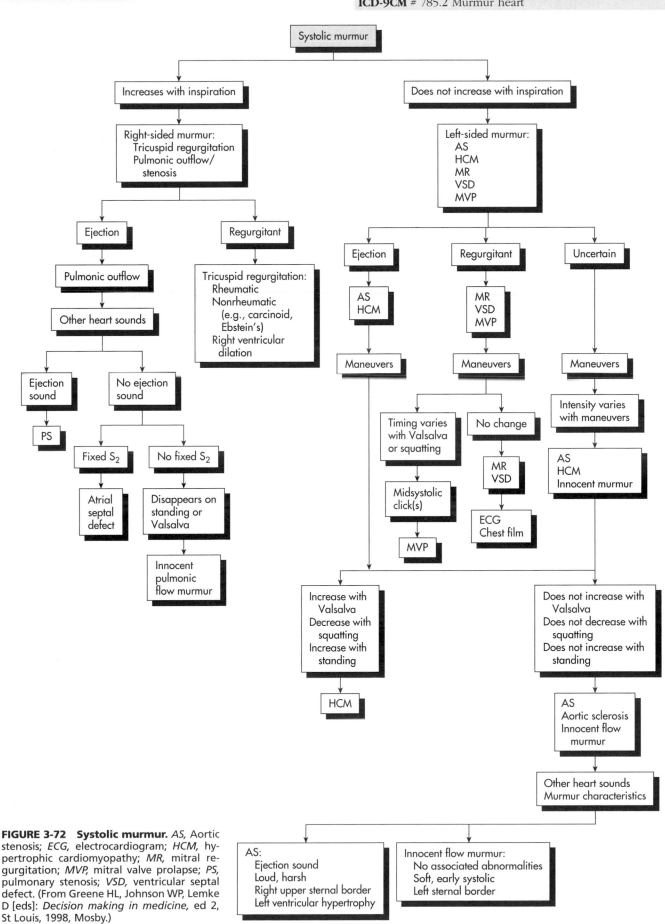

FIGURE 3-72 Systolic murmur. *AS,* Aortic stenosis; *ECG,* electrocardiogram; *HCM,* hypertrophic cardiomyopathy; *MR,* mitral regurgitation; *MVP,* mitral valve prolapse; *PS,* pulmonary stenosis; *VSD,* ventricular septal defect. (From Greene HL, Johnson WP, Lemke D [eds]: *Decision making in medicine,* ed 2, St Louis, 1998, Mosby.)

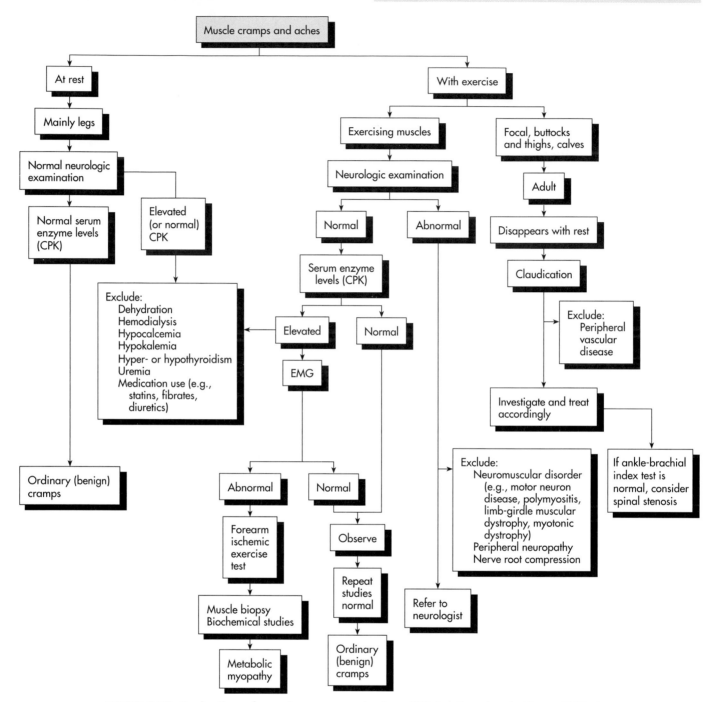

FIGURE 3-73 Evaluation of muscle cramps and aches. *CPK,* Creatine phosphokinase; *EMG,* electromyography. (Adapted from Greene HL, Johnson WP, Lemcke D [eds]: *Decision making in medicine,* ed 2, St Louis, 1998, Mosby.)

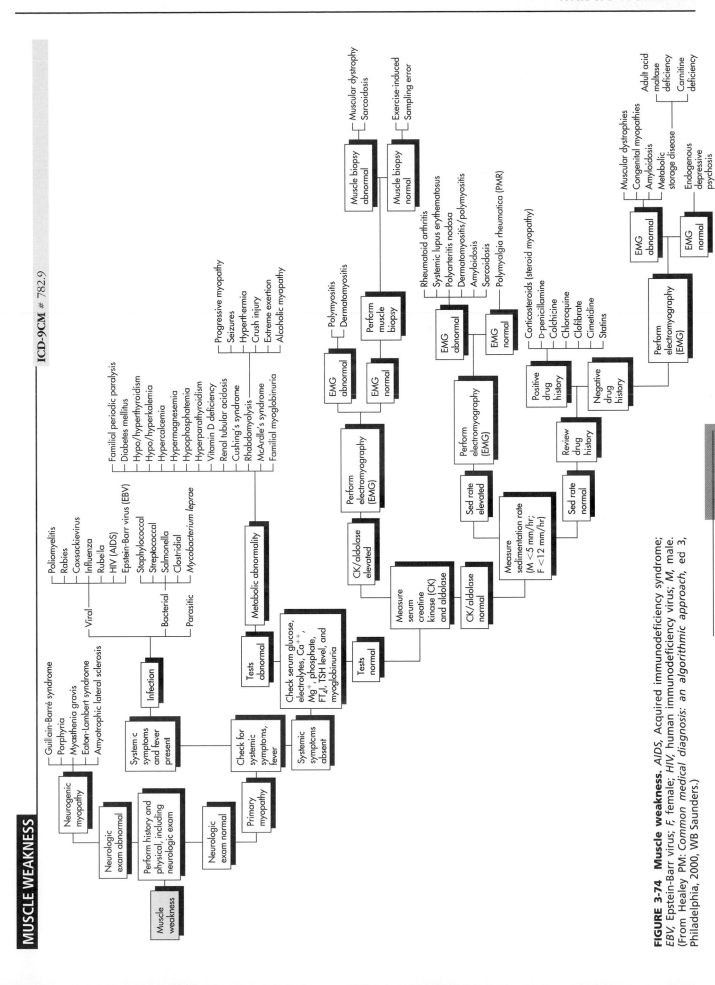

FIGURE 3-74 Muscle weakness. *AIDS,* Acquired immunodeficiency syndrome; *EBV,* Epstein-Barr virus; *F,* female; *HIV,* human immunodeficiency virus; *M,* male. (From Healey PM: *Common medical diagnosis: an algorithmic approach,* ed 3, Philadelphia, 2000, WB Saunders.)

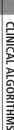

ICD-9CM # 238.7

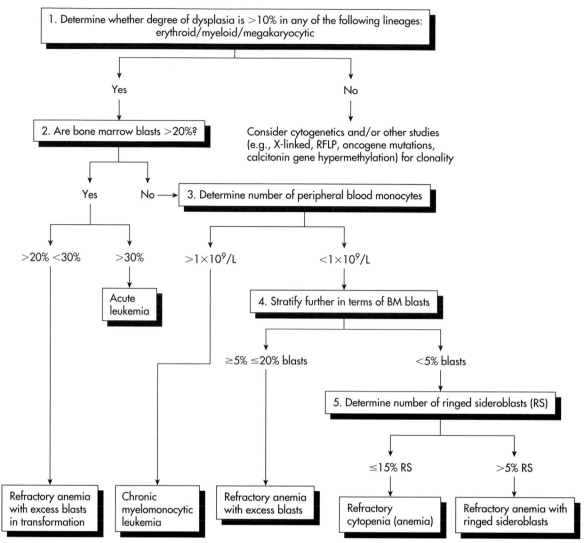

FIGURE 3-75 Myelodysplastic syndromes. *BM blasts,* Bone marrow blastocyst; *RFLP,* restriction fragment length polymorphism. (From Abeloff MD: *Clinical oncology,* ed 2, New York, 2000, Churchill Livingstone.)

MYOCARDIAL ISCHEMIA, SUSPECTED

ICD-9CM # 411.89 Myocardial Ischemia, acute without MI
414.8 Myocardial Ischemia, chronic
411.1 Angina, stable
413 Angina pectoris

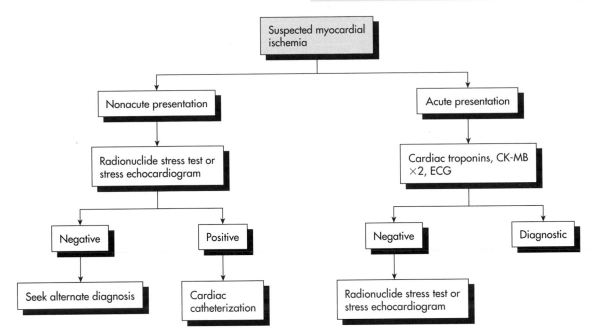

FIGURE 3-78   Myocardial Ischemia, suspected. *CK-MB,* Myocardial muscle creatine kinase isoenzyme, *ECG,* electrocardiogram.

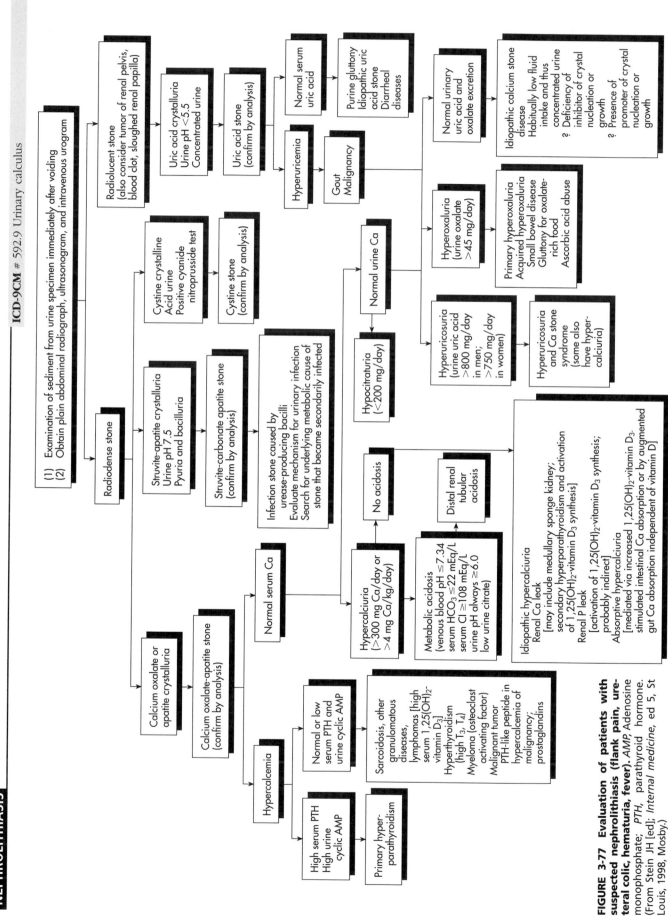

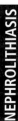

FIGURE 3-77 **Evaluation of patients with suspected nephrolithiasis (flank pain, ureteral colic, hematuria, fever).** *AMP,* Adenosine monophosphate; *PTH,* parathyroid hormone. (From Stein JH [ed]: *Internal medicine,* ed 5, St Louis, 1998, Mosby.)

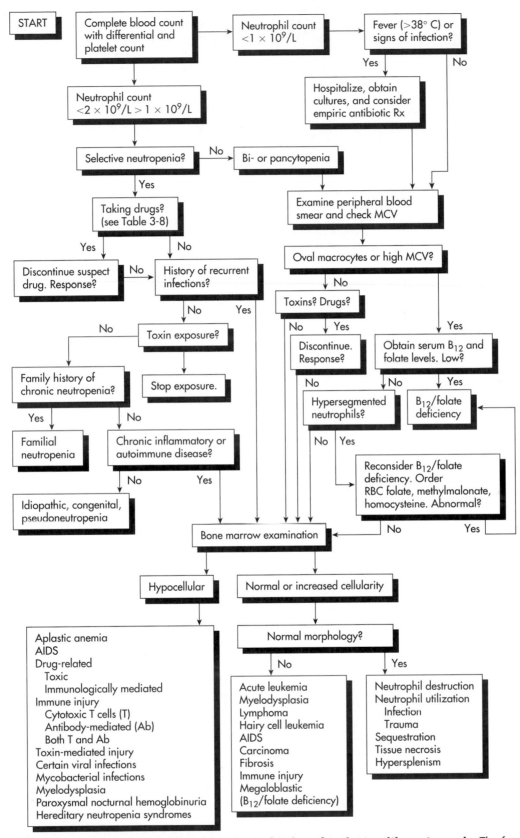

FIGURE 3-78 A practical algorithm for the evaluation of patients with neutropenia. The fundamental diagnostic principle is that for patients with severe neutropenia or for those with bicytopenia or pancytopenia, bone marrow examination will likely be necessary unless the following diagnoses are made: (1) a nutritional (folate or vitamin B_{12}) deficiency or (2) drug- or toxin-induced neutropenia in a patient whose neutropenia resolves after discontinuation of the offending agent. *AIDS,* Acquired immunodeficiency syndrome; *MCV,* mean corpuscular volume; *RBC,* red blood cell. (From Goldman L, Ausiello D [eds]: *Cecil textbook of medicine,* ed 22, Philadelphia, 2004, WB Saunders.)

ICD-9CM # 269.9

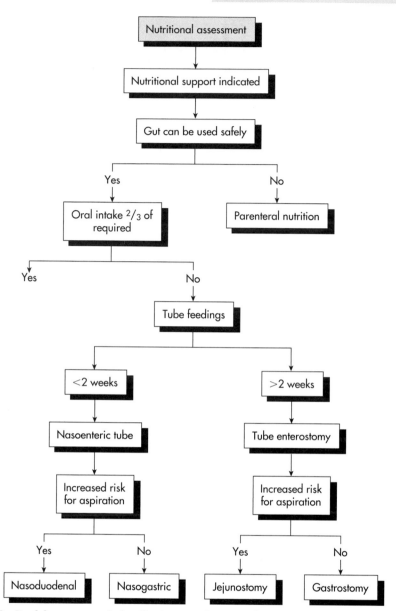

FIGURE 3-79 Decision approach for the type and route of nutritional support. (From Goldman L, Ausiello D [eds]: *Cecil textbook of medicine,* ed 22, Philadelphia, 2004, WB Saunders.)

BOX 3-5	**Indications for the Use of Enteral Nutrition in Adult Medical Patients**

Protein-energy malnutrition with anticipated significantly decreased oral intake for at least 7 days
Anticipated significantly decreased oral intake for 10 days
Severe dysphagia
Massive small bowel resection (used in combination with total parenteral nutrition)
Low-output (<500 mL/day) enterocutaneous fistula

From Goldman L, Ausiello D (eds): *Cecil textbook of medicine,* ed 22, Philadelphia, 2004, WB Saunders.

PAIN CONTROL

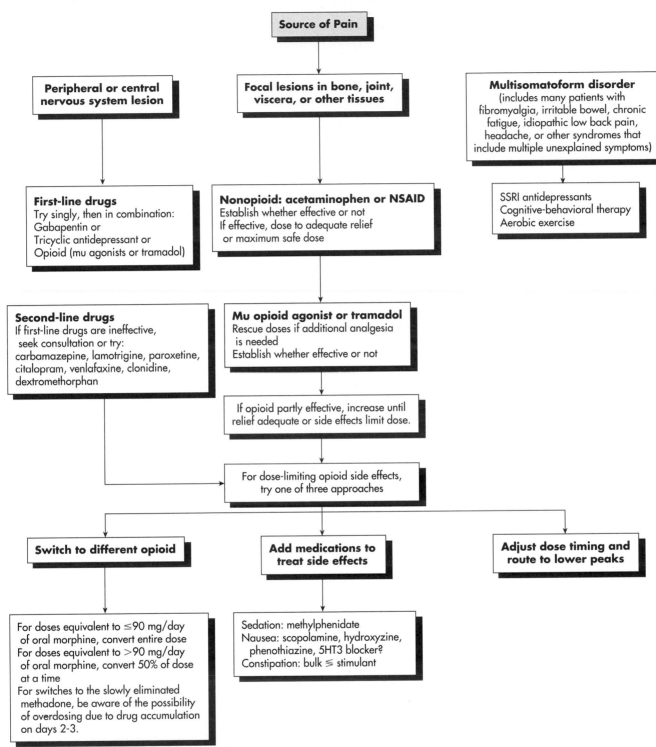

FIGURE 3-80 Algorithm for the treatment of pain. *COX,* Cyclooxygenase; *NSAID,* nonsteroidal anti-inflammatory drug; *SSRI,* selective serotonin reuptake inhibitor. (From Goldman L, Ausiello D [eds]: *Cecil textbook of medicine,* ed 22, Philadelphia, 2004, WB Saunders.)

ICD-9CM # 789.36

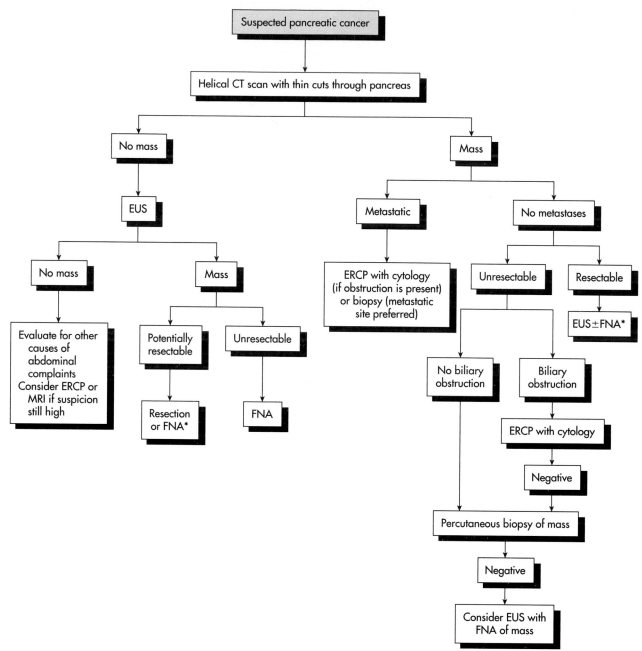

FIGURE 3-81 Diagnostic algorithm for pancreatic cancer. Intraoperative fine-needle aspiration (FNA) if found inoperable during surgery. *CT,* Computed tomographic scan; *ERCP,* endoscopic retrograde cholangiopancreatography; *EUS,* endoscopic ultrasonography; *MRI,* magnetic resonance imaging. (From Goldman L, Ausiello D [eds]: *Cecil textbook of medicine,* ed 22, Philadelphia, 2004, WB Saunders.)

ICD-9CM # 332.0 Idiopathic Parkinson's disease
332.1 Parkinson's disease, secondary

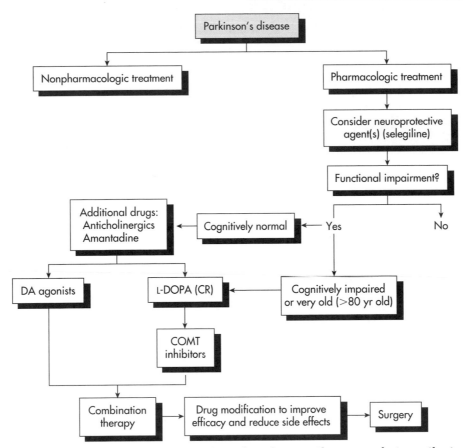

FIGURE 3-82 Diagrammatic representation of a therapeutic approach to patients with parkinsonism. *COMT,* Catechol-*O*-methyl transferase; *CR,* controlled release; *DA,* dopamine. (Adapted from Goldman L, Ausiello D [eds]: *Cecil textbook of medicine,* ed 22, Philadelphia, 2004, WB Saunders.)

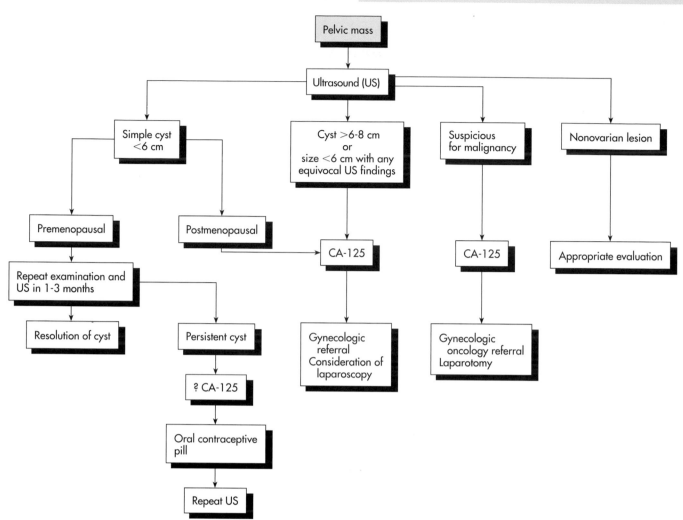

FIGURE 3-83   Approach to the patient with a pelvic mass. *US,* Ultrasound. (From Carlson KJ et al: *Primary care of women,* ed 2, St Louis, 2002, Mosby.)

PERIPHERAL NEUROPATHY

ICD-9CM # 356.9 Peripheral nerve neuropathy
355.10 Lower extremity neuropathy
354.11 Upper extremity neuropathy

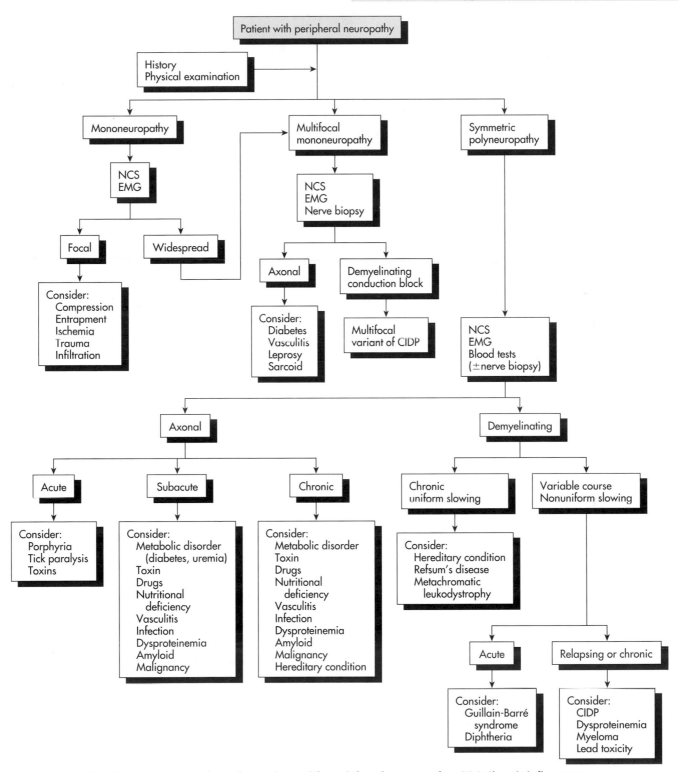

FIGURE 3-84 Approach to the patient with peripheral neuropathy. *CIDP,* Chronic inflammatory demyelinating polyradioneuropathy; *EMG,* electromyogram; *NCS,* nerve conduction studies. (From Greene HL, Johnson WP, Lemcke DL: *Decision making in medicine,* ed 2, St Louis, 1988, Mosby.)

ICD-9CM # 511.9 Pleural effusion, unspecified

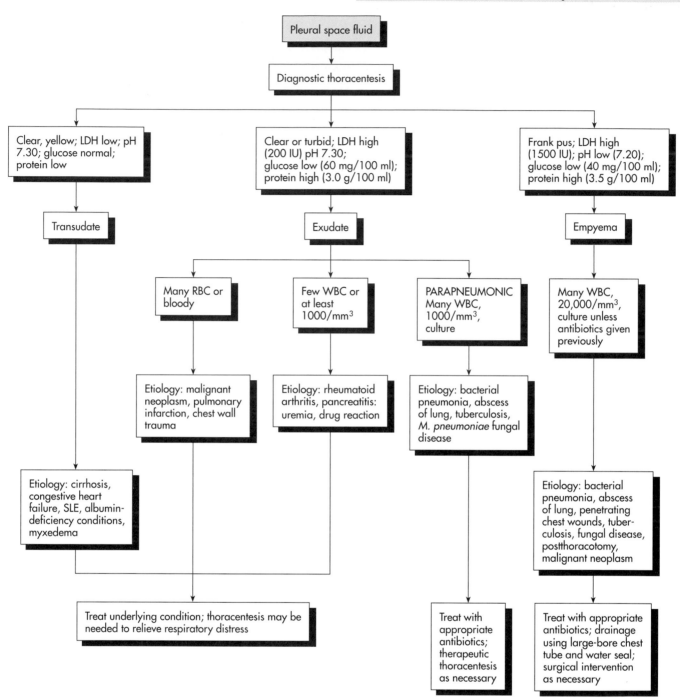

FIGURE 3-85 Evaluation, common etiologies, and management of pleural effusion and empyema. *LDH,* Lactate dehydrogenase; *RBC,* red blood cells; *SLE,* systemic lupus erythematosus; *WBC,* white blood cells. (From Kassirer J [ed]: *Current therapy in adult medicine,* ed 4, St Louis, 1998, Mosby.)

PREOPERATIVE EVALUATION, PATIENT WITH CORONARY HEART DISEASE

ICD-9CM # 411.89 Coronary insufficiency, acute
411.8 Coronary insufficiency, chronic
411.1 Coronary insufficiency or intermediate syndrome

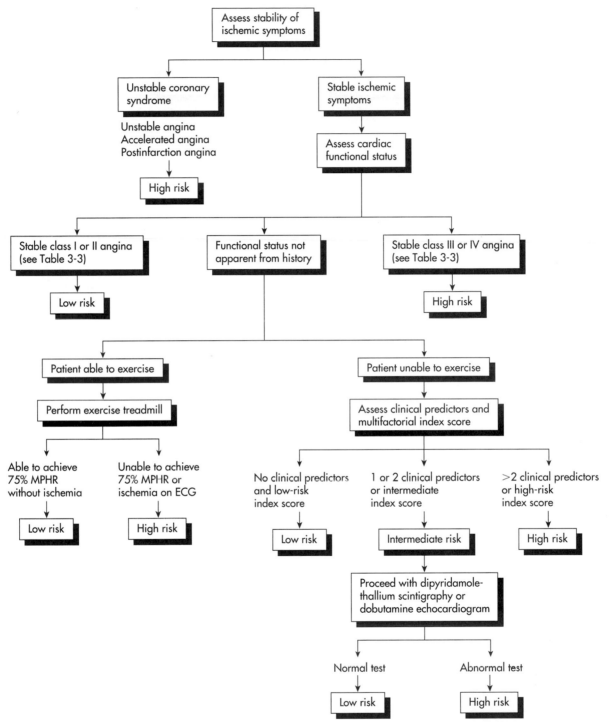

FIGURE 3-86 Preoperative evaluation of patients with known or suspected coronary artery disease. (From Goldman L, Braunwald E [eds]: *Primary cardiology*, Philadelphia, 1998, WB Saunders.)

TABLE 3-3 New York Heart Association Functional Classification

Class I	No limitation	Ordinary physical activity does not cause symptoms
Class II	Slight limitation	Comfortable at rest Ordinary physical activity causes symptoms
Class III	Marked limitation	Comfortable at rest Less than ordinary activity causes symptoms
Class IV	Inability to carry on any physical activity	Symptoms present at rest

From Ferri FF: *Ferri's clinical advisor,* St Louis, 2006, Mosby.

ICD-9CM # 185

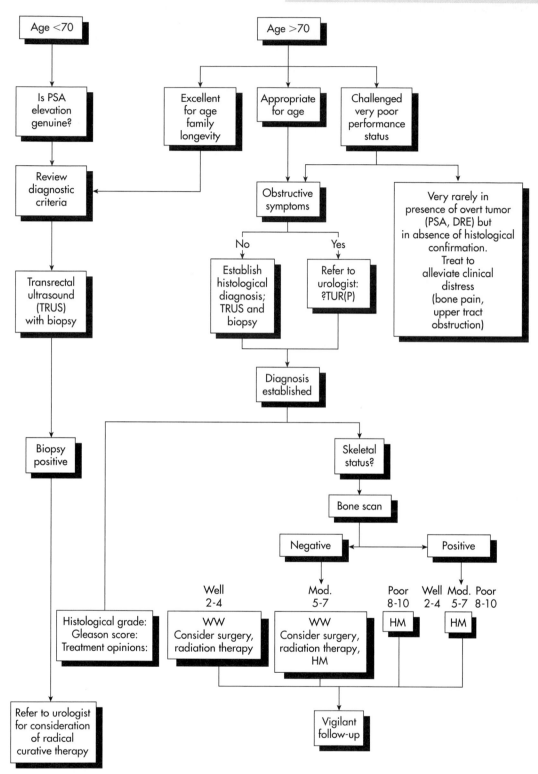

FIGURE 3-87   Assessment and treatment of a patient with prostate cancer suspected on the grounds of a digital rectal exam and PSA. *WW,* Watchful waiting; *HM,* hormonal manipulation; *PSA,* prostate specific antigen. (Modified from Tallis RC, Fillit HM [eds]: *Brocklehurst's textbook of geriatric medicine and gerontology,* ed 6, London, 2003, Churchill Livingstone.)

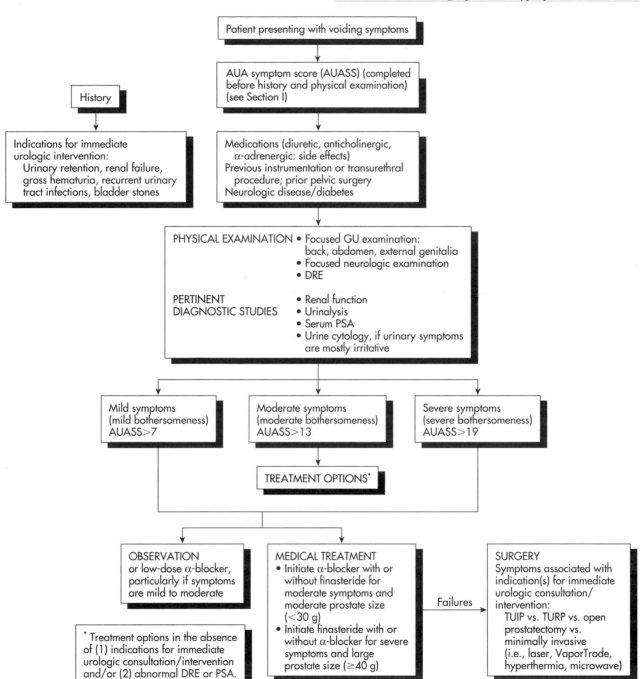

Patient presenting with voiding symptoms

AUA symptom score (AUASS) (completed before history and physical examination) (see Section I)

History

Indications for immediate urologic intervention:
Urinary retention, renal failure, gross hematuria, recurrent urinary tract infections, bladder stones

Medications (diuretic, anticholinergic, α-adrenergic: side effects)
Previous instrumentation or transurethral procedure; prior pelvic surgery
Neurologic disease/diabetes

PHYSICAL EXAMINATION • Focused GU examination: back, abdomen, external genitalia
• Focused neurologic examination
• DRE

PERTINENT DIAGNOSTIC STUDIES
• Renal function
• Urinalysis
• Serum PSA
• Urine cytology, if urinary symptoms are mostly irritative

Mild symptoms (mild bothersomeness) AUASS>7

Moderate symptoms (moderate bothersomeness) AUASS>13

Severe symptoms (severe bothersomeness) AUASS>19

TREATMENT OPTIONS*

OBSERVATION
or low-dose α-blocker, particularly if symptoms are mild to moderate

* Treatment options in the absence of (1) indications for immediate urologic consultation/intervention and/or (2) abnormal DRE or PSA.

MEDICAL TREATMENT
• Initiate α-blocker with or without finasteride for moderate symptoms and moderate prostate size (<30 g)
• Initiate finasteride with or without α-blocker for severe symptoms and large prostate size (≥40 g)

Failures

SURGERY
Symptoms associated with indication(s) for immediate urologic consultation/ intervention:
TUIP vs. TURP vs. open prostatectomy vs. minimally invasive (i.e., laser, VaporTrode, hyperthermia, microwave)

FIGURE 3-88 Critical pathway for patients with benign prostatic hypertrophy. *AUA,* American Urological Association; *DRE,* digital rectal examination; *GU,* genitourinary; *PSA,* prostate-specific antigen; *TUIP,* transurethral incision of the prostate; *TURP,* transurethral resection of the prostate. (From Nseyo UO [ed]: *Urology for primary care physicians,* Philadelphia, 1999, WB Saunders.)

ICD-9CM # 791.0

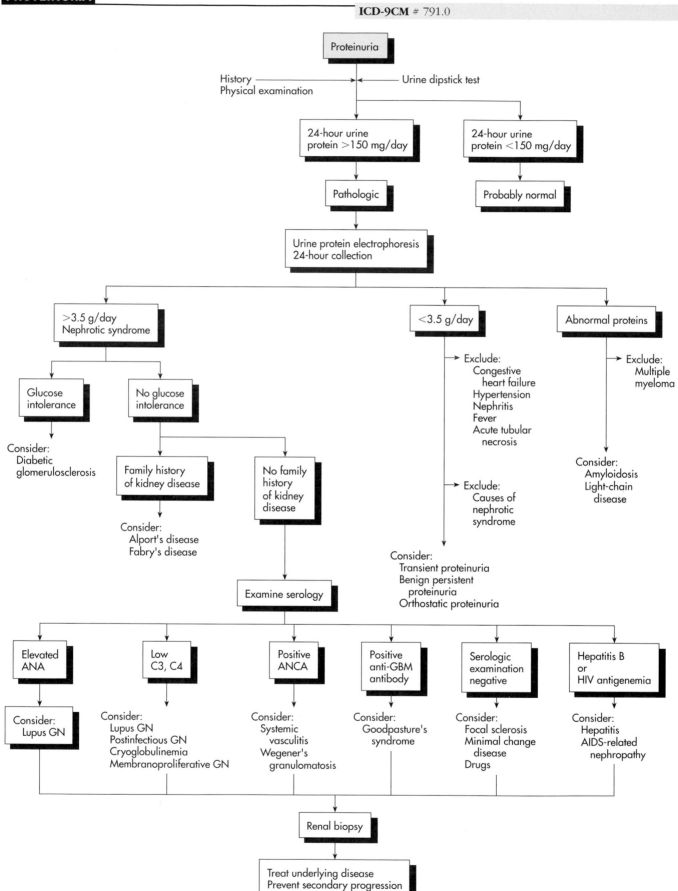

FIGURE 3-89 Proteinuria. *AIDS,* Acquired immunodeficiency syndrome; *ANA,* antinuclear antibody; *ANCA,* antineutrophil cytoplasmic autoantibody; *anti-GBM,* anti–glomerular basement membrane; *GN,* glomerulonephritis. (From Greene HL, Johnson WP, Lemcke D [eds]: *Decision making in medicine,* ed 2, St Louis, 1998, Mosby.)

PRURITUS, GENERALIZED

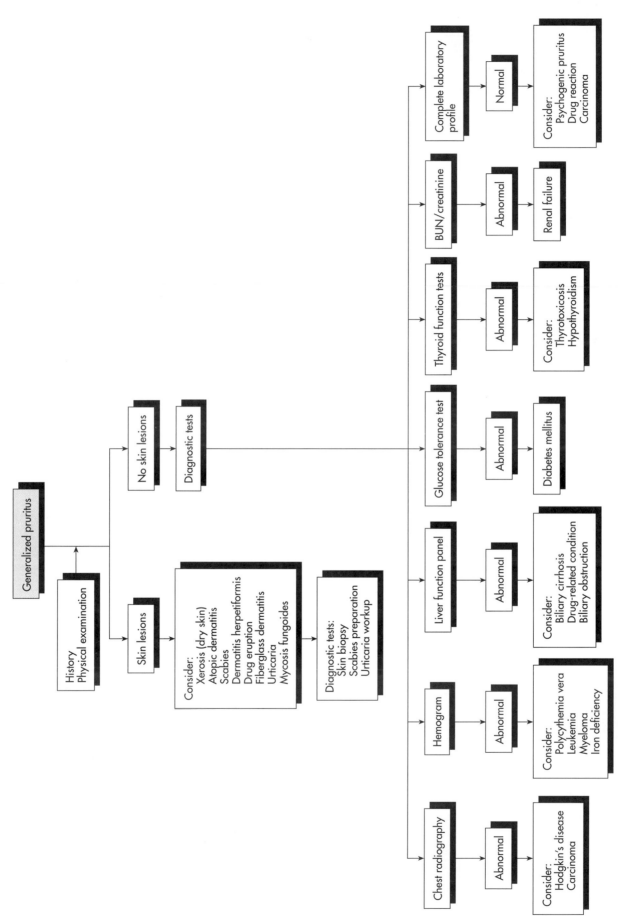

FIGURE 3-90 Evaluation of generalized pruritus. *BUN,* Blood urea nitrogen. (From Greene HL, Johnson WP, Lemcke D [eds]: *Decision making in medicine,* ed 2, St Louis, 1998, Mosby.)

ICD-9CM # 415.1

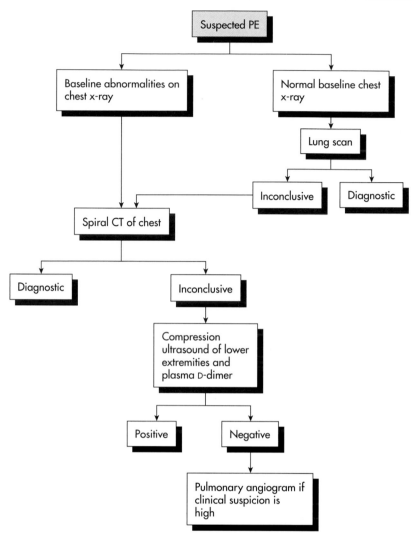

FIGURE 3-91   Pulmonary embolism. *CT,* Computed tomography; *PE,* pulmonary embolism. (From Ferri FF: *Ferri's clinical advisor*, St Louis, 2006, Mosby.)

ICD-9CM # 518.89

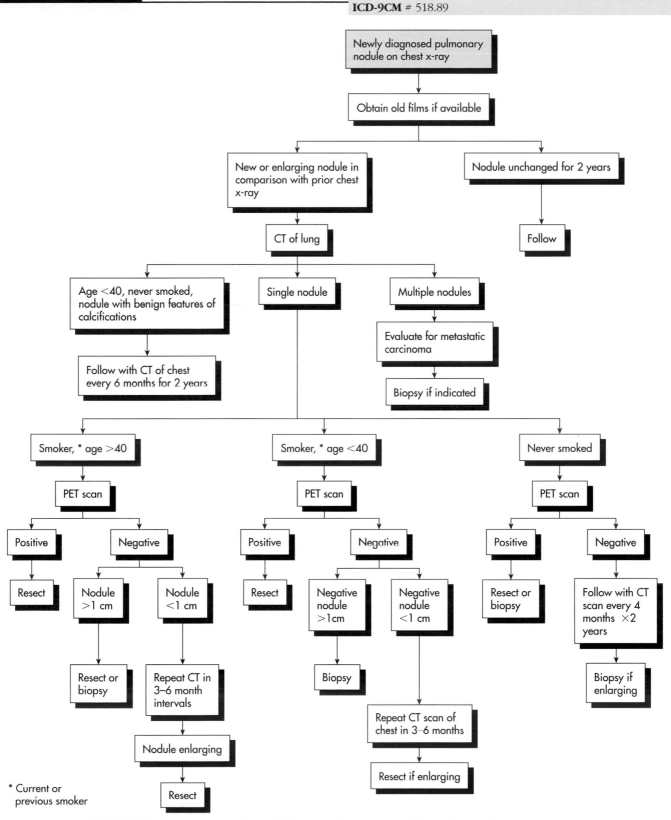

FIGURE 3-92 Pulmonary nodule. *CT,* Computed tomography; *PET,* positron emission tomography. (From Ferri FF: *Ferri's clinical advisor,* St Louis, 2006, Mosby.)

ICD-9CM # 379.93

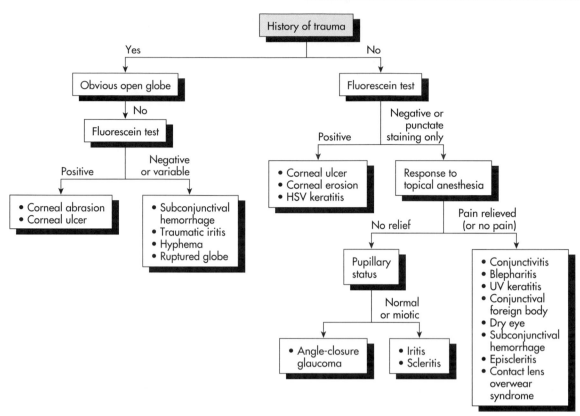

FIGURE 3-93 **Algorithm showing diagnostic procedure for the acute red eye.** *HSV,* Herpes simplex virus; *UV,* ultraviolet. (From Auerbach PS: *Wilderness medicine,* ed 4, St Louis, 2001, Mosby.)

ICD-9CM # 584.9 Acute renal failure, unspecified

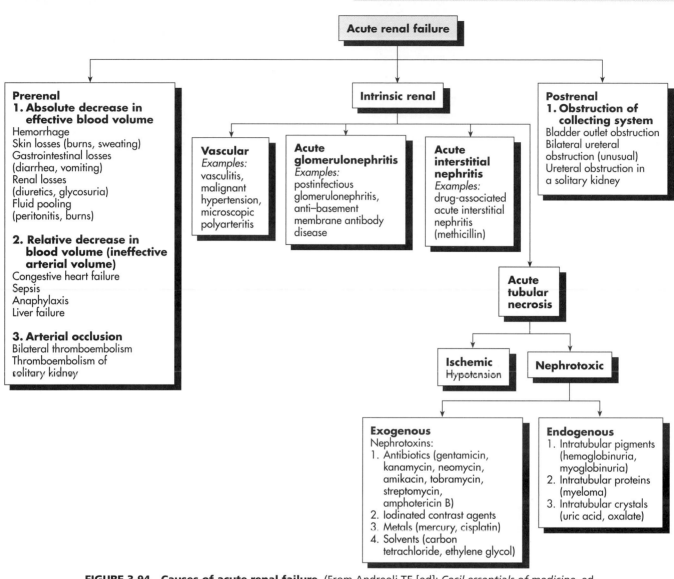

Acute renal failure

Prerenal
1. Absolute decrease in effective blood volume
Hemorrhage
Skin losses (burns, sweating)
Gastrointestinal losses (diarrhea, vomiting)
Renal losses (diuretics, glycosuria)
Fluid pooling (peritonitis, burns)

2. Relative decrease in blood volume (ineffective arterial volume)
Congestive heart failure
Sepsis
Anaphylaxis
Liver failure

3. Arterial occlusion
Bilateral thromboembolism
Thromboembolism of solitary kidney

Intrinsic renal

Vascular
Examples: vasculitis, malignant hypertension, microscopic polyarteritis

Acute glomerulonephritis
Examples: postinfectious glomerulonephritis, anti–basement membrane antibody disease

Acute interstitial nephritis
Examples: drug-associated acute interstitial nephritis (methicillin)

Postrenal
1. Obstruction of collecting system
Bladder outlet obstruction
Bilateral ureteral obstruction (unusual)
Ureteral obstruction in a solitary kidney

Acute tubular necrosis

Ischemic
Hypotension

Nephrotoxic

Exogenous
Nephrotoxins:
1. Antibiotics (gentamicin, kanamycin, neomycin, amikacin, tobramycin, streptomycin, amphotericin B)
2. Iodinated contrast agents
3. Metals (mercury, cisplatin)
4. Solvents (carbon tetrachloride, ethylene glycol)

Endogenous
1. Intratubular pigments (hemoglobinuria, myoglobinuria)
2. Intratubular proteins (myeloma)
3. Intratubular crystals (uric acid, oxalate)

FIGURE 3-94 Causes of acute renal failure. (From Andreoli TE [ed]: *Cecil essentials of medicine,* ed 4, Philadelphia, 1997, WB Saunders.)

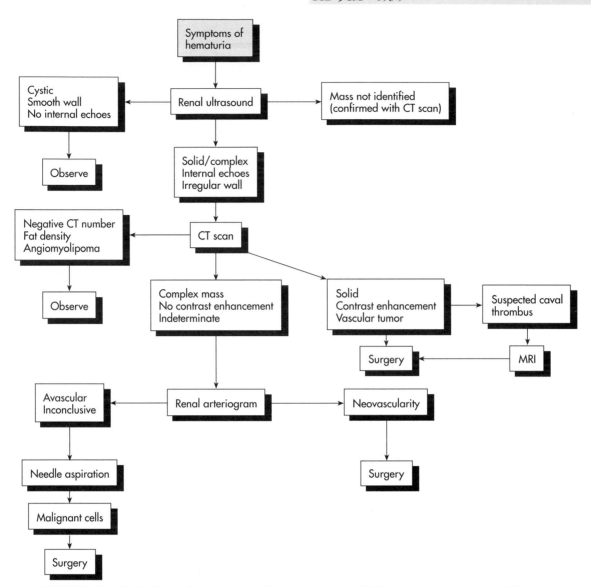

FIGURE 3-95 Evaluation of a patient with a renal mass. *CT,* Computed tomography; *MRI,* magnetic resonance imaging. (Modified from Williams RD: Tumors of the kidney, ureter, and bladder. In Goldman L, Ausiello D [eds]: *Cecil textbook of medicine,* ed 22, Philadelphia, 2004, WB Saunders.)

RESPIRATORY DISTRESS

ICD-9CM # 786.09 Respiratory distress NOS
518.82 Respiratory distress, acute

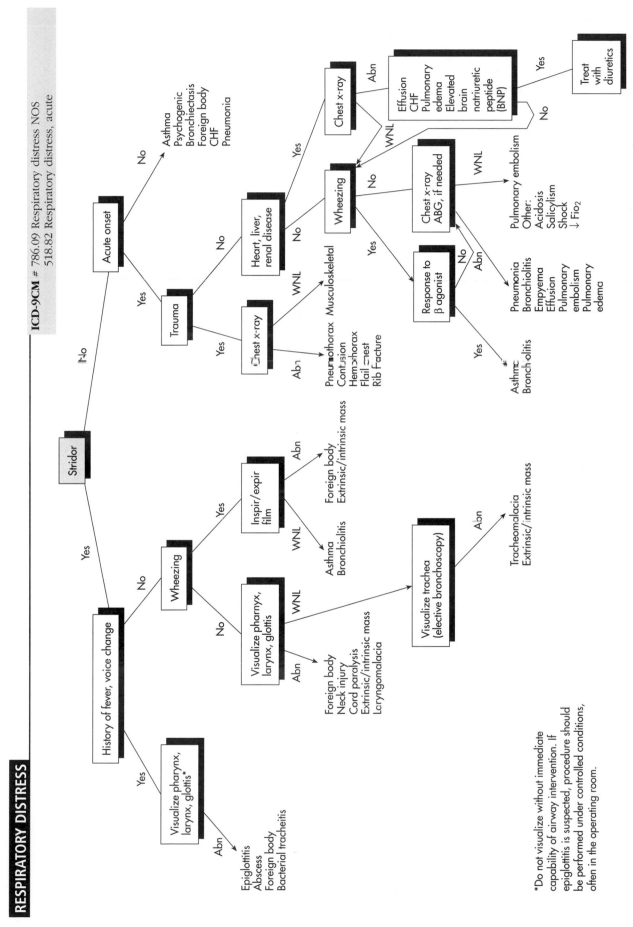

FIGURE 3-96 Respiratory distress. *ABG,* Arterial blood gas; *Abn,* abnormal; *CHF,* congestive heart failure; *WNL,* within normal limits. (Adapted from Barkin RM, Rosen P: *Emergency pediatrics,* St Louis, 1999, Mosby.)

*Do not visualize without immediate capability of airway intervention. If epiglottitis is suspected, procedure should be performed under controlled conditions, often in the operating room.

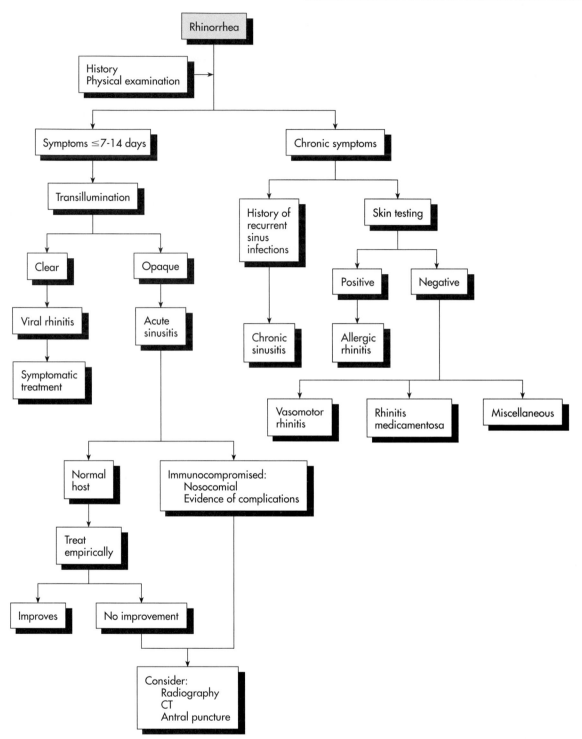

FIGURE 3-97   Approach to a patient with rhinorrhea. *CT,* Computed tomography. (From Noble J [ed]: *Primary care medicine,* ed 3, St Louis, 2001, Mosby.)

SEXUAL DYSFUNCTION

ICD-9CM # 309.2 Sexual disorder (psychosexual)
V41.7 Sexual function problem

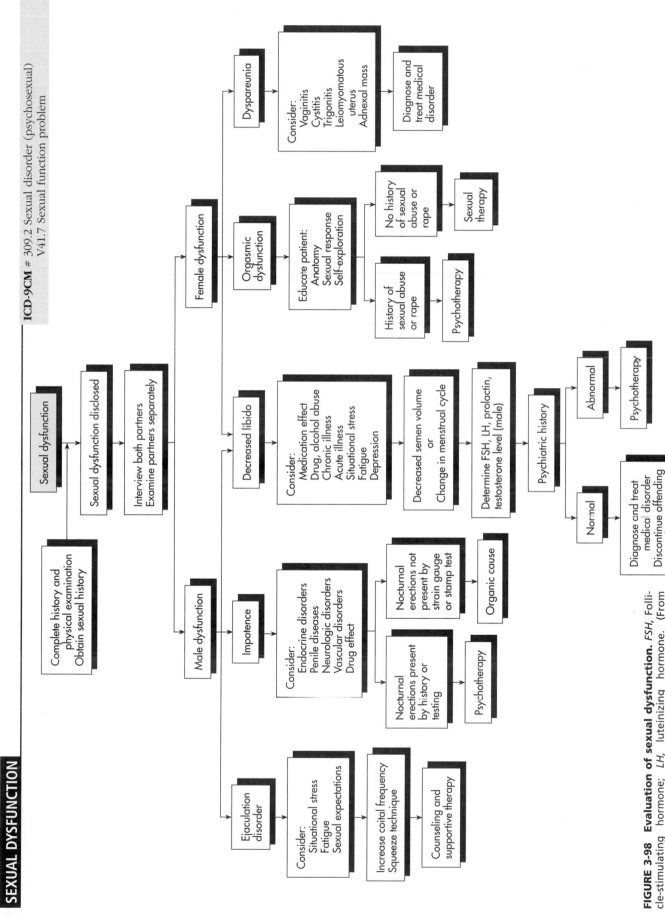

FIGURE 3-98 Evaluation of sexual dysfunction. *FSH,* Follicle-stimulating hormone; *LH,* luteinizing hormone. (From Greene HL, Johnson WP, Lemcke D [eds]: *Decision making in medicine,* ed 2, St Louis, 1998, Mosby.)

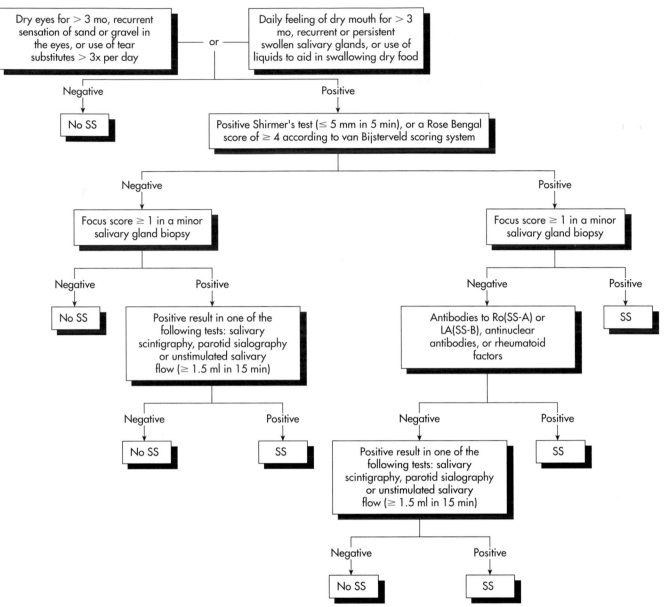

FIGURE 3-99 Algorithm for the diagnosis of Sjögren's syndrome. (From Tzoufas AG, Mout-sopoulos HM: Sjögren's syndrome. In Klippel JH, Dieppe P [eds]: *Rheumatology,* ed 2, London, 1998, Mosby, with permission.)

ICD-9CM # 780.50 Sleep disorder, unspecified cause

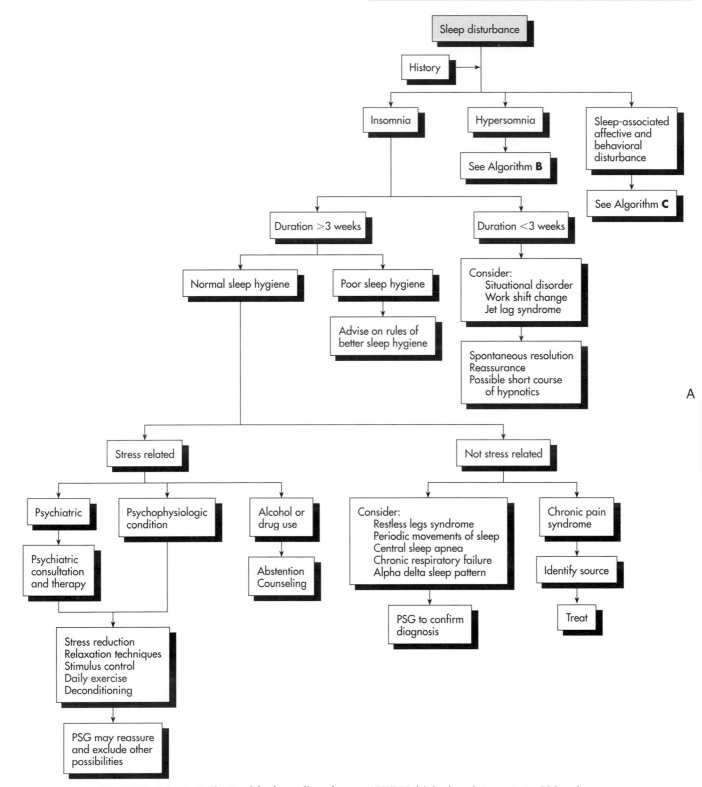

FIGURE 3-100   A, Patient with sleep disturbance. *MSLT,* Multiple sleep latency tests; *PSG,* polysomnography. (From Greene HL, Johnson WP, Lemcke D [eds]: *Decision making in medicine,* ed 2, St Louis, 1998, Mosby.)

Continued on following page

Section III

CLINICAL ALGORITHMS

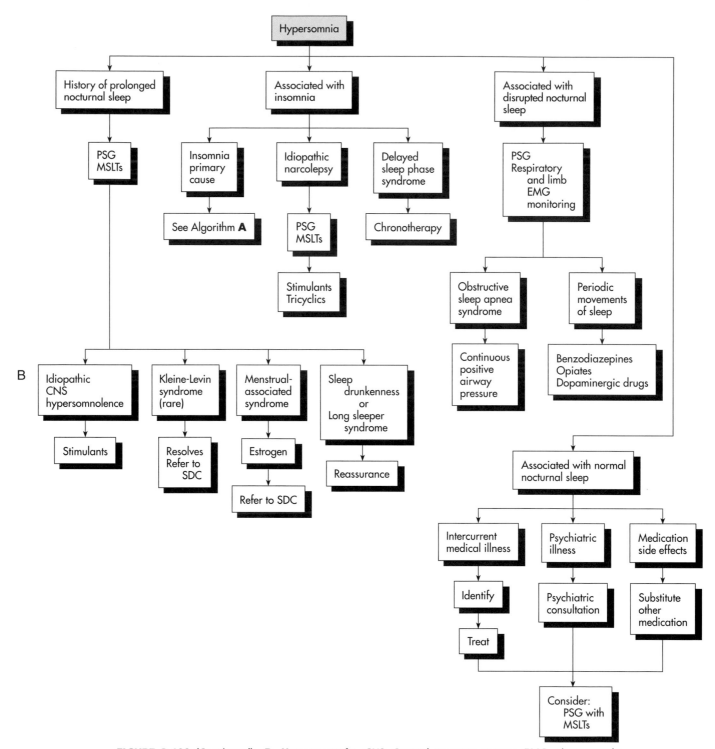

FIGURE 3-100 (Continued) **B, Hypersomnia.** *CNS,* Central nervous system; *EMG,* electromyelogram; *MSLTs,* multiple sleep latency tests; *PSG,* polysomnography; *SDC,* sleep disorders clinic.

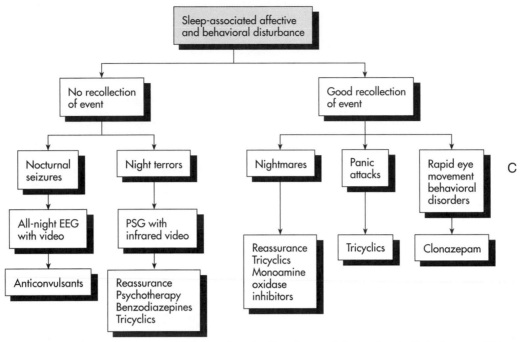

FIGURE 3-100 (Continued) **C, Sleep-associated affective and behavioral disturbance.** *EEG, Electroencephalogram; PSG, polysomnography.*

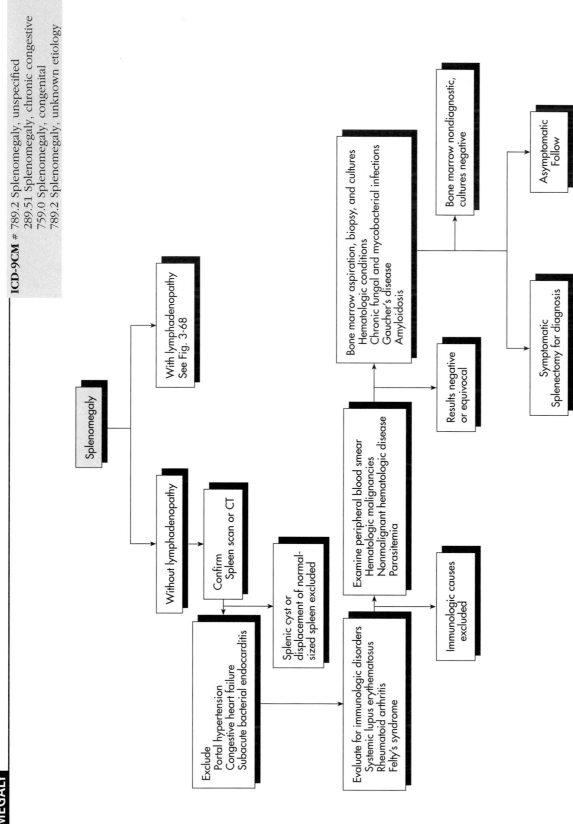

ICD-9CM # 789.2 Splenomegaly, unspecified
289.51 Splenomegaly, chronic congestive
759.0 Splenomegaly, congenital
789.2 Splenomegaly, unknown etiology

Splenomegaly

With lymphadenopathy
See Fig. 3-68

Without lymphadenopathy

Confirm
Spleen scan or CT

Exclude
Portal hypertension
Congestive heart failure
Subacute bacterial endocarditis

Splenic cyst or
displacement of normal-
sized spleen excluded

Evaluate for immunologic disorders
Systemic lupus erythematosus
Rheumatoid arthritis
Felty's syndrome

Immunologic causes
excluded

Examine peripheral blood smear
Hematologic malignancies
Nonmalignant hematologic disease
Parasitemia

Results negative
or equivocal

Bone marrow aspiration, biopsy, and cultures
Hematologic conditions
Chronic fungal and mycobacterial infections
Gaucher's disease
Amyloidosis

Bone marrow nondiagnostic,
cultures negative

Symptomatic
Splenectomy for diagnosis

Asymptomatic
Follow

FIGURE 3-101 Clinical approach to patient with splenomegaly. *CT,* Computed tomography. (From Stein JH [ed]: *Internal medicine,* ed 5, St Louis, 1998, Mosby.)

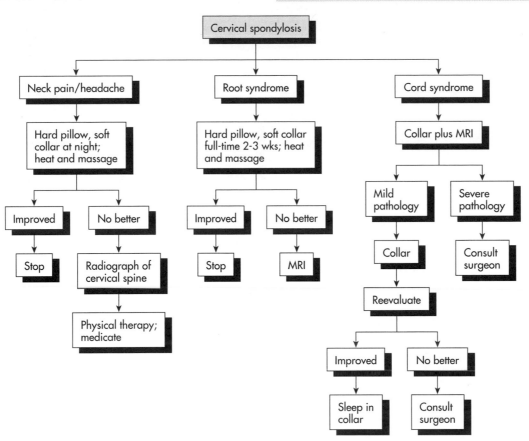

FIGURE 3-102 Algorithm for the treatment of cervical spondylosis. *MRI,* Magnetic resonance imaging. (From Ronthal M, Rachlin JR: Cervical spondylosis. In Johnson RT, Griffin JW [eds]: *Current therapy in neurologic disease,* ed 5, St Louis, 1997, Mosby.)

ICD-9CM # 436

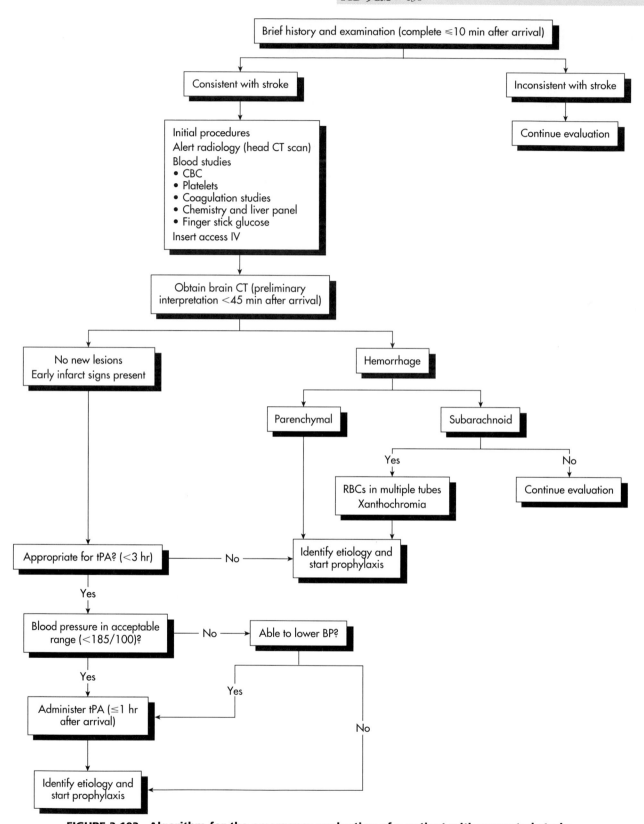

FIGURE 3-103 Algorithm for the emergency evaluation of a patient with suspected stroke.
BP, Blood pressure; *CBC,* complete blood count; *CT,* computed tomography; *RBCs,* red blood cells; *tPA,* tissue plasminogen activator. (From Goldman L, Ausiello D [eds]: *Cecil textbook of medicine,* ed 22, Philadelphia, 2004, WB Saunders.)

ICD-9CM # 720.2

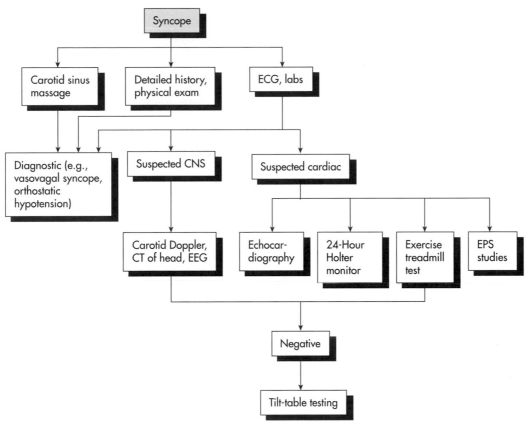

FIGURE 3-104   Syncope evaluation. *CNS*, Central nervous system; *CT*, computed tomography; *ECG*, electrocardiograph; *EEG*, electroencephalograph; *EPS*, electrophysiologic. (From Ferri FF: *Ferri's best test: a practical guide to clinical laboratory medicine and diagnostic imaging*, Philadelphia, 2004, Elsevier Mosby.)

BOX 3-6   Syncope

Diagnostic imaging
Best test
None. Diagnostic imaging should be guided by history and physical exam
Ancillary tests
Echocardiography is useful in patients with a heart murmur to r/o aortic stenosis, hypertrophic cardiomyopathy, or atrial myxoma
If seizure is suspected, CT of head and EEG is indicated
Spiral CT of chest or ventilation/perfusion scan if PE is suspected

Lab evaluation
Best test
None
Ancillary tests
Routine blood tests rarely yield diagnostically useful information and should be done only when specifically suggested by history and physical exam
CBC, lytes, BUN, creatinine
Serum calcium, magnesium
ABGs
ECG
Cardiac troponins, isoenzymes if history of chest pain before syncope
Toxicology screen in selected patients
Cardiac stress test
Electrophysiologic (EPS) studies

From Ferri FF: *Ferri's best test: a practical guide to clinical laboratory medicine and diagnostic imaging*, Philadelphia, 2004, Elsevier Mosby.
ABG, Arterial blood gas; *BUN*, blood urea nitrogen; *CBC*, complete blood count; *CT*, computed tomography; *ECG*, electrocardiograph; *EEG*, electroencephalograph.

ICD-9CM # 427.2 Paroxysmal tachycardia
427.0 Supraventricular paroxysmal tachycardia
427.89 Atrial tachycardia

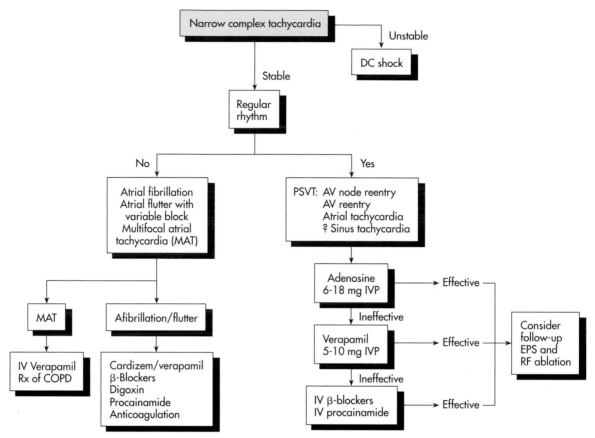

FIGURE 3-105 Evaluation and management of narrow complex tachycardia. *AV,* Atrioventricular; *COPD,* chronic obstructive pulmonary disease; *EPS,* electrophysiologic studies; *IV,* intravenous; *IVP,* intravenous push; *PSVT,* paroxysmal supraventricular tachycardia; *RF,* radiofrequency. (From Driscoll CE et al: *The family practice desk reference,* ed 3, St Louis, 1996, Mosby.)

ICD-9CM # 427.2 Paroxysmal tachycardia
427.0 Supraventricular paroxysmal tachycardia
427.42 Ventricular flutter
427.1 Ventricular paroxysmal tachycardia
427.89 Atrial tachycardia

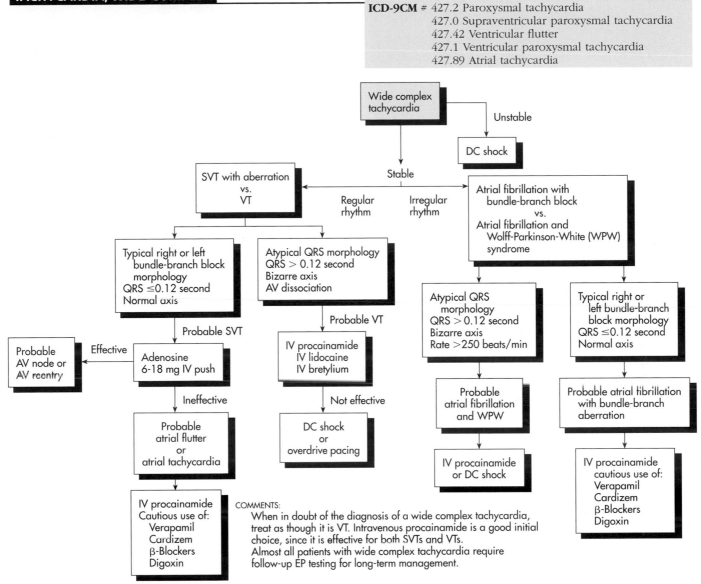

FIGURE 3-106 Evaluation and management of wide complex tachycardia. *AV,* Atrioventricular; *EP,* electrophysiologic; *IV,* intravenous; *SVT,* supraventricular tachycardia; *VT,* ventricular tachycardia. (From Driscoll CE et al: *The family practice desk reference,* ed 3, St Louis, 1996, Mosby.)

Section III

CLINICAL ALGORITHMS

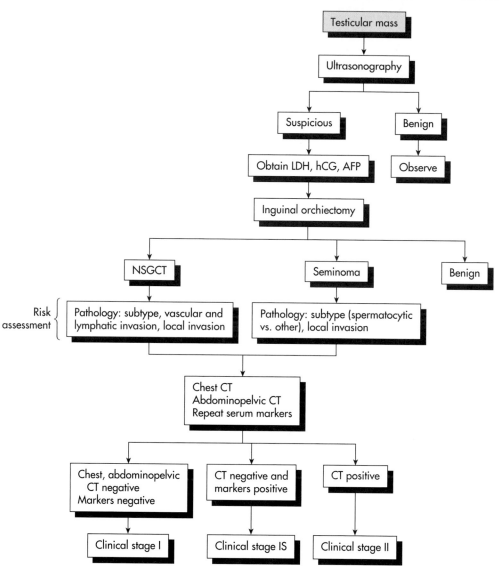

ICD-9CM # 186.9 Testicular neoplasm
M906/3 (seminoma)
M9101/3 (embryonal carcinoma or teratoma)
M9100/3 (choriocarcinoma)

FIGURE 3-107   Diagnosis, staging, and risk assessment of patients with testicular germ cell tumor. *AFP,* Alpha-fetoprotein; *CT,* computed tomography; *hCG,* human chorionic gonadotropin; *LDH,* lactic dehydrogenase; *NSGCT,* nonseminoma germ cell tumor. (From Abeloff MD: *Clinical oncology,* ed 2, New York, 2000, Churchill Livingstone.)

ICD-9CM # 287.3 Congenital or primary
            287.4 Secondary
            287.5 Thrombocytopenia NOS

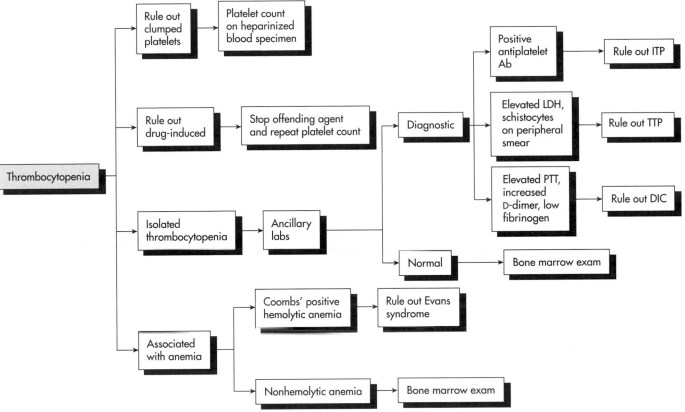

FIGURE 3-108 Evaluation of thrombocytopenia. *DIC,* Disseminated intravascular coagulation; *ITP,* idiopathic thrombocytopenic purpura; *LDH,* lactic dehydrogenase; *PPT,* partial thromboplastin time; *TTP,* thrombotic thrombocytopenic purpura. (From Ferri FF: *Ferri's best test: a practical guide to clinical laboratory medicine and diagnostic imaging,* Philadelphia, 2004, Elsevier Mosby.)

BOX 3-7   Thrombocytopenia

Diagnostic imaging	Lab evaluation
Best test	**Best test**
None	Bone marrow exam
Ancillary test	**Ancillary tests**
CT of abdomen if splenomegaly is present	CBC, PT, PTT
	LDH
	HIV, ANA
	Antiplatelet Ab
	D-dimer
	Coombs' tests

From Ferri FF: *Ferri's best test: a practical guide to clinical laboratory medicine and diagnostic imaging,* Philadelphia, 2004, Elsevier Mosby.
   ANA, Antibody to nuclear antigens; *CBC,* complete blood count; *CT,* computed tomography; *HIV,* human immunodeficiency virus; *LDH,* lactic dehydrogenase; *PT,* prothrombin time; *PTT,* partial thromboplastin time.

ICD-9CM # 289.9

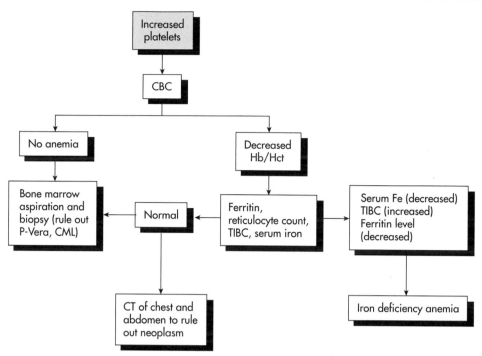

FIGURE 3-109 **Thrombocytosis diagnosis.** *CBC,* Complete blood count; *CML,* chronic myelogenous leukemia; *CT,* computed tomography; *Fe,* iron; *Hb/Hct,* hemoglobin/hematocrit; *TIBC,* total iron-binding capacity. (From Ferri FF: *Ferri's best test: a practical guide to clinical laboratory medicine and diagnostic imaging,* Philadelphia, 2004, Elsevier Mosby.)

BOX 3-8 **Thrombocytosis**	
Diagnostic imaging	**Lab evaluation**
Best test	*Best test*
None	Bone marrow exam
Ancillary test	*Ancillary tests*
CT of chest and abdomen	CBC
	Reticulocyte count
	Stool for OB ×3
	Serum ferritin, TIBC, iron

From Ferri FF: *Ferri's best test: a practical guide to clinical laboratory medicine and diagnostic imaging,* Philadelphia, 2004, Elsevier Mosby.
  CBC, Complete blood count; *CT,* computed tomography; *OB,* occult blood; *TIBC,* total iron-binding capacity.

ICD-9CM # 241.0 Nodule, thyroid

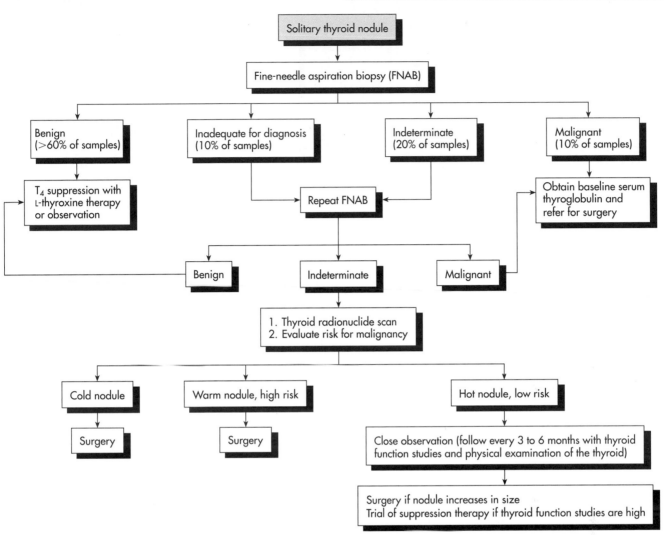

FIGURE 3-110 Diagnostic evaluation of solitary thyroid nodule. High risk for malignancy: nodule >2 cm, age <40 yr, male sex, regional lymphadenopathy, fixation to adjacent tissues, history of prior head and neck irradiation. (From Ferri F: *Practical guide to the care of the medical patient*, ed 6, St Louis, 2004, Mosby.)

ICD-9CM # V77.0

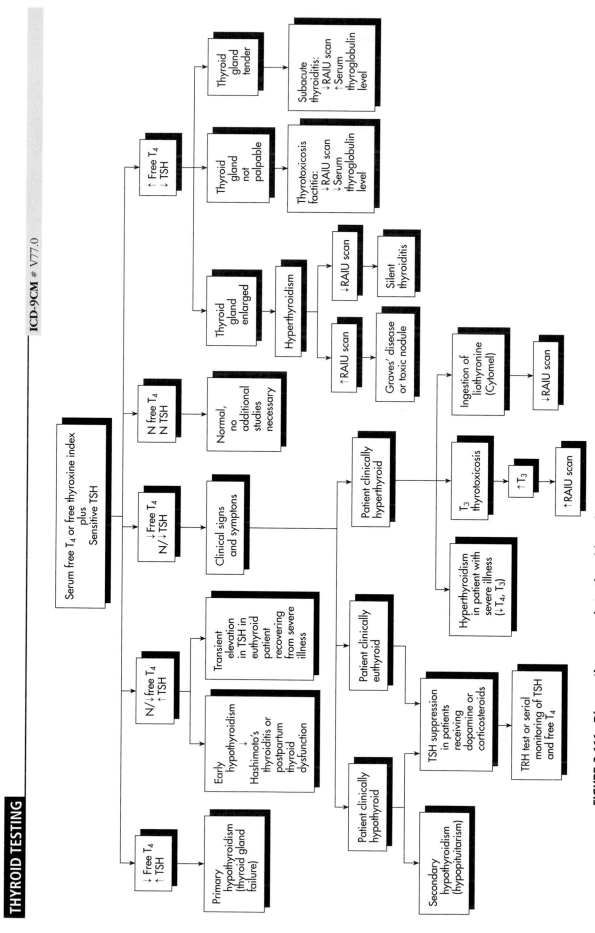

FIGURE 3-111 Diagnostic approach to thyroid testing. *N*, Normal; *RAIU*, radioactive iodine uptake; *TRH*, thyrotropin-releasing hormone; *TSH*, thyroid-stimulating hormone. (From Ferri FF: *Practical guide to the care of the medical patient*, ed 6, St Louis, 2004, Mosby.)

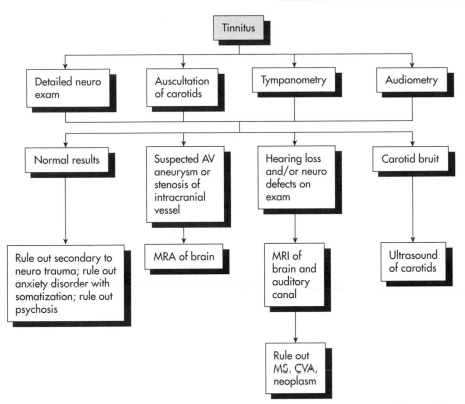

FIGURE 3-112 Tinnitus evaluation. *AV,* Atrioventricular; *CVA,* cerebrovascular accident; *MRA,* magnetic resonance angiography; *MRI,* magnetic resonance imaging; *MS,* multiple sclerosis. (From Ferri FF: *Ferri's best test: a practical guide to clinical laboratory medicine and diagnostic imaging,* Philadelphia, 2004, Elsevier Mosby.)

BOX 3-9 **Tinnitus**	
Diagnostic imaging	**Lab evaluation**
Best test	*Best test*
None	None
Ancillary tests	*Ancillary tests*
Carotid Doppler ultrasound	CBC
MRI of brain and auditory canals	Lipid panel
Brain MRA	

From Ferri FF: *Ferri's best test: a practical guide to clinical laboratory medicine and diagnostic imaging,* Philadelphia, 2004, Elsevier Mosby.
    CBC, Complete blood count; *MRA,* magnetic resonance angiography; *MRI,* magnetic resonance imaging.

ICD-9CM # 435.9 Unspecified transient cerebral ischemia

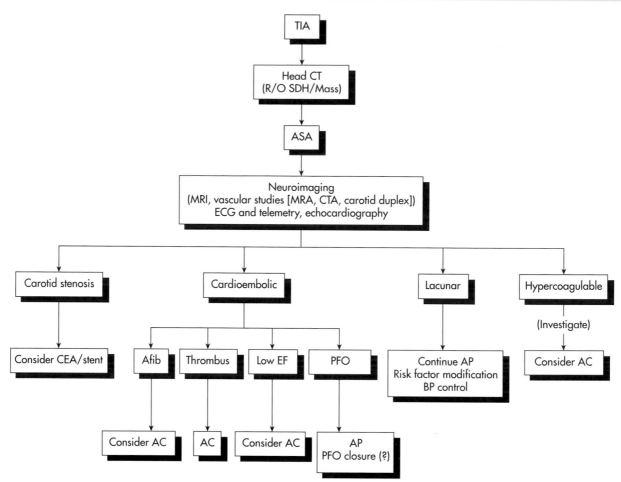

FIGURE 3-113   **Transient ischemic attack.** *AC,* Anticoagulation; *AP,* antiplatelet; *ASA,* aspirin; *BP,* blood pressure; *CEA,* carotid endarterectomy; *EF,* ejection fraction; *PFO,* patent foramen ovale.

ICD-9CM # 780.09

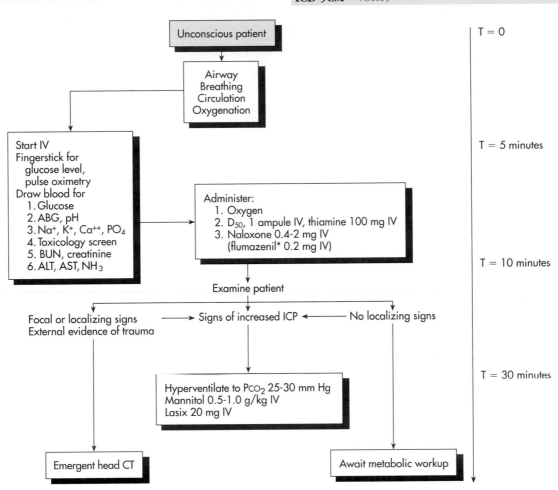

* Use of flumazenil should not be considered routine because
it can precipitate seizures in certain subsets of patients.

FIGURE 3-114 Approach to the unconscious patient. *ABG,* Arterial blood gas; *ALT,* alanine amino-transferase; *AST,* aspartate aminotransferase; *BUN,* blood urea nitrogen; *CT,* computed tomography; *ICP,* intracranial pressure. (Modified from Johnson RT, Griffin JW: *Current therapy in neurologic disease,* ed 5, St Louis, 1997, Mosby.)

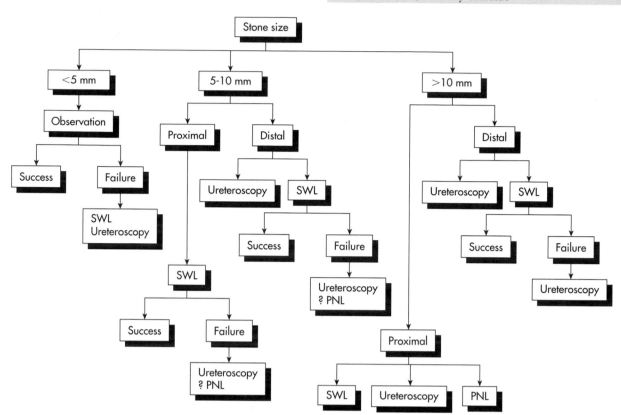

FIGURE 3-115 Management of ureteral calculi. *PNL,* Percutaneous nephrostolithotomy; *SWL,* shock wave lithotripsy. (From Noble J: *Primary care medicine,* ed 3, St Louis, 2001, Mosby.)

URINARY TRACT INFECTION

ICD-9CM # 595.0 Acute cystitis
595.3 Trigonitis
595.2 Chronic cystitis
590.1 Acute pyelonephritis
590.0 Chronic pyelonephritis
590.8 Nonspecific pyelonephritis

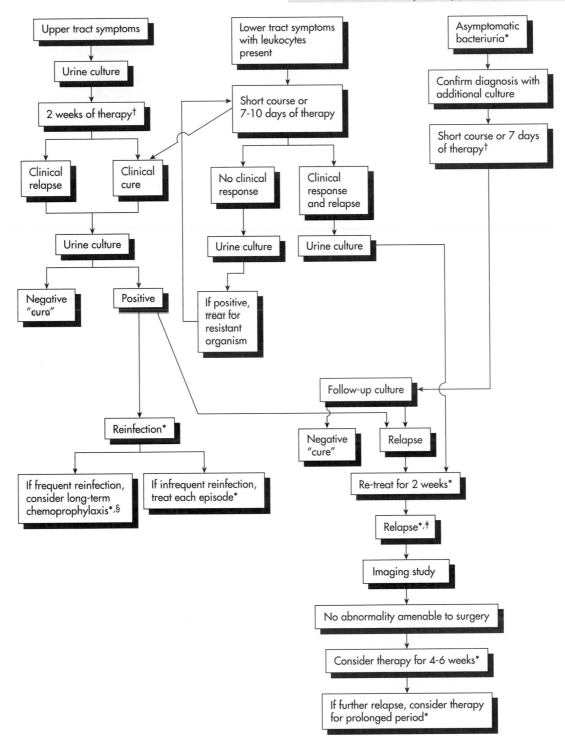

* Consider no therapy in patients without obstructive uropathy or symptoms of urinary tract infection.
† Consider imaging studies in all males with correction of significant lesions.
‡ Evaluate men for chronic bacterial prostatitis.
§ Consider imaging studies after three to four reinfections in women.

FIGURE 3-116 Approach to the management of urinary tract infection. (Adapted from Mandell GL: *Mandell, Douglas, and Bennett's principles and practice of infectious diseases,* ed 5, New York, 2000, Churchill Livingstone.)

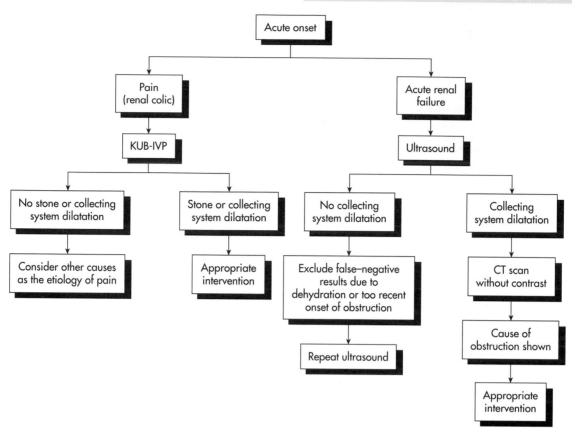

FIGURE 3-117 **Scheme of a diagnostic approach to urinary tract obstruction.** *CT,* Computed tomography; *IVP,* intravenous pyelography; *KUB,* kidney, ureter, bladder (a flat film of the abdomen without contrast medium). (From Goldman L, Ausiello D [eds]: *Cecil textbook of medicine,* ed 22, Philadelphia, 2004, WB Saunders.)

BOX 3-10   Diagnostic Tests Used in Obstructive Uropathy

Upper Urinary Tract Obstruction
Sonography (ultrasound)
Plain films of the abdomen (KUB)
Excretory or intravenous pyelography
Retrograde pyelography
Isotopic renography
Computed tomography
Magnetic resonance imaging
Pressure flow studies (the Whitaker test)

Lower Urinary Tract Obstruction
Some of the tests listed above
Cystoscopy
Voiding cystourethrogram
Retrograde urethrography
Urodynamic tests
   Debimetry
   Cystometrography
   Electromyography
   Urethral pressure profile

From Klahr S: Obstructive uropathy. In Jacobson HR, Striker GE, Klahr S (eds). *The principles and practice of nephrology,* Toronto, 1991, BC Decker, pp 432-441. Reproduced by permission of Mosby-Year Book.
   KUB, Kidneys, ureter, bladder.

URTICARIA

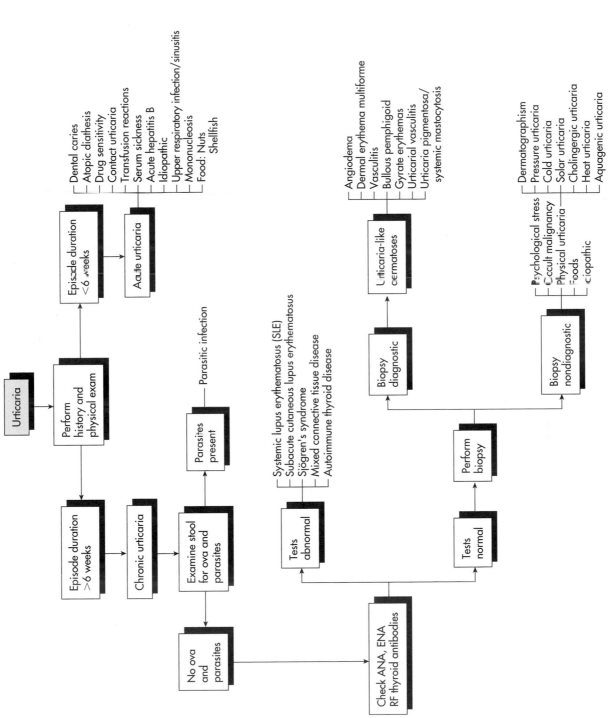

FIGURE 3-118   Evaluation of urticaria. *ANA,* Antibody to nuclear antigens; *ENA,* extractable nuclear antigens; *RF,* rheumatoid factor. (From Healy PM, Jacobson EJ: *Common medical diagnoses,* ed 3, Philadelphia, 2000, WB Saunders.)

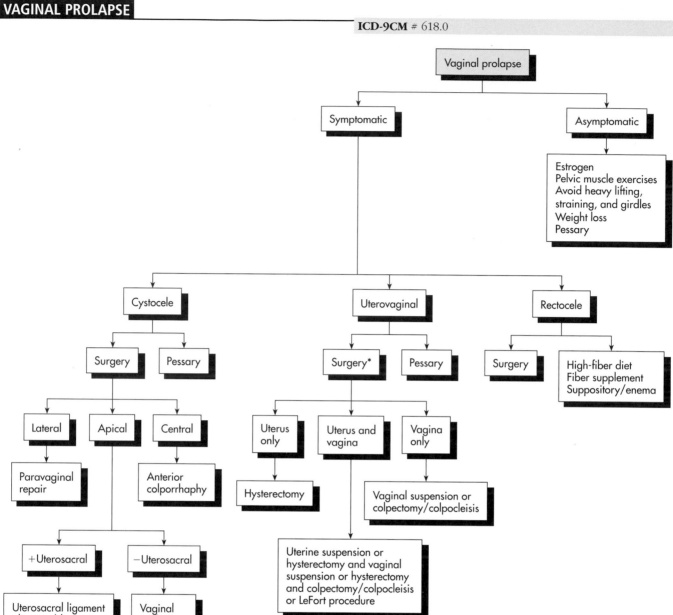

FIGURE 3-119 Management of vaginal prolapse. (From Zuspan FP [ed]: *Handbook of obstetrics, gynecology, and primary care,* St Louis, 1998, Mosby.)

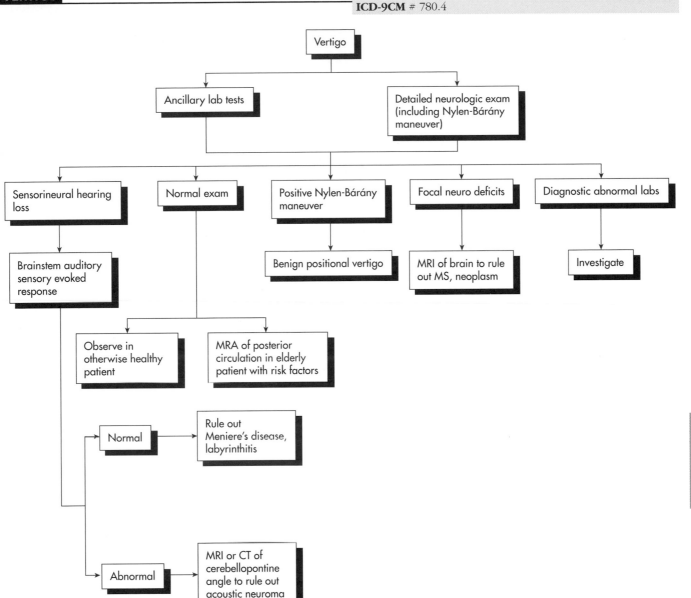

FIGURE 3-120 **Vertigo evaluation.** *CT,* Computed tomography; *MRA,* magnetic resonance arteriography; *MRI,* magnetic resonance imaging; *MS,* multiple sclerosis. (From Ferri FF: *Ferri's best test: a practical guide to clinical laboratory medicine and diagnostic imaging,* Philadelphia, 2004, Elsevier Mosby.)

BOX 3-11   **Vertigo**

Diagnostic imaging
Best test
MRI of brain
Ancillary tests
MRA of posterior circulation
CT of cerebellopontine region if MRI is contraindicated

Lab evaluation
Best test
None
Ancillary tests
CBC with differential
Serum glucose, creatinine, ALT, electrolytes

From Ferri FF: *Ferri's best test: a practical guide to clinical laboratory medicine and diagnostic imaging,* Philadelphia, 2004, Elsevier Mosby.
   Alt, Alanine aminotransferase; *CBC,* complete blood count; *CT,* computed tomography; *MRA,* magnetic resonance arteriography; *MRI,* magnetic resonance imaging.

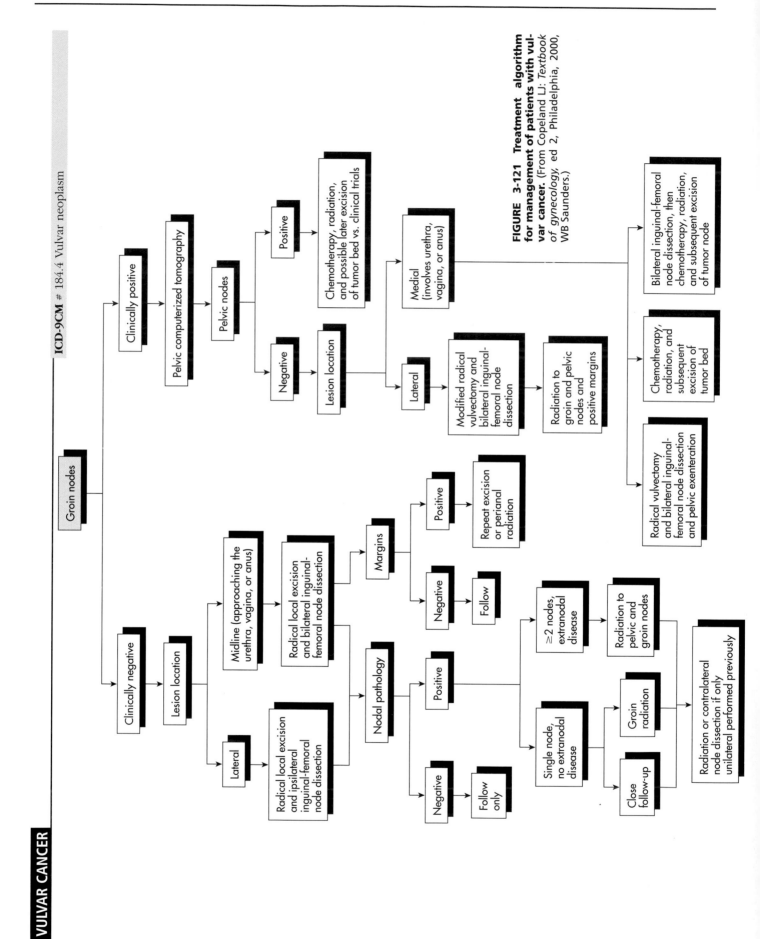

ICD-9CM # 184.4 Vulvar neoplasm

FIGURE 3-121 Treatment algorithm for management of patients with vulvar cancer. (From Copeland LJ: *Textbook of gynecology*, ed 2, Philadelphia, 2000, WB Saunders.)

WEIGHT GAIN

ICD-9CM # 783.1 Abnormal weight gain
278.00 Obesity

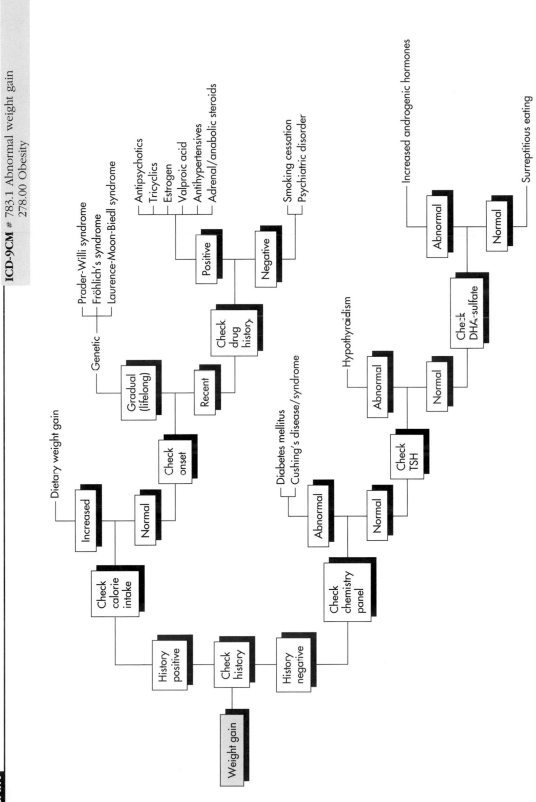

FIGURE 3-122 Weight gain. *DHA,* Dehydroepiandrosterone; *TSH,* thyroid-stimulating hormone. (From Healey PM: *Common medical diagnosis: an algorithmic approach,* ed 3, Philadelphia, 2000, WB Saunders.)

ICD-9CM # 783.21

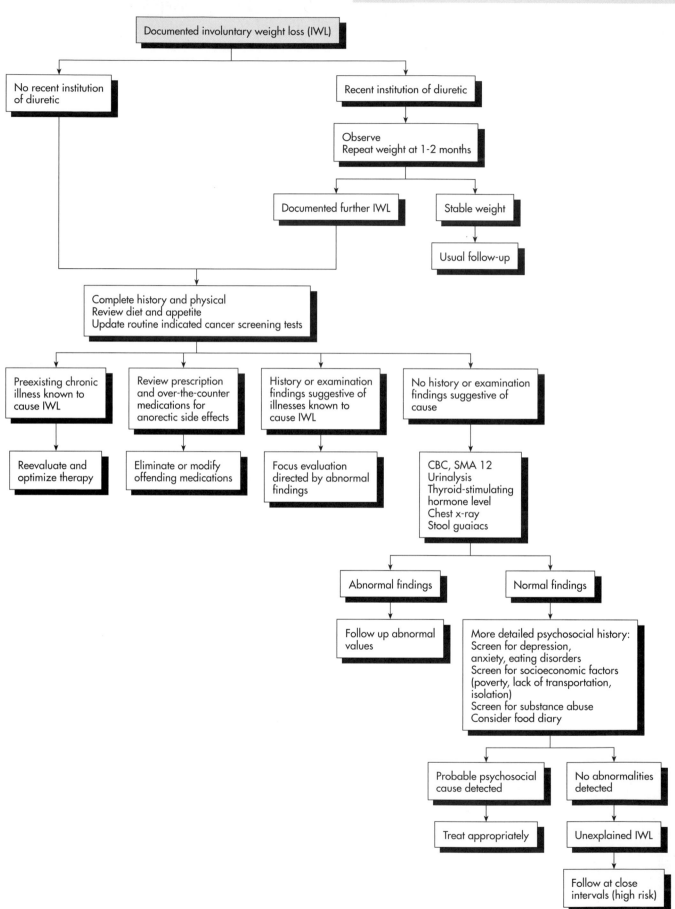

FIGURE 3-123 **Involuntary weight loss.** *CBC,* Complete blood count. (From Greene HL, Johnson WP, Lemcke D [eds]: *Decision making in medicine,* ed 2, St Louis, 1998, Mosby.)

Laboratory Tests and Interpretation of Results

This section contains more than 150 commonly performed laboratory tests. In general, the tests are approached with the following format:

1. Laboratory test
2. Normal range in adult patients
3. Common abnormalities, such as positive test, increased or decreased value
4. Causes of abnormal result

The normal ranges may differ slightly, depending on the laboratory. The reader should be aware of the "normal range" of the particular laboratory performing the test. Every attempt has been made to present current laboratory test data, with emphasis on practical considerations.

ACETYLCHOLINE RECEPTOR (ACHR) ANTIBODY

Normal: <0.03 nmol/L

Elevated in: Myasthenia gravis. Changes in AChR concentration correlate with the clinical severity of myasthenia gravis following therapy and during therapy with prednisone and immunosuppressants. False-positive AChR antibody results may be found in patients with Eaton-Lambert syndrome.

ACID-BASE REFERENCE VALUES; *see* Tables 4-1 and 4-2.

ACID PHOSPHATASE (serum)

Normal range: 0-5.5 U/L

Elevated in: Carcinoma of prostate, other neoplasms (breast, bone), Paget's disease, osteogenesis imperfecta, malignant invasion of bone, Gaucher's disease, multiple myeloma, myeloproliferative disorders, benign prostatic hypertrophy, prostatic palpation or surgery, hyperparathyroidism, liver disease, chronic renal failure, idiopathic thrombocytopenic purpura, bronchitis

ALANINE AMINOTRANSFERASE (ALT, SGPT)

Normal range: 0-35 U/L

Elevated in: Liver disease (hepatitis, cirrhosis), hepatic congestion, infectious mononucleosis, myocardial infarction, myocarditis, severe muscle trauma, dermatomyositis/polymyositis, muscular dystrophy, drugs (antibiotics, narcotics, antihypertensive agents, heparin, labetalol, statins, NSAIDs, amiodarone, chlorpromazine, phenytoin), malignancy, renal and pulmonary infarction, convulsions, shock liver

ALBUMIN (serum)

Normal range: 4-6 g/dl

Elevated in: Dehydration (relative increase)

Decreased in: Liver disease, nephrotic syndrome, poor nutritional status, rapid IV hydration, protein-losing enteropathies (inflammatory bowel disease), severe burns, neoplasia, chronic inflammatory diseases, prolonged immobilization, lymphomas, hypervitaminosis A, chronic glomerulonephritis

---

TABLE 4-1   **Commonly Used Acid-Base Reference Values for Arterial and Venous Plasma or Serum (Averaged from Various Sources)**

	ARTERIAL		VENOUS	
	Conventional Units	SI Units*	Conventional Units	SI Units*
pH	7.40 (7.35-7.45)	7.40 (7.35-7.45)	7.37 (7.32-7.42)	7.37 (7.32-7.42)
Pco_2	40 mm Hg (35-45)	5.33 kPa (4.67-6.10)	45 mm Hg (45-50)	6.10 kPa (5.33-6.67)
Po_2	80-100 mm Hg	10.66-13.33 kPa	40 mm Hg (37-43)	5.33 kPa (4.93-5.73)
HCO3 (CO_2 combining power)	24 mEq/L (20-28)	24 mmol/L (20-28)	26 mEq/L (22-30)	26 mmol/L (22-30)
CO_2 content	25 mEq/L (22-28)	25 mmol/L (22-28)	27 mEq/L (24-30)	27 mmol/L (24-30)

From Ravel R: *Clinical laboratory medicine,* ed 6, St Louis, 1995, Mosby.
*International system.

TABLE 4-2   **Summary of Laboratory Findings in Primary Uncomplicated Respiratory and Metabolic Acid-Base Disorders***

Disorder	Pco_2	pH	Base Excess
Acute primary respiratory hypoactivity (respiratory acidosis)	Increase	Decrease	Normal/positive
Acute primary respiratory hyperactivity (respiratory alkalosis)	Decrease	Increase	Normal/negative
Uncompensated metabolic acidosis	Normal	Decrease	Negative
Uncompensated metabolic alkalosis	Normal	Increase	Positive
Partially compensated metabolic acidosis	Decrease	Decrease	Negative
Partially compensated metabolic alkalosis	Increase	Increase	Positive
Chronic primary respiratory hypoactivity (compensated respiratory acidosis)	Increase	Normal	Positive
Fully compensated metabolic alkalosis	Increase	Normal	Positive
Chronic primary respiratory hyperactivity (compensated respiratory alkalosis)	Decrease	Normal	Negative
Fully compensated metabolic acidosis	Decrease	Normal	Negative

From Ravel R: *Clinical laboratory medicine,* ed 6, St Louis, 1995, Mosby.
*Base excess results refer to negative (−) values more than 22 and positive (+) values more than +2.

ALDOLASE (serum)

Normal range: 0-6 U/L
Elevated in: Muscular dystrophy, rhabdomyolysis, dermatomyositis/polymyositis, trichinosis, acute hepatitis and other liver diseases, myocardial infarction, prostatic carcinoma, hemorrhagic pancreatitis, gangrene, delirium tremens, burns
Decreased in: Loss of muscle mass, late stages of muscular dystrophy

ALDOSTERONE

Normal range: Recumbent: 50-150 ng/L
Upright: 150-300 ng/L
Elevated in: Primary aldosteronism, secondary aldosteronism, pseudoprimary aldosteronism
Decreased in: Patient with hypertension: diabetes mellitus, Turner's syndrome, acute alcohol intoxication, excess secretion of deoxycorticosterone, corticosterone, and 18-hydroxycorticosterone
Patient without hypertension: Addison's disease, hypoaldosteronism resulting from renin deficiency, isolated aldosterone deficiency

ALKALINE PHOSPHATASE (serum)

Normal range: 30-120 U/L
Elevated in:
LIVER AND BILIARY TRACT ORIGIN
Extrahepatic bile duct obstruction
Intrahepatic biliary obstruction
Liver cell acute injury
Liver passive congestion
Drug-induced liver cell dysfunction
Space-occupying lesions
Primary biliary cirrhosis
Sepsis
BONE ORIGIN (OSTEOBLAST HYPERACTIVITY)
Metastatic tumor with osteoblastic reaction
Fracture healing
Paget's disease of bone
CAPILLARY ENDOTHELIAL ORIGIN
Granulation tissue formation (active)
OTHER
Thyrotoxicosis
Benign transient hyperphosphatasemia
Primary hyperparathyroidism
Decreased in: Hypothyroidism, pernicious anemia, hypophosphatemia, hypervitaminosis D, malnutrition

ALT; *see* ALANINE AMINOTRANSFERASE

AMMONIA (serum)

Normal range: 10-80 μg/dl
Elevated in: Hepatic failure, hepatic encephalopathy, portacaval shunt, drugs (diuretics, polymyxin B, methicillin)
Decreased in: Drugs (neomycin, lactulose, tetracycline), renal failure

AMYLASE (serum)

Normal range: 0-130 U/L
Elevated in: Acute pancreatitis, pancreatic neoplasm, abscess, pseudocyst, ascites, macroamylasemia, perforated peptic ulcer, intestinal obstruction, intestinal infarction, acute cholecystitis, appendicitis, salivary gland inflammation, peritonitis, burns, diabetic ketoacidosis, renal insufficiency, drugs (morphine), carcinomatosis (of lung, esophagus, ovary), acute ethanol ingestion,

mumps, prostate tumors, post–endoscopic retrograde cholangiopancreatography
Decreased in: Advanced chronic pancreatitis, hepatic necrosis, cystic fibrosis

ANA; *see* ANTINUCLEAR ANTIBODY

ANCA; *see* ANTINEUTROPHIL CYTOPLASMIC ANTIBODY

ANION GAP

Normal range: 9-14 mEq/L
Elevated in: Lactic acidosis, ketoacidosis (diabetes, alcoholic starvation), uremia (chronic renal failure), ingestion of toxins (paraldehyde, methanol, salicylates, ethylene glycol), hyperosmolar nonketotic coma, antibiotics (carbenicillin)
Decreased in: Hypoalbuminemia, severe hypermagnesemia, IgG myeloma, lithium toxicity, laboratory error (falsely decreased sodium or overestimation of bicarbonate or chloride), hypercalcemia of parathyroid origin, antibiotics (e.g., polymyxin)

ANTICARDIOLIPIN ANTIBODY (ACA)

Normal range: Negative: Test includes detection of IgG, IgM, and IgA antibody to phospholipid, cardiolipin
Present in: Antiphospholipid antibody syndrome, chronic hepatitis C

ANTICOAGULANT; *see* CIRCULATING ANTICOAGULANT

ANTI-DNA

Normal range: Absent
Present in: Systemic lupus erythematosus, chronic active hepatitis, infectious mononucleosis, biliary cirrhosis

ANTIMITOCHONDRIAL ANTIBODY

Normal range: <1:20 titer
Elevated in: Primary biliary cirrhosis (85% to 95%), chronic active hepatitis (25% to 30%), cryptogenic cirrhosis (25% to 30%)

ANTINEUTROPHIL CYTOPLASMIC ANTIBODY (ANCA)

Positive test: Cytoplasmic pattern (cANCA): positive in Wegener's granulomatosis
Perinuclear pattern (pANCA): positive in inflammatory bowel disease, primary biliary cirrhosis, primary sclerosing cholangitis, autoimmune chronic active hepatitis, crescenteric glomerulonephritis

ANTINUCLEAR ANTIBODY (ANA)

Normal range: <1:20 titer
Positive test: Systemic lupus erythematosus (more significant if titer >1:160), drugs (phenytoin, ethosuximide, primidone, methyldopa, hydralazine, carbamazepine, penicillin, procainamide, chlorpromazine, griseofulvin, thiazides), chronic active hepatitis, age over 60 years (particularly age over 80 years), rheumatoid arthritis, scleroderma, mixed connective tissue disease, necrotizing vasculitis, Sjögren's syndrome, tuberculosis, pulmonary interstitial fibrosis. Table 4-3 describes diseases associated with ANA subtypes. Fig. 4-1 illustrates various fluorescent ANA test patterns.

ANTI-RNP ANTIBODY; *see* EXTRACTABLE NUCLEAR ANTIGEN

ANTI-SM (ANTI-SMITH) ANTIBODY; *see* EXTRACTABLE NUCLEAR ANTIGEN

ANTI-SMOOTH MUSCLE ANTIBODY; *see* SMOOTH MUSCLE ANTIBODY

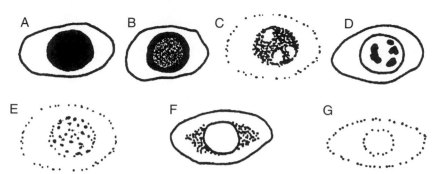

FIGURE 4-1 Fluorescent antinuclear antibody test patterns (HEP-2 cells). A, Solid (homogeneous). **B,** Peripheral (rim). **C,** Speckled. **D,** Nucleolar. **E,** Anticentromere. **F,** Antimitochondrial. **G,** Normal (non-reactive). (From Ravel R [ed]: *Clinical laboratory medicine,* ed 6, St Louis, 1995, Mosby.)

TABLE 4-3 Disease-Associated ANA Subtypes

Nuclear Location	Disease(s)
"Native" DNA (dsDNA, or dsDNA/ssDNA complex)	SLE (60%-70%; range, 35%-75%) —also PSS (5%-55%), MCTD (11%-25%), RA (5%-40%), DM (5%-25%), SS (5%)
sNP	SLE (50%) —also other collagen diseases
DNP (DNA-histone complex)	SLE (52%) —also MCTD (8%), RA (3%)
Histones	Drug-induced SLE (95%) —also SLE (30%), RA (15%-24%)
ENA	
Sm	SLE (30%-40%; range, 28%-40%) —also MCTD (0%-8%)
RNP (U1-RNP)	MCTD (in high titer without any other ANA subtype present: 95%-100%) —also SLE (26%-50%), PSS (11%-22%), RA (10%), SS (3%)
SS-A (Ro)*	SS without RA (60%-70%) —also SLE (26%-50%), neonatal SLE (over 95%), PSS (30%), MCTD (50%), SS with RA (9%), PBC (15%-19%)
SS-B (La)	SS without RA (40%-60%) —also SLE (5%-15%), SS with RA (5%)
Scl-70*	PSS (15%-43%)
Centromere*	CREST syndrome (70%-90%; range 57%-96%) —also PSS (4%-20%), PBC (12%)
Nucleolar	PSS (scleroderma) (54%-90%) —also SLE (25%-26%), RA (9%)
RAP (RANA)	SS with RA (60%-76%) —also SS without RA (5%)
Jo-1	Polymyositis (30%)
PM-1	Polymyositis or PMS/PSS overlap syndrome (60%-90%) —also DM (17%)
ssDNA	SLE (60%-70%) —also CAH, infectious mononucleosis, RA, chronic GN, chronic infections, PBC

Cytoplasmic Location	Disease(s)
Mitochondrial	Primary biliary cirrhosis (90%-100%) —also CAH (7%-30%), cryptogenic cirrhosis (30%), acute hepatitis, viral hepatitis (3%), other liver diseases (0%-20%), SLE (5%), SS and PSS (8%)
Microsomal†	Chronic active hepatitis (60%-80%), Hashimoto's thyroiditis (97%)
Ribosomal	SLE (5%-12%)
Smooth muscle‡	Chronic active hepatitis (60%-91%) —also cryptogenic cirrhosis (28%), acute hepatitis, viral hepatitis (5%-87%), infectious mononucleosis (81%), MS (40%-50%), malignancy (67%), PBC (10%-50%)

From Ravel R: *Clinical laboratory medicine,* ed 6, St Louis, 1995, Mosby.
CAH, Chronic active hepatitis; *DM,* dermatomyositis; *GN,* glomerulonephritis; *MS,* multiple sclerosis; *PBC,* primary biliary cirrhosis; *SS,* Sjögren's syndrome.
*Not detected using rat or mouse liver or kidney tissue method.
†Not detected by cultured cell method.
‡Detected by cultured cells but better with rat or mouse tissue.

ANTISTREPTOLYSIN O TITER (Streptozyme, ASLO titer)

Normal range for adults: <160 Todd units

Elevated in: Streptococcal upper airway infection, acute rheumatic fever, acute glomerulonephritis, increased levels of β-lipoprotein

NOTE: A fourfold increase in titer between acute and convalescent specimens is diagnostic of streptococcal upper airway infection regardless of the initial titer.

ARTERIAL BLOOD GASES

Normal range: Po$_2$: 75-100 mm Hg
Pco$_2$: 35-45 mm Hg
HCO$_3$: 24-28 mEq/L
pH: 7.35-7.45

Abnormal values: Acid-base disturbances (see the following)

METABOLIC ACIDOSIS

Metabolic acidosis with increased AG (AG acidosis)

Lactic acidosis
Ketoacidosis (diabetes mellitus, alcoholic ketoacidosis)
Uremia (chronic renal failure)
Ingestion of toxins (paraldehyde, methanol, salicylate, ethylene glycol)
High-fat diet (mild acidosis)

Metabolic acidosis with normal AG (hyperchloremic acidosis)

Renal tubular acidosis (including acidosis of aldosterone deficiency)
Intestinal loss of HCO$_3^-$ (diarrhea, pancreatic fistula)
Carbonic anhydrase inhibitors (e.g., acetazolamide)
Dilutional acidosis (as a result of rapid infusion of bicarbonate-free isotonic saline)
Ingestion of exogenous acids (ammonium chloride, methionine, cystine, calcium chloride)
Ileostomy
Ureterosigmoidostomy
Drugs: amiloride, triamterene, spironolactone, β-blockers

RESPIRATORY ACIDOSIS

Pulmonary disease (COPD, severe pneumonia, pulmonary edema, interstitial fibrosis)
Airway obstruction (foreign body, severe bronchospasm, laryngospasm)
Thoracic cage disorders (pneumothorax, flail chest, kyphoscoliosis)
Defects in muscles of respiration (myasthenia gravis, hypokalemia, muscular dystrophy)
Defects in peripheral nervous system (amyotrophic lateral sclerosis, poliomyelitis, Guillain-Barré syndrome, botulism, tetanus, organophosphate poisoning, spinal cord injury)
Depression of respiratory center (anesthesia, narcotics, sedatives, vertebral artery embolism or thrombosis, increased intracranial pressure)
Failure of mechanical ventilator

METABOLIC ALKALOSIS

It is divided into chloride-responsive (urinary chloride <15 mEq/L) and chloride-resistant forms (urinary chloride level >15 mEq/L)

Chloride-responsive

Vomiting
Nasogastric (NG) suction
Diuretics
Posthypercapnic alkalosis
Stool losses (laxative abuse, cystic fibrosis, villous adenoma)
Massive blood transfusion
Exogenous alkali administration

Chloride-resistant

Hyperadrenocorticoid states (Cushing's syndrome, primary hyperaldosteronism, secondary mineralocorticoidism [licorice, chewing tobacco])
Hypomagnesemia
Hypokalemia
Bartter's syndrome

RESPIRATORY ALKALOSIS

Hypoxemia (pneumonia, pulmonary embolism, atelectasis, high-altitude living)
Drugs (salicylates, xanthines, progesterone, epinephrine, thyroxine, nicotine)
Central nervous system (CNS) disorders (tumor, cerebrovascular accident [CVA], trauma, infections)
Psychogenic hyperventilation (anxiety)
Hepatic encephalopathy
Gram-negative sepsis
Hyponatremia
Sudden recovery from metabolic acidosis
Assisted ventilation

ARTHROCENTESIS FLUID

Interpretation of results:

1. **Color:** Normally it is clear or pale yellow; cloudiness indicates inflammatory process or presence of crystals, cell debris, fibrin, or triglycerides.
2. **Viscosity:** Normally it has a high viscosity because of hyaluronate; when fluid is placed on a slide, it can be stretched to a string >2 cm in length before separating (low viscosity indicates breakdown of hyaluronate [lysosomal enzymes from leukocytes] or the presence of edema fluid).
3. **Mucin clot:** Add 1 ml of fluid to 5 ml of a 5% acetic acid solution and allow 1 minute for the clot to form; a firm clot (does not fragment on shaking) is normal and indicates the presence of large molecules of hyaluronic acid (this test is nonspecific and infrequently done).
4. **Glucose:** Normally it approximately equals serum glucose level; a difference of more than 40 mg/dl is suggestive of infection.
5. **Protein:** Total protein concentration is <2.5 g/dl in the normal synovial fluid; it is elevated in inflammatory and septic arthritis.
6. **Microscopic examination for crystals:**
   a. Gout: Monosodium urate crystals
   b. Pseudogout: Calcium pyrophosphate dihydrate crystals

ASLO TITER: *see* ANTISTREPTOLYSIN O TITER

ASPARTATE AMINOTRANSFERASE (AST, SGOT)

Normal range: 0-35 U/L

Elevated in:

HEART

Acute myocardial infarction
Pericarditis (active: some cases)

LIVER

Hepatitis virus, Epstein-Barr, or cytomegalovirus infection
Active cirrhosis
Liver passive congestion or hypoxia
Alcohol or drug-induced liver dysfunction
Space-occupying lesions (active)
Fatty liver
Extrahepatic biliary obstruction (early)
Drug-induced

SKELETAL MUSCLE

Acute skeletal muscle injury
Muscle inflammation (infectious or noninfectious)
Muscular dystrophy (active)
Recent surgery
Delirium tremens

KIDNEY
Acute injury or damage
Renal infarct
OTHER
Intestinal infarction
Shock
Cholecystitis
Acute pancreatitis
Hypothyroidism
Heparin therapy (60%-80% of cases)

B-TYPE NATRIURETIC PEPTIDE

Normal range: Up to 100 pg/mL
Elevated in: Heart failure. This test is useful in the emergency department setting to differentiate heart failure patients from those with chronic obstructive pulmonary disease presenting with dyspnea.

BILIRUBIN, DIRECT (conjugated bilirubin)

Normal range: 0-0.2 mg/dl
Elevated in: Hepatocellular disease, biliary obstruction, drug-induced cholestasis, hereditary disorders (Dubin-Johnson syndrome, Rotor's syndrome)

BILIRUBIN, INDIRECT (unconjugated bilirubin)

Normal range: 0-1.0 mg/dl
Elevated in: A. Increased bilirubin production (if normal liver, serum unconjugated bilirubin is usually less than 4 mg/100 ml)
1. Hemolytic anemia
   a. Acquired
   b. Congenital
2. Resorption from extravascular sources
   a. Hematomas
   b. Pulmonary infarcts
3. Excessive ineffective erythropoiesis
   a. Congenital (congenital dyserythropoietic anemias)
   b. Acquired (pernicious anemia, severe lead poisoning; if present, bilirubinemia is usually mild)

B. Defective hepatic unconjugated bilirubin clearance (defective uptake or conjugation)
1. Severe liver disease
2. Gilbert's syndrome
3. Crigler-Najjar type I or II
4. Drug-induced inhibition
5. Portacaval shunt
6. Congestive heart failure
7. Hyperthyroidism (uncommon)

BILIRUBIN, TOTAL

Normal range: 0-1.0 mg/dl
Elevated in: Liver disease (hepatitis, cirrhosis, cholangitis, neoplasm, biliary obstruction, infectious mononucleosis), hereditary disorders (Gilbert's disease, Dubin-Johnson syndrome), drugs (steroids, diphenylhydantoin, phenothiazines, penicillin, erythromycin, clindamycin, captopril, amphotericin B, sulfonamides, azathioprine, isoniazid, 5-aminosalicylic acid, allopurinol, methyldopa, indomethacin, halothane, procainamide, tolbutamide, labetalol), hemolysis, pulmonary embolism or infarct, hepatic congestion secondary to congestive heart failure

BLEEDING TIME (modified Ivy method)

Normal range: 2 to 9½ min
Elevated in: Thrombocytopenia, capillary wall abnormalities, platelet abnormalities (Bernard-Soulier disease, Glanzmann's disease), drugs (aspirin, warfarin, antiinflammatory medications, streptokinase, urokinase, dextran, β-lactam antibiotics, moxalactam), disseminated intravascular coagulation, cirrhosis, uremia, myeloproliferative disorders, von Willebrand's disease

BUN; *see* UREA NITROGEN

C3; *see* COMPLEMENT C3

C4; *see* COMPLEMENT C4

CALCIUM (serum)

Normal range: 8.8-10.3 mg/dl
ELEVATED
RELATIVELY COMMON
Neoplasia (noncutaneous)
  Bone primary
  Myeloma
  Acute leukemia
  Nonbone solid tumors
  Breast
  Lung
  Squamous nonpulmonary
  Kidney
Neoplasm secretion of parathyroid hormone-related protein (PTHrP, "ectopic PTH")
Primary hyperparathyroidism
Thiazide diuretics
Tertiary (renal) hyperparathyroidism
Idiopathic
Spurious (artifactual) hypercalcemia
Dehydration
Serum protein elevation
Laboratory technical problem
RELATIVELY UNCOMMON
Neoplasia (less common tumors)
Sarcoidosis
Hyperthyroidism
Immobilization (mostly seen in children and adolescents)
Diuretic phase of acute renal tubular necrosis
Vitamin D intoxication
Milk-alkali syndrome
Addison's disease
Lithium therapy
Idiopathic hypercalcemia of infancy
Acromegaly
Theophylline toxicity
• Table 4-4 describes the laboratory differential diagnosis of hypercalcemia.
DECREASED
Artifactual
Hypoalbuminemia
Hemodilution
Primary hypoparathyroidism
Pseudohypoparathyroidism
Vitamin D–related
Vitamin D deficiency
Malabsorption
Renal failure
Magnesium deficiency
Sepsis
Chronic alcoholism
Tumor lysis syndrome
Rhabdomyolysis
Alkalosis (respiratory or metabolic)
Acute pancreatitis
Drug-induced hypocalcemia
Large doses of magnesium sulfate
Anticonvulsants
Mithramycin
Gentamicin
Cimetidine
• Table 4-5 describes the laboratory differential diagnosis of hypocalcemia.

Section IV

LABORATORY TESTS AND INTERPRETATION

TABLE 4-4   Laboratory Differential Diagnosis of Hypercalcemia

Diagnosis	PLASMA TESTS					URINE TESTS			Comments
	Ca	PO$_4$	PTH	25(OH)D	1,25(OH)$_2$D	cAMP	TmP/GFR	Ca	
Primary hyper-parathyroidism	↑	N/↓	↑	N	N/↑	↑	↓	↑	Parathyroid adenoma most common
MEN I									Parathyroid hyperplasia; also includes pituitary and pancreatic neoplasms
MEN IIa									Parathyroid hyperplasia; also includes medullary thyroid carcinoma and pheochromocytoma
MEN IIb									Parathyroid disease uncommon, primarily medullary thyroid carcinoma and pheochromocytoma
FHH	↑	N	N/↑	N	N	N/↑	N/↓	↓↓	Autosomal dominant inheritance; hypercalcemia present within first decade; benign
Malignancy									
Solid tumor—humoral	↑	N/↓	↓	N	N	↑	↓	↑↑	Primarily epidermoid tumors; PTH-related protein(s) is mediator
Solid tumor—osteolytic	↑	N/↑	↓	N	N	↓	↑	↑↑	
Lymphoma	↑	N/↑	↓	N/↓	↑	↓	↑	↑↑	
Granulomatous disease	↑	N/↑	↓	N/↓	↑↑	↓	↑	↑↑	Sarcoid most common etiology
Vitamin D intoxication	↑	N/↑	↓	↑↑	N	↓	↑	↑↑	
Hyperthyroidism	↑	N	↓	N	N	N	N	↑↑	Plasma concentrations of T4 and/or T$_3$ are elevated

From Moore WT, Eastman RC: *Diagnostic endocrinology*, ed 2, St Louis, 1996, Mosby.
Ca, Calcium; *cAMP,* cyclic adenosine monophosphate; *FHH,* familial hypocalciuric hypercalcemia; *GFR,* glomerular filtration rate; *MEN,* multiple endocrine neoplasia; *25(OH)D,* 25 hydroxyvitamin D; *PO$_4$,* phosphate; *PTH,* parathormone; *T$_3$,* triiodothyronine; *T$_4$,* thyroxine; *TmP,* renal threshold for phosphorus.

CARCINOEMBRYONIC ANTIGEN (CEA)
Normal range: Nonsmokers: 0-2.5 ng/ml
Smokers: 0-5 ng/ml
Elevated in: Colorectal carcinomas, pancreatic carcinomas, and metastatic disease (usually produce higher elevations: >20 ng/ml) Carcinomas of the esophagus, stomach, small intestine, liver, breast, ovary, lung, and thyroid (usually produce lesser elevations) Benign conditions (smoking, inflammatory bowel disease, hypothyroidism, cirrhosis, pancreatitis, infections) (usually produce levels <10 ng/ml)

CAROTENE (serum)
Normal range: 50-250 μg/dl
Elevated in: Carotenemia, chronic nephritis, diabetes mellitus, hypothyroidism, nephrotic syndrome, hyperlipidemia
Decreased in: Fat malabsorption, steatorrhea, pancreatic insufficiency, lack of carotenoids in diet, high fever, liver disease

CEA; *see* CARCINOEMBRYONIC ANTIGEN

CEREBROSPINAL FLUID (CSF)
Interpretation of results:
1. Appearance of the fluid
   a. Clear: normal.
   b. Yellow color (xanthochromia) in the supernatant of centrifuged CSF within 1 hour or less after collection is usually the result of previous bleeding (subarachnoid hemorrhage); it may also be caused by increased CSF protein, melanin from meningeal melanosarcomas, or carotenoids.
   c. Pinkish color is usually the result of a bloody tap; the color generally clears progressively from tubes 1 to 4 (the supernatant is usually crystal clear in traumatic taps).
   d. Turbidity usually indicates the presence of leukocytes (bleeding introduces approximately 1 WBC/500 RBCs into the CSF).
2. CSF pressure: elevated pressure can be seen with meningitis, meningoencephalitis, mass lesions, and intracerebral bleeding.
3. Cell count: in the adult the CSF is normally free of cells (although up to 5 mononuclear cells/mm^3 is considered normal); the presence of granulocytes is never normal.
   a. Neutrophils: seen in bacterial meningitis, early viral meningoencephalitis, and early tuberculosis (TB) meningitis.
   b. Increased lymphocytes: TB meningitis, viral meningoencephalitis, syphilitic meningoencephalitis, fungal meningitis.
4. Protein: serum proteins are generally too large to cross the normal blood-CSF barrier; however, increased CSF protein is seen with meningeal inflammation, traumatic tap, increased CNS synthesis, tissue degeneration, obstruction to CSF circulation, and Guillain-Barré syndrome.
5. Glucose
   a. Decreased glucose is seen with bacterial meningitis, TB meningitis, fungal meningitis, subarachnoid hemorrhage, and some cases of viral meningitis.
   b. A mild increase in CSF glucose can be seen in patients with very elevated serum glucose levels.
Table 4-6 describes cerebrospinal fluid findings in central nervous system disorders.

TABLE 4-5　Laboratory Differential Diagnosis of Hypocalcemia

DIAGNOSIS	PLASMA TESTS					URINE TESTS					COMMENTS
	Ca	PO4	PTH	25(OH)D	1,25(OH)2D	cAMP	cAMP AFTER PTH	TmP/GFR	TmP/GFR AFTER PTH	Ca	
Hypoparathyroidism	↓	↑	N/↓	N	↓	↓	↑↑	↑	↓↓	N/↓	Deficiency of PTH
Pseudohypoparathyroidism Type I	↓	↑	↑↑	N	↓	↓	NC	↑	↑	N/↓	Resistance to PTH; patients may have Albright's hereditary osteodystrophy and resistance to multiple hormones
Type II	↓	N	↑↑	N	↓	↓	↑	↑	↑	N/↓	Renal resistance to cAMP
Vitamin D deficiency	↓	N/↓	↑↑	↓↓	N/↓	↑	↑	↓	↓	↓↓	Deficient supply (e.g., nutrition) or absorption (e.g., pancreatic insufficiency) of vitamin D
Vitamin D–dependent rickets Type I	↓	N/↓	↑↑	N	↓	↑		↓		↓↓	Deficient activity of renal 25(OH)D-1a-hydroxylase
Type II	↓	N/↓	↑↑	N	↑↑	↑		↓		↓↓	Resistance to 1,25(OH)2D

From Moore WT, Eastman RC. *Diagnostic endocrinology*, ed 2, St Louis, 1996, Mosby.
Ca, Calcium; *cAMP*, cyclic adenosine monophosphate; *FHH*, familial hypocalciuric hypercalcemia; *GFR*, glomerular filtration rate; *MEN*, multiple endocrine neoplasia; *NC*, no change or small increase; *(OH)D*, hydroxycalciferol D; *PO₄*, phosphate; *PTH*, parathyroid hormone; *T₃*, triiodothyronine; *T₄*, thyroxine; *TmP*, renal threshold for phosphorus.

Section IV

LABORATORY TESTS AND INTERPRETATION

TABLE 4-6   Cerebrospinal Fluid Findings in Central Nervous System Disorders

Condition	Pressure (mm H₂O)	Leukocytes (mm³)	Protein (mg/dL)	Glucose (mg/dL)	Comments
Normal	50-80	<5, ≥75% lymphocytes	20-45	>50 (or 75% serum glucose)	
Common Forms of Meningitis					
Acute bacterial meningitis	Usually elevated (100-300)	100-10,000 or more; usually 300-2000; PMNs predominate	Usually 100-500	Decreased, usually <40 (or <66% serum glucose)	Organisms usually seen on Gram stain and recovered by culture. Latex agglutination of CSF usually positive
Partially treated bacterial meningitis	Normal or elevated	5-10,000; PMNs usual but mononuclear cells may predominate if pretreated for extended period of time	Usually 100-500	Normal or decreased	Organisms may be seen on Gram stain. Latex agglutination CSF may be positive. Pretreatment may render CSF sterile
Viral meningitis or meningoencephalitis	Normal or slightly elevated (80-150)	Rarely >1000 cells. Eastern equine encephalitis and lymphocytic choriomeningitis (LCM) may have cell counts of several thousand. PMNs early but mononuclear cells predominate through most of the course	Usually 50-200	Generally normal; may be decreased to <40 in some viral diseases, particularly mumps (15%-20% of cases)	HSV encephalitis is suggested by focal seizures or by focal findings on CT or MRI scans or EEG. Enteroviruses and HSV infrequently recovered from CSF. HSV and enteroviruses may be detected by PCR of CSF
Uncommon Forms of Meningitis					
Tuberculous meningitis	Usually elevated	10-500; PMNs early, but lymphocytes predominate through most of the course	100-3000; may be higher in presence of block	<50 in most cases; decreases with time if treatment is not provided	Acid-fast organisms almost never seen on smear. Organisms may be recovered in culture of large volumes of CSF. *Mycobacterium tuberculosis* may be detected by PCR of CSF
Fungal meningitis	Usually elevated	5-500; PMNs early but mononuclear cells predominate through most of the course. Cryptococcal meningitis may have no cellular inflammatory response	25-500	<50; decreases with time if treatment is not provided	Budding yeast may be seen. Organisms may be recovered in culture. Cryptococcal antigen (CSF and serum) may be positive in cryptococcal infection
Syphilis (acute) and leptospirosis	Usually elevated	50-500; lymphocytes predominate	50-200	Usually normal	Positive CSF serology. Spirochetes not demonstrable by usual techniques of smear or culture; darkfield examination may be positive
Amebic (*Naegleria*) meningoencephalitis	Elevated	1000-10,000 or more; PMNs predominate	50-500	Normal or slightly decreased	Mobile amebae may be seen by hanging-drop examination of CSF at room temperature

	Pressure	Leukocytes	Protein	Glucose	Comments
Brain and Parameningeal Abscesses					
Brain abscess	Usually elevated (100–300)	5–200; CSF rarely acellular; lymphocytes predominate; if abscess ruptures into ventricle, PMNs predominate and cell count may reach >100,000	75–500	Normal unless abscess ruptures into ventricular system	No organisms on smear or culture unless abscess ruptures into ventricular system
Subdural empyema	Usually elevated (100–300)	100–5000; PMNs predominate	100–500	Normal	No organisms on smear or culture of CSF unless meningitis also present; organisms found on tap of subdural fluid
Cerebral epidural abscess	Normal to slightly elevated	10–500; lymphocytes predominate	50–200	Normal	No organisms on smear or culture of CSF
Spinal epidural abscess	Usually low, with spinal block	10–100; lymphocytes predominate	50–400	Normal	No organisms on smear or culture of CSF
Chemical (drugs, dermoid cysts, myelography dye)	Usually elevated	100–1000 or more; PMNs predominate	50–100	Normal or slightly decreased	Epithelial cells may be seen within CSF by use of polarized light in some children with dermoids
Noninfectious Causes					
Sarcoidosis	Normal or elevated slightly	0–100; mononuclear	40–100	Normal	No specific findings
Systemic lupus erythematosus with CNS involvement	Slightly elevated	0–500; PMNs usually predominate; lymphocytes may be present	100	Normal or slightly decreased	No organisms on smear or culture. LE preparation may be positive. Positive neuronal and ribosomal P protein antibodies in CSF
Tumor, leukemia	Slightly elevated to very high	0–100 or more; mononuclear or blast cells	50–1000	Normal to decreased (20–40)	Cytology may be positive

From Behrman RE: *Nelson textbook of pediatrics*, ed 16, Philadelphia, 2000, WB Saunders.
CSF, Cerebrospinal fluid; *EEG,* electroencephalogram; *HSV,* herpes simplex virus; *PCR,* polymerase chain reaction; *PMN,* polymorphonuclear neutrophils.

Section IV

LABORATORY TESTS AND INTERPRETATION

CERULOPLASMIN (serum)

Normal range: 20-35 mg/dl

Elevated in: Estrogens, neoplastic diseases (leukemias, Hodgkin's lymphoma, carcinomas), inflammatory states, systemic lupus erythematosus, primary biliary cirrhosis, rheumatoid arthritis

Decreased in: Wilson's disease (values often <10 mg/dl), nephrotic syndrome, advanced liver disease, malabsorption, total parenteral nutrition

CHOLESTEROL, HIGH-DENSITY LIPOPROTEIN; *see* HIGH-DENSITY LIPOPROTEIN CHOLESTEROL

CHOLESTEROL, LOW-DENSITY LIPOPROTEIN; *see* LOW-DENSITY LIPOPROTEIN CHOLESTEROL

CHOLESTEROL, TOTAL

Normal range: Varies with age

Generally <200 mg/dl

Elevated in: Primary hypercholesterolemia, biliary obstruction, diabetes mellitus, nephrotic syndrome, hypothyroidism, primary biliary cirrhosis, high-cholesterol diet, myocardial infarction, drugs (steroids, phenothiazines)

Decreased in: Starvation, malabsorption, sideroblastic anemia, thalassemia, abetalipoproteinemia, hyperthyroidism, Cushing's syndrome, hepatic failure, multiple myeloma, polycythemia vera, chronic myelocytic leukemia, myeloid metaplasia, Waldenström's macroglobulinemia, myelofibrosis

CIRCULATING ANTICOAGULANT (lupus anticoagulant)

Normal: Negative

Detected in: Systemic lupus erythematosus, drug-induced lupus, long-term phenothiazine therapy, multiple myeloma, ulcerative colitis, rheumatoid arthritis, hemophilia, neoplasms, chronic inflammatory states, AIDS, nephrotic syndrome

NOTE: The name is a misnomer because these patients are prone to hypercoagulability and thrombosis.

CK; *see* CREATINE KINASE

CLOSTRIDIUM DIFFICILE TOXIN ASSAY (stool)

Normal: Negative

Detected in: Antibiotic-associated diarrhea and pseudomembranous colitis

COAGULATION FACTORS; *see* Table 4-7 for characteristics of coagulation factors

Factor reference ranges:

V: >10%

VII: >10%

VIII: 50% to 170%

IX: 60% to 136%

X: >10%

XI: 50% to 150%

XII: >30%

• Table 4-8 describes screening laboratory results in coagulation factor deficiencies.

COMPLEMENT

Normal range: C3: 70-160 mg/dl

C4: 20-40 mg/dl

Abnormal values:

DECREASED C3: Active SLE, immune complex disease, acute glomerulonephritis, inborn C3 deficiency, membranoproliferative glomerulonephritis, infective endocarditis, serum sickness, autoimmune/chronic active hepatitis

---

TABLE 4-7   **Characteristics of Coagulation Factors**

Factor	Descriptive Name	Source	Approximate Half-Life (hr)	Function
I	Fibrinogen	Liver	120	Substrate for fibrin clot (CP)
II	Prothrombin	Liver (VKD)	60	Serine protease (CP)
V	Proaccelerin, labile factor	Liver	12-36	Cofactor (CP)
VII	Serum prothrombin conversion accelerator, proconvertin	Liver (VKD)	6	(?) Serine protease (EP)
VIII	Antihemophilic factor or globulin	Endothelial cells and (?) elsewhere	12	Cofactor (IP)
IX	Plasma thromboplastin component, Christmas factor	Liver (VKD)	24	Serine protease (IP)
X	Stuart-Prower factor	Liver (VKD)	36	Serine protease (CP)
XI	Plasma thromboplastin antecedent	(?) Liver	40-84	Serine protease (IP)
XII	Hageman factor	(?) Liver	50	Serine protease contact activation (IP)
XIII	Fibrin-stabilizing factor	(?) Liver	96-180	Transglutaminase (CP)
Prekallikrein	Fletcher factor	(?) Liver	?	Serine protease contact activation (IP)
High-molecular-weight kininogen	Fitzgerald factor, Flaujeac or Williams factor	(?) Liver	?	Cofactor, contact activation (IP)

From Noble J (ed): *Primary care medicine,* ed 3, St Louis, 2001, Mosby.

CP, Common pathway; *EP,* extrinsic pathway; *IP,* intrinsic pathway; *VKD,* vitamin K dependent.

TABLE 4-8 Screening Laboratory Results in Coagulation Factor Deficiencies

Deficient Factor	Frequency	PT	PTT	TT
I (fibrinogen)	Rare	↑	↑	↑
II (prothrombin)	Very rare	↑	↑	↑
V 1:1,000,000	↑	↑	NL	
VII	1:500,000	↑	NL	NL
VIII	1:5000 (male)	NL	↑	NL
IX	1:30,000 (male)	NL	↑	NL
X 1:500,000	↑	↑	NL	
XI	Rare*	NL	↑	NL
XII† or HMWK† or PK†	Rare	NL	↑	NL
XIII	Rare	NL	NL	NL

From Andreoli TE (ed): *Cecil essentials of medicine,* ed 5, Philadelphia, 2001, WB Saunders.

↑, Increased over normal range; *HMWK,* high-molecular-weight kininogen; *NL,* normal; *PK,* prekallikrein; *PT,* prothrombin time; *PTT,* partial thromboplastin time; *TT,* thrombin time.

*Except in those of Ashkenazi Jewish descent (approximately 4% are heterozygous for factor XI deficiency).

†Not associated with clinical bleeding.

DECREASED C4: Immune complex disease, active SLE, infective endocarditis, inborn C4 deficiency, hereditary angioedema, hypergammaglobulinemic states, cryobulinemic vasculitis Table 4-9 describes complement deficiency states.

COMPLETE BLOOD COUNT (CBC)

White blood cells 3200-9800 mm³ (3.2-9.8 × 10⁹/L)
Red blood cells
Male: 4.3 5.9 × 10⁶/mm³ (4.3-5.9 × 10¹²/L)
Female: 3.5-5 × 10⁶/mm³ (3.5-5 × 10¹²/L)
Hemoglobin
Male: 13.6-17.7 g/dl (136-172 g/L)
Female: 12-15 g/dl (120-150 g/L)
Hematocrit
Male: 39% to 49% (0.39-0.49)
Female: 33% to 43% (0.33-0.43)
Mean corpuscular volume (MCV): 76-100 μm³ (76-100 fL)
Mean corpuscular hemoglobin (MCH): 27-33 pg (27-33 pg)
Mean corpuscular hemoglobin concentration (MCHC): 33-37 g/dl (330-370 g/L)
Red blood cell distribution width index (RDW): 11.5% to 14.5%
Platelet count: 130-400 × 10³/mm³ (130-400 × 10⁹/L)
Differential:
2-6 stabs (bands, early mature neutrophils)
60-70 segs (mature neutrophils)
1-4 eosinophils
0-1 basophils
2-8 monocytes
25-40 lymphocytes

CONJUGATED BILIRUBIN; *see* BILIRUBIN, DIRECT

COOMBS, DIRECT

Normal: Negative
Positive: Autoimmune hemolytic anemia, transfusion reactions, drugs (α-methyldopa, penicillins, tetracycline, sulfonamides, levodopa, cephalosporins, quinidine, insulin)
False positive: May be seen with cold agglutinins

COOMBS, INDIRECT

Normal: Negative
Positive: Acquired hemolytic anemia, incompatible cross-matched blood, anti-Rh antibodies, drugs (methyldopa, mefenamic acid, levodopa)

COPPER (serum)

Normal range: 70-140 μg/dl (11-22 μmol/L)
Decreased in: Wilson's disease, malabsorption, malnutrition, nephrosis, total parenteral nutrition, acute leukemia in remission
Elevated in: Aplastic anemia, biliary cirrhosis, systemic lupus erythematosus, hemochromatosis, hyperthyroidism, hypothyroidism, infection, iron deficiency anemia, leukemia, lymphoma, pernicious anemia, rheumatoid arthritis

CORTISOL, PLASMA

Normal range: Varies with time of collection (circadian variation):
8 AM: 4-19 μg/dl (110-520 nmol/L)
4 PM: 2-15 μg/dl (50-410 nmol/L)
Elevated in: Ectopic adrenocorticotropic hormone production (i.e., oat cell carcinoma of lung), loss of normal diurnal variation, chronic renal failure, iatrogenic, stress, adrenal, or pituitary hyperplasia or adenomas
Decreased in: Primary adrenocortical insufficiency, anterior pituitary hypofunction, secondary adrenocortical insufficiency, adrenogenital syndromes

C-PEPTIDE

Elevated in: Insulinoma, sulfonylurea administration
Decreased in: Insulin-dependent diabetes mellitus, factitious insulin administration

CPK; *see* CREATINE KINASE

C-REACTIVE PROTEIN

Normal range: 6.8-820 μg/dl (68-8200 μg/L)
Elevated in: Rheumatoid arthritis, rheumatic fever, inflammatory bowel disease, bacterial infections, myocardial infarction, inflammatory and neoplastic diseases

C-REACTIVE PROTEIN, HIGH SENSITIVITY (hs-CRP, Cardio-CRP)

is a new test used as a cardiac risk marker. It is increased in patients with silent atherosclerosis years before a cardiovascular event and is independent of cholesterol level and other lipoproteins. It can be used to help stratify cardiac risk.

TABLE 4-9 Complement Deficiency States

Component	Number of Reported Patients	Mode of Inheritance	Functional Defects	Disease Associations
Classic pathway				
C1qrs	31	ACD	Impaired IC handling, delayed C' activation, impaired immune response	CVD, 48%; infection (encaps bact), 22%; both, 18%; healthy, 12%
C4	21	ACD		
C2	109	ACD		
Alternative pathway				
D	3	ACD	Impaired C' activation in absence of specific antibody	Infection (meningococcal), 74%; healthy, 26%
P	70	XL		
Junction of classic and alternative pathways				
C3	19	ACD	Impaired IC handling, opson/phag; granulocytosis, CTX, immune response, and absent SBA	CVD, 79%; recurrent infection (encaps bact), 71%
Terminal components				
C5	27	ACD	Impaired CTX; absent SBA	Infection (*Neisseria,* primarily meningococcal), 58%; CVD, 4%
C6	77	ACD	Absent SBA	Both, 1%
C7	73	ACD		Healthy, 25%
C8	73	ACD		
C9	165	ACD	Impaired SBA	Healthy, 91%; infection, 9%
Plasma proteins regulating C' activation				
C1-INH	Many	AD, Acq	Uncontrolled generation of an inflammatory mediator on C' activation	Hereditary angioedema
H	13	ACD	Uncontrolled AP activation → low C3	CVD, 40%; CVD plus infection (encaps bact), 40%; healthy, 20%
I	14	ACD	Uncontrolled AP activation → low C3	Infection (encaps bact), 100%
Membrane proteins regulating C' activation				
Decay-accelerating factor Homologous restriction factor CD59	Many	Acq	Impaired regulation of C3b and C8 deposited on host RBC; PMN, platelets → cell lysis	Paroxysmal nocturnal hemoglobinuria
CR3	>20	ACD	Impaired PMN adhesive functions (i.e., margination), CTX, C3bi-mediated opson/phag	Infection (*Staphylococcus aureus, Pseudomonas* spp.), 100%
Autoantibodies				
C3 nephritic factors	>59	Acq	Stabilize AP, convertase → low C3	MPGN, 41%; PLD, 25%; infection (encaps bact), 16%; MPGN plus PLD, 10%; PLD plus infection, 5%; MPGN plus PLD plus infection, 3%; MPGN plus infection, 2%
C4 nephritic factor		Acq	Stabilize CP, C3 convertase → low C3	Glomerulonephritis, 50%; CVD, 50%

From Mandell GL: *Mandell, Douglas, and Bennett's principles and practice of infectious diseases,* ed 5, New York, 2000, Churchill Livingstone.
ACD, Autosomal codominant; *Acq,* acquired; *AD,* autosomal dominant; *AP,* alternative pathway; *C',* complement; *CP,* classic pathway; *CTX,* chemotaxis; *CVD,* collagen-vascular disease; *encaps bact,* encapsulated bacteria; *IC,* immune complex, *MPGN,* membranoproliferative glomerulonephritis; *PLD,* partial lipodystrophy; *PMN,* polymorphonuclear neutrophil; *RBC,* red blood cells; *SBA,* serum bactericidal activity; *XL,* X-linked.

Interpretation of results:

Cardio-CRP result (mg/L)	RISK
≤0.6	Lowest risk
0.7-1.1	Low risk
1.2-1.9	Moderate risk
2.0-3.8	High risk
3.9-4.9	Highest risk
≥5.0	Results may be confounded by acute inflammatory disease. If clinically indicated, a repeat test should be performed in 2 or more weeks.

CREATINE KINASE (CK, CPK)

Normal range: 0-130 U/L

Elevated in: Myocardial infarction, myocarditis, rhabdomyolysis, myositis, crush injury/trauma, polymyositis, dermatomyositis, vigorous exercise, muscular dystrophy, myxedema, seizures, malignant hyperthermia syndrome, IM injections, cerebrovascular accident, pulmonary embolism and infarction, acute dissection of aorta

Decreased in: Steroids, decreased muscle mass, connective tissue disorders, alcoholic liver disease, metastatic neoplasms

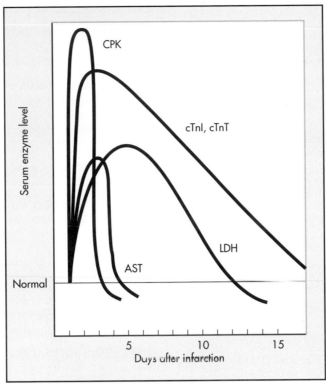

FIGURE 4-2   **Evaluation of creatine kinase elevation.** *CPK,* Creatine phosphokinase. (From Greene HL, Johnson WP, Lemcke D [eds]: *Decision making in medicine,* ed 2, St Louis, 1998, Mosby.)

CREATINE KINASE ISOENZYMES

CK-BB: Elevated in: cerebrovascular accident, subarachnoid hemorrhage, neoplasms (prostate, gastrointestinal tract, brain, ovary, breast, lung), severe shock, bowel infarction, hypothermia, meningitis

CK-MB: Elevated in: myocardial infarction (MI), myocarditis, pericarditis, muscular dystrophy, cardiac defibrillation, cardiac surgery, extensive rhabdomyolysis, strenuous exercise (marathon runners), mixed connective tissue disease, cardiomyopathy, hypothermia

NOTE: CK-MB exists in the blood in two subforms. MB_2 is released from cardiac cells and converted in the blood to MB_1. Rapid assay of CK-MB subforms can detect MI (CK-MB_2 $\geq$1.0 U/L, with a ratio of CK-MB_2/CK-MB_1 $\geq$1.5) within 6 hours of onset of symptoms.

Fig. 4-2 illustrates the time course of CK, AST, troponins, and LDH activity after acute MI.

CK-MM: Elevated in: crush injury, seizures, malignant hyperthermia syndrome, rhabdomyolysis, myositis, polymyositis, dermatomyositis, vigorous exercise, muscular dystrophy, IM injections, acute dissection of aorta

CREATININE (serum)

Normal range: 0.6-1.2 mg/dl

Elevated in: Renal insufficiency (acute and chronic), decreased renal perfusion (hypotension, dehydration, congestive heart failure), urinary tract infection, rhabdomyolysis, ketonemia

Drugs (antibiotics [aminoglycosides, cephalosporins], hydantoin, diuretics, methyldopa)

Falsely elevated in: Diabetic ketoacidosis, administration of some cephalosporins (e.g., cefoxitin, cephalothin)

Decreased in: Decreased muscle mass (including amputees and older persons), prolonged debilitation

CREATININE CLEARANCE

Normal range: 75-124 ml/min. Box 4-1 describes a formula for calculation of creatinine clearance.

The Cockcroft-Gault formula to calculate creatinine clearance is described in Box 4-2.

Elevated in: Exercise

Decreased in: Renal insufficiency, drugs (cimetidine, procainamide, antibiotics, quinidine)

BOX 4-1   **Calculation of the Creatinine Clearance**

$Ccr = U_{cr} \times V/P_{cr}$
where C_{cr} = clearance of creatinine (ml/min)
   U_{cr} = urine creatinine (mg/dl)
   V = volume of urine (ml/min) (for 24-hr volume: divide by 1440)
   P_{cr} = plasma creatinine (mg/dl)

Normal range: 95 to 105 ml/min/1.75 m^2

BOX 4-2   **Cockroft-Gault Formula to Calculate Creatinine Clearance (Ccr)**

$$C_{cr} = \frac{(140 - \text{age in year}) \times (\text{lean body weight in kg})}{S_{cr} \text{ in mg/dl} - 72}$$

For women multiply final value by 0.85

CRYOGLOBULINS (serum)

Normal range: Not detectable
Present in: Collagen-vascular diseases, chronic lymphocytic leukemia, hemolytic anemias, multiple myeloma, Waldenström's macroglobulinemia, chronic active hepatitis, Hodgkin's disease

CSF; *see* CEREBROSPINAL FLUID

D-DIMER

Normal range: <0.3 mcg/mL
Elevated in: DVT, pulmonary embolism, high levels of rheumatoid factor, activation of coagulation and fibrolytic system from any cause
D-dimer assay by ELISA assists in the diagnosis of DVT and pulmonary embolism. This test has significant limitations because it can be elevated whenever the coagulation and fibrinolytic systems are activated and can also be falsely elevated with high rheumatoid factor levels.

D-XYLOSE ABSORPTION

Normal range: 21% to 31% excreted in 5 hr
Decreased in: Malabsorption syndrome

D-XYLOSE ABSORPTION TEST

Normal range:
URINE: ≥ 4 g/5 hours (5-hour urine collection in adults > 12 years (25 g dose)
SERUM: ≥ 25 mg/dl (adult, 1 h, 25 g dose, normal renal function)
Normal results: In patients with malabsorption, normal results suggest pancreatic disease as an etiology of the malabsorption.
Abnormal results: Celiac disease, Crohn's disease, tropical sprue, surgical bowel resection, AIDS. False-positives can occur with decreased renal function, dehydration/hypovolemia, surgical blind loops, decreased gastric emptying, vomiting.

ELECTROPHORESIS, HEMOGLOBIN; *see* HEMOGLOBIN ELECTROPHORESIS

ELECTROPHORESIS, PROTEIN; *see* PROTEIN ELECTROPHORESIS

ENA-COMPLEX; *see* EXTRACTABLE NUCLEAR ANTIGEN

ENDOMYSIAL ANTIBODIES

Normal: Not detected
Present in: Celiac disease, dermatitis herpetiformis

EPSTEIN-BARR VIRUS SEROLOGY

Normal range: IgG anti VCA <1:10 or negative
Abnormal: IgG anti VCA >1:10 or positive indicates either current or previous infection
IgM anti VCA >1:10 or positive indicates current or recent infection
Anti-EBNA ≥1.5 or positive indicates previous infection
Table 4-10 and Fig. 4-3 describe test interpretation.

ERYTHROCYTE SEDIMENTATION RATE (ESR; Westergren)

Normal range: Male: 0-15 mm/hr
Female: 0-20 mm/hr
Elevated in: Collagen-vascular diseases, infections, myocardial infarction, neoplasms, inflammatory states (acute phase reactant), hyperthyroidism, hypothyroidism, rouleaux formation
Decreased in: Sickle cell disease, polycythemia, corticosteroids, spherocytosis, anisocytosis, hypofibrinogenemia, increased serum viscosity

ERYTHROPOIETIN (EP)

Normal: 3.7-16.0 IU/L by radioimmunoassay
Erythropoietin is a glycoprotein secreted by the kidneys that stimulates RBC production by acting on erythroid-committed stem cells.
Increased in: Extremely high: generally seen in patients with severe anemia (Hct <25, <7) such as in cases of aplastic anemia, severe hemolytic anemia, hematologic cancers. Very high: patients with mild to moderate anemia (Hct 25-35, Hb 7-10); high: patients with mild anemia (e.g., AIDS, myelodysplasia). Erythropoietin can be inappropriately elevated in patients with malignant neoplasms, renal cysts, postrenal transplant, meningioma, hemangioblastoma, and leiomyoma.
Decreased in: Renal failure, polycythemia vera, autonomic neuropathy

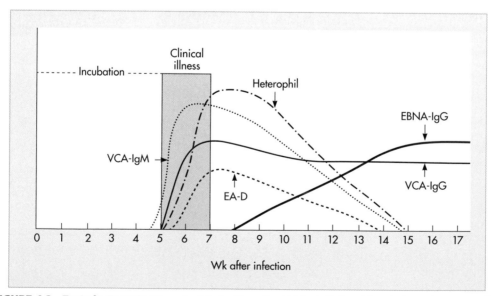

FIGURE 4-3 Tests in Epstein-Barr viral infection. See Table 4-10 for abbreviations. (From Ravel R: *Clinical laboratory medicine,* ed 6, St Louis, 1995, Mosby.)

TABLE 4-10   **Antibody Tests in Epstein-Barr Viral Infection**

	Appearance	Peak	Disappears
Heterophil Ab	3-5 days after onset of Sx (range, 0-21 days)	During second wk after onset of Sx (1-4 wk)	2-3 mo after onset of Sx (still found at 1 yr in 20% of cases)
VCA-IgM	Beginning of Sx (1 wk before to 1 wk after Sx begins)	During first wk after onset of Sx (0-21 days)	2-3 mo after onset of Sx (1-6 mo)
VCA-IgG	3 days after onset of Sx (0-2 wk)	During second wk after onset of Sx (1-3 wk)	Decline to lower level, then persists for life
EBNA-IgG	3 wk after onset of Sx (1-4 wk)	8 mo after appearance (3-12 mo)	Lifelong
EA-D	5 days after onset of Sx (during first 1-2 wk after onset of Sx)	14-21 days after onset of Sx (1-4 wk)	9 wk after appearance (2-6 mo)
(EBNA-IgM)	(Same as VCA-IgM)	(Same as VCA-IgM)	(Same as VCA-IgM)

From Ravel R: *Clinical laboratory medicine*, ed 6, St Louis, 1995, Mosby.
Ab, Antibody; *EA*, early antigen; *EBNA*, Epstein-Barr virus nuclear antigen; *Sx*, symptoms; *VCA*, viral capsid antigen.

ESTRADIOL (serum)

***Normal range:* FEMALE, POSTMENOPAUSAL:** 0-30 pg/ml
MALE, ADULT: 10-50 pg/ml
Decreased in: Ovarian failure
Elevated in: Tumors of ovary, testis, adrenal, or nonendocrine sites (rare)

ESTROGEN

Normal range:

Serum:	Males:	20-80 pg/ml
	Females:	Follicular: 60-200 pg/ml
		Luteal: 160-400 pg/ml
		Postmenopausal: <130 pg/ml
Urine:	Males:	4-23 µg/g creatinine
	Females:	Follicular: 7-65 µg/g creatinine
		Midcycle: 32-104 µg/g creatinine
		Luteal: 8-135 µg/g creatinine

Elevated in: Hyperplasia of adrenal cortex, ovarian tumors producing estrogen, granulosa and thecal cell tumors, testicular tumors
Decreased in: Menopause

ETHANOL (blood)

Normal range: Negative (values <10 mg/dl are considered negative)
Ethanol is metabolized at 10-25 mg/dl/hour. Levels ≥80 mg/dl are considered evidence of impairment for driving. Fatal blood concentration is considered to be >400 mg/dl.

EXTRACTABLE NUCLEAR ANTIGEN (ENA complex, anti-RNP antibody, anti-Sm, anti-Smith)

Normal: Negative
Present in: Systemic lupus erythematosus, rheumatoid arthritis, Sjögren's syndrome, mixed connective tissue disease

FECAL FAT, QUANTITATIVE (72-hr collection)

Normal range: 2-6 g/24 hr
Elevated in: Malabsorption syndrome

FERRITIN (serum)

Normal range: 18-300 ng/ml
Elevated in: Hyperthyroidism, inflammatory states, liver disease (ferritin elevated from necrotic hepatocytes), neoplasms (neuroblastomas, lymphomas, leukemia, breast carcinoma), iron replacement therapy, hemochromatosis, hemosiderosis
Decreased in: Iron deficiency anemia

α-1 FETOPROTEIN

Normal range: 0-20 ng/ml
Elevated in: Hepatocellular carcinoma (usually values >1000 ng/ml), germinal neoplasms (testis, ovary, mediastinum, retroperitoneum), liver disease (alcoholic cirrhosis, acute hepatitis, chronic active hepatitis), basal cell carcinoma, breast carcinoma, pancreatic carcinoma, gastric carcinoma, esophageal atresia

FOLATE (folic acid)

Normal range: Plasma: 2-10 ng/ml
Red blood cells: 140-960 ng/ml
Decreased in: Folic acid deficiency (inadequate intake, malabsorption), alcoholism, drugs (methotrexate, trimethoprim, phenytoin, oral contraceptives, Azulfidine), vitamin B_{12} deficiency (defective red cell folate absorption), hemolytic anemia
Elevated in: Folic acid therapy

FREE T$_4$; see T$_4$, FREE

FREE THYROXINE INDEX

Normal range: 1.1-4.3
INCREASED THYROXINE OR FREE THYROXINE VALUES
Laboratory error
Primary hyperthyroidism (T_4/T_3 type)
Severe thyroxine-binding globulin elevation
Excess therapy of hypothyroidism
Excessive dose of levothyroxine
Active thyroiditis (subacute, painless, early active Hashimoto's disease)
Familial dysalbuminemic hyperthyroxinemia (some FT_4 kits, especially analog types)
Peripheral resistance to T_4 syndrome
Amiodarone or propranolol
Factitious hyperthyroidism
Jod-Basedow (iodine-induced) hyperthyroidism
Severe nonthyroid illness
T_4 sample drawn 2-4 hr after levothyroxine dose
Struma ovarii
Pituitary thyroid-stimulating hormone–secreting tumor
Certain x-ray contrast media (Telepaque and Oragrafin)
Acute porphyria
Heparin effect (some T_4 and FT_4 kits)
Amphetamine, heroin, methadone, and phencyclidine abuse
Perphenazine or 5-fluorouracil
Antithyroid or anti-IgG heterophil (HAMA) autoantibodies
"T_4" hyperthyroidism

Hyperemesis gravidarum; about 50% of patients

High altitudes

DECREASED THYROXINE OR FREE THYROXINE VALUES

Laboratory error

Primary hypothyroidism

Severe nonthyroid illness*

Lithium therapy

Severe thyroxine-binding globulin decrease (congenital, disease, or drug-induced) or severe albumin decrease*

Dilantin, Depakene, or high-dose salicylate drugs*

Pituitary insufficiency

Large doses of inorganic iodide (e.g., saturated solution of potassium iodide)

Moderate or severe iodine deficiency

Cushing's syndrome

High-dose glucocorticoid drugs

Addison's disease; some patients (30%)

Heparin effect (a few FT_4 kits)

Desipramine or amiodarone drugs

Acute psychiatric illness

GLUCOSE, FASTING

Normal range: 70-110 mg/dl

Elevated in: Diabetes mellitus, stress, infections, myocardial infarction, cerebrovascular accident, Cushing's syndrome, acromegaly, acute pancreatitis, glucagonoma, hemochromatosis, drugs (glucocorticoids, diuretics [thiazides, loop diuretics]), glucose intolerance

Decreased in: Sulfonylurea therapy, insulin therapy, reactive hypoglycemia (e.g., s/b subtotal gastrectomy), starvation, insulinoma, glycogen storage disorders, severe liver disease or renal disease, ethanol-induced hypoglycemia, mesenchymal tumors that secrete insulin-like hormones

GLUCOSE, POSTPRANDIAL

Normal range: <140 mg/dl

Elevated in: Diabetes mellitus, glucose intolerance

Decreased in: Postgastrointestinal resection, reactive hypoglycemia

GLUCOSE TOLERANCE TEST

Normal values above fasting:

30 min: 30-60 mg/dl

60 min: 20-50 mg/dl

120 min: 5-15 mg/dl

180 min: fasting level or below

Abnormal in: Glucose intolerance, diabetes mellitus, Cushing's syndrome, acromegaly, pheochromocytoma

γ-GLUTAMYL TRANSFERASE (GGT)

Normal range: 0-30 U/L

Elevated in: Chronic alcoholic liver disease, neoplasms (hepatoma, metastatic disease to the liver, carcinoma of the pancreas), systemic lupus erythematosus, congestive heart failure, trauma, nephrotic syndrome, sepsis, cholestasis, drugs (phenytoin, barbiturates)

GLYCATED (GLYCOSYLATED) HEMOGLOBIN (HbA₁c)

Normal range: 4.0% to 6.7%

Elevated in: Uncontrolled diabetes mellitus (glycated hemoglobin levels reflect the level of glucose control over the preceding 120 days), lead toxicity, alcoholism, iron deficiency anemia, hypertriglyceridemia

Decreased in: Hemolytic anemias, decreased red blood cell survival, acute or chronic blood loss, chronic renal failure, insulinoma, congenital spherocytosis, hemoglobin S, C, and D diseases

HAM TEST (acid serum test)

Normal: Negative

Positive in: Paroxysmal nocturnal hemoglobinuria

False positive in: Hereditary or acquired spherocytosis, recent transfusion with aged red blood cells, aplastic anemia, myeloproliferative syndromes, leukemia, hereditary dyserythropoietic anemia type II

HAPTOGLOBIN (serum)

Normal range: 50-220 mg/dl

Elevated in: Inflammation (acute phase reactant), collagen-vascular diseases, infections (acute phase reactant), drugs (androgens), obstructive liver disease

Decreased in: Hemolysis (intravascular more than extravascular), megaloblastic anemia, severe liver disease, large tissue hematomas, infectious mononucleosis

HDL; *see* HIGH-DENSITY LIPOPROTEIN CHOLESTEROL

HELICOBACTER PYLORI (serology, stool antigen)

Normal range: Not detected

Detected in: *H. pylori* infection. Positive serology can indicate current or past infection. Positive stool antigen test indicates acute infection (sensitivity and specificity >90%). Stool testing should be delayed at least 4 weeks after eradication therapy.

HEMATOCRIT

Normal range: Male: 39% to 49%

Female: 33% to 43%

Elevated in: Polycythemia vera, smoking, chronic obstructive pulmonary disease, high altitudes, dehydration, hypovolemia

Decreased in: Blood loss (gastrointestinal, genitourinary) anemia

HEMOGLOBIN

Normal range: Male: 13.6-17.7 g/dl

Female: 12.0-15.0 g/dl

Elevated in: Hemoconcentration, dehydration, polycythemia vera, chronic obstructive pulmonary disease, high altitudes, false elevations (hyperlipemic plasma, white blood cells >50,000/mm³), stress

Decreased in: Hemorrhage (gastrointestinal, genitourinary) anemia

HEMOGLOBIN A₁c, *see* GLYCATED HEMOGLOBIN

HEMOGLOBIN ELECTROPHORESIS

Normal range:

HbA₁: 95%-98%

HbA₂: 1.5%-3.5%

HbF: <2%

HbC: absent

HbS: absent

HEMOGLOBIN, GLYCATED; *see* GLYCATED HEMOGLOBIN

HEMOGLOBIN, GLYCOSYLATED; *see* GLYCATED HEMOGLOBIN

HEPATITIS A ANTIBODY

Normal: Negative

Present in: Viral hepatitis A; can be IgM or IgG (if IgM, acute hepatitis A; if IgG, previous infection with hepatitis A)

See Fig. 4-4 for serologic tests in HAV infection.

HAV-IGM ANTIBODY

Appearance

About the same time as clinical symptoms (3-4 wk after exposure, range 14-60 days), or just before beginning of AST/ALT elevation (range 10 days before–7 days after)

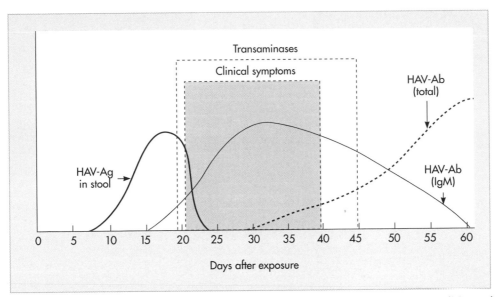

FIGURE 4-4　Serologic tests in HAV infection. (From Ravel R: *Clinical laboratory medicine,* ed 6, St Louis, 1995, Mosby.)

Peak
About 3-4 wk after onset of symptoms (1 6 wk)
Becomes Nondetectable
3-4 mo after onset of symptoms (1-6 mo). In a few cases HAV-IgM antibody can persist as long as 12-14 mo.
HAV-TOTAL ANTIBODY
Appearance
About 3 wk after IgM becomes detectable (therefore about the middle of clinical symptom period to early convalescence)
Peak
About 1-2 mo after onset
Becomes Nondetectable
Remains elevated for life, but can slowly fall somewhat

HEPATITIS A VIRAL INFECTION

Best all-purpose test(s) to diagnose acute HAV infection = HAV-Ab (IgM)
Best all-purpose test(s) to demonstrate past HAV infection/immunity = HAV-Ab (total)

HEPATITIS B SURFACE ANTIGEN (HBSAG)

Normal: Not detected
Detected in: Acute viral hepatitis type B, chronic hepatitis B
Appearance
2-6 wk after exposure (range 6 days–6 mo); 5%-15% of patients are negative at onset of jaundice
Peak
1-2 wk before to 1-2 wk after onset of symptoms
Becomes Nondetectable
1-3 mo after peak (range 1 wk-5 mo)

HEPATITIS B VIRAL INFECTION

Figs. 4-5, 4-6, and 4-7 illustrate antigens and antibodies in hepatitis B infection.
HB$_S$
-Ag
HB$_S$Ag: shows current active HBV infection.
Persistence over 6 mo indicates carrier/chronic HBV infection.

HBV nucleic acid probe: present before and longer than HB$_S$Ag. More reliable marker for increased infectivity than HB$_S$Ag and/or HB$_e$Ag.
-Ab
HB$_S$Ab-total: shows previous healed HBV infection and evidence of immunity.
HB$_C$
-Ab
HB$_C$Ab-IgM: shows either acute or very recent infection by HBV. In convalescent phase of acute HBV, may be elevated when HB$_S$Ag has disappeared (core window).
Negative HB$_C$Ab-IgM with positive HB$_S$Ag suggests either very early acute HBV or carrier/chronic HBV.
HB$_C$Ab-total: only useful to show past HBV infection if HB$_S$Ag and HB$_C$Ab-IgM are both negative.
HB$_E$
-Ag
HB$_e$-AbAg: when present, especially without HB$_C$Ab, suggests increased patient infectivity.
HB$_e$Ab-total: when present, suggests less patient infectivity.
I.　HB$_S$Ag positive, HB$_C$Ab negative*
　　About 5% (range 0%-17%) of patients with early-stage HBV acute infection (HB$_C$Ab rises later)
II.　HB$_S$Ag positive, HB$_C$Ab positive, HB$_S$Ab negative
　　a. Most of the clinical symptom stage
　　b. Chronic HBV carriers without evidence of liver disease ("asymptomatic carriers")
　　c. Chronic HBV hepatitis (chronic persistent type or chronic active type)
III.　HB$_S$Ag negative, HB$_C$Ab positive,* HB$_S$Ab negative
　　a. Late clinical symptom stage or early convalescence stage (core window)
　　b. Chronic HBV infection with HB$_S$Ag below detection levels with current tests
　　c. Old previous HBV infection
IV.　HB$_S$Ag negative, HB$_C$Ab positive, HB$_S$Ab positive
　　a. Late convalescence to complete recovery
　　b. Old infection

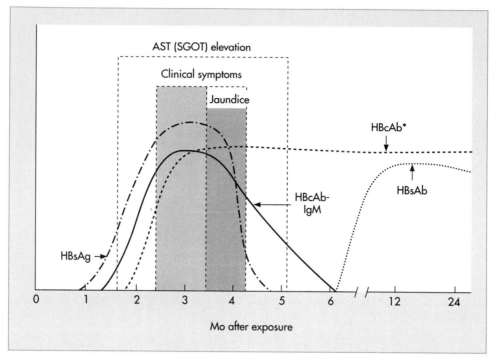

FIGURE 4-5   HBV surface antigen-antibody and core antibodies (note "core window"). *HB$_C$Ab = HB$_C$Ab-IgM + HBCAb-IgG (combined). (From Ravel R: *Clinical laboratory medicine,* ed 6, St Louis, 1995, Mosby.)

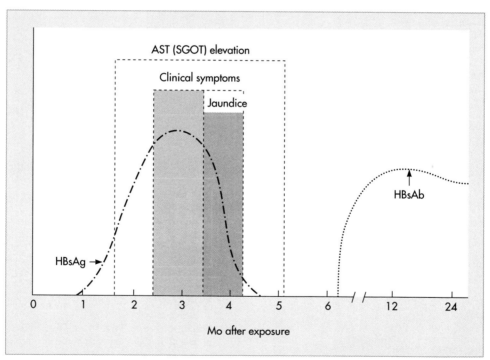

FIGURE 4-6   HBV surface antigen and antibody (HB$_S$Ag and HB$_S$Ab-total). (From Ravel R: *Clinical laboratory medicine,* ed 6, St Louis, 1995, Mosby.)

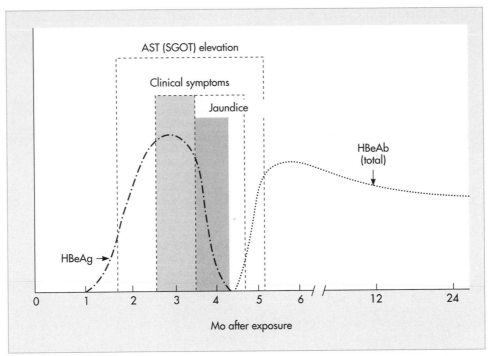

FIGURE 4-7   HBV e antigen and antibody. (From Ravel R: *Clinical laboratory medicine*, ed 6, St Louis, 1995, Mosby.)

HEPATITIS C VIRAL INFECTION

Fig. 4-8 illustrates antigens and antibodies in hepatitis C infection.
HCV
-Ag
HCV nucleic acid probe: shows current infection by HCV (especially using PCR amplification).
-Ab
HCV-Ab (IgG): current, convalescent, or old HCV infection.

HAV
-Ag
HAV-Ag by EM: shows presence of virus in stool early in infection.
-Ab
HAV-Ab (IgM): current or recent HAV infection.
HAV-Ab (total): convalescent or old HAV infection.

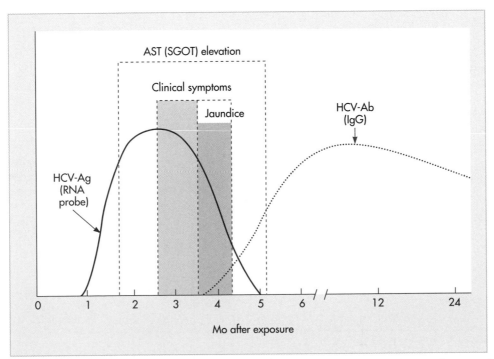

FIGURE 4-8   HCV antigen and antibody. (From Ravel R: *Clinical laboratory medicine*, ed 6, St Louis, 1995, Mosby.)

HIGH-DENSITY LIPOPROTEIN (HDL) CHOLESTEROL

Normal range:
Male: 45-70 mg/dl
Female: 45-90 mg/dl
Increased in: Use of gemfibrozil, statins, fenofibrate, nicotinic acid, estrogens, regular aerobic exercise, small (1 oz) daily alcohol intake
Decreased in: Deficiency of apoproteins, liver disease, probucol ingestion, Tangier disease
NOTE: A cholesterol/HDL ratio >4.0 is associated with increased risk of coronary artery disease.

5-HYDROXYINDOLE-ACETIC ACID, URINE; *see* URINE 5-HYDROXYINDOLE-ACETIC ACID

IMMUNOGLOBULINS

Normal range:
IgA: 50-350 mg/dl
IgD: <6 mg/dl
IgE: <25 μg/dl
IgG: 800-1500 mg/dl
IgM: 45-150 mg/dl
Elevated in:
IgA: lymphoproliferative disorders, Berger's nephropathy, chronic infections, autoimmune disorders, liver disease
IgE: allergic disorders, parasitic infections, immunologic disorders, IgE myeloma
IgG: chronic granulomatous infections, infectious diseases, inflammation, myeloma, liver disease
IgM: primary biliary cirrhosis, infectious diseases (brucellosis, malaria), Waldenström's macroglobulinemia, liver disease
Decreased in:
IgA: nephrotic syndrome, protein-losing enteropathy, congenital deficiency, lymphocytic leukemia, ataxia-telangiectasia, chronic sinopulmonary disease
IgE: hypogammaglobulinemia, neoplasm (breast, bronchial, cervical), ataxia-telangiectasia
IgG: congenital or acquired deficiency, lymphocytic leukemia, phenytoin, methylprednisolone, nephrotic syndrome, protein-losing enteropathy
IgM: congenital deficiency, lymphocytic leukemia, nephrotic syndrome

INTERNATIONAL NORMALIZED RATIO (INR)

The INR is a comparative rating of prothrombin time (PT) ratios. The INR represents the observed PT ratio adjusted by the International Reference Thromboplastin. It provides a universal result indicative of what the patient's PT result would have been if measured using the primary World Health Organization International Reference reagent. For proper interpretation of INR values, the patient should be on stable anticoagulant therapy.
Recommended INR ranges:
Proximal deep vein thrombosis: 2-3
Pulmonary embolism: 2-3
Transient ischemic attacks: 2-3
Atrial fibrillation: 2-3
Mechanical prosthetic valves: 3-4.5
Recurrent venous thromboembolic disease: 3-4.5

IRON-BINDING CAPACITY, TOTAL (TIBC)

Normal range: 250-460 μg/dl
Elevated in: Iron deficiency anemia, polycythemia, hepatitis, weight loss
Decreased in: Anemia of chronic disease, hemochromatosis, chronic liver disease, hemolytic anemias, malnutrition (protein depletion)
Table 4-11 describes TIBC and serum iron abnormalities.

LACTATE DEHYDROGENASE (LDH)

Normal range: 50-150 U/L
Elevated in: Infarction of myocardium, lung, kidney
Diseases of cardiopulmonary system, liver, collagen, central nervous system
Hemolytic anemias, megaloblastic anemias, transfusions, seizures, muscle trauma, muscular dystrophy, acute pancreatitis, hypotension, shock, infectious mononucleosis, inflammation, neoplasia, intestinal obstruction, hypothyroidism

LACTATE DEHYDROGENASE ISOENZYMES

Normal range:
LDH_1: 22% to 36% (cardiac, red blood cell)
LDH_2: 35% to 46% (cardiac, red blood cell)
LDH_3: 13% to 26% (pulmonary)
LDH_4: 3% to 10% (striated muscle, liver)
LDH_5: 2% to 9% (striated muscle, liver)

TABLE 4-11   Serum Iron and Total Iron-Binding Capacity Patterns

SI↓	TIBC↓	Chronic diseases
		Uremia
SI↓	TIBC↑	Chronic iron deficiency anemia
SI↑	TIBC↓	Hemachromatosis
		Iron therapy overload (TIBC may be normal)
		Hemolytic anemia; thalassemia; lead poisoning; megaloblastic anemia; aplastic, pyridoxine deficiency, or other sideroblastic anemias
SI↑	TIBC↑	Oral contraceptives
		Acute hepatitis (some report TIBC is low normal)
		Chronic hepatitis (some patients)
SI↑	TIBC NL	B_{12} or folate deficiency
SI↓	TIBC NL	Chronic iron deficiency (some patients)
		Acute infection, surgery, tissue damage
SI NL	TIBC↑	B_{12}/folate deficiency plus iron deficiency

From Ravel R: *Clinical laboratory medicine*, ed 6, St Louis, 1995, Mosby.
NL, Normal; *SI,* serum iron; *TIBC,* total iron-binding capacity.

Normal ratios:
$LDH_1 < LDH_2$
$LDH_5 < LDH_4$
Abnormal values:
$LDH_1 > LDH_2$: myocardial infarction (can also be seen with hemolytic anemias, pernicious anemia, folate deficiency, renal infarct)
$LDH_5 > LDH_4$: liver disease (cirrhosis, hepatitis, hepatic congestion)

LAP SCORE; *see* LEUKOCYTE ALKALINE PHOSPHATASE

LDH; *see* LACTATE DEHYDROGENASE

LDL; *see* LOW-DENSITY LIPOPROTEIN CHOLESTEROL

LEGIONELLA TITER

Normal:
Negative
Positive in:
Legionnaire's disease (presumptive: $\geq 1:256$ titer; definitive: fourfold titer increase to $\geq 1:128$)

LEUKOCYTE ALKALINE PHOSPHATASE

Normal range: 13-100
Elevated in: Leukemoid reactions, neutrophilia secondary to infections (except in sickle cell crisis—no significant increase in LAP score), Hodgkin's disease, polycythemia vera, hairy cell leukemia, aplastic anemia, Down's syndrome, myelofibrosis
Decreased in: Acute and chronic granulocytic leukemia, thrombocytopenic purpura, paroxysmal nocturnal hemoglobinuria, hypophosphatemia, collagen disorders

LEUKOCYTE COUNT; *see* COMPLETE BLOOD COUNT

LIPASE

Normal range: 0-160 U/L
Elevated in: Acute pancreatitis, perforated peptic ulcer, carcinoma of pancreas (early stage), pancreatic duct obstruction, bowel infarction, intestinal obstruction

LIPOPROTEIN CHOLESTEROL, HIGH-DENSITY; *see* HIGH-DENSITY LIPOPROTEIN CHOLESTEROL

LIPOPROTEIN CHOLESTEROL, LOW-DENSITY; *see* LOW-DENSITY LIPOPROTEIN CHOLESTEROL

LOW-DENSITY LIPOPROTEIN (LDL) CHOLESTEROL

Normal range:
50-130 mg/dl
LDL cholesterol
<100   Optimal
100-129   Near or above optimal
130-159   Borderline high
160-189   High
≥ 190 Very high

LUPUS ANTICOAGULANT; *see* CIRCULATING ANTICOAGULANT

LYME DISEASE ANTIBODY TITER

Normal range: Negative
Positive result: Fig. 4-9 illustrates the usual serologic response in Lyme disease.
A serologic test is not necessary or helpful for several days after a tick bite, because it is only 40%-50% sensitive in this stage and a negative test does not rule out the diagnosis.

LYMPHOCYTES

Normal range:
15% to 40%:   Total lymphocyte count = 800-2600/mm³
              Total T lymphocyte = 800-2200/mm³
              CD4 lymphocytes = ≥ 400/mm³
              CD8 lymphocytes = 200-800/mm³
              Normal CD4/CD8 ratio is 2.0
Elevated in: Chronic infections, infectious mononucleosis and other viral infections, chronic lymphocytic leukemia, Hodgkin's disease, ulcerative colitis, hypoadrenalism, idiopathic thrombocytopenia
Decreased in: AIDS, bone marrow suppression from chemotherapeutic agents or chemotherapy, aplastic anemia, neoplasms, steroids, adrenocortical hyperfunction, neurologic disorders (multiple sclerosis, myasthenia gravis, Guillain-Barré syndrome)
CD4 lymphocytes are calculated as total white blood cells × % lymphocytes × % lymphocytes stained with CD4. They are decreased in AIDS and other immune dysfunction.
Table 4-12 describes various lymphocyte abnormalities in peripheral blood.

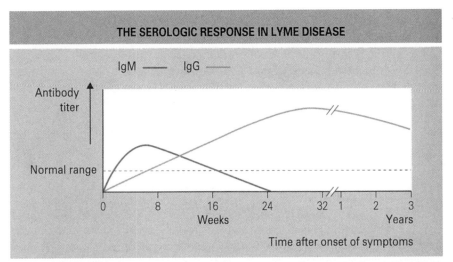

FIGURE 4-9   IgM and IgG response in Lyme disease. (From Ravel R: *Clinical laboratory medicine,* ed 6, St Louis, 1995, Mosby.)

Section IV

LABORATORY TESTS AND INTERPRETATION

TABLE 4-12 Differential Diagnosis of Abnormal Lymphocytes in Peripheral Blood

Lymphocyte Type	Usual Disease Association	Cytologic Features	Laboratory Features	Clinical Features
Small lymphocyte	Chronic lymphocytic leukemia	B-cell surface markers with low concentration of surface immunoglobulin, CD5 antigen	Hypogammaglobulinemia in 50%; positive direct Coombs' test in 15%; on node biopsy, diffuse, well-differentiated lymphocytic infiltrate	Elderly adults; presentation runs gamut from asymptomatic with lymphocytosis only to bulky disease with adenopathy, splenomegaly, and "packed" bone marrow
Atypical lymphocyte	Infectious mononucleosis, other viral illnesses	Suppressor T-cell markers	Heterophil agglutinin; positive serology for Epstein-Barr virus, cytomegalovirus, toxoplasma, HBsAg	Pharyngitis, fever, adenopathy, rash, splenomegaly, palatal petechiae, jaundice
Plasmacytoid lymphocyte	Waldenström's macroglobulinemia	Cytoplasmic IgM, periodic acid–Schiff (PAS) positivity	IgM paraprotein, rouleaux, cryoglobulins	Adenopathy, splenomegaly, absence of bone lesions, hyperviscosity syndrome, cryopathic phenomena
Lymphoblast	Acute lymphoblastic leukemia (ALL)	Terminal transferase positivity, common ALL antigen, B- or T-precursor markers	Anemia, granulocytopenia, thrombocytopenia, hyperuricemia, diffuse bone marrow infiltration	Peak incidence in childhood, acute onset, bone pain frequent
Lymphosarcoma cell	Lymphocytic lymphoma	B-cell surface markers with high concentration of monoclonal surface immunoglobulin	Nodular or diffuse, poorly differentiated lymphocytic lymphoma on node biopsy, patchy, peritrabecular bone marrow involvement	Middle-aged to older adults, generalized adenopathy, constitutional symptoms
Sézary cell	Cutaneous lymphomas	T-lymphocyte surface markers	Skin biopsy is diagnostic	Exfoliative erythroderma, cutaneous plaques or tumors
Hairy cell	Hairy cell leukemia	B-lymphocyte markers, cytoplasmic projections, tartrate-resistant acid phosphatase, interleukin-2 receptors, CD11 antigen	Pancytopenia	Middle-aged males, moderate to marked splenomegaly without adenopathy
Prolymphocyte	Prolymphocytic leukemia	B-cell surface markers with high concentration of surface immunoglobulin, CD5 negative	Marked lymphocytosis (frequently $>100 \times 10^9/L$)	Elderly adults, massive splenomegaly, minimum adenopathy, poor response to therapy

From Stein JH (ed): *Internal medicine*, ed 5, St Louis, 1998, Mosby.

MAGNESIUM (serum)
Normal range: 1.8-3.0 mg/dl
CAUSES OF HYPERMAGNESEMIA
I. Decreased renal excretion
    A. Renal failure—glomerular filtration rate less than 30 ml/min
    B. Hyperparathyroidism
    C. Hypothyroidism
    D. Addison's disease
    E. Lithium intoxication
    F. Familial hypocalciuric hypercalcemia
II. Other causes: usually in association with decrease in glomerular filtration rate
    A. Endogenous loads
        1. Diabetic ketoacidosis
        2. Severe tissue injury—burns
    B. Exogenous loads
        1. Gastrointestinal
            a. Magnesium-containing laxatives and antacids
            b. High-dose vitamin D analogs

CAUSES OF HYPOMAGNESEMIA
Alcohol abuse
Diuretic use
Renal losses
Acute and chronic renal failure
Postobstructive diuresis
Acute tubular necrosis
Chronic glomerulonephritis
Chronic pyelonephritis
Interstitial nephropathy
Renal transplantation
Gastrointestinal losses
Chronic diarrhea
Nasogastric suctioning
Short bowel syndrome
Protein calorie malnutrition
Bowel fistula
Total parenteral nutrition
Acute pancreatitis
Endocrine

Diabetes mellitus
Hyperaldosteronism
Hyperthyroidism
Hyperparathyroidism
Acute intermittent porphyria
Drugs
Aminoglycosides
Amphotericin
β-Agonists
Cisplatin
Cyclosporine
Diuretics
Foscarnet
Pentamidine
Theophylline
Familial hypomagnesemia
Maternal hypothyroidism
Maternal hyperparathyroidism

MEAN CORPUSCULAR VOLUME (MCV)

Normal range: 76-100 μm^3 (76-100 fL)

See Tables 4-13 and 4-14 for descriptions of MCV abnormalities.

NEUTROPHIL COUNT

Normal range: 50% to 70%

Subsets

Stabs (bands, early mature neutrophils): 2% to 6%

Segs (mature neutrophils): 60% to 70%

Elevated in: Acute bacterial infections, acute myocardial infarction, stress, neoplasms, myelocytic leukemia

Decreased in: Viral infections, aplastic anemias, immunosuppressive drugs, radiation therapy to bone marrow, agranulocytosis, drugs (antibiotics, antithyroidals, clopidogrel), lymphocytic and monocytic leukemias

- Table 4-15 describes various drugs that can cause neutropenia.

TABLE 4-13 Some Causes of Increased Mean Corpuscular Volume (Macrocytosis)

Causes	% of all Macrocytosis Patients*	% of Macrocytosis in Each Disease†
Common		
Folate or B_{12} deficiency	20-30 (5-50)‡	80-90 (4-100)
Chronic liver disease	15-20 (6-28)	25-30 (8-65)
Chronic alcoholism	10-12 (3-15)	60 (26-90)
Cytotoxic chemotherapy	10-15 (2-20)	30-40 (13-82)
Cardiorespiratory abnormality	8 (7-9.5)	?
Reticulocytosis	6-7 (0-15)	Depends on severity
Myelodysplastic syndromes	Frequent over age 40 yr	>60 in RAEB and RARS
Unexplained	25 (22.5-27)	—
Less Common	<4%	
Noncytotoxic drugs		
Zidovudine		
Phenytoin		30 (14-50)
Azathioprine		
Hypothyroidism		20-30 (8-55)
Chronic leukemia/myelofibrosis		
Radiotherapy for malignancy		
Chronic renal disease (occasional patients)		
Distance-runner macrocytosis (some persons)		
Down syndrome		
Artifactual (e.g., cold agglutinins)		

From Ravel R: *Clinical laboratory medicine,* ed 6, St Louis, 1995, Mosby.

RAEB, Refractory anemia with excessive blasts; *RARS,* refractory anemia with ring sideroblasts (formerly called IASA, or idiopathic acquired sideroblastic anemia).

*Percentage of all patients with macrocytosis.

†Percentage of patients with each condition listed who have macrocytosis.

‡Numbers in parentheses are literature range.

TABLE 4-14 Some Causes of Decreased Mean Corpuscular Volume (Microcytosis)

Common	Less Common
Chronic iron deficiency	Some cases of polycythemia
α- or β-thalassemia (minor)	Some cases of lead poisoning
Anemia of chronic disease	Some cases of congenital spherocytosis
	Some cases of sideroblastic anemia
	Certain abnormal Hbs (Hb E, Hb Lepore)

From Ravel R: *Clinical laboratory medicine,* ed 6, St Louis, 1995, Mosby.

TABLE 4-15   **Drugs That Cause Neutropenia**

Antiarrhythmics
    Tocainide, procainamide, propranolol, quinidine

Antibiotics
    Chloramphenicol, penicillins, sulfonamides, p-aminosalicylic acid (PAS), rifampin, vancomycin, isoniazid, nitrofurantoin

Antimalarials
    Dapsone, quinine, pyrimethamine

Anticonvulsants
    Phenytoin, mephenytoin, trimethadione, ethosuximide, carbamazepine

Hypoglycemic agents
    Tolbutamide, chlorpropamide

Antihistamines
    Cimetidine, brompheniramine, tripelennamine

Antihypertensives
    Methyldopa, captopril

Antiinflammatory agents
    Aminopyrine, phenylbutazone, gold salts, ibuprofen, indomethacin

Antithyroid agents
    Propylthiouracil, methimazole, thiouracil

Diuretics
    Acetazolamide, hydrochlorothiazide, chlorthalidone

Phenothiazines
    Chlorpromazine, promazine, prochlorperazine

Immunosuppressive agents
    Antimetabolites

Cytotoxic agents
    Alkylating agents, antimetabolites, anthracyclines, Vinca alkaloids, cisplatin, hydroxyurea, dactinomycin

Other agents
    Recombinant interferons, allopurinol, ethanol, levamisole, penicillamine, zidovudine, streptokinase, carbamazepine, clopidogrel, ticlopidine

Modified from Goldman L, Ausiello D (eds): *Cecil textbook of medicine,* ed 22, Philadelphia, 2004, WB Saunders.

NOREPINEPHRINE

Normal range: 0-600 pg/ml
Elevated in: Pheochromocytomas, stress, vigorous exercise, certain foods (bananas, chocolate, coffee, tea, vanilla)

5′-NUCLEOTIDASE

Normal range: 2-16 IU/L
Elevated in: Biliary obstruction, metastatic neoplasms to liver, primary biliary cirrhosis, renal failure, pancreatic carcinoma, chronic active hepatitis

OSMOLALITY (serum)

Normal range: 280-300 mOsm/kg
It can also be estimated by the following formula:
$2([Na] + [K]) + glucose/18 + BUN/2.8$
Elevated in: Dehydration, hypernatremia, diabetes insipidus, uremia, hyperglycemia, mannitol therapy, ingestion of toxins (ethylene glycol, methanol, ethanol), hypercalcemia, diuretics
Decreased in: Syndrome of inappropriate diuretic hormone secretion, hyponatremia, overhydration, Addison's disease, hypothyroidism

PARACENTESIS FLUID

Testing and evaluation of results:
1. Process the fluid as follows:
    a. Tube 1: LDH, glucose, albumin.
    b. Tube 2: protein, specific gravity.
    c. Tube 3: cell count and differential.
    d. Tube 4: save until further notice.
2. Draw serum LDH, protein, albumin.

3. Gram stain, AFB stain, bacterial and fungal cultures, amylase, and triglycerides should be ordered only when clearly indicated; bedside inoculation of blood-culture bottles with ascitic fluid improves sensitivity in detecting bacterial growth.
4. If malignant ascites is suspected, consider a carcinoembryonic antigen level on the paracentesis fluid and cytologic evaluation.
5. In suspected spontaneous bacterial peritonitis (SBP) the incidence of positive cultures can be increased by injecting 10 to 20 ml of ascitic fluid into blood culture bottles.
6. Peritoneal effusion can be subdivided as exudative or transudative based on its characteristics.
7. The serum-ascites albumin gradient (serum albumin level-ascitic fluid albumin level) correlates directly with portal pressure and can also be used to classify ascite. Patients with gradients $\geq$1.1 g/dl have portal hypertension, and those with gradients <1.1 g/dl do not; the accuracy of this method is >95%.
8. An ascitic fluid polymorphonuclear leukocyte count >500/μl is suggestive of SBP.
9. A blood-ascitic fluid albumin gradient.

PARTIAL THROMBOPLASTIN TIME (PTT), ACTIVATED PARTIAL THROMBOPLASTIN TIME (APTT)

Normal range: 25-41 sec
Elevated in: Heparin therapy, coagulation factor deficiency (I, II, V, VIII, IX, X, XI, XII), liver disease, vitamin K deficiency, disseminated intravascular coagulation, circulating anticoagulant, warfarin therapy, specific factor inhibition (PCN reaction, rheumatoid arthritis), thrombolytic therapy, nephrotic syndrome
NOTE: Useful to evaluate the intrinsic coagulation system.

PH, BLOOD
Normal values:
Arterial: 7.35-7.45
Venous: 7.32-7.42
For abnormal values refer to "Arterial Blood Gases."

PHOSPHATASE, ACID; *see* ACID PHOSPHATASE

PHOSPHATASE, ALKALINE; *see* ALKALINE
PHOSPHATASE

PHOSPHATE (serum)
Normal range: 2.5-5 mg/dl
DECREASED
Parenteral hyperalimentation
Diabetic acidosis
Alcohol withdrawal
Severe metabolic or respiratory alkalosis
Antacids that bind phosphorus
Malnutrition with refeeding using low-phosphorus nutrients
Renal tubule failure to reabsorb phosphate (Fanconi's syndrome; congenital disorder; vitamin D deficiency)
Glucose administration
Nasogastric suction
Malabsorption
Gram-negative sepsis
Primary hyperparathyroidism
Chlorothiazide diuretics
Therapy of acute severe asthma
Acute respiratory failure with mechanical ventilation
INCREASED
Renal failure
Severe muscle injury
Phosphate-containing antacids
Hypoparathyroidism
Tumor lysis syndrome

PLATELET COUNT
Normal range: 130-400 $\times$ 10^3/mm^3
Elevated in:
REACTIVE THROMBOCYTOSIS
Infections or inflammatory states—vasculitis, allergic reactions, etc.
Surgery and tissue damage—myocardial infarction, pancreatitis, etc.
Postsplenectomy state
Malignancy—solid tumors, lymphoma
Iron deficiency anemia, hemolytic anemia, acute blood loss
Uncertain etiology
Rebound effect after chemotherapy or immune thrombocytopenia
Renal disorders—renal failure, nephrotic syndrome
MYELOPROLIFERATIVE DISORDERS
Chronic myeloid leukemia
Primary thrombocythemia
Polycythemia vera
Idiopathic myelofibrosis
Decreased:
A. Increased destruction
  1. Immunologic
    a. Drugs: quinine, quinidine, digitalis, procainamide, thiazide diuretics, sulfonamides, phenytoin, aspirin, penicillin, heparin, gold, meprobamate, sulfa drugs, phenylbutazone, NSAIDs, methyldopa, cimetidine, furosemide, INH, cephalosporins, chlorpropamide, organic arsenicals, chloroquine
    b. Idiopathic thrombocytopenic purpura
    c. Transfusion reaction: transfusion of platelets with platelet antigen HPA-1a (PL^{A1}) in recipients without PL^{A1}
    d. Vasculitis (e.g., systemic lupus erythematosus)

    e. Autoimmune hemolytic anemia
    f. Lymphoreticular disorders (e.g., chronic lymphocytic leukemia)
  2. Nonimmunologic
    a. Prosthetic heart valves
    b. Thrombotic thrombocytopenic purpura
    c. Sepsis
    d. Disseminated intravascular coagulation
    e. Hemolytic-uremic syndrome
    f. Giant cavernous hemangioma
B. Decreased production
  1. Abnormal marrow
    a. Marrow infiltration (e.g., leukemia, lymphoma, fibrosis)
    b. Marrow suppression (e.g., chemotherapy, alcohol, radiation)
  2. Hereditary disorders
    a. Wiskott-Aldrich syndrome: X-linked disorder characterized by thrombocytopenia, eczema, and repeated infections
    b. May-Hegglin anomaly: increased megakaryocytes but ineffective thrombopoiesis
  3. Vitamin deficiencies (e.g., vitamin B$_{12}$, folic acid)
C. Splenic sequestration, hypersplenism
D. Dilutional, secondary to massive transfusion

POTASSIUM (serum)
Normal range: 3.5-5 mEq/L
CAUSES OF HYPERKALEMIA
I. Pseudohyperkalemia
  A. Hemolysis of sample
  B. Thrombocytosis
  C. Leukocytosis
  D. Laboratory error
II. Increased potassium intake and absorption
  A. Potassium supplements (oral and parenteral)
  B. Dietary—salt substitutes
  C. Stored blood
  D. Potassium-containing medications
III. Impaired renal excretion
  A. Acute renal failure
  B. Chronic renal failure
  C. Tubular defect in potassium secretion
    1. Renal allograft
    2. Analgesic nephropathy
    3. Sickle cell disease
    4. Obstructive uropathy
    5. Interstitial nephritis
    6. Chronic pyelonephritis
    7. Potassium-sparing diuretics
    8. Miscellaneous (lead, systemic lupus erythematosus, pseudohypoaldosteronism)
  D. Hypoaldosteronism
    1. Primary (Addison's disease)
    2. Secondary
      a. Hyporeninemic hypoaldosteronism (type IV RTA)
      b. Drug-induced
        (1) Nonsteroidal antiinflammatory medications
        (2) ACE inhibitors
        (3) Heparin
        (4) Cyclosporine
IV. Transcellular shifts
  A. Acidosis
  B. Hypertonicity
  C. Insulin deficiency
  D. Drugs
    1. β-blockers
    2. Digitalis toxicity
    3. Succinylcholine

E. Exercise
F. Hyperkalemic periodic paralysis
V. Cellular injury
  A. Rhabdomyolysis
  B. Severe intravascular hemolysis
  C. Acute tumor lysis syndrome
  D. Burns and crush injuries

CAUSES OF HYPOKALEMIA

I. Decreased intake
  A. Decreased dietary potassium
  B. Impaired absorption of potassium
  C. Clay ingestion
  D. Kayexalate
II. Increased loss
  A. Renal
    1. Hyperaldosteronism
      a. Primary
        1. Conn's syndrome
        2. Adrenal hyperplasia
      b. Secondary
        1. Congestive heart failure
        2. Cirrhosis
        3. Nephrotic syndrome
        4. Dehydration
      c. Bartter's syndrome
    2. Glycyrrhizic acid (licorice, chewing tobacco)
    3. Excessive adrenal corticosteroids
      a. Cushing's syndrome
      b. Steroid therapy
      c. Adrenogenital syndrome
    4. Renal tubular defects
      a. Renal tubular acidosis
      b. Obstructive uropathy
      c. Salt-wasting nephropathy
    5. Drugs
      a. Diuretics
      b. Aminoglycosides
      c. Mannitol
      d. Amphotericin
      e. Cisplatin
      f. Carbenicillin
  B. Gastrointestinal
    1. Vomiting
    2. Nasogastric suction
    3. Diarrhea
    4. Malabsorption
    5. Ileostomy
    6. Villous adenoma
    7. Laxative abuse
  C. Increased losses from the skin
    1. Excessive sweating
    2. Burns
III. Transcellular shifts
  A. Alkalosis
    1. Vomiting
    2. Diuretics
    3. Hyperventilation
    4. Bicarbonate therapy
  B. Insulin
    1. Exogenous
    2. Endogenous response to glucose
  C. β_2-Agonists (albuterol, terbutaline, epinephrine)
  D. Hypokalemia periodic paralysis
    1. Familial
    2. Thyrotoxic
IV. Miscellaneous

  A. Anabolic state
  B. Intravenous hyperalimentation
  C. Treatment of megaloblastic anemia
  D. Acute mountain sickness

PROSTATE-SPECIFIC ANTIGEN (PSA)

Normal range: 0-4 ng/ml
Table 4-16 describes age-specific reference ranges for PSA.
Elevated in: Benign prostatic hypertrophy, carcinoma of prostate, postrectal examination, prostate trauma
Factors affecting serum PSA are described in Table 4-17.
  NOTE: Measurement of free PSA is useful to assess the probability of prostate cancer in patients with normal digital rectal examination and total PSA between 4 and 10 ng/ml. In these patients, the global risk of prostate cancer is 25%; however, if the free PSA is >25%, the risk of prostate cancer decreases to 8%, whereas if the free PSA is <10%, the risk of cancer increases to 56%. Free PSA is also useful to evaluate the aggressiveness of prostate cancer. A low free PSA percentage generally indicates a high-grade cancer, whereas a high free PSA percentage is generally associated with a slower growing tumor or BPH.
Decreased in: Finasteride therapy, dutasteride therapy, saw palmetto use, bedrest, antiandrogens

TABLE 4-16 Age-Specific Reference Ranges for PSA

	SERUM PSA (NG/ML)		
Age (yr)	Whites	Japanese	African American
40-49	0-2.5	0-2.0	0-2.0
50-59	0-3.5	0-3.0	0-4.0
60-69	0-4.5	0-4.0	0-4.5
70-79	0-6.5	0-5.0	0-5.5

From Nseyo UO (ed): *Urology for primary care physicians,* Philadelphia, 1999, WB Saunders.
PSA, Prostate-specific antigen.

TABLE 4-17 Factors Affecting Serum Prostate-Specific Antigen (PSA)

Factors Affecting Serum PSA	Duration of Effect
Prostate size	Not applicable
Recent ejaculation	6-48 hours
Prostate manipulation	
Vigorous massage	1 week
Cystoscopy	1 week
Prostate biopsy	4-6 weeks
Prostatitis	
Acute	3-6 months
Chronic	Unknown
Prostate cancer	Not applicable
Drugs: finasteride (Proscar)*	3-6 months

From Nseyo UO (ed): *Urology for primary care physicians,* Philadelphia, 1999, WB Saunders.
*Lowers PSA for as long as patient is on the medication.

PROTEIN (serum)

Normal range: 6-8 g/dl

Elevated in: Dehydration, multiple myeloma, Waldenström's macroglobulinemia, sarcoidosis, collagen-vascular diseases

Decreased in: Malnutrition, low-protein diet, overhydration, malabsorption, severe burns, neoplasms, chronic diseases, cirrhosis, nephrosis

PROTEIN ELECTROPHORESIS (serum)

Normal range: Albumin: 60% to 75%

α-1: 1.7% to 5%
α-2: 6.7% to 12.5%
β: 8.3% to 16.3%
γ: 10.7% to 20%
Albumin: 3.6-5.2 g/dl
α-1: 0.1-0.4 g/dl
α-2: 0.4-1 g/dl
β: 0.5-1.2 g/dl
γ: 0.6-1.6 g/dl

Elevated in: Albumin: dehydration

α-1: neoplastic diseases, inflammation
α-2: neoplasms, inflammation, infection, nephrotic syndrome
β: hypothyroidism, biliary cirrhosis, diabetes mellitus
γ: *see* IMMUNOGLOBULINS

Decreased in: Albumin: malnutrition, chronic liver disease, malabsorption, nephrotic syndrome, burns, systemic lupus erythematosus

α-1: emphysema (α-1 antitrypsin deficiency), nephrosis
α-2: hemolytic anemias (decreased haptoglobin), severe hepatocellular damage
β: hypocholesterolemia, nephrosis
γ: *see* IMMUNOGLOBULINS

Fig. 4-10 describes serum protein electrophoretic patterns.

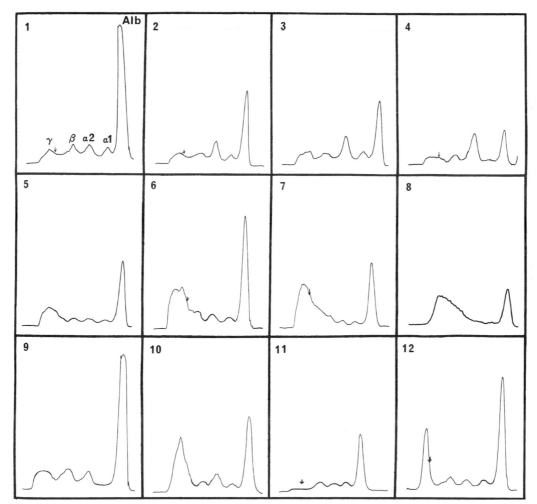

FIGURE 4-10   **Typical serum protein electrophoretic patterns.** *1,* Normal (*arrow* near γ region indicates serum application point). *2,* Acute reaction pattern. *3,* Acute reaction or nephrotic syndrome. *4,* Nephrotic syndrome. *5,* Chronic inflammation, cirrhosis, granulomatous diseases, rheumatoid-collagen group. *6,* Same as 5, but g elevation is more pronounced. There is also partial (but not complete) β-γ fusion. *7,* Suggestive of cirrhosis but could be found in the granulomatous diseases or the rheumatoid-collagen group. *8,* Characteristic pattern of cirrhosis. *9,* α-1 Antitrypsin deficiency with mild γ elevation suggesting concurrent chronic disease. *10,* Same as 5, but the γ elevation is marked. The configuration of the γ peak superficially mimics that of myeloma, but is more broad-based. There are superimposed acute reaction changes. *11,* Hypogammaglobulinemia or light-chain myeloma. *12,* Myeloma, Waldenström's macroglobulinemia, idiopathic or secondary monoclonal gammopathy. (From Ravel R: *Clinical laboratory medicine,* ed 6, St Louis, 1995, Mosby.)

PROTHROMBIN TIME (PT)

Normal range: 10-12 sec

Elevated in: Liver disease, oral anticoagulants (warfarin), heparin, factor deficiency (I, II, V, VII, X), disseminated intravascular coagulation, vitamin K deficiency, afibrinogenemia, dysfibrinogenemia, drugs (salicylate, chloral hydrate, diphenylhydantoin, estrogens, antacids, phenylbutazone, quinidine, antibiotics, allopurinol, anabolic steroids)

Decreased in: Vitamin K supplementation, thrombophlebitis, drugs (glutethimide, estrogens, griseofulvin, diphenhydramine)

PROTOPORPHYRIN (free erythrocyte)

Normal range: 16-36 μg/dl of red blood cells

Elevated in: Iron deficiency, lead poisoning, sideroblastic anemias, anemia of chronic disease, hemolytic anemias, erythropoietic protoporphyria

PSA; *see* PROSTATE-SPECIFIC ANTIGEN

PT; *see* PROTHROMBIN TIME

PTT; *see* PARTIAL THROMBOPLASTIN TIME

RDW; *see* RED BLOOD CELL DISTRIBUTION WIDTH

RED BLOOD CELL (RBC) COUNT

Normal range: Male: 4.3-$5.9 \times 10^6/mm^3$
Female: 3.5-$5 \times 10^6/mm^3$

Elevated in: Polycythemia vera, smokers, high altitude, cardiovascular disease, renal cell carcinoma and other erythropoietin-producing neoplasms, stress, hemoconcentration/dehydration

Decreased in: Anemias, hemolysis, chronic renal failure, hemorrhage, failure of marrow production

RED BLOOD CELL DISTRIBUTION WIDTH (RDW)

Measures variability of red cell size (anisocytosis)

Normal range: 11.5-14.5

Normal RDW and:

ELEVATED MEAN CORPUSCULAR VOLUME (MCV): aplastic anemia, preleukemia

NORMAL MCV: normal, anemia of chronic disease, acute blood loss or hemolysis, chronic lymphocytic leukemia (CLL), chronic myelocytic leukemia, nonanemic enzymopathy or hemoglobinopathy

DECREASED MCV: anemia of chronic disease, heterozygous thalassemia

Elevated RDW and:

ELEVATED MCV: vitamin B_{12} deficiency, folate deficiency, immune hemolytic anemia, cold agglutinins, CLL with high count, liver disease

NORMAL MCV: early iron deficiency, early vitamin B_{12} deficiency, early folate deficiency, anemic globinopathy

DECREASED MCV: iron deficiency, red blood cell fragmentation, HbH disease, thalassemia intermedia

RED BLOOD CELL FOLATE; *see* FOLATE, RED BLOOD CELL

RETICULOCYTE COUNT

Normal range: 0.5% to 1.5%

Elevated in: Hemolytic anemia (sickle cell crisis, thalassemia major, autoimmune hemolysis), hemorrhage, postanemia therapy (folic acid, ferrous sulfate, vitamin B_{12}), chronic renal failure

Decreased in: Aplastic anemia, marrow suppression (sepsis, chemotherapeutic agents, radiation), hepatic cirrhosis, blood transfusion, anemias of disordered maturation (iron deficiency anemia, megaloblastic anemia, sideroblastic anemia, anemia of chronic disease)

RHEUMATOID FACTOR

Normal: Negative

Present in titer >1:20

RHEUMATIC DISEASES

Rheumatoid arthritis

Sjögren's syndrome

Systemic lupus erythematosus

Polymyositis/dermatomyositis

Mixed connective tissue disease

Scleroderma

INFECTIOUS DISEASES

Subacute bacterial endocarditis

Tuberculosis

Infectious mononucleosis

Hepatitis

Syphilis

Leprosy

Influenza

MALIGNANCIES

Lymphoma

Multiple myeloma

Waldenström's macroglobulinemia

Postradiation or postchemotherapy

MISCELLANEOUS

Normal adults, especially the elderly

Sarcoidosis

Chronic pulmonary disease (interstitial fibrosis)

Chronic liver disease (chronic active hepatitis, cirrhosis)

Mixed essential cryoglobulinemia

Hypergammaglobulinemic purpura

RNP; *see* EXTRACTABLE NUCLEAR ANTIGEN

SEDIMENTATION RATE; *see* ERYTHROCYTE SEDIMENTATION RATE

SGOT; *see* ASPARTATE AMINOTRANSFERASE

SGPT; *see* ALANINE AMINOTRANSFERASE

SMOOTH MUSCLE ANTIBODY

Normal: Negative

Present in: Chronic acute hepatitis (≥1:80), primary biliary cirrhosis (≤1:80), infectious mononucleosis

SODIUM (serum)

Normal range: 135-147 mEq/L

HYPONATREMIA

A. Sodium and water depletion (deficit hyponatremia)
1. Loss of gastrointestinal secretions with replacement of fluid but not electrolytes
   a. Vomiting
   b. Diarrhea
   c. Tube drainage
2. Loss from skin with replacement of fluids but not electrolytes
   a. Excessive sweating
   b. Extensive burns
3. Loss from kidney
   a. Diuretics
   b. Chronic renal insufficiency (uremia) with acidosis
4. Metabolic loss
   a. Starvation with acidosis
   b. Diabetic acidosis
5. Endocrine loss
   a. Addison's disease
   b. Sudden withdrawal of long-term steroid therapy
6. Iatrogenic loss from serous cavities
   a. Paracentesis or thoracentesis

B. Excessive water (dilution hyponatremia)
   1. Excessive water administration
   2. Congestive heart failure
   3. Cirrhosis
   4. Nephrotic syndrome
   5. Hypoalbuminemia (severe)
   6. Acute renal failure with oliguria
C. Inappropriate antidiuretic hormone (IADH) syndrome
D. Intracellular loss (reset osmostat syndrome)
E. False hyponatremia (actually a dilutional effect)
   1. Marked hypertriglyceridemia*
   2. Marked hyperproteinemia*
   3. Severe hyperglycemia

HYPERNATREMIA

Dehydration is the most frequent overall clinical finding in hypernatremia.
   1. Deficient water intake (either orally or intravenously)
   2. Excess kidney water output (diabetes insipidus, osmotic diuresis)
   3. Excess skin water output (excess sweating, loss from burns)
   4. Excess gastrointestinal tract output (severe protracted vomiting or diarrhea without fluid therapy)
   5. Accidental sodium overdose
   6. High-protein tube feedings

SYNOVIAL FLUID ANALYSIS

Table 4-18 describes the classification and interpretation of synovial fluid analysis.

T₃ (triiodothyronine)

Normal range: 75-220 ng/dl
Abnormal values:
A. Elevated in hyperthyroidism (usually earlier and to a greater extent than serum T₄).
B. Useful in diagnosing:
   1. T₃ hyperthyroidism (thyrotoxicosis): increased T₃, normal FTI.

2. Toxic nodular goiter: increased T₃, normal or increased T₄.
3. Iodine deficiency: normal T₃, possibly decreased T₄.
4. Thyroid replacement therapy with liothyronine (Cytomel): normal T₄, increased T₃ if patient is symptomatically hyperthyroid.

Not ordered routinely but indicated when hyperthyroidism is suspected and serum free T₄ or FTI inconclusive.

T₃ (triiodothyronine); *see* Table 4-19 for T₃ abnormalities

T₃ RESIN UPTAKE (T₃RU)

Normal range:
25% to 35%
Abnormal values:
Increased in hyperthyroidism. T₃ resin uptake (T₃RU or RT₃U) measures the percentage of free T₄ (not bound to protein); it does not measure serum T₃ concentration; T₃RU and other tests that reflect thyroid hormone binding to plasma protein are also known as *thyroid hormone-binding ratios* (THBR).

T₄, SERUM T₄, AND FREE (free thyroxine)

Normal range:
0.8-2.8 ng/dl
Abnormal values:
Serum thyroxine (T₄)
Elevated in:
1. Graves' disease
2. Toxic multinodular goiter
3. Toxic adenoma
4. Iatrogenic and factitious
5. Transient hyperthyroidism.
   a. Subacute thyroiditis
   b. Hashimoto's thyroiditis
   c. Silent thyroiditis
6. Rare causes: hypersecretion of TSH (e.g., pituitary neoplasms), struma ovarii, ingestion of large amounts of iodine in a patient with preexisting thyroid hyperplasia or adenoma

TABLE 4-18 Classification and Interpretation of Synovial Fluid Analysis

Group	Diseases	Appearance	Viscosity	Mucin Clot	WBC/MM³	%PMN	Glucose (mg/dl) (Blood–Synovial Fluid)	Protein (g/dl)
Normal	—	Clear	↑	Firm	<200	<25	<10	<2.5
I (noninflammatory)	Osteoarthritis, aseptic necrosis, traumatic arthritis, erythema nodosum, osteochondritis dissecans	Clear, yellow (may be xanthochromic if traumatic arthritis)	↑	Firm	↑ Up to 10,000	<25	<10	<2.5
II (inflammatory)	Crystal-induced arthritis, rheumatoid arthritis, Reiter's syndrome, collagen-vascular disease, psoriatic arthritis, serum sickness, rheumatic fever	Clear, yellow, turbid	↓	Friable	↑↑ Up to 100,000	40-90	<40	.2.5
III (septic)	Bacterial (staphylococcal, gonococcal, tuberculosis)	Turbid	↓/↑	Friable	↑↑↑ Up to 5 million	40-100	20-100	.2.5

↑, Elevated; ↑↑, markedly high; ↓, decreased; *PMN,* polymorphonuclear leukocytes. Note that there is considerable overlap in the numbers listed above.

TABLE 4-19　**Findings in Thyroid Function Tests in Various Clinical Conditions**

Condition	T_4	FT_4I	T_3	FT_3I	TSH	TSI	TRH Stimulation
Hyperthyroidism							
Graves' disease	↑	↑	↑	↑	↓	+	↓
Toxic nodular goiter	↑	↑	↑	↑	↓	−	↓
Pituitary TSH-secreting tumors	↑	↑	↑	↑	↑	−	↓
T3 thyrotoxicosis	N	N	↑	↑	↓	+, −	↓
T4 thyrotoxicosis	↑	↑	N	N	↓	+, −	↓
Hypothyroidism							
Primary	↓	↓	↓	↓	↑	+, −	↑
Secondary	↓	↓	↓	↓	↓, N	−	↓
Tertiary	↓	↓	↓	↓	↓, N	−	N
Peripheral unresponsiveness	↑, N	↑, N	↑, N	↑	↑, N	−	N, ↑

From Tilton RC, Barrows A: *Clinical laboratory medicine,* St Louis, 1992, Mosby.
N, Normal; ↑, increased; ↓, decreased; +, − variable.

(Jod-Basedow phenomenon), carcinoma of thyroid, amiodarone therapy of arrhythmias.

Serum thyroxine test measures both circulating thyroxine bound to protein (represents >99% of circulating T_4) and unbound (free) thyroxine. Values vary with protein binding; changes in the concentration of T_4 secondary to changes in thyroxine-binding globulin (TBG) can be caused by the following:

Increased TBG (↑T_4)
Estrogens
Acute infectious hepatitis
Familial
Fluorouracil, clofibrate, heroin, methadone

Decreased TBG (↓T_4)
Androgens, glucocorticoids
Nephrotic syndrome, cirrhosis
Acromegaly
Hypoproteinemia
Familial
Phenytoin, ASA and other NSAIDs, high-dose penicillin, asparaginase
Chronic debilitating illness

To eliminate the suspected influence of protein binding on thyroxine values, two additional tests are available: T_3 resin uptake and serum free thyroxine.

T_4, FREE (free thyroxine)

Normal range: 0.8-2.8 ng/dl
Elevated in: Graves' disease, toxic multinodular goiter, toxic adenoma, iatrogenic and factitious causes, transient hyperthyroidism

Serum free T_4 directly measures unbound thyroxine. Free T_4 can be measured by equilibrium dialysis (gold standard of free T_4 assays) or by immunometric techniques (influenced by serum levels of lipids, proteins, and certain drugs). The free thyroxine index (FTI) can also be easily calculated by multiplying T_4 times T_3RU and dividing the result by 100; the FTI corrects for any abnormal T_4 values secondary to protein binding: $FTI = T_4 \times T_3RU/100$.
Normal values equal 1.1 to 4.3.

TESTOSTERONE (total testosterone)

Normal range: (Variable with age and sex)
Serum/plasma:　　Males: 280-1100 ng/dl
　　　　　　　　Females: 15-70 ng/dl
Urine:　　　　　Males: 50-135 μg/day
　　　　　　　　Females: 2-12 μg/day
Elevated in: Testicular tumors, ovarian masculinizing tumors
Decreased in: Hypogonadism

THORACENTESIS FLUID

Testing and evaluation of results:
1. Pleural effusion fluid should be differentiated in exudate or transudate. The initial laboratory studies should be aimed only at distinguishing an exudate from a transudate.
   a. Tube 1: protein, LDH, albumin.
   b. Tubes 2, 3, 4: save the fluid until further notice. In selected patients with suspected empyema, a pH level may be useful (generally ≤7.0). See following for proper procedure to obtain a pH level from pleural fluid.
   NOTE: Do not order further tests until the presence of an exudate is confirmed on the basis of protein and LDH determinations (Section III, Fig. 3-70); however, if the results of protein and LDH determinations cannot be obtained within a reasonable time (resulting in unnecessary delay), additional laboratory tests should be ordered at the time of thoracentesis.
2. A serum/effusion albumin gradient of ≤1.2 g/dl is indicative of exudative effusions, especially in patients with congestive heart failure (CHF) treated with diuretics.
3. Note the appearance of the fluid:
   a. A grossly hemorrhagic effusion can be a result of a traumatic tap, neoplasm, or an embolus with infarction.
   b. A milky appearance indicates either of the following:
      (1) Chylous effusion: caused by trauma or tumor invasion of the thoracic duct; lipoprotein electrophoresis of the effusion reveals chylomicrons and triglyceride levels >115 mg/dl.
      (2) Pseudochylous effusion: often seen with chronic inflammation of the pleural space (e.g., TB, connective tissue diseases).
4. If transudate, consider CHF, cirrhosis, chronic renal failure, and other hypoproteinemic states and perform subsequent workup accordingly.
5. If exudate, consider ordering these tests on the pleural fluid:
   a. Cytologic examination for malignant cells (for suspected neoplasm).
   b. Gram stain, cultures (aerobic and anaerobic), and sensitivities (for suspected infectious process).
   c. AFB stain and cultures (for suspected TB).
   d. pH: a value < 7.0 suggests parapneumonic effusion or empyema; a pleural fluid pH must be drawn anaerobically and iced immediately; the syringe should be pre-rinsed with 0.2 ml of 1:1000 heparin.
   e. Glucose: a low glucose level suggests parapneumonic effusions and rheumatoid arthritis.

f. Amylase: a high amylase level suggests pancreatitis or ruptured esophagus.

g. Perplexing pleural effusions are often a result of malignancy (e.g., lymphoma, malignant mesothelioma, ovarian carcinoma), TB, subdiaphragmatic processes, prior asbestos exposure, and postcardiac injury syndrome.

THYROID-STIMULATING HORMONE (TSH)

Normal range: 2-11 μU/ml

CONDITIONS THAT INCREASE SERUM THYROID-STIMULATING HORMONE VALUES

Laboratory error
Primary hypothyroidism
Synthroid therapy with insufficient dose
Lithium or amiodarone; some patients
Hashimoto's thyroiditis in later stage
Large doses of inorganic iodide (e.g., SSKI)
Severe nonthyroid illness in recovery phase
Iodine deficiency (moderate or severe)
Addison's disease
TSH specimen drawn in evening (peak of diurnal variation)
Pituitary TSH-secreting tumor
Therapy of hypothyroidism (3-6 wk after beginning therapy [range, 1-8 wk]; sometimes longer when pretherapy TSH is over 100 μU/ml)
Acute psychiatric illness
Peripheral resistance to T_4 syndrome
Antibodies (e.g., HAMA) interfering with monoclonal sandwich method of TSH assay
Telepaque (iopanoic acid) and Oragrafin (ipodate) x-ray contrast media
Amphetamines
High altitudes

CONDITIONS THAT DECREASE SERUM THYROID-STIMULATING HORMONE VALUES

Laboratory error
T_4/T_3 toxicosis (diffuse or nodular etiology)
Excessive therapy for hypothyroidism
Active thyroiditis (subacute, painless, or early active Hashimoto's disease)
Multinodular goiter containing areas of autonomy
Severe nonthyroid illness (especially acute trauma, dopamine, or glucocorticoid)
T_3 toxicosis
Pituitary insufficiency
Cushing's syndrome (and some patients on high-dose glucocorticoid)
Jod-Basedow (iodine-induced) hyperthyroidism
Thyroid-stimulating hormone drawn 2-4 hr after levothyroxine dose
Postpartum transient toxicosis
Factitious hyperthyroidism
Struma ovarii
Radioimmunoassay, surgery, or antithyroid drug therapy for hyperthyroidism 4-6 wk (range 2 wk–2 yr) after the treatment
Interleukin-2 drugs (3%-6% of cases) or α-interferon therapy (1% of cases)
Hyperemesis gravidarum
Amiodarone therapy

THYROXINE (T_4)

Normal range: 4-11 μg/dl

TIBC; *see* IRON-BINDING CAPACITY

TRANSFERRIN

Normal range: 170-370 mg/dl
Elevated in: Iron deficiency anemia, viral hepatitis

Decreased in: Nephrotic syndrome, liver disease, hereditary deficiency, protein malnutrition, neoplasms, chronic inflammatory states, chronic illness, thalassemia, hemochromatosis, hemolytic anemia

TRIGLYCERIDES

Normal range: <150 mg/dl
Elevated in: Hyperlipoproteinemias (types I, IIb, III, IV, V), hypothyroidism, estrogens, acute myocardial infarction, pancreatitis, alcohol intake, nephrotic syndrome, diabetes mellitus, glycogen storage disease
Decreased in: Malnutrition, congenital abetalipoproteinemias, drugs (e.g., gemfibrozil, fenofibrate, nicotinic acid, clofibrate)

TRIIODOTHYRONINE; *see* T_3

TROPONINS, SERUM

Normal range: 0-0.4 ng/ml (negative). If there is clinical suspicion of evolving acute MI or ischemic episode, repeat testing in 5-6 hours is recommended.
Indeterminate: 0.05-0.49 ng/ml. Suggest further tests. In a patient with unstable angina and this troponin I level, there is an increased risk of a cardiac event in the near future.
Strong probability of acute MI: ≥0.05 ng/ml
CARDIAC TROPONIN T (CTNT) is a highly sensitive marker for myocardial injury for the first 48 hours after MI and for up to 5-7 days (see Fig. 4-2, under "Creatine Kinase Isoenzymes"). It may be also elevated in renal failure, chronic muscle disease, and trauma.
CARDIAC TROPONIN I (CTNI) is highly sensitive and specific for myocardial injury (≥CK-MB) in the initial 8 hours, peaks within 24 hours, and lasts up to 7 days. With progressively higher levels of cTnI, the risk of mortality increases because the amount of necrosis increases.

TSH; *see* THYROID-STIMULATING HORMONE

TT; *see* THROMBIN TIME

TUBERCULIN TEST (PPD)

Abnormal results: *see* Boxes 4-3 and 4-4 for interpretation

UNCONJUGATED BILIRUBIN; *see* BILIRUBIN, INDIRECT

UREA NITROGEN, BLOOD (BUN)

Normal range: 8-18 mg/dl
Box 4-5 describes factors affecting BUN level independent of renal function.
Elevated in: Drugs (aminoglycosides and other antibiotics, diuretics, lithium, corticosteroids), dehydration, gastrointestinal bleeding, decreased renal blood flow (shock, congestive heart failure, myocardial infarction), renal disease (glomerulonephritis, pyelonephritis, diabetic nephropathy), urinary tract obstruction (prostatic hypertrophy)
Decreased in: Liver disease, malnutrition, overhydration, acromegaly, celiac disease

URIC ACID (serum)

Normal range: 2-7 mg/dl
Elevated in: Renal failure, gout, excessive cell lysis (chemotherapeutic agents, radiation therapy, leukemia, lymphoma, hemolytic anemia), hereditary enzyme deficiency (hypoxanthine-guanine-phosphoribosyl transferase), acidosis, myeloproliferative disorders, diet high in purines or protein, drugs (diuretics, low doses of ASA, ethambutol, nicotinic acid), lead poisoning, hypothyroidism, Addison's disease, nephrogenic diabetes insipidus, active psoriasis, polycystic kidneys
Decreased in: Drugs (allopurinol, high doses of ASA, probenecid, warfarin, corticosteroid), deficiency of xanthine

BOX 4-3 **PPD Reaction Size Considered "Positive" (Intracutaneous 5 TU Mantoux Test at 48 hr)**

5 mm or More
HIV infection or risk factors for HIV
Close recent contact with active TB case
Persons with chest x-ray consistent with healed TB
10 mm or More
Foreign-born persons from countries with high TB prevalence in Asia, Africa, and Latin America
IV drug users
Medically underserved low-income population groups (including Native Americans, Hispanics, and blacks)

Residents of long-term care facilities (nursing homes, mental institutions)
Medical conditions that increase risk for TB (silicosis, gastrectomy, undernourished, diabetes mellitus, high-dose corticosteroids or immunosuppression Rx, leukemia or lymphoma, other malignancies)
Employees of long-term care facilities, schools, child-care facilities, health care facilities
15 mm or More
All others not already listed

TB, Tuberculosis; *TU,* tuberculin units.

BOX 4-4 **Factors Associated with False-Negative Tuberculin Tests**

Technical Errors
Improper administration
Inaccurate reading
Loss of potency of antigen
Patient-Related Factors (Anergy)
Age (elderly)
Nutritional status

Medications—corticosteroids, immunosuppressive agents
Severe tuberculosis
Coexisting diseases
  HIV infection
  Viral illness or vaccination
  Lymphoreticular malignancies
  Sarcoidosis
  Solid tumors

Lepromatous leprosy
Sjögren's syndrome
Ataxia telangiectasia
Uremia
Primary biliary cirrhosis
Systemic lupus erythematosus
Severe systemic disease of any etiology

From Stein JH (ed): *Internal medicine,* ed 4, St Louis, 1994, Mosby.

BOX 4-5 **Factors Affecting Blood Urea Nitrogen Level Independent of Renal Function**

Disproportionate Increase in Blood Urea Nitrogen
Volume depletion "prerenal azotemia"
Gastrointestinal hemorrhage
Corticosteroid or cytotoxic agents
High-protein diet
Obstructive uropathy

Sepsis
Catabolic states tissue breakdown
Disproportionate Decrease in Blood Urea Nitrogen
Low-protein diet
Liver disease

From Andreoli TE (ed): *Cecil essentials of medicine,* ed 5, Philadelphia, 2001, WB Saunders.

oxidase, syndrome of inappropriate antidiuretic hormone secretion, renal tubular deficits (Fanconi's syndrome), alcoholism, liver disease, diet deficient in protein or purines, Wilson's disease, hemochromatosis

URINALYSIS

Normal range:
Color: light straw
Appearance: clear
Ketones: absent
pH: 4.5-8 (average, 6)
Protein: absent
Glucose: absent
Specific gravity: 1.005-1.030
Occult blood absent
Microscopic examination:
Red blood cells: 0-5 (high-power field)
White blood cells: 0-5 (high-power field)
Bacteria (spun specimen): absent
Casts: 0-4 hyaline (low-power field)
Abnormalities in the microscopic examination of urine are described in Table 4-20.

URINE 5-HYDROXYINDOLE-ACETIC ACID (urine 5-HIAA)

Normal range: 2-8 mg/24 hr

Elevated in: Carcinoid tumors, after ingestion of certain foods (bananas, plums, tomatoes, avocados, pineapples, eggplant, walnuts), drugs (monoamine oxidase inhibitors, phenacetin, methyldopa, glycerol guaiacolate, acetaminophen, salicylates, phenothiazines, imipramine, methocarbamol, reserpine, methamphetamine)

URINE VANILLYLMANDELIC ACID (VMA)

Normal range: <6.8 mg/24 hr
Elevated in: Pheochromocytoma, drugs (isoproterenol, methocarbamol, levodopa, sulfonamides, chlorpromazine), severe stress, after ingestion of bananas, chocolate, vanilla, tea, coffee
Decreased in: Drugs (monoamine oxidase inhibitors, reserpine, guanethidine, methyldopa)

VDRL

Normal range: Negative
Positive test: Syphilis, other treponemal diseases (yaws, pinta, bejel)
  NOTE: A false-positive test may be seen in patients with systemic lupus erythematosus and other autoimmune diseases, infectious mononucleosis, HIV, atypical pneumonia, malaria, leprosy, typhus fever, rat-bite fever, relapsing fever.
  NOTE: See Table 4-21 for interpretation of serologic tests for syphilis.

TABLE 4-20 **Microscopic Examination of the Urine**

Finding	Associations
Casts	
Red blood cell	Glomerulonephritis, vasculitis
White blood cell	Interstitial nephritis, pyelonephritis
Epithelial cell	Acute tubular necrosis, interstitial nephritis, glomerulonephritis
Granular	Renal parenchymal disease (nonspecific)
Waxy, broad	Advanced renal failure
Hyaline	Normal finding in concentrated urine
Fatty	Heavy proteinuria
Cells	
Red blood cell	Urinary tract infection, urinary tract inflammation
White blood cell	Urinary tract infection, urinary tract inflammation
Eosinophil	Acute interstitial nephritis
(Squamous) epithelial cell	Contaminants
Crystals	
Uric acid	Acid urine, acute uric acid nephropathy, hyperuricosuria
Calcium phosphate	Alkaline urine
Calcium oxalate	Acid urine, hyperoxaluria, ethylene glycol poisoning
Cystine	Cystinuria
Sulfur	Sulfa-containing antibiotics

From Andreoli TE (ed): *Cecil essentials of medicine,* ed 5, Philadelphia, 2001, WB Saunders.

TABLE 4-21 **Interpretation of Serologic Tests for Syphilis***

FINDING

Nontreponemal Tests	Treponemal Tests	Interpretation of Finding: Is Syphilis Present?*
Nonreactive	Nonreactive	Early primary syphilis is not ruled out by negative serologic tests.
		Early syphilis is present in 13%-30% of patients who have a negative microhemagglutination–*Treponema pallidum* test; in about 30% of patients who present with chancre but have a nonreactive reagin test; and in about 10% of patients who have a negative FTA-ABS test.
		Late syphilis is present in a very small fraction of patients.
		Adequately treated syphilis in remote past may produce these results, but treponemal tests usually remain reactive.
	Reactive	Observed in about 10% of patients with chancre. The treponemal tests may turn positive shortly before the reagin tests. Reagin tests repeated after several days are generally positive.
		In adequately treated early syphilis, the reagin test may return to nonreactive within 1-2 yr, whereas the treponemal tests generally do not.
		Late syphilis is not ruled out by a negative reagin test. The sensitivity of the reagin tests is lower than that of treponemal tests in untreated late syphilis.
		In secondary syphilis, rarely, a highly reactive serum appears negative when tested undiluted with a reagin test because flocculation is inhibited by relative antibody excess. Not reported to occur with treponemal tests. Quantitative reagin tests are positive.
		False-positive treponemal tests occur in 40% of patients with Lyme disease.
Reactive	Nonreactive borderline (FTA-ABS)	Finding is not diagnostic of syphilis but constitutes a classic biologic false-positive reaction.
		Not diagnostic of syphilis: most patients (90%) with this pattern do not develop clinical or serologic evidence of syphilis. Repeat test is indicated. Chronic borderline results are associated with a variety of conditions other than syphilis.
	Beaded (FTA-ABS)	Not diagnostic of syphilis. Seen with collagen-vascular disease.
	Reactive	Findings diagnostic of syphilis or other treponemal disease.
		In adequately treated syphilis, one would expect (1) a sustained fourfold drop in titer of reagin test, although reagin test may remain positive after adequate therapy; (2) treponemal tests remain positive after adequate therapy.
		Concurrent false-positive results on both nontreponemal and treponemal tests could occur in rare instances. It may be impossible to rule out syphilis in an individual with this test profile.

From Stein JH (ed): *Internal medicine,* ed 4, St Louis, 1994, Mosby.
FTA-ABS, Fluorescent treponemal antibody, absorbed.
*Serologic data must always be interpreted in the light of a total clinical evaluation. Diagnosis based on serologic criteria alone is fraught with error. Serologic tests apparently in conflict with clinical diagnosis should be confirmed by repetition or possibly referral to a reference laboratory.

VITAMIN B₁₂

Normal:

190-900 ng/ml

Causes of Vitamin B_{12} deficiency:

1. Pernicious anemia (antibodies against intrinsic factor and gastric parietal cells)
2. Dietary (strict lacto-ovovegetarians, food faddists)
3. Malabsorption (achlorhydria, gastrectomy, ileal resection, pancreatic insufficiency, drugs [omeprazole, cholestyramine])

Falsely low levels occur in patients with severe folate deficiency, in patients using high doses of ascorbic acid, and when cobalamin levels are measured after nuclear medicine studies (radioactivity interferes with cobalamin radioimmunoassay).

Falsely high or normal levels in patients with cobalamin deficiency can occur in severe liver disease and chronic granulocytic leukemia.

The absence of anemia or macrocytosis does not exclude the diagnosis of cobalamin deficiency.

WBC; *see* COMPLETE BLOOD COUNT

WHITE BLOOD COUNT; *see* COMPLETE BLOOD COUNT

Clinical Preventive Services

*Data modified from US Preventive Services Task Force: Guide to clinical preventive services: report of the US Preventive Services Task Force, ed 2, Washington, DC, 1996 (revised 2001), US Department of Health and Human Services. Text downloaded from Internet site: http://text.nlm.nih.gov

PART A • THE PERIODIC HEALTH EXAMINATION

TABLE 5-1 Ages 65 and Older

Interventions considered
and recommended for the
Periodic Health Examination

Leading causes of death
  Heart diseases
  Malignant neoplasms (lung, colorectal, breast)
  Cerebrovascular disease
  Chronic obstructive pulmonary disease
  Pneumonia and influenza

INTERVENTIONS FOR THE GENERAL POPULATION

Screening

Blood pressure
Height and weight
Fecal occult blood test[1] and/or colonoscopy
Mammogram ± clinical breast exam[2] (women ≤69 yr)
Papanicolaou (Pap) test (women)[3]
Vision screening
Assess for hearing impairment
Assess for problem drinking

Counseling

Substance use
Tobacco cessation
Avoid alcohol/drug use while driving, swimming, boating, etc.*

Diet and exercise
Limit fat and cholesterol; maintain caloric balance; emphasize
  grains, fruits, vegetables
Adequate calcium intake (women)
Regular physical activity*

Injury prevention
Lap/shoulder belts

Motorcycle and bicycle helmets*
Fall prevention*
Safe storage/removal of firearms*
Smoke detector*
Set hot water heater to <120°-130° F
CPR training for household members

Dental health
Regular visits to dental care provider*
Floss, brush with fluoride toothpaste daily*

Sexual behavior
STD prevention: avoid high-risk sexual behavior*; use condoms

Immunizations
Pneumococcal vaccine
Influenza[1]
Tetanus-diphtheria (Td) boosters

INTERVENTIONS FOR HIGH-RISK POPULATIONS

Population	*Potential Interventions (See detailed high-risk definitions)*
Institutionalized persons	PPD (HR1); hepatitis A vaccine (HR2); amantadine/rimantadine (HR4)
Chronic medical conditions; TB contacts; low income; immigrants; alcoholics	PPD (HR1)
Persons ≥75 yr, or ≥70 yr with risk factors for falls	Fall prevention intervention (HR5)
Cardiovascular disease risk factors	Consider lipid screening (HR6)
Family hx of skin cancer; nevi; fair skin, eyes, hair	Avoid excess/midday sun, use protective clothing* (HR7)
Native Americans/Alaska Natives	PPD (HR1); hepatitis A vaccine (HR2)
Travelers to developing countries	Hepatitis A vaccine (HR2); hepatitis B vaccine (HR8)
Blood product recipients	HIV screen (HR3); hepatitis B vaccine (HR8)
High-risk sexual behavior	Hepatitis A vaccine (HR2); HIV screen (HR3); hepatitis B vaccine (HR8); RPR/VDRL (HR9)
Injection or street drug use	PPD (HR1); hepatitis A vaccine (HR2); HIV screen (HR3); hepatitis B vaccine (HR8); RPR/VDRL (HR9); advice to reduce infection risk (HR10)
Health care/lab workers	PPD (HR1); hepatitis A vaccine (HR2); amantadine/rimantadine (HR4); hepatitis B vaccine (HR8)
Persons susceptible to varicella	Varicella vaccine (HR11)
Men aged 65 to 75 who have ever smoked	Ultrasound of abdominal aorta (HR12)

[1]Annually. [2]Mammogram q1-2 yr, or mammogram q1-2 yr with annual clinical breast exam. [3]All women who are or have been sexually active and who have a cervix.
  Consider discontinuation of testing after age 65 yr if previous regular screening with consistently normal results.
*The ability of clinician counseling to influence this behavior is unproven.

HR1: HIV positive, close contacts of persons with known or suspected TB, health care workers, persons with medical risk factors associated with TB, immigrants from countries with high TB prevalence, medically underserved low-income populations (including homeless), alcoholics, injection drug users, and residents of long-term care facilities.

HR2: Persons living in, traveling to, or working in areas where the disease is endemic and where periodic outbreaks occur (e.g., countries with high or intermediate endemicity; certain Alaska Native, Pacific Island, Native American, and religious communities); men who have sex with men; injection or street drug users. Consider for institutionalized persons and workers in these institutions, and day-care, hospital, and laboratory workers. Clinicians should also consider local epidemiology and consider HIV screening in the general population.

HR3: Men who had sex with men after 1975; past or present injection drug use; persons who exchange sex for money or drugs, and their sex partners; injection drug–using, bisexual, or HIV-positive sex partner currently or in the past; blood transfusion during 1978-1985; persons seeking treatment for STDs. Clinicians should also consider local epidemiology.

HR4: Consider for persons who have not received influenza vaccine or are vaccinated late; when the vaccine may be ineffective due to major antigenic changes in the virus; for unvaccinated persons who provide home care for high-risk persons; to supplement protection provided by vaccine in persons who are expected to have a poor antibody response; and for high-risk persons in whom the vaccine is contraindicated.

HR5: Persons aged 75 years and older; or aged 70-74 with one or more additional risk factors including use of certain psychoactive and cardiac medications (e.g., benzodiazepines, anti-hypertensives); use of ≥ 4 prescription medications; impaired cognition, strength, balance, or gait. Intensive individualized home-based multifactorial fall prevention intervention is recommended in settings where adequate resources are available to deliver such services.

HR6: Clinicians should consider fasting lipid panel screening on a case-by-case basis for persons aged 65-75, especially in those with additional risk factors (e.g., smoking, diabetes, or hypertension).

HR7: Persons with a family or personal history of skin cancer, a large number of moles, atypical moles, poor tanning ability, or light skin, hair, and eye color.

HR8: Blood product recipients (including hemodialysis patients), persons with frequent occupational exposure to blood or blood products, men who have sex with men, injection drug users and their sex partners, persons with multiple recent sex partners, persons with other STDs (including HIV), travelers to countries with endemic hepatitis B.

HR9: Persons who exchange sex for money or drugs and their sex partners; persons with other STDs (including HIV); and sexual contacts of persons with active syphilis. Clinicians should also consider local epidemiology.

HR10: Persons who continue to inject drugs.

HR11: Healthy adults without a history of chickenpox or previous immunization. Consider serologic testing for presumed susceptible adults.

HR12: Consider ultrasound of abdominal aorta to screen for abdominal aortic aneurysm in all men aged 65 to 75 who have ever smoked.

PART B • IMMUNIZATIONS AND CHEMOPROPHYLAXIS

Immunizations for Adults

TABLE 5-2, A   Recommended Adult Immunization Schedule—United States

Vaccine[23]	Age group (yrs) ≥65
Tetanus, diphtheria (Td)[4]	1 dose booster every 10 years*
Influenza	1 dose annually†
Pneumococcal (polysaccharide)	1 dose§¶
Hepatitis B[4]	3 doses (0, 1–2, 4–6 months)**
Hepatitis A	2 doses (0, 6–12 months)††
Measles, mumps, rubella (MMR)[4]	1 dose if MMR vaccination history is unreliable; 2 doses for persons with occupational or other indications§§
Varicella[4]	2 doses (0, 4–8 weeks) for persons who are susceptible¶¶
Meningococcal (polysaccharide)	1 dose***

☐ For all persons in this age group   ☐ For persons with medical/ exposure indications   ■ Catch-up on childhood vaccinations

[1]Approved by the Advisory Committee on Immunization Practices and accepted by the American College of Obstetricians and Gynecologists (ACOG) and the American Academy of Family Physicians (AAFP).

[2]This schedule indicates recommended age groups for routine administration of currently licensed vaccines for persons aged ≥19 years. Licensed combination vaccine may be used whenever any components of the combination are indicated and the vaccine's other components are not contraindicated. Health-care providers should consult manufacturers' package inserts for detailed recommendations.

[3]Additional information regarding these vaccines and contraindications for vaccination is available from the National Immunization Hotline (telephone, 800-232-2522 [English] or 800-232-0233 [Spanish] or at http://www.cdc.gov/nip.

[4]Covered by the Vaccine Injury Compensation Program. Information on how to file a claim is available at http://www.hrsa.gov/osp/vicp or by telephone, 800-338-2382. Vaccine injury claims are filed with U.S. Court of Federal Claims, 717 Madison Place, N.W., Washington, D.C. 20005; telephone, 202-219-9657.

*Tetanus and diphtheria (Td). Adults should receive a primary series of Td. A primary series for adults is 3 doses: the first 2 doses administered at least 4 weeks apart and the third dose, 6–12 months after the second. Administer 1 dose if the person received the primary series and the last vaccination was ≥10 years previously. In addition, information is available regarding administration of Td as prophylaxis in wound management (1). The American College of Physicians Task Force on Adult Immunization supports a second option for Td use in adults: a single Td booster at age 50 years for persons who have completed the full pediatric series, including the teenage/young adult booster.

†Influenza vaccination. Medical indications: chronic disorders of the cardiovascular or pulmonary systems including asthma; chronic metabolic diseases including diabetes mellitus, renal dysfunction, hemoglobinopathies, or immunosuppression (including immunosuppression caused by medications or by human immunodeficiency virus [HIV]) requiring medical follow-up or hospitalization during the preceding year. Occupational indications: health-care workers (HCWs). Other indications: residents of nursing homes and other long-term-care facilities; persons likely to transmit influenza to persons at high risk (e.g., in-home caregivers to persons with medical indications; household contact and out-of-home caregivers for children aged ≤23 months, or children with asthma or other indicator conditions for influenza vaccination; household members and caregivers for elderly and adults with high-risk conditions); and anyone who wishes to be vaccinated.

§Pneumococcal polysaccharide vaccination. Medical indications: chronic disorders of the pulmonary system, excluding asthma, cardiovascular diseases, diabetes mellitus, chronic liver diseases (including liver disease as a result of alcohol abuse [e.g., cirrhosis]), chronic renal failure or nephrotic syndrome, functional or anatomic asplenia (e.g., sickle cell disease or splenectomy), immunosuppressive conditions (e.g., HIV infection, leukemia, lymphoma, multiple myeloma, Hodgkin's disease, generalized malignancy, and organ or bone marrow transplantation), chemotherapy with alkylating agents, antimetabolites, or long-term systemic corticosteroids. Geographic/other indications: Alaska Natives and certain American Indian populations. Other indications: residents of nursing homes and other long-term-care facilities (4).

¶Revaccination with pneumococcal polysaccharide vaccine. One-time revaccination after 5 years for persons with chronic renal failure or nephrotic syndrome, functional or anatomic asplenia (e.g., sickle cell disease or splenectomy), immunosuppressive conditions (e.g., HIV infection, leukemia, lymphoma, multiple myeloma, Hodgkin's disease, generalized malignancy, and organ or bone marrow transplantation), chemotherapy with alkylating agents, antimetabolites, or long-term systemic corticosteroids. For persons aged ≥65 years, one-time revaccination if they were vaccinated ≥5 years previously and were aged <65 years at the time of primary vaccination (4).

Continued on following page

**Hepatitis B (HepB) vaccine. *Medical indications:* hemodialysis patients, patients who receive clotting-factor concentrates. *Occupational indications:* HCWs and public-safety workers who have exposure to blood in the workplace, persons in training in schools of medicine, dentistry, nursing, laboratory technology, and other allied health professions. *Behavioral indications:* injection-drug users, persons with more than one sex partner during the previous 6 months, persons with a recently acquired sexually transmitted disease (STD), all clients in STD clinics, men who have sex with men (MSM). *Other indications:* household contacts and sex partners of persons with chronic Hepatitis B virus (HBV) infection, clients and staff of institutions for the developmentally disabled, international travelers to countries with high or intermediate prevalence of chronic HBV infection for >6 months, and inmates of correctional facilities (5).

††Hepatitis A (HepA) vaccine. For the combined HepA-HepB vaccine, use 3 doses (at 0, 1, and 6 months). *Medical indications:* persons with clotting-factor disorders or chronic liver disease. *Behavioral indications:* MSM, users of injecting and noninjecting illegal drugs. *Occupational indications:* persons working with Hepatitis A virus (HAV)-infected primates or with HAV in a research laboratory setting. *Other indications:* persons traveling to or working in countries that have high or intermediate endemicity of HAV (6).

§§Measles, Mumps, Rubella (MMR) vaccination. *Measles component:* adults born before 1957 might be considered immune to measles. Adults born in or after 1957 should receive at least 1 dose of MMR unless they have a medical contraindication, documentation of at least 1 dose, or other acceptable evidence of immunity. A second dose of MMR is recommended for adults who 1) were exposed recently to measles or were in an outbreak setting, 2) were previously vaccinated with killed measles vaccine, 3) were vaccinated with an unknown vaccine during 1963–1967, 4) are students in postsecondary educational institutions, 5) work in health-care facilities, or 6) plan to travel internationally. *Mumps component:* 1 dose of MMR should be adequate for protection. *Rubella component:* Administer 1 dose of MMR to women whose rubella vaccination history is unreliable.

¶¶Varicella vaccination. Recommended for all persons who do not have reliable clinical history of varicella infection, or serologic evidence of varicella zoster virus (VZV) infection who might be at high risk for exposure or transmission. This includes HCWs and family contacts of immunocompromised persons, those who live or work in environments where transmission is likely (e.g., teachers of young children, day-care employees, and residents and staff members in institutional settings), persons who live or work in environments where VZV transmission can occur (e.g., inmates and staff members of correctional institutions, and military personnel) adults living in households with children, and international travelers who are not immune to infection. Approximately 95% of U.S.-born adults are immune to VZV (8,9).

***Meningococcal vaccine (quadrivalent polysaccharide for serogroups A, C, Y, and W-135). Consider vaccination for persons with medical indications: adults with terminal complement component deficiencies or with anatomic or functional asplenia. Other indications: travelers to countries where meningitis is hyperendemic or epidemic (e.g., the "meningitis belt" of sub-Saharan Africa, Mecca, or Saudi Arabia). Revaccination at 3–5 years may be indicated for persons at high risk for infection (e.g., persons residing in areas in which disease is epidemic). Physicians need not initiate discussion of the meningococcal quadrivalent polysaccharide vaccine as part of routine medical care.

References

1. CDC. Diphtheria, tetanus, and pertussis: recommendations for vaccine use and other preventive measures. Recommendations of the Immunization Practices Advisory Committee (ACIP). MMWR 1991;40(No. RR-10).
2. CDC. Prevention and control of influenza: recommendations of the Advisory Committee for Immunization Practices. MMWR 2003;52(No. RR-8).
3. CDC. Using live, attenuated influenza vaccine for prevention and control of influenza: supplemental recommendations of the Advisory Committee on Immunization Practices (ACIP). MMWR 2003;52(No. RR-13).
4. CDC. Prevention of pneumococcal disease: recommendations of the Advisory Committee on Immunization Practices (ACIP). MMWR 1997;47(No. RR-8).
5. CDC. Hepatitis B virus: a comprehensive strategy for eliminating transmission in the United States through universal childhood vaccination. Recommendations of the Immunization Practices Advisory Committee (ACIP). MMWR 1991;40(No. RR-13).
6. CDC. Prevention of hepatitis A through active or passive immunization: recommendations of the Advisory Committee on Immunization Practices (ACIP). MMWR 1999;48(No. RR-12).
7. CDC. Prevention of varicella: recommendations of the Advisory Committee on Immunization Practices (ACIP). MMWR 1996;45(No. RR-11).
8. CDC. Prevention of varicella: updated recommendations of the Advisory Committee on Immunization Practices (ACIP). MMWR 1999;48(No. RR-6).
9. *MMRW Morb Mortal Wkly Rep* 52, 2003.

TABLE 5-2, B   Recommended Adult Immunization Schedule for Adults with Medical Conditions— United States

Medical condition	Vaccine						
	Tetanus-diphtheria (Td)*	Influenza†	Pneumo-coccal (polysac-charide)§¶	Hepatitis B**	Hepatitis A††	Measles, mumps, rubella (MMR)§§	Varicella¶¶
Diabetes, heart disease, chronic pulmonary disease, and chronic liver disease, including chronic alcoholism		A	B		C		
Congenital immunodeficiency, leukemia, lymphoma, generalized malignancy, therapy with alkylating agents, antimetabolites, radiation, or large amounts of corticosteroids			D				E
Renal failure/end-stage renal disease and patients receiving hemodialysis or clotting factor concentrates			D	F			
Asplenia, including elective splenectomy and terminal complement-component deficiencies		G	D,H,I				
Human immunodeficiency virus (HIV) infection			D,J			K	

☐ For all persons in this group   ▨ For persons with medical/exposure indications   ▨ Catch-up on childhood vaccinations   ■ Contraindicated

From *MMWR Morb Mortal Wkly Rep* 52, 2003.

A. Although chronic liver disease and alcoholism are not indicator conditions for influenza vaccination, administer 1 dose annually if the patient is aged >50 years, has other indications for influenza vaccine, or requests vaccination.

B. Asthma is an indicator condition for influenza but not for pneumococcal vaccination.

C. For all persons with chronic liver disease.

D. For persons aged <65 years, revaccinate once after ≥5 years have elapsed since initial vaccination.

E. Persons with impaired humoral but not cellular immunity may be vaccinated (*9*).

F. For hemodialysis patients use special formulation of vaccine (40 μg/ml) or two 1.0 ml 20 μg doses administered at one site. Vaccinate early in the course of renal disease. Assess antibody titers to hepatitis B surface antigen (anti-HBs) levels annually. Administer additional doses if anti-HBs levels decline to ≤10 mlU/ml.

G. No data have been reported specifically on risk for severe or complicated influenza infections among persons with asplenia. However, influenza is a risk factor for secondary bacterial infections that might cause severe disease in asplenics.

H. Administer meningococcal vaccine and consider *Haemophilus influenzae* type b vaccine.

I. In the event of elective splenectomy, vaccinate >2 weeks before surgery.

J. Vaccinate as close to diagnosis as possible when CD4 cell counts are highest.

K. Withhold MMR or other measles-containing vaccines from HIV-infected persons with evidence of severe immunosuppression.
   Please refer to Table 5-2A for footnote explanations.

TABLE 5-3   Immunizing Agents and Immunization Schedules for Health-Care Workers (HCWs)*

Generic Name	Primary Schedule and Booster(s)	Indications	Major Precautions and Contraindications	Special Considerations
Immunizing Agents Strongly Recommended for Health-Care Workers				
Hepatitis B (HB) recombinant vaccine	Two doses IM 4 wk apart; third dose 5 mo after second; booster doses not necessary.	**Preexposure:** HCWs at risk for exposure to blood or body fluids.	Previous anaphylactic reaction to common baker's yeast is a contraindication to vaccination.	The vaccine produces neither therapeutic nor adverse effects on HBV-infected persons. Prevaccination serologic screening is not indicated for persons being vaccinated because of occupational risk. HCWs who have contact with patients or blood should be tested 1-2 mo after vaccination to determine serologic response.
Hepatitis B immune globulin (HBIG)	0.06 ml/kg IM as soon as possible after exposure. A second dose of HBIG should be administered 1 mo later if the HB vaccine series has not been started.	**Postexposure prophylaxis:** For persons exposed to blood or body fluids containing HBsAg and who are not immune to HBV infection—0.06 ml/kg IM as soon as possible (but no later than 7 days after exposure).		
Influenza vaccine (inactivated whole-virus and split-virus vaccines)	Annual vaccination with current vaccine. Administered IM.	HCWs who have contact with patients at high risk for influenza or its complications; HCWs who work in chronic care facilities; HCWs with high-risk medical conditions or who are aged ≥65 yr.	History of anaphylactic hypersensitivity to egg ingestion.	
Measles live-virus vaccine	One dose SC; second dose at least 1 mo later.	HCWs† born during or after 1957 who do not have documentation of having received two doses of live vaccine on or after the first birthday **or** a history of physician-diagnosed measles or serologic evidence of immunity. Vaccination should be considered for all HCWs who lack proof of immunity, including those born before 1957.	Immunocompromised persons,‡ including HIV-infected persons who have evidence of severe immunosuppression; anaphylaxis after gelatin ingestion or administration of neomycin; recent administration of immune globulin.	MMR is the vaccine of choice if recipients are likely to be susceptible to rubella and/or mumps as well as to measles. Persons vaccinated during 1963-1967 with a killed measles vaccine alone, killed vaccine followed by live vaccine, or with a vaccine of unknown type should be revaccinated with two doses of live measles virus vaccine.
Mumps live-virus vaccine	One dose SC; no booster	HCWs† believed to be susceptible can be vaccinated. Adults born before 1957 can be considered immune.	Immunocompromised persons‡; history of anaphylactic reaction after gelatin ingestion or administration of neomycin	MMR is the vaccine of choice if recipients are likely to be susceptible to measles and rubella as well as to mumps.

Modified from *MMWR Morb Mortal Wkly Rep* 46(RR-18), 1998.

HBsAg, Hepatitis B surface antigen; *HBV,* hepatitis B virus; *HIV,* human immunodeficiency virus; *IM,* intramuscular; *MMR,* measles, mumps, rubella vaccine; *SC,* subcutaneous.

*Persons who provide health care to patients or work in institutions that provide patient care (e.g., physicians, nurses, emergency medical personnel, dental professionals and students, medical and nursing students, laboratory technicians, hospital volunteers, and administrative and support staff in health-care institutions).

†All HCWs (i.e., medical or nonmedical, paid or volunteer, full time or part time, student or nonstudent, with or without patient-care responsibilities) who work in health-care institutions (e.g., inpatient and outpatient, public and private) should be immune to measles, rubella, and varicella.

‡Persons immunocompromised because of immune deficiency diseases, HIV infection, leukemia, lymphoma, or generalized malignancy or immunosuppressed as a result of therapy with corticosteroids, alkylating drugs, antimetabolites, or radiation.

TABLE 5-3   Immunizing Agents and Immunization Schedules for Health-Care Workers (HCWs)*
(Continued)

Generic Name	Primary Schedule and Booster(s)	Indications	Major Precautions and Contraindications	Special Considerations
Hepatitis A vaccine	Two doses of vaccine either 6-12 mo apart (HAVRIX), or 6 mo apart (VAQTA)	Not routinely indicated for HCWs in the United States. Persons who work with HAV-infected primates or with HAV in a research laboratory setting should be vaccinated.	History of anaphylactic hypersensitivity to alum or, for HAVRIX, the preservative 2-phenoxyethanol. The risk associated with vaccination should be weighed against the risk for hepatitis A in women who may be at high risk for exposure to HAV.	
Meningococcal polysaccharide vaccine (tetravalent A, C, W135, and Y)	One dose in volume and by route specified by manufacturer; need for boosters unknown	Not routinely indicated for HCWs in the United States.		
Typhoid vaccine, IM, SC, and oral	IM vaccine: One 0.5-ml dose, booster 0.5 ml every 2 yr. SC vaccine: two 0.5 ml doses, ≥4 wk apart, booster 0.5 ml SC or 0.1 ID every 3 yr if exposure continues *Oral vaccine:* Four doses on alternate days. The manufacturer recommends revaccination with the entire four-dose series every 5 yr	Workers in microbiology laboratories who frequently work with *Salmonella typhi*	Severe local or systemic reaction to a previous dose. Ty21a (oral) vaccine should not be administered to immunocompromised persons† or to persons receiving antimicrobial agents.	Vaccination should not be considered an alternative to the use of proper procedures when handling specimens and cultures in the laboratory.
Vaccinia vaccine (smallpox)	One dose administered with a bifurcated needle; boosters administered every 10 yr	Laboratory workers who directly handle cultures with vaccinia, recombinant vaccinia viruses, or orthopox viruses that infect humans	The vaccine is contraindicated in persons with eczema or a history of *eczema* and in immunocompromised persons† and their household contacts.	Vaccination may be considered for HCWs who have direct contact with contaminated dressings or other infectious material from volunteers in clinical studies involving recombinant vaccinia virus.
Other Vaccine-Preventable Diseases				
Tetanus and diphtheria (toxoids [Td])	Two IM doses 4 wk apart; third dose 6-12 mo after second dose; booster every 10 yr	All adults	History of a neurologic reaction or immediate hypersensitivity reaction after a previous dose. History of severe local (Arthus-type) reaction after a previous dose. Such persons should not receive further routine or emergency doses of Td for 10 yr.	Tetanus prophylaxis in wound management‡

*Persons who provide health care to patients or work in institutions that provide patient care (e.g., physicians, nurses, emergency medical personnel, dental professionals and students, medical and nursing students, laboratory technicians, hospital volunteers, and administrative and support staff in health-care institutions).
†All HCWs (i.e., medical or nonmedical, paid or volunteer, full time or part time, student or nonstudent, with or without patient-care responsibilities) who work in health-care institutions (e.g., inpatient and outpatient, public and private) should be immune to measles, rubella, and varicella.
‡Persons immunocompromised because of immune deficiency diseases, HIV infection, leukemia, lymphoma or generalized malignancy or immunosuppressed as a result of therapy with corticosteroids, alkylating drugs, antimetabolites, or radiation.

Continued on following page

TABLE 5-3 Immunizing Agents and Immunization Schedules for Health-Care Workers (HCWs)* *(Continued)*

Generic Name	Primary Schedule and Booster(s)	Indications	Major Precautions and Contraindications	Special Considerations
Pneumococcal polysaccharide vaccine (23 valent)	One dose, 0.5 ml, IM or SC; revaccination recommended for those at highest risk ≥5 yr after the first dose	Adults who are at increased risk of pneumococcal disease and its complications because of underlying health conditions; older adults, especially those age ≥65 who are healthy	Previous recipients of any type of pneumococcal polysaccharide vaccine who are at highest risk for fatal infection or antibody loss may be revaccinated ≥5 yr after the first dose.	
Rubella live-virus vaccine	One dose SC; no booster	Indicated for HCWs,† both men and women, who do not have documentation of having received live vaccine on or after their first birthday **or** laboratory evidence of immunity. Adults born before 1957 can be considered immune.	Immunocompromised persons†; history of anaphylactic reaction after administration of neomycin	MMR is the vaccine of choice if recipients are likely to be susceptible to measles or mumps, as well as to rubella.
Varicella zoster live-virus vaccine	Two 0.5-ml doses SC 4-8 wk apart if ≥13 yr of age	Indicated for HCWs† who do not have either a reliable history of varicella or serologic evidence of immunity	Immunocompromised persons,‡ history of anaphylactic reaction following receipt of neomycin or gelatin. Avoid salicylate use for 6 wk after vaccination.	Vaccine is available from the manufacturer for certain patients with acute lymphocytic leukemia (ALL) in remission. Because 71%-93% of persons without a history of varicella are immune, serologic testing before vaccination is likely to be cost-effective.
Varicella-zoster immune globulin (VZIG)	Persons <50 kg: 125 μ/10 kg IM; persons ≥50 kg: 625 μ§	Persons known or likely to be susceptible (particularly those at high risk for complications) who have close and prolonged exposure to a contact case or to an infectious hospital staff worker or patient		Serologic testing may help in assessing whether to administer VZIG. If use of VZIG prevents varicella disease, patient should be vaccinated subsequently.

BCG Vaccination

Generic Name	Primary Schedule and Booster(s)	Indications	Major Precautions and Contraindications	Special Considerations
Bacille Calmette-Guérin (BCG) vaccine (tuberculosis)	One percutaneous dose of 0.3 ml; no booster dose recommended	Should be considered only for HCWs in areas where multidrug tuberculosis is prevalent, a strong likelihood of infection exists, and where comprehensive infection control precautions have failed to prevent TB transmission to HCWs	Should not be administered to immunocompromised persons‡	In the United States tuberculosis-control efforts are directed toward early identification, treatment of cases, and preventive therapy with isoniazid.

Other Immunobiologics That Are or May Be Indicated for Health-Care Workers

Generic Name	Primary Schedule and Booster(s)	Indications	Major Precautions and Contraindications	Special Considerations
Immune globulin (hepatitis A)	**Postexposure**—One IM dose of 0.02 ml/kg administered ≤2 wk after exposure	Indicated for HCWs exposed to feces of infectious patients	Contraindicated in persons with IgA deficiency; do not administer within 2 wk after MMR vaccine, or 3 wk after varicella vaccine. Delay administration of MMR vaccine for ≥3 mo and varicella vaccine ≥5 mo after administration of IG	Administer in large muscle mass (deltoid, gluteal).

Modified from *MMWR Morb Mortal Wkly Rep* 46(RR-18), 1998.
§Some experts recommend 125 μ/10 kg regardless of total body weight.

TABLE 5-4   Recommendations for Persons with Medical Conditions Requiring Special Vaccination Considerations

Condition	Td	MMR	Varicella	HBV[b]	HAV	Pneumovax[a]	Influenza[b]	HbCV	Meningococcal	IPV	Other live vaccines[c]	Other Killed Vaccines[d]
HIV infection	Rou	Rou/Contr[e]	Contr[f]	Rou[g]	Rou	Rec	Rec	Cons	Rou	Rou	Contr	Rou
Severe immuno-compromise[h]	Rou	Contr	Contr[f]	Rou[g]	Rou	Rec	Rec	Rou[i]	Rou	Rou	Contr	Rou
Renal failure	Rou	Rou	Rou	Rec[g]	Rou	Rec	Rec	Rou	Rou	Rou	Rou	Rou
Diabetes	Rou	Rou	Rou	Rou	Rou	Rec	Rec	Rou	Rou	Rou	Rou	Rou
Chronic liver disease	Rou	Rou	Rou	Rou	Rec	Rec	Rec	Rou	Rou	Rou	Rou	Rou
Cardiac disease	Rou	Rou	Rou	Rou	Rou	Rec	Rec	Rou	Rou	Rou	Rou	Rou
Pulmonary disease	Rou	Rou	Rou	Rou	Rou	Rec	Rec	Rou	Rou	Rou	Rou	Rou
Alcoholism	Rou	Rou	Rou	Rou	Rou	Rec	Rec	Rou	Rou	Rou	Rou	Rou
Functional/anatomic asplenia	Rou	Rou	Rou	Rou	Rou	Rec[j]	Rec	Rec[j]	Rec[j]	Rou	Rou	Rou
Terminal complement deficiency	Rou	Rou	Rou	Rou	Rou	Rou	Rou	Rou	Rec	Rou	Rou	
Clotting factor disorders	Rou	Rou	Rou	Rec	Rec	Rou	Rou	Rou	Rou	Rou	Rou	Rou

Modified and updated from *MMWR Morb Mortal Wkly Rep* 42(RR-4):16 and 17, 1993.

Cons, Consider vaccination; *Contr*, contraindicated; *Rec*, recommended; *Rou*, routine as outlined for all adults.

[a]Pneumovax should be repeated in 5 years for patients in whom vaccine is recommended. Asthma without chronic obstructive pulmonary disease is not an indication for the vaccine.

[b]Influenza vaccine should also be given to caregivers and household members.

[c]Includes bacille Calmette-Guérin, vaccinia, oral typhoid, yellow fever (if exposure cannot be avoided, persons with HIV can be given yellow fever vaccine; see text).

[d]Includes rabies (check postvaccination titers in HIV or severely immunocompromised persons), Lyme, inactivated typhoid, cholera, plague, and anthrax.

[e]For asymptomatic, nonseverely immunocompromised persons with human immunodeficiency virus (HIV), MMR can be used; it is contraindicated in severely immunocompromised persons. MMR can be considered in symptomatic HIV patients without severe immunocompromise.

[f]Varicella can be given to household members and caregivers, but if varicella-like rash develops after vaccination, contact should be avoided.

[g]Recommended for persons with severe chronic renal failure approaching or already receiving dialysis, and higher doses should be given. Antibody titers should be measured after vaccination in these patients and in those with HIV or severe immunocompromise (who may require higher doses) to ensure adequate response. Yearly titers should be measured in dialysis patients.

[h]Severe immunocompromise can result from congenital immunodeficiency, leukemia, lymphoma, malignancy, organ transplant, chemotherapy, radiation therapy, or high-dose corticosteroids.

[i]Only for persons with Hodgkin's disease.

[j]Give at least 2 weeks in advance of elective splenectomy.

TABLE 5-5, A Guidelines for Spacing of Live and Inactivated Antigens

Antigen Combination	Recommended Minimum Interval Between Doses
≥2 inactivated	None; can be administered simultaneously or at any interval between doses
Inactivated and live	None; can be administered simultaneously or at any interval between doses
≥2 live parenteral*	4-week minimum interval, if not administered simultaneously

From *MMWR Morb Mortal Wkly Rep* 51(RR-2), 2002.
*Live oral vaccines (e.g., Ty21a typhoid vaccine, oral polio vaccine) can be administered simultaneously or at any interval before or after inactivated or live parenteral vaccines.

TABLE 5-5, B Guidelines for Administering Antibody-Containing Products* and Vaccines

Simultaneous Administration

Combination	Recommended Minimum Interval Between Doses
Antibody-containing products and inactivated antigen	None; can be administered simultaneously at different sites or at any time between doses
Antibody-containing products and live antigen	Should not be administered simultaneously,† if simultaneous administration of measles-containing vaccine or varicella vaccine is unavoidable, administer at different sites and revaccinate or test for seroconversion after the recommended interval

Nonsimultaneous Administration

Product Administered		Recommended Minimum Interval Between Doses
First	**Second**	
Antibody-containing products	Inactivated antigen	None
Inactivated antigen	Antibody-containing products	None
Antibody-containing products	Live antigen	Dose-related‡
Live antigen	Antibody-containing products	2 weeks

From *MMWR Morb Mortal Wkly Rep* 51(RR-2), 2002.
*Blood products containing substantial amounts of immunoglobulin, including intramuscular and intravenous immune globulin, specific hyperimmune globulin (e.g., hepatitis B immune globulin, tetanus immune globulin, varicella zoster immune globulin, and rabies immune globulin), whole blood, packed red cells, plasma, and platelet products.
†Yellow fever and oral Ty21a typhoid vaccines are exceptions to these recommendations. These live attenuated vaccines can be administered at any time before, after, or simultaneously with an antibody-containing product without substantially decreasing the antibody response.
‡The duration of interference of antibody-containing products with the immune response to the measles component of measles-containing vaccine, and possibly varicella vaccine, is dose-related.

TABLE 5-6 Guide to Contraindications and Precautions[a] to Commonly Used Vaccines

Vaccine	True Contraindications and Precautions[a]	Untrue (Vaccines Can Be Administered)
General for all vaccines, including diphtheria and tetanus toxoids; adult tetanus-diphtheria toxoid (Td); inactivated poliovirus vaccine (IPV); measles-mumps-rubella vaccine (MMR); hepatitis A vaccine; hepatitis B vaccine; varicella vaccine; pneumococcal conjugate vaccine (PCV); influenza vaccine; and pneumococcal polysaccharide vaccine (PPV)	**Contraindications** Serious allergic reaction (e.g., anaphylaxis) after a previous vaccine dose Serious allergic reaction (e.g., anaphylaxis) to a vaccine component **Precautions** Moderate or severe acute illness with or without fever	Mild acute illness with or without fever Mild to moderate local reaction (i.e., swelling, redness, soreness); low-grade or moderate fever after previous dose Lack of previous physical examination in well-appearing person Current antimicrobial therapy Convalescent phase of illness Recent exposure to an infectious disease History of penicillin allergy, other nonvaccine allergies, relatives with allergies, receiving allergen extract immunotherapy
DTaP	**Contraindications** Severe allergic reaction after a previous dose or to a vaccine component **Precautions** Moderate or severe acute illness with or without fever	Temperature of <40.5° C, fussiness or mild drowsiness after a previous dose of diphtheria toxoid-tetanus toxoid-pertussis vaccine (DTP)/DTaP Family history of seizures Stable neurologic conditions (e.g., cerebral palsy, well-controlled convulsions, developmental delay)
DT, Td	**Contraindications** Severe allergic reaction after a previous dose or to a vaccine component **Precautions** Guillain-Barré syndrome ≤6 wk after previous dose of tetanus toxoid-containing vaccine Moderate or severe acute illness with or without fever	
IPV	**Contraindications** Severe allergic reaction to previous dose or vaccine component **Precautions** Moderate or severe acute illness with or without fever	
MMR[b]	**Contraindications** Severe allergic reaction after a previous dose or to a vaccine component Known severe immunodeficiency (e.g., hematologic and solid tumors; congenital immunodeficiency; long-term immunosuppressive therapy,[c] or severely symptomatic human immunodeficiency virus [HIV] infection) **Precautions** Recent (≤11 mo) receipt of antibody-containing blood product (specific interval depends on product) History of thrombocytopenia or thrombocytopenic purpura Moderate or severe acute illness with or without fever	Positive tuberculin skin test Simultaneous TB skin testing[d] Immunodeficient family member or household contact Asymptomatic or mildly symptomatic HIV infection Allergy to eggs
Hib	**Contraindications** Severe allergic reaction after a previous dose or to a vaccine component Age <6 wk **Precaution** Moderate or severe acute illness with or without fever	
Hepatitis B	**Contraindications** Severe allergic reaction after a previous dose or to a vaccine component **Precautions** Moderate or severe acute illness with or without fever	Autoimmune disease (e.g., systemic lupus erythematosus or rheumatoid arthritis)
Hepatitis A	**Contraindications** Severe allergic reaction after a previous dose or to a vaccine component **Precautions** Moderate or severe acute illness with or without fever	

Continued on following page

TABLE 5-6 **Guide to Contraindications and Precautions[a] to Commonly Used Vaccines** *(Continued)*

Vaccine	True Contraindications and Precautions[a]	Untrue (Vaccines Can Be Administered)
Varicella[b]	**Contraindications** Severe allergic reaction after a previous dose or to a vaccine component Substantial suppression of cellular immunity **Precautions** Recent (≤11 mo) receipt of antibody-containing blood product (specific interval depends on product) Moderate or severe acute illness with or without fever	Immunodeficient family member or household contact[e] Asymptomatic or mildly symptomatic HIV infection Humoral immunodeficiency (e.g., agammaglobulinemia)
PCV	**Contraindications** Severe allergic reaction after a previous dose or to a vaccine component **Precaution** Moderate or severe acute illness with or without fever	
Influenza	**Contraindications** Severe allergic reaction to previous dose or vaccine component, including egg protein **Precautions** Moderate or severe acute illness with or without fever	Nonsevere (e.g., contact) allergy to latex or thimerosal Concurrent administration of Coumadin or aminophylline
PPV	**Contraindications** Severe allergic reaction after a previous dose or to a vaccine component **Precaution** Moderate or severe acute illness with or without fever	

From *MMWR Morb Mortal Wkly Rep* 51(RR-2), 2002.

[a]Events or conditions listed as precautions should be reviewed carefully. Benefits and risks of administering a specific vaccine to a person under these circumstances should be considered. If the risk from the vaccine is believed to outweigh the benefit, the vaccine should not be administered. If the benefit of vaccination is believed to outweigh the risk, the vaccine should be administered.

[b]MMR and varicella vaccines can be administered on the same day. If not administered on the same day, these vaccines should be separated by ≥28 days.

[c]Substantially immunosuppressive steroid dose is considered to be ≥2 weeks of daily receipt of 20 mg or 2 mg/kg body weight of prednisone or equivalent.

[d]Measles vaccination can suppress tuberculin reactivity temporarily. Measles-containing vaccine can be administered on the same day as tuberculin skin testing. If testing cannot be performed until after the day of MMR vaccination, the test should be postponed for ≥4 weeks after the vaccination. If an urgent need exists to skin test, do so with the understanding that reactivity might be reduced by the vaccine.

[e]If a vaccinee experiences a presumed vaccine-related rash 7-25 days after vaccination, avoid direct contact with immunocompromised persons for the duration of the rash.

TABLE 5-7　Vaccinations for International Travel

Disease*	Areas Affected†	Prophylaxis Recommended	Ideal Time Between Last Vaccine Dose and Travel
Tetanus	All	All travelers; vaccine series/booster.	Probably 30 days for series Anamnestic response to booster
Varicella	All	All travelers; antibody titer, reported illness, or vaccine series.	7-14 days
Hepatitis B	5%-20% of population are carriers in Africa, Middle East except Israel, all Southeast Asia, Amazon basin, Haiti, and Dominican Republic; 2%-5% of population are carriers in south-central and southwest Asia, Israel, Japan, Americas, Russia, and eastern and southern Europe.	Travelers for more than 6 mo in close contact with population or for less time but with high-risk activities (close household contact, seeking dental or medical care, sex); vaccine series.	Probably 30 days
Hepatitis A	Developing countries.	Travelers to rural areas; eating and drinking in settings of poor sanitation; vaccine or pooled immune globulin (IG).	Vaccine, 30 days Pooled IG, 2 days
Influenza	Tropics throughout the year; Southern Hemisphere from April to September.	Travelers for whom vaccine is otherwise indicated; give current vaccine and revaccinate in fall as usual.	7-14 days
Meningococcus*	Sub-Saharan Africa "belt" (Senegal to Ethiopia) from December to June; required for pilgrims to Saudi Arabia during Haj; epidemics reported in other African nations, India, Nepal, and Mongolia.	All travelers; vaccine.	7-10 days
Rabies	Endemic dog rabies exists in Mexico, El Salvador, Guatemala, Peru, Colombia, Ecuador, India, Nepal, Philippines, Sri Lanka, Thailand, and Vietnam.	Travelers staying for more than 30 days or at high risk of exposure to domestic or wild animals; vaccine series/booster.	7-14 days
Poliomyelitis	Developing countries not in Western Hemisphere; at risk all year in tropics; in temperate zones, incidence increases in summer and fall.	All travelers; vaccine series/booster.	Parenteral vaccine series, 28 day (see text) Anamnestic response to booster
Typhoid fever	Many countries in Asia, Africa, Central America, and South America.	Travelers with prolonged stay in rural areas with poor sanitation; vaccine series/booster.	Oral vaccine, 7 days Parenteral vaccine, probably 14 days
Yellow fever*	North and central South America, forest-savannah zones of Africa; some countries in Africa, Asia, and Middle East require travelers from endemic areas to be vaccinated.	All travelers; vaccine/booster at approved yellow fever vaccination center.	10 days
Japanese encephalitis	Seasonally in most areas of Asia, Indian subcontinent, and western Pacific islands; in temperate zones, incidence increases in summer and early fall; in tropics, year-round incidence.	Travelers staying for more than 30 days in high-risk rural areas; staying outdoors during transmission season; vaccine series.	10 days
Cholera*	Certain undeveloped countries.	If required by local authorities, one dose usually suffices; primary series only for those living in high-risk areas under poor sanitary conditions or those with compromised gastric defense mechanisms (achlorhydria, antacid therapy, previous ulcer surgery); booster every 6 mo.	Probably 30 days
Plague	Africa, Asia, and Americas in rural mountainous or upland areas.	Travelers whose research or field activities bring them in contact with rodents; vaccine series/booster; consider taking tetracycline (500 mg four times a day) for chemoprophylaxis (inferred from clinical experience in treating plague).	Probably 30 days

From Noble J: *Primary care medicine,* ed 3, St Louis, 2001, Mosby.

*Only yellow fever vaccine is required for entry by any country; cholera vaccine may be required by some local authorities; and meningococcus vaccine is required for pilgrims to Mecca, Saudia Arabia, during Haj. However, it is important to follow CDC recommendations for all vaccines to prevent disease. If a required vaccine is contraindicated or withheld for any reason, attempts should be made to obtain a waiver from the country's consulate or embassy.

†Because areas affected can change, and for more specific details, consult CDC's traveler's hotline.

TABLE 5-8 **Recommended Doses of Currently Licensed Hepatitis B Vaccines**

Population Group	Recombivax HB* Dose in μg (Dose in ml)	Engerix-B* Dose in mg (Dose in ml)
Adults ≥20 yr	10 (1.0)	20 (1.0)
Dialysis patients and other immunocompromised persons	40†	40‡

Modified from *MMWR Morb Mortal Wkly Rep* 40(RR-13):7, 1991.
*Both vaccines are routinely administered in a three-dose series at 0, 1, and 6 mo. Engerix-B is also licensed for a four-dose series administered at 0, 1, 2, and 12 mo.
†Special formulation.
‡Two 1.0-ml doses administered at one site in a four-dose schedule at 0, 1, 2, and 6 mo.

ENDOCARDITIS PROPHYLAXIS

BOX 5-1 **Cardiac Conditions Associated with Endocarditis**

Endocarditis Prophylaxis Recommended
High-Risk Category
Prosthetic cardiac valves, including bioprosthetic and homograft valves
Previous bacterial endocarditis
Complex cyanotic congenital heart disease (e.g., single ventricle states, transposition of the great arteries, tetralogy of Fallot)
Surgically constructed systemic pulmonary shunts or conduits
Moderate-Risk Category
Most other congenital cardiac malformations (other than above and below)
Acquired valvar dysfunction (e.g., rheumatic heart disease)
Hypertrophic cardiomyopathy
Mitral valve prolapse with valvar regurgitation and/or thickened leaflets

Endocarditis Prophylaxis Not Recommended
Negligible-Risk Category (No Greater Risk Than the General Population)
Isolated secundum atrial septal defect
Surgical repair of atrial septal defect, ventricular defect, or patent ductus arteriosus (without residua beyond 6 mos)
Previous coronary artery bypass graft surgery
Mitral valve prolapse without valvar regurgitation
Physiologic, functional, or innocent heart murmurs
Previous Kawasaki disease without valvar dysfunction
Previous rheumatic fever without valvar dysfunction
Cardiac pacemakers (intravascular and epicardial) and implanted defibrillators

From Dajani AS et al: *JAMA* 277:1794-1801, 1997.

BOX 5-2 **Dental Procedures and Endocarditis Prophylaxis**

Endocarditis Prophylaxis Recommended*
Dental extractions
Periodontal procedures including surgery, scaling and root planing, probing, and recall maintenance
Dental implant placement and reimplantation of avulsed teeth
Endodontic (root canal) instrumentation of surgery only beyond the apex
Subgingival placement of antibiotic fibers or strips
Initial placement of orthodontic bands—but not brackets
Intraligamentary local anesthetic injections
Prophylactic cleaning of teeth or implants where bleeding is anticipated

Endocarditis Prophylaxis Not Recommended
Restorative dentistry† (operative and prosthodontic) with or without retraction cord‡
Local anesthetic injections (nonintraligamentary)
Intracanal endodontic treatment; postplacement and buildup
Placement of rubber dams
Postoperative suture removal
Placement of removable prosthodontic or orthodontic appliances
Taking of oral impressions
Fluoride treatments
Taking of oral radiographs
Orthodontic appliance adjustment
Shedding of primary teeth

From Dajani AS et al: *JAMA* 277:1794-1801, 1997.
*Prophylaxis is recommended for patients with high- and moderate-risk cardiac conditions.
†This includes restoration of decayed teeth (filling cavities) and replacement of missing teeth.
‡Clinical judgment may indicate antibiotic use in selected circumstances that may create significant bleeding.

BOX 5-3   Other Procedures and Endocarditis Prophylaxis

Endocarditis Prophylaxis Recommended
Respiratory tract
Tonsillectomy and/or adenoidectomy
Surgical operations that involve respiratory mucosa
Bronchoscopy with a rigid bronchoscope
Gastrointestinal Tract*
Sclerotherapy for esophageal varices
Esophageal stricture dilation
Endoscopic retrograde cholangiography* with biliary obstruction
Biliary tract surgery
Surgical operations that involve intestinal mucosa
Genitourinary Tract
Prostatic surgery
Cystoscopy
Urethral dilation

Endocarditis Prophylaxis Not Recommended
Respiratory Tract
Endotracheal intubation
Bronchoscopy with a flexible bronchoscope, with or without biopsy†
Tympanostomy tube insertion

Gastrointestinal Tract
Transesophageal echocardiography†
Endoscopy with or without gastrointestinal biopsy†
Genitourinary Tract
Vaginal hysterectomy†
Vaginal delivery†
Cesarean section
In uninfected tissue:
    Urethral catheterization
    Uterine dilation and curettage
    Therapeutic abortion
    Sterilization procedures
    Insertion or removal of intrauterine devices
Other
Cardiac catheterization, including balloon angioplasty
Implanted cardiac pacemakers, implanted defibrillators, and coronary stents
Incision or biopsy of surgically scrubbed skin
Circumcision

From Dajani AS et al: *JAMA* 277:1794-1801, 1997.
  *Prophylaxis is recommended for high-risk patients; optional for medium-risk patients.
  †Prophylaxis is optional for high-risk patients.

TABLE 5-9   Prophylactic Regimens for Dental, Oral, Respiratory Tract, or Esophageal Procedures

Situation	Agent	Regimen
Standard general prophylaxis	Amoxicillin	2.0 g
Unable to take oral medications	Ampicillin	2.0 g intramuscularly (IM) or intravenously (IV)
Allergic to penicillin	Clindamycin *or*	600 mg
	Cephalexin* or cefadroxil* *or*	2.0 g
	Azithromycin or clarithromycin	500 mg
Allergic to penicillin and unable to take oral medications	Clindamycin *or*	600 mg
	Cefazolin*	1.0 g

From Dajani AS et al: *JAMA* 277:1794-1801, 1997.
*Cephalosporins should not be used in individuals with immediate-type hypersensitivity reaction (urticaria, angioedema, or anaphylaxis) to penicillins.

TABLE 5-10   Prophylactic Regimens for Genitourinary/Gastrointestinal (Excluding Esophageal) Procedures

Situation	Agents	Regimen*
High-risk patients	Ampicillin plus gentamicin	Ampicillin 2.0 g intramuscularly (IM) or intravenously (IV) plus gentamicin 1.5 mg/kg (not to exceed 120 mg) within 30 min of starting the procedure; 6 hr later, ampicillin 1 g IM/IV or amoxicillin 1 g orally (PO)
High-risk patients allergic to ampicillin	Vancomycin plus gentamicin	Vancomycin 1.0 g IV over 1-2 hr plus gentamicin 1.5 mg/kg IV/IM (not to exceed 120 mg); complete injection/infusion within 30 min of starting the procedure
Moderate-risk patients	Amoxicillin or ampicillin	Amoxicillin 2.0 g PO 1 hr before procedure, or ampicillin 2.0 g IV/IV within 30 min of starting the procedure
Moderate-risk patients allergic to ampicillin/amoxicillin	Vancomycin	Vancomycin 1.0 g IV over 1-2 hr; complete infusion within 30 min of starting the procedure

From Dajani AS et al: *JAMA* 277:1794-1801, 1997.
*No second dose of vancomycin or gentamicin is recommended.

TABLE 5-11 Recommended Daily Dosage of Influenza Antiviral Medications for Treatment and Prophylaxis

Antiviral Agent	65 Years and Older
Amantadine[a]	
Treatment	100 mg or less per day
Prophylaxis	100 mg or less per day
Rimantadine[b]	
Treatment[c]	100 or 200[d] mg per day
Prophylaxis	100 or 200[d] mg per day
Zanamivir[e,f]	
Treatment	10 mg bid
Oseltamivir	
Treatment[g]	75 mg bid
Prophylaxis	75 mg per day

Modified from *MMWR Morb Mortal Wkly Rep* 50(RR-4):1, 2001.

NA, Not applicable.

[a]The drug package insert should be consulted for dosage recommendations for administering amantadine to persons with creatinine clearance of 50 ml or less per min per 1.73m².

[b]A reduction in dosage to 100 mg per day of rimantadine is recommended for persons who have severe hepatic dysfunction or those with creatinine clearance of 10 ml or less per min. Other persons with less severe hepatic or renal dysfunction taking 100 mg per day of rimantadine should be observed closely, and the dosage should be reduced or the drug discontinued, if necessary.

[c]Only approved for treatment in adults.

[d]Elderly residents of nursing homes should be administered only 100 mg per day of rimantadine. A reduction in dosage of 100 mg per day should be considered for all persons 65 yr of age or older if they experience side effects when taking 200 mg per day.

[e]Zanamivir is administered via inhalation by using a plastic device included in the package with the medication. Patients will benefit from instruction and demonstration of correct use of the device.

[f]Zanamivir is not approved for prophylaxis.

[g]A reduction in the dose of oseltamivir is recommended for persons with creatinine clearance of less than 30 ml per min.

TABLE 5-12 Recommended Postexposure Prophylaxis for Exposure to Hepatitis B Virus

Vaccination and Antibody Response Status of Exposed Workers*	TREATMENT		
	Source HBsAg Positive	Source HBsAg Negative	Source Unknown or Not Available for Testing
Unvaccinated	HBIG† × 1 and initiate HB vaccine series‡	Initiate HB vaccine series	Initiate HB vaccine series
Previously vaccinated			
Known responder§	No treatment	No treatment	No treatment
Known nonresponder‖	HBIG × 1 and initiate revaccination or HBIG × 2¶	No treatment	If known high-risk source, treat as if source were HBsAg positive
Antibody response unknown	Test exposed person for anti-HBs¶ 1. If adequate,§ no treatment is necessary 2. If inadequate,‖ administer HBIG × 1 and vaccine booster	No treatment	Test exposed person for anti-HBs 1. If adequate,‡ no treatment is necessary 2. If inadequate,‡ administer vaccine booster and recheck titer in 1-2 mo

Anti-HBs, Antibody to HBsAg; *HB,* hepatitis B; *HBIG,* hepatitis B immune globulin; *HBsAg,* hepatitis B surface antigen.

*Persons who have previously been infected with HBV are immune to reinfection and do not require postexposure prophylaxis.

†Hepatitis B immune globulin; dose is 0.06 ml/kg intramuscularly.

‡Hepatitis B vaccine.

§A responder is a person with adequate levels of serum antibody to HBsAg (i.e., anti-HBs ≥10 mIU/ml).

‖A nonresponder is a person with inadequate response to vaccination (i.e., serum anti-HBs <10 mIU/ml).

¶The option of giving one dose of HBIG and reinitiating the vaccine series is preferred for nonresponders who have not completed a second 3-dose vaccine series. For persons who previously completed a second vaccine series but failed to respond, two doses of HBIG are preferred.

TABLE 5-13 Recommended HIV Postexposure Prophylaxis for Percutaneous Injuries

	INFECTION STATUS OF SOURCE				
Exposure Type	HIV-Positive Class 1*	HIV-Positive Class 2*	Source of Unknown HIV Status†	Unknown Source‡	HIV-Negative
Less severe§	Recommend basic 2-drug PEP	Recommend expanded 3-drug PEP	Generally, no PEP warranted; however, consider basic 2-drug PEP‖ for source with HIV risk factors††	Generally, no PEP warranted; however, consider basic 2-drug PEP‖ in settings where exposure to HIV-infected persons is likely	No PEP warranted
More severe#	Recommend expanded 3-drug PEP	Recommend expanded 3-drug PEP	Generally, no PEP warranted; however, consider basic 2-drug PEP‖ for source with HIV risk factors¶	Generally, no PEP warranted; however, consider basic 2-drug PEP‖ in settings where exposure to HIV-infected persons is likely	No PEP warranted

HIV, Human immunodeficiency virus; PEP, postexposure prophylaxis (see Box 5-7).
*HIV-Positive, Class 1—asymptomatic HIV infection or known low viral load (e.g., <1500 RNA copies/ml). HIV-Positive, Class 2—symptomatic HIV infection, acquired immunodeficiency syndrome, acute seroconversion, or known high viral load. If drug resistance is a concern, obtain expert consultation. Initiation of PEP should not be delayed pending expert consultation, and, because expert consultation alone cannot substitute for face-to-face counseling, resources should be available to provide immediate evaluation and follow-up care for all exposures.
†Source of unknown HIV status (e.g., deceased source person with no samples available for HIV testing).
‡Unknown source (e.g., a needle from a sharps disposal container).
§Less severe (e.g., solid needle and superficial injury).
‖The designation "consider PEP" indicates that PEP is optional and should be based on an individualized decision between the exposed person and the treating clinician.
¶If PEP is offered and taken and the source is later determined to be HIV-negative, PEP should be discontinued.
#More severe (e.g., large-bore hollow needle, deep puncture, visible blood on device, or needle used in patient's artery or vein).

TABLE 5-14 Recommended HIV Postexposure Prophylaxis for Mucous Membrane Exposures and Nonintact Skin[a] Exposures

	INFECTION STATUS OF SOURCE				
Exposure Type	HIV-Positive Class 1[b]	HIV-Positive Class 2[b]	Source of Unknown HIV Status[c]	Unknown Source[d]	HIV-Negative
Small volume[e]	Consider basic 2-drug PEP[f]	Recommend basic 2-drug PEP	Generally, no PEP warranted; however, consider basic 2-drug PEP[f] for source with HIV risk factors[g]	Generally, no PEP warranted; however, consider basic 2-drug PEP[f] in settings where exposure to HIV-infected persons is likely	No PEP warranted
Large volume[h]	Recommend basic 2-drug PEP	Recommend expanded 3-drug PEP	Generally, no PEP warranted; however, consider basic 2-drug PEP[f] for source with HIV risk factors[g]	Generally, no PEP warranted; however, consider basic 2-drug PEP[f] in settings where exposure to HIV-infected persons is likely	No PEP warranted

HIV, Human immunodeficiency virus; PEP, postexposure prophylaxis (see Box 5-7).
[a]For skin exposures, follow-up is indicated only if there is evidence of compromised skin integrity (e.g., dermatitis, abrasion, or open wound).
[b]HIV-Positive, Class 1—asymptomatic HIV infection or known low viral load (e.g., <1,500 RNA copies/mL). HIV-Positive, Class 2—symptomatic HIV infection, acquired immunodeficiency syndrome, acute seroconversion, or known high viral load. If drug resistance is a concern, obtain expert consultation. Initiation of PEP should not be delayed pending expert consultation, and, because expert consultation alone cannot substitute for face-to-face counseling, resources should be available to provide immediate evaluation and follow-up care for all exposures.
[c]Source of unknown HIV status (e.g., deceased source person with no samples available for HIV testing).
[d]Unknown source (e.g., splash from inappropriately disposed blood).
[e]Small volume (i.e., a few drops).
[f]The designation, "consider PEP," indicates that PEP is optional and should be based on an individualized decision between the exposed person and the treating clinician.
[g]If PEP is offered and taken and the source is later determined to be HIV-negative, PEP should be discontinued.
[h]Large volume (i.e., major blood splash).

BOX 5-4   Situations for Which Expert* Consultation for HIV Postexposure Prophylaxis Is Advised

- Delayed (i.e., later than 24-36 hr) exposure report
  — the interval after which there is no benefit from postexposure prophylaxis (PEP) is undefined
- Unknown source (e.g., needle in sharps disposal container or laundry)
  — decide use of PEP on a case-by-case basis
  — consider the severity of the exposure and the epidemiologic likelihood of HIV exposure
  — do not test needles or other sharp instruments for HIV
- Resistance of the source virus to antiretroviral agents
  — influence of drug resistance on transmission risk is unknown
  — selection of drugs to which the source person's virus is unlikely to be resistant is recommended, if the source person's virus is known or suspected to be resistant to ≥1 of the drugs considered for the PEP regimen
  — resistance testing of the source person's virus at the time of the exposure is not recommended
- Toxicity of the initial PEP regimen
  — adverse symptoms, such as nausea and diarrhea are common with PEP
  — symptoms often can be managed without changing the PEP regimen by prescribing antimotility and/or antiemetic agents
  — modification of dose intervals (i.e., administering a lower dose of drug more frequently throughout the day, as recommended by the manufacturer), in other situations, might help alleviate symptoms

HIV, Human immunodeficiency virus.
*Local experts and/or the National Clinicians' Postexposure Prophylaxis Hotline (PEPline [1-888-448-4911]).

BOX 5-5   Occupational Exposure Management Resources

National Clinicians' Postexposure Prophylaxis Hotline (PEPline)
Run by University of California–San Francisco/San Francisco General Hospital staff; supported by the Health Resources and Services Administration Ryan White CARE Act, HIV/AIDS Bureau, AIDS Education and Training Centers, and CDC.

Phone: (888) 448-4911
Internet: http://www.ucsf.edu/hivcntr

Needlestick!
A website to help clinicians manage and document occupational blood and body fluid exposures. Developed and maintained by the University of California, Los Angeles (UCLA), Emergency Medicine Center, UCLA School of Medicine, and funded in party by CDC and the Agency for Healthcare Research and Quality.

Internet: http://www.needlestick.mednet.ucla.edu

Hepatitis Hotline

Phone: (888) 443-7232
Internet: http://www.cdc.gov/ncidod/diseases/hepatitis/index.htm

Reporting to CDC: Occupationally acquired HIV infections and failures of PEP.

Phone: (800) 893-0485

Food and Drug Administration
Report unusual or severe toxicity to antiretroviral agents.

Phone: (800) 332-1088
Address:
  MedWatch
  HF-2, FDA
  5600 Fishers Lane
  Rockville, MD 20857
Internet: http://www.fda.gov/medwatch

HIV/AIDS Treatment Information Service

Internet: http://www.hivatis.org

BOX 5-6   Management of Occupational Blood Exposures

Provide immediate care to the exposure site:
- Wash wounds and skin with soap and water
- Flush mucous membranes with water

Determine risk associated with exposure:
- Type of fluid (e.g., blood, visibly bloody fluid, other potentially infectious fluid or tissue, and concentrated virus)
- Type of exposure (i.e., percutaneous injury, mucous membrane or nonintact skin exposure, and bites resulting in blood exposure)

Evaluate exposure source:
- Assess the risk of infection using available information
- Test known sources for HBsAg, anti-HCV, and HIV antibodies (consider using rapid testing)
- For unknown sources, assess risk of exposure to HBV, HCV, or HIV infection
- Do not test discarded needles or syringes for virus contamination

Evaluate the exposed person:
- Assess immune status for HBV infection (i.e., by history of hepatitis B vaccination and vaccine response)

Give PEP for exposures posing risk of infection transmission:
- HBV: See Table 5-13
- HCV: PEP not recommended
- HIV: See Tables 5-14 and 5-15
  — Initiate PEP as soon as possible, preferably within hours of exposure
  — Seek expert consultation if viral resistance is suspected
  — Administer PEP for 4 wk if tolerated

Perform follow-up testing and provide counseling:
- Advise exposed persons to seek medical evaluation for any acute illness occurring during follow-up

HBV exposures
- Perform follow-up anti-HBs testing in persons who receive hepatitis B vaccine
  — Test for anti-HBs 1-2 mo after last dose of vaccine
  — Anti-HBs response to vaccine cannot be ascertained if HBIG was received in the previous 3-4 mo

HCV exposures
- Perform baseline and follow-up testing for anti-HCV and alanine aminotransferase (ALT) 4-6 mo after exposures
- Perform HCV RNA at 4-6 wk if earlier diagnosis of HCV infection desired
- Confirm repeatedly reactive anti-HCV enzyme immunoassays (EIAs) with supplemental tests

HIV exposures
- Perform HIV-antibody testing for at least 6 mo postexposure (e.g., at baseline, 6 wk, 3 mo, and 6 mo)
- Perform HIV antibody testing if illness compatible with an acute retroviral syndrome occurs
- Advise exposed persons to use precautions to prevent secondary transmission during the follow-up period
- Evaluate exposed persons taking PEP within 72 hr after exposure and monitor for drug toxicity for at least 2 wk

HBIG, Hepatitis B immune globulin; *HBsAg,* hepatitis B surface antigen; *HBV,* hepatitis B virus; *HCV,* hepatitis C virus; *HIV,* human immunodeficiency virus; *PEP,* postexposure prophylaxis; *RNA,* ribonucleic acid.

BOX 5-7   **Basic and Expanded HIV Postexposure Prophylaxis Regimens**

Basic Regimen

- **Zidovudine (Retrovir; ZDV; AZT) and Lamivudine (Epivir; 3TC); available as Combivir**
  — ZDV: 600 mg per day, in two or three divided doses
  — 3TC: 150 mg bid

Advantages
  — ZDV is associated with decreased risk of HIV transmission in the CDC case-control study of occupational HIV infection
  — ZDV has been used more than the other drugs for PEP in HCP
  — Serious toxicity is rare when used for PEP
  — Side effects are predictable and manageable with antimotility and antiemetic agents
  — Can be given as a single tablet (Combivir) bid

Disadvantages
  — Side effects are common and might result in low adherence
  — Source patient virus might have resistance to this regimen
  — Potential for delayed toxicity (oncogenic) is unknown

Alternative Basic Regimens

- **Lamivudine (3TC) and Stavudine (Zerit; d4T)**
  — 3TC: 150 mg bid
  — d4T: 40 mg (if body weight is <60 kg, 30 mg) bid

Advantages
  — Well tolerated in patients with HIV infection, resulting in good adherence
  — Serious toxicity appears to be rare
  — Twice daily dosing might improve adherence

Disadvantages
  — Source patient virus might be resistant to this regimen
  — Potential for delayed toxicity (oncogenic/teratogenic) is unknown

- **Didanosine (Videx, chewable/dispersable buffered tablet; Videx EC, delayed-release capsule; ddI) and Stavudine (d4T)**
  — ddI: 400 mg (if body weight is <60 kg, 125 mg bid) daily, on an empty stomach
  — d4T: 40 mg (if body weight is <60 kg, 30 mg bid) bid

Advantages
  — Likely effective against HIV strains from source patients who are taking ZDV and 3TC

Disadvantages
  — ddI is difficult to administer and unpalatable.
  — Chewable/dispersable buffered tablet formulation of ddI interferes with absorption of some drugs (e.g., quinolone antibiotics, and indinavir).
  — Serious toxicity (e.g., neuropathy, pancreatitis, or hepatitis) can occur. Fatal and nonfatal pancreatitis has occurred in HIV-positive, treatment-naive patients. Patients taking ddI and d4T should be carefully assessed and closely monitored for pancreatitis, lactic acidosis, and hepatitis.
  — Side effects are common; anticipate diarrhea and low adherence.
  — Potential for delayed toxicity (oncogenic/teratogenic) is unknown.

Expanded Regimen
Basic regimen plus one of the following:

- **Indinavir (Crixivan; IDV)**
  — 800 mg every 8 hr, on an empty stomach

Advantages
  — Potent HIV inhibitor

Disadvantages
  — Serious toxicity (e.g., nephrolithiasis) can occur; must take 8 glasses of fluid per day
  — Hyperbilirubinemia common
  — Requires acid for absorption and cannot be taken simultaneously with ddI in chewable/dispersable buffered tablet formulation (doses must be separated by at least 1 hr)
  — Concomitant use of astemizole, terfenadine, dihydroergotamine, ergotamine, ergonovine, methylergonovine, rifampin, cisapride, St. John's Wort, lovastatin, simvastatin, pimozide, midazolam, or triazolam is not recommended
  — Potential for delayed toxicity (oncogenic/teratogenic) is unknown

- **Nelfinavir (Viracept; NFV)**
  — 750 mg tid, with meals or snack, or
  — 1250 mg bid, with meals or snack

Advantages
  — Potent HIV inhibitor
  — Twice dosing per day might improve adherence

Disadvantages
  — Concomitant use of astemizole, terfenadine, dihydroergotamine, ergotamine, ergonovine, methylergonovine, rifampin, cisapride, St. John's Wort, lovastatin, simvastatin, pimozide, midazolam, or triazolam is not recommended
  — Might accelerate the clearance of certain drugs
  — Potential for delayed toxicity (oncogenic) is unknown

| BOX 5-7 | **Basic and Expanded HIV Postexposure Prophylaxis Regimens** *(Continued)* |

- **Efavirenz (Sustiva; EFV)**
  — 600 mg daily, at bedtime
Advantages
  — Does not require phosphorylation before activation and might be active earlier than other antiretroviral agents (NOTE: this might be only a theoretical advantage of no clinical benefit)
  — One dose daily might improve adherence
Disadvantages
  — Drug is associated with rash (early onset) that can be severe and might rarely progress to Stevens-Johnson syndrome.
  — Differentiating between early drug-associated rash and acute seroconversion can be difficult and cause extraordinary concern for the exposed person.
  — Nervous system side effects (e.g., dizziness, somnolence, insomnia, and/or abnormal dreaming) are common. Severe psychiatric symptoms are possible (dosing before bedtime might minimize these side effects).
  — Concomitant use of astemizole, cisapride, midazolam, triazolam, ergot derivatives, or St. John's Wort is not recommended because inhibition of the metabolism of these drugs could create the potential for serious and/or life-threatening adverse events (e.g., cardiac arrhythmias, prolonged sedation, or respiratory depression).
  — Potential for oncogenic toxicity is unknown.

- **Abacavir (Ziagen; ABC); available as Trizivir, a combination of ZDV, 3TC, and ABC**
  — 300 mg bid
Advantages
  — Potent HIV inhibitor
  — Well tolerated in patients with HIV infection
Disadvantages
  — Severe hypersensitivity reactions can occur, usually within the first 6 wk of treatment
  — Potential for delayed toxicity (oncogenic) is unknown

Antiretroviral Agents for Use as PEP Only with Expert Consultation
- **Retonavir (Norvir; RTV)**
Disadvantages
  — Difficult to take (requires dose escalation)
  — Poor tolerability
  — Many drug interactions

- **Saquinavir (Fortovase, soft-gel formulation; SQV)**
Disadvantages
  — Bioavailability is relatively poor, even with new formulation

- **Amprenavir (Agenerase; AMP)**
Disadvantages
  — Dosage consists of eight large pills taken bid
  — Many drug interactions

- **Delavirdine (Rescriptor; DLV)**
Disadvantages
  — Drug is associated with rash (early onset) that can be severe and progress to Stevens-Johnson syndrome
  — Many drug interactions

- **Lopinavir/Ritonavir (Kaletra)**
  — 400/100 mg bid
Advantages
  — Potent HIV inhibitor
  — Well tolerated in patients with HIV infection
Disadvantages
  — Concomitant use of flecainide, propafenone, astemizole, terfenadine, dihydroergotamine, ergotamine, ergonovine, methyler-gonovine, rifampin, cisapride, St. John's Wort, lovastatin, simvastatin, pimozide, midazolam, or triazolam is not recommended because inhibition of the metabolism of these drugs could create the potential for serious and/or life-threatening adverse events (e.g., cardiac arrhythmias, prolonged sedation, or respiratory depression)
  — May accelerate the clearance of certain drugs
  — Potential for delayed toxicity (oncogenic) is unknown

Antiretroviral Agents Generally Not Recommended for Use as PEP
- **Nevirapine (Viramune; NVP)**
  — 200 mg daily for 2 wk, then 200 mg bid
Disadvantages
  — Associated with severe hepatotoxicity (including at least one case of liver failure requiring liver transplantation in an exposed person taking PEP)
  — Associated with rash (early onset) that can be severe and progress to Stevens-Johnson syndrome
  — Differentiating between early drug-associated rash and acute seroconversion can be difficult and cause extraordinary concern for the exposed person
  — Concomitant use of St. John's Wort is not recommended because this might result in suboptimal antiretroviral drug concentrations

PART C • DISCONTINUATION CONSIDERATIONS

TABLE 5-15 Discontinuation Considerations in Preventive Health Screening

Hyperlipidemia	When patient and physician agree that therapy would not be warranted
Colorectal Cancer	When early detection is unlikely to prolong life (5-7 more yr)
	Little evidence to recommend screening in patients >80 yr
Breast Cancer	Until a woman has a life expectancy of 8 to 10 yr
Cervical Cancer	At age 65 if previous tests have been consistently normal
Prostate Cancer	When patient's life expectancy is <10 yr or after age 75 for men with average health

Adapted from Takahashi PY et al: Preventive health care in the elderly population: a guide for practicing physicians, *Mayo Clin Proc* 79:416-427, 2004.

Systems of Geriatric Care

INTRODUCTION

The term *advance directive* refers to designating treatment preferences when one is alert and competent that would go into effect if the person should become unable to make medical decisions on her or his own behalf. Authority for advance directives was relegated to the states by the U.S. Supreme Court in Cruzan vs. Director in 1990 and by Congress in the Patient Self-Determination Act of 1991. Written advance directives generally fall into three categories: living will, power of attorney for health care, and health care proxy. All 50 states and the District of Columbia have statutes that address the creation of one or more form of document. In practice, all states accept duly executed advance directives from other states, and many states have specific statutes noting the acceptance of out-of-state forms. As of 2004, 38 states had Default Surrogate Consent Statutes that address the incapacitated individual with no advance directive and a few states had nonhospital Do Not Resuscitate statutes. A more recent variation is the psychiatric advance directives (PAD). Descriptions of the available advance directives are listed.

ADVANCE DIRECTIVE DOCUMENTS

LIVING WILL

A living will is a written document that specifies what types of medical treatment are desired should an individual become incapacitated. A living will can be general or very specific. More specific living wills may include information regarding an individual's desire for such services as analgesia, antibiotics, hydration, feeding, cardiopulmonary resuscitation, and the use of life-support equipment. A living will is the most advantageous advance directive for individuals who do not have anyone in their life whom they want to entrust with responsibility for making their health care decisions. The major limitation of a living will is that it is a static document and one cannot anticipate all of the possible scenarios that may be encountered. Many states stipulate that living wills can go into effect only when an individual is terminally ill. Some states further limit the living will by requiring the provision of fluids and nutrition, unless there is a specific statement in the living will of the wish to withhold fluids and nutrition.

HEALTH CARE PROXY

This is a legal document in which an individual designates another person to make health care decisions if he or she is rendered incapable of making his or her wishes known. The health care proxy has, in essence, the same rights to request or refuse treatment that the individual would have if capable of making and communicating decisions. It has the major advantage of being flexible, allowing the proxy to make different decisions as conditions change. An alternate proxy is generally included in the execution of the document in case the primary designee is not capable of fulfilling his or her role as proxy (e.g., death, incapacity). These are generally very simple forms to complete. In most states where they exist, they apply whenever the individual is incapacitated, not just when terminally ill.

DURABLE POWER OF ATTORNEY FOR HEALTH CARE

A number of states have provisions for a document called a durable power of attorney for health care. These are comparable in function to the health care proxy, in which an agent (and alternate agents) are appointed by the individual to make decisions on the individual's behalf in the event that he or she is no longer capable of doing so. A durable power of attorney for health care generally does not require an attorney to be carried out. It should be pointed out that this is different from a power of attorney that addresses legal and financial issues. A financial power of attorney would allow the designee to make bank transactions, sign Social Security checks, etc., whereas a durable power of attorney for health care applies only to health care decisions. Like a health care proxy, the durable power of attorney for health care is a flexible vehicle and generally applies even when there is no terminal illness.

DEFAULT SURROGATE CONSENT STATUTES

In the United States, four of every five adults have no advance directive. Thus, it is common for the situation to arise in which an individual is not capable of making his or her own health care decisions and there is no written advance directive. Some states allow for the validity of verbal statements in the absence of written documents. As of July 2004, 38 states had passed Default Surrogate Consent statutes. These statutes establish the right of certain individuals to act as surrogate health care decision makers in the event that a person is incapable of making health care decisions and has not executed an advanced directive. Each state's statute is different, but most establish a priority order for designation of the surrogate decision maker. The most common prioritization identifies the spouse as the primary surrogate with the following persons in decreasing priority order: adult child, parent, sibling, adult grandchild, and close friend. Some states make provisions for other persons including partners, health professionals, clergy, and beneficiaries, among others.

DO NOT ATTEMPT RESUSCITATION (DNAR) OR DO NOT RESUSCITATE (DNR) ORDER

Some states have a special advance directive that is called a Do Not Attempt Resuscitation (DNAR) or Do Not Resuscitate (DNR) Order. The nonhospital DNR is intended for emergency medical service (EMS) teams, who are usually required to provide every possible life-sustaining service. Even though families expecting a death are advised to call other sources for help when the patient worsens, a moment of uncertainty sometimes results in a 911 call and unwanted measures that prolong death. The nonhospital DNAR or nonhospital DNR Order offers a way for patients to refuse the full resuscitation effort even if EMS is called. It generally must be signed by both the patient and the doctor.

PSYCHIATRIC ADVANCE DIRECTIVE

A psychiatric advance directive is a document in which persons can describe the kind of mental health treatment they want to receive if they cannot make decisions for themselves in the future. This can include a person's wishes about medications, electroconvulsive treatment (ECT), or admission to a hospital. As of April 2005, 21 states had passed laws outlining provisions for psychiatric advance directives or health care power of attorneys for mental health treatment.

PRACTICAL CONSIDERATIONS

Encouraging patients to execute advance directives should constitute a routine component of providing health maintenance in primary care. The crisis situation is not the best time to begin discussions on the issue. It is far preferable to institute such discussions when there is ample time to allow for a full discussion of the issues between the patient and his or her family and friends and the physician. However, in a busy office practice there is not sufficient time to devote to an advance directive discussion with each patient. By adopting the readiness to change model (developed for counseling on smoking cessation), one can target the intervention at those who are ready for the discussion and not waste time in lengthy discussions with persons who are precontemplative (i.e., not ready to consider the issue). Simply asking the question, "Have you given any thought to how you want to be cared for near the end of life, if you could no longer speak for yourself?" can identify a patient's level of readiness to deal with the issues. For those who are precontemplative, make a brief statement that this an important issue to consider and provide them a patient information brochure. When the patient is ready (contemplative) then an office-based discussion is warranted. In the likely event that a patient does not complete a written advance directive, but is able to identify a preferred surrogate decision maker, this should be documented in the patient's chart. Depending on the quality of evidence required in a given state, such documentation may serve as sufficient evidence of a patient's wishes.

If patients have completed an advance directive, a copy should be kept with their other important documents and one copy should be placed in their medical record in their primary care physician's office. Providing a copy to any surrogate, proxy, or agent is also an important step. It should be noted that in most states an advance directive remains valid until revoked and that it can be revoked at any time. A lawyer is not necessary for the completion of an advance directive.

SUGGESTED READINGS

American Bar Association (ABA): The ABA provides a list of state and generally accepted advance directive forms at www.abanet.org/aging/

Basanta WE: Advance directives and life-sustaining treatment: a legal primer, *Hematol Oncol Clin North Am* 16(6):1381-1396, 2002.

Derse AR: Limitation of treatment at the end-of-life: withholding and withdrawal, *Clin Geriatr Med* 21(1):223-238, 2005.

Emanuel LL: Advance directives and advancing age, *J Am Geriatr Soc* 52(4):641-642, 2004.

Westley C, Briggs LA: Using the stages of change model to improve communication about advance care planning, *Nurs Forum* 39(3):5-12, 2004.

AUTHOR: **JOHN B. MURPHY, M.D.**

INTRODUCTION

Assisted living consists of non–nursing home residential long-term care settings licensed by states. There has been dramatic growth in the number of assisted living facilities in the past 15 years and it is estimated that there are currently as many as 50,000 assisted living facilities operating nationwide. It is further estimated that 1.3 million persons live in assisted living settings. There are a wide variety of designations including board and care, domiciliary care, adult foster care, sheltered housing, residential care, and congregate care. These facilities vary from small family-run settings operating out of a home to large campuses operated by national organizations. Table A1-1 lists names for a variety of different types of facilities and general characteristics of each class of facility.

SERVICES

Although the state definitions for assisted living facilities are very diverse and inconsistent, there are some similarities in the services offered in most facilities. Typical services include room and board; 24-hour supervision; housekeeping; maintenance and laundry services; some assistance with activities of daily living (ADL) and instrumental activities of daily living (IADL); limited medical services, often assistance with medications; and structured activities and recreation. Group home settings often serve residents with chronic mental illness or mental retardation and usually have staff-to-resident ratios that are higher than in other assisted living settings.

TARGET POPULATION

The population living in assisted living settings is diverse. Although this population has some overlap with nursing home populations, the assisted living population is less disabled. Common characteristics of the residents are a need for assistance with ADL and IADL, cognitive deficits, and generally less social support in the community.

FINANCING

Reimbursement for assisted living is largely out-of-pocket, but there are a growing number of states providing support through their Medicaid programs. Depending on the nature of an individual's health insurance program or long-term care insurance policy, costs may be reimbursed, but very few individuals have such coverage. Care in an assisted living facility is generally less expensive than in a nursing home but there is also usually less care provided. Regulations for assisted living are likely to be less stringent than in nursing homes, allowing for more efficient (not necessarily better) operations. Costs vary with the residence, room size, and the types of services needed by the residents. Across the nation, daily basic fees range from approximately $15 to $200—generally less than the cost of home health services and nursing home care. A basic assisted living fee may cover all services or there may be additional charges for special services. Most assisted living residences charge month-to-month rates, but a few residences require long-term arrangements.

PHYSICIAN'S ROLE IN ASSISTED LIVING SETTINGS

Most patients living in assisted living settings receive their medical care in physician offices and in most states there is no requirement that an assisted living facility have a medical director. The criteria for billing for physician home visits in an assisted living setting are the same as for persons living in private homes (e.g., homebound); however, the CPT codes are different and the payment level is currently lower than for home visits. If there is a medical office established in the assisted living setting the billing is based on outpatient billing codes not nursing home codes.

SUGGESTED READINGS

Eleazer P: Community based care. In Cobbs E, Duthie E, Murphy JB (eds): *Geriatric Review Syllabus,* ed 5, Malden, MA, 2003, Blackwell, pp 93-100.

The National Center for Assisted Living (NCAL): http://www.ncal.org/consumer/finding.htm

Sloane P, Boustani M: Institutional care. In Ham R, Sloane P, Warshaw G (eds): *Primary Care Geriatrics,* ed 4, St. Louis, 2002, Mosby, pp 199-215.

AUTHOR: **JOHN B. MURPHY, M.D.**

TABLE A1-1 Assisted Living Facilities and Their Characteristics

Names/Types of Facilities	Characteristics
Personal Care Homes Homes for Adults Board and Care Domiciliary Care Adult Foster Care Senior Group Homes	Facilities using these names tend to be smaller (fewer than 10 individuals) and less expensive. Many of these are in traditional homes in residential neighborhoods. Shared bathrooms, bedrooms, and living spaces are the norm.
Residential Care Facilities Assisted Living Facilities Adult Congregate Living	Facilities within this grouping tend to be larger, more expensive, and specifically designed to house the frail elderly or persons with disabilities, with an emphasis on independence and privacy. Most offer private rooms or apartments along with large common areas for activities and meals.
Continuing Care Retirement Communities Life Care Facilities	These are usually large complexes that offer a variety of options ranging from independent living to skilled-nursing home care. These facilities are specifically designed to provide lifetime care within one community. Facilities within this category tend to be the most expensive option.

INTRODUCTION

- Motor vehicle accidents among older drivers have been increasing steadily since 1980, particularly for those 85 and older.
- Motor vehicle injuries are the leading cause of injury-related death among those age 65 to 74 years and are second only to falls for those 75 to 84 years.
- The fatality rate per mile driven is higher for older drivers than any group aside from male drivers under 25.
- Older driver involvement in fatal crashes is expected to increase by 155% by 2030, accounting for 54% of the total projected increases in fatal crashes among all drivers.
- The responsibility for identifying impaired drivers increasingly falls to medical professionals.

ETIOLOGY

- Vision
  - Safe driving requires good visual acuity and adequate visual fields.
  - Impairments caused by conditions that increase in prevalence with age (e.g., macular degeneration, glaucoma, cataracts, stroke).
- Cognition
  - Safe driving requires adequate memory, attention, visual processing, and executive functioning.
  - Impairments caused by conditions that increase in prevalence with age (e.g., stroke, Alzheimer's dementia).
- Physical function
  - Safe driving requires adequate strength and flexibility as well as intact neurologic function (e.g., proprioception, reaction time).
  - Impairments caused by conditions that increase in prevalence with increasing age (e.g., rheumatologic conditions, peripheral neuropathies, stroke, deconditioning).

DIAGNOSIS

History—confirm with family member
- Motor vehicle accidents and moving violations
- Copilot phenomenon (physically able/cognitively impaired driver, directed by physically impaired/cognitively able passenger)
- Past medical conditions
  - Stroke
  - Diabetes (vision, peripheral neuropathy)
  - Macular degeneration, glaucoma, cataracts
  - Neurologic—stroke, TIA, dementia, seizures, neuropathy
- Medications—sedative-hypnotics, narcotic analgesics, sedating antidepressants, antihistamines, and alcohol

Physical
- Visual testing—acuity and visual field testing
- Cognitive assessment
  - Mini-Mental State Exam (memory and attention deficits)
  - Clock drawing (executive function)
- Functional assessment—musculoskeletal and neurologic exams

INTERVENTIONS

Reversible impairments:
- Stop/taper high-risk medications.
- Treat musculoskeletal and rheumatologic conditions.
- Physical therapy and exercise for deconditioning.
- Cataract removal and refraction.

Irreversible impairments:
- Possibly unsafe driver
  - Refer for driver simulator testing (if available).
  - Refer to agency specializing in road-testing older drivers.
  - Refer to motor vehicle department for routine road test.
- Clearly unsafe driver
  - Refer to motor vehicle department noting concern.

LEGAL ISSUES

Jurisdiction
- Dealt with on state level

Liability
- Some states mandate reporting.
- Case law suggests there is risk in not reporting patients who have impairments.
- Some states have statutes granting immunity to physicians who report in good faith.
- Where statutes do not exist case law suggests physicians are immune if they report in good faith.
- At the very least, instruct the patient (or family where appropriate) to stop driving and self-report to the registry of motor vehicles.

SUGGESTED READINGS

American Medical Association: Physician's guide to assessing and counseling older drivers, June 2003: www.ama-assn.org/go/olderdrivers

Freund B et al: Clock drawing and driving cars, *J Gen Intern Med* 20:240-244, 2005.

Grabowski D, Campbell AB, Morrisey MA: Elderly licensure laws and motor vehicle fatalities, *JAMA* 291:2840-2846, 2004.

Hogan DB: Which older patients are competent to drive? *Can Fam Physician* 51:362-368, 2005.

AUTHOR: **JOHN B. MURPHY, M.D.**

INTRODUCTION

When physicians prescribe home care services for Medicare beneficiaries, they must certify that the patient is (1) homebound; (2) in need of intermittent skilled nursing care or physical, speech, or occupational therapy; and (3) under the physician's ongoing care. By signing a standard authorization form approved for home care services by the Centers for Medicare & Medicaid Services (CMS), the physician verifies that the patient has met the three eligibility criteria and that the physician will review the home care plan periodically but no less than every 2 months and recertify the patient if appropriate. Even though physicians may not have firsthand knowledge that the home care services they prescribe are appropriate and necessary, prescribers of home care need to know that the federal government's position is that "when a physician signs a Medicare certification form, there is an implied representation that all the rules are complied with." In fact, the official form for the home care plan contains a statement that "misrepresentation, falsification or information concealment may be subject to fine, imprisonment or civil penalty."

The eligibility criteria for home care are stringent because the intent of the Medicare program is generally to cover acute care rather than long-term care or preventive care. However, the clinical reality for many patients is that their chronic conditions exacerbate and improve over time, causing them to shift in and out of home care eligibility. These changes in condition complicate the physician's role in determining patients' eligibility for home care services covered by Medicare. This topic discusses the role of the physician in authorizing and monitoring home care services given CMS regulations.

THE HOMEBOUND CRITERIA

If the federal Medicare program defined home confinement literally, patients who visit doctors in their offices while receiving home care would not be, strictly speaking, confined to their home. Fortunately, CMS does not define home confinement literally. Currently, patients need not be bedridden, but "there should exist a normal inability to leave home and leaving their homes would require a considerable and taxing effort." For practical purposes, Medicare considers patients homebound if they lack the ability to leave their place of residence independently; however, such patients may leave their home with the aid of assistive devices (e.g., canes, crutches, walkers, wheelchairs), special transportation (e.g., ambulance, van), or another person (e.g., family member). Still, not all patients who use canes are eligible for home care. Medicare also expects that absences from the home be infrequent or relatively short in duration (e.g., a trip to the hairdresser or to church), and that in most instances absences from the home be for the purpose of medical treatment. Patients may also be considered homebound if leaving the home is medically contraindicated.

The criteria for home confinement are rather subjective. Therefore, how physicians, home care agencies, patients, and CMS define home confinement may differ. For example, in a review of claims for home care in New York and Texas, CMS found that 40% of the claims were improperly billed, with the majority of improper billings resulting from patients failing to meet home confinement criteria. Box A1-1 lists clinical situations that would qualify patients for meeting the Medicare criteria for home confinement.

SKILLED SERVICES REQUIREMENT

A frail person who is homebound is not considered eligible for home care unless criteria for intermittent skilled care are also met. The criteria for skilled care are even more ambiguous than those for home confinement. Skilled care is care that must be provided by a registered nurse, or physical, occupational, or speech therapist. However, just because a service is provided by

one of these health professionals does not necessarily mean the service is a skilled service. To be considered a skilled service, a nurse must be required to provide it because of "its complexity" and "the patient condition." The service must also meet "accepted standards of medical and nursing practice." A diagnosis alone is rarely adequate documentation of the need for skilled services. Rather, the relation between a patient's diagnosis, symptoms, and functional status must justify the complexity of services. In addition, the need for skilled services must be intermittent, meaning that the services are required less frequently than 7 days per week, but at least once every 60 days.

CMS provides a list of examples that do and do not meet this requirement (Table A1-2). The documentation in the medical record should describe the patient's condition and the complexity of required services and include an assessment of the risk of complications or deterioration should such skilled services become unavailable. These same principles of medical documentation apply for physical, occupational, and speech therapy.

THE PHYSICIAN AS GATEKEEPER

The home care gatekeeping role may be appropriate for primary care physicians in many cases. However, nurses, therapists, or social workers may sometimes be better suited to determine home care eligibility because of the nature of the patient's condition or because, unlike physicians, they routinely make house calls.

Without firsthand knowledge of the patient's homebound status, physicians should not certify the patient in a perfunctory manner as confined to home. Physicians should take the time to assess the patient's functional status and need for skilled services before prescribing home care services. In some cases, the physician who prescribes home care has no doubt that the patient meets the Medicare criteria for home confinement. Examples include a patient with a dense hemiparesis, a patient with advanced dementia, or a patient who recently underwent major surgery. These patients are incapable of leaving their home independently or have a medical contraindication to do so; if they have a need for intermittent skilled care, they meet the Medicare criteria for in-home care.

For many patients, however, physicians may not know whether they are eligible to be certified for home care. For example, a diabetic patient with a foot ulcer who is capable of driving her car may benefit greatly from home care for wound

---

BOX A1-1 Examples of Homebound Cases According to Medicare Criteria

1. Restricted mobility from a disease process such as unsteady gait, draining wounds, or pain.
2. Poor cardiac reserve, shortness of breath, or activity intolerance as a result of an unstable or exacerbated disease process.
3. Bed- or wheelchair-bound patients who require physical assistance to move any distance.
4. Patients who require caregiver help with assistive devices such as a cane, walker, wheelchair, or other special device to leave home.
5. A tracheostomy, abdominal drains, colostomy, Foley catheter, or nasogastric tube that restricts ambulation.
6. Psychotic ideation, confusion, or impaired mental status that restricts functional abilities outside the home.
7. Fluctuating blood pressures or blood sugar levels that may cause syncope.
8. Patients who cannot ambulate stairs or uneven surfaces without assistance of caregiver.
9. Postoperative patients for whom the physician has restricted patient activity.
10. Patients who are legally blind or cannot drive.

management and diabetic teaching by a visiting nurse, but her physician knows or should know that she is able to drive to her doctor's office to receive the wound care and teaching. She is not eligible for home care services. Patients who need physical therapy or daily monitoring of vital signs following hospital discharge may not meet the eligibility criteria for home confinement if they can travel independently to their doctor's office or to a rehabilitation facility. Yet, physicians prescribe home care in such situations without much afterthought because wound care, diabetic teaching, gait training, and blood pressure checks are performed by nurses or physical or occupational therapists. In each of these cases, for the patient to receive outpatient nursing care, usually available only through home care agencies, the office-based primary care physician who does not employ a nurse will prescribe home care and certify that patient as home confined, which may be a misrepresentation of the patient's status.

Thus physicians are sometimes placed in conflicting roles as advocates for their patients and as gatekeepers for CMS eligibility criteria for home care. This conflict is even more pronounced when patients have chronic conditions such as congestive heart failure or chronic obstructive pulmonary disease and only meet criteria for skilled services during episodes of exacerbation. Yet, in-home services for those conditions have been shown to reduce exacerbations and hospitalizations.

Physicians should always pay sufficient attention to home care certification and plan-of-care forms completed by home care agency staff and mailed to physicians for signature. Physicians should not rely solely on the recertification plan-of-care forms sent to them as the forms may not contain adequate information about the patient's functional status and condition. Physicians should demand that these forms document not only patients' current needs for skilled care, but also the reasons for their homebound status. Copies of these forms should be entered into the medical record and used to justify the in-home skilled services provided. Physicians also should not allow long periods to go by (e.g., 6 months for a stable patient) without seeing patients who receive home care services; this may require house calls for some patients. Patients whose chronic diseases are unstable (e.g., those with cardiopulmonary conditions) may require more frequent updates, not only to provide good care, but also to verify that they remain eligible for needed home care services. Inability to carry out activities of daily life, cognitive impairment, and urinary incontinence correlate with the need of in-home services. Given that an assessment of functional status is an integral component of geriatric care, the medical record can and should contain up-to-date functional assessments that can be used to justify patients' home confinement and need for skilled services.

SUGGESTED READING

Wachtel TJ, Gifford DR: Eligibility for home care certification: the doctor's job? *J Gen Intern Med* 13:705-709, 1998.

AUTHOR: **TOM J. WACHTEL, M.D.**

TABLE A1-2　Clinical Vignettes Related to Medicare Home Care Eligibility Criteria

Vignette	Home Confined	Skilled Care Need	Meets Medicare Eligibility Criteria
Patient with unsteady gait who requires assistance for ambulation and whose blood pressure is 190/110	Yes	Yes	Yes
Patient with a dense hemiparesis who is bed- or chairbound and who has a pressure ulcer	Yes	Yes	Yes
Patient with severe peripheral neuropathy and blindness who is wheelchair dependent for mobility and whose diabetes is well controlled with insulin	Yes	No	No
Patient with advanced Alzheimer's dementia, incontinent of urine, and living in his daughter's home. No other medical problem.	Yes	No	No
Patient with a draining venous ulcer who is able to walk and drive her car independently	No	Yes	No
Patient with severe emphysema and cor pulmonale who is ambulatory and stable on home oxygen therapy and medication	No	No	No

INTRODUCTION

Hospice is a term that is used for a number of entities and activities. Hospice is a benefit offered by Medicare, most Medicaid programs, and many private insurers. Hospice refers to palliative care provided near the end of life and to a physical place where end of life care is provided. For the purpose of this discussion the focus will be on the Medicare benefit and the services provided under the Medicare hospice benefit. In 1983, Congress enacted the hospice benefit within the Medicare program. Because of an aging of the population, a greater understanding of the place of palliative care in the continuum of care, and growth in the number and quality of hospice organizations, there has been considerable growth in the number of persons enrolled in hospice since the inception of the benefit. That growth has been most dramatic in the past 10 years, which has seen annual hospice admissions rise from 200,000 to almost 1,000,000. Under Medicare, hospice is a program of care delivered by a Medicare-approved hospice. Reasonable and necessary medical and support services for the management of a terminal illness are furnished under a plan-of-care established by the beneficiary's attending physician and the hospice team. Over 90% of services are provided in the beneficiaries' homes. Respite and general inpatient services are also provided when socially or medically necessary. Although most physicians think of hospice and palliation with cancer diagnoses, many other conditions are also appropriate for hospice care. National data show that 50.5% of hospice patients die from cancer. The top five noncancer diagnoses are end-stage heart disease, dementia, lung disease, end-stage kidney disease, and end-stage liver disease. The common thread is that their physicians feel the patients are unlikely to survive more than 6 months if their disease runs its natural course. National data also suggest that the referral to hospice is often much later in the course of an illness than is appropriate.

ELIGIBILITY

Hospice care is available under Medicare in the following circumstances:

- The patient is eligible for Medicare Hospital Insurance (Part A).
- The patient's doctor and the hospice medical director certify that the patient is terminally ill with 6 months or less to live if the disease runs its expected course.
- The patient signs a statement choosing hospice care instead of standard Medicare benefits for the terminal illness.
- The patient receives care from a Medicare-approved hospice program.

Hospice care is a benefit under the hospital insurance program. To be eligible to elect hospice care under Medicare, an individual must be entitled to Part A of Medicare and be certified as being terminally ill. An individual is considered terminally ill if the medical prognosis is that the individual's life expectancy is 6 months or less if the illness runs its normal course. Section §1814(a)(7) of the Social Security Act specifies that certification of terminal illness for hospice benefits shall be based on the clinical judgment of the hospice physician and the individual's attending physician (if he or she has one) or the medical director regarding the normal course of the individual's illness. Once a patient enters a hospice program the first certification is for 90 days. The first recertification is also for 90 days, and all subsequent recertifications are for 60 days. Recertifications require only a single physician signature. A physician can discharge a patient from a hospice program, and patients can revoke or transfer hospice programs at any time. Predicting of life expectancy is not always exact. The fact that a beneficiary lives longer than expected in itself is not cause to terminate benefits.

Once the initial election is processed, the beneficiary remains in hospice status until death or until the patient elects to terminate hospice. While on hospice an individual must waive all rights to Medicare payments for the duration of the election of hospice care for the following services:

- Hospice care provided by a hospice other than the hospice designated by the individual (unless provided under arrangements made by the designated hospice)
- Any Medicare services that are related to the treatment of the terminal condition for which hospice care was elected or a related condition or services that are equivalent to hospice care, except for services provided by:
  - The designated hospice (either directly or under arrangement)
  - Another hospice under arrangements made by the designated hospice
  - The individual's attending physician, if that physician is not an employee of the designated hospice or receiving compensation from the hospice for those services

Medicare services for a condition completely unrelated to the terminal condition for which hospice was elected remain available to the patient if he or she is eligible for such care.

COVERED SERVICES

Once enrolled in a hospice, the hospice is financially responsible for all diagnostic and therapeutic services related to the terminal disease. This may include palliative treatments, medications, therapies, and any respite or medically related admissions. For conditions totally unrelated to the hospice diagnosis, a patient can be admitted to a hospital, treated at an outpatient facility, or cared for at a physician's office under traditional Medicare.

Medicare covers:

- Physicians' services
- Nursing care (intermittent with 24-hour on call)
- Medical appliances and supplies related to the terminal illness
- Outpatient drugs for symptom management and pain relief
- Short-term acute inpatient care, including respite care,
- Home health aide and homemaker services
- Physical therapy, occupational therapy, and speech/language pathology services
- Medical social services
- Counseling, including dietary and spiritual counseling
- Bereavement services

It should be noted that these services are provided as part of symptom control or to enable the individual to maintain activities of daily living and basic functional skills and not as part of a curative care plan.

There are four levels of hospice care

- Routine home care
- Continuous home care
- Respite care
- General inpatient care

Routine home care is provided as medically necessary and involves at least nursing care and social service with overall direction by a hospice medical director. The frequency and intensity of service depend on medical needs, but usually increase over time. Continuous home care is 8 or more hours daily, provided to a patient in crisis, with at least 50% of that care performed by licensed nurses. Respite care involves admission to an institution (skilled nursing facility [SNF] or other) for up to 5 days when needed to allow the family a temporary break from their caregiving duties. General inpatient care (GIP) is provided by the hospice under contract with a facility (SNF or other) and is for short-term provision of intensive, aggressive management of acute symptoms, which cannot be provided in another setting. In addition, GIP may be provided when a beneficiary's home support system has acutely deteriorated, and short-term placement is required while arranging a more permanent placement option. Nursing home residents are eligible for hospice within their long-term care facility under the same eligibility criteria described previously.

PHYSICIAN'S ROLE IN HOSPICE

The hospice medical director provides administrative and general oversight of the program. The patient's hospice attending physician (who can also be the medical director) is reimbursed for all hands-on care. If the attending physician is salaried by the hospice, the hospice bills Part A. If the attending physician is not employed by the hospice, the Part B carrier is billed using regular evaluation and management (E & M) codes with the modifier GV (not employed by hospice). The attending physician is listed in the Medicare common working file. Physicians covering for the attending physician should use locum tenens rules (modifier GV with Q5 or Q6 as appropriate). For non-hospice-related conditions and services, the physician uses regular E & M codes plus the modifier GW (service not related to the hospice patient's terminal condition). The primary medical attending physician continues to bill Medicare directly for services and may bill under comprehensive procedural technology (CPT) code 99375 for phone management of the hospice patient if it exceeds 30 minutes per month. Consultations (e.g., with an oncologist) related to the terminal illness must be paid for by the hospice and require prior authorization by the hospice program. Unauthorized testing or treatment for the terminal illness is not covered by Medicare and becomes the patient's responsibility. Treatment of disease unrelated to the terminal illness may be independently covered by Medicare, including reimbursement of attending and consulting physician fees. This is more likely to occur for the patient who enrolls in hospice early in the course of his or her illness.

SUGGESTED READINGS

Fried T et al: Older persons' preferences for site of terminal care, *Ann Intern Med* 131:109-112, 1999.

Lorenz K, Lynn J: Care of the dying patient. In Hazzard W et al: *Principles of Geriatric Medicine and Gerontology,* ed 5, New York, 2003, McGraw-Hill, pp 323-334.

Pinderhughes S, Morrison R: Palliative care. In Cobbs E, Duthie E, Murphy JB (eds): *Geriatric Review Syllabus,* ed 5, Malden, MA, 2003, Blackwell, pp 105-115.

Potash J, Horst P: Palliative care at the end of life. In Ham R, Sloane P, Warshaw G (eds): *Primary Care Geriatrics,* ed 4, St. Louis, 2002, Mosby, pp 229-242.

AUTHOR: **JOHN B. MURPHY, M.D.**

INTRODUCTION

A growing number of people in the U.S. are homebound. Some live at home; others live in congregate housing arrangements such as elderly housing, independent living, assisting living, boarding houses, and group homes.

House calls refer to the provision of physician services to patients in their home. House calls are generally provided in lieu of office-based medical care for selected patients. This care may be delivered as part of an interdisciplinary care team, as in home health care following a hospitalization, but more commonly as ongoing care to patients who are homebound. House calls can also be exceptionally helpful in providing the physician with a better understanding of the patient's home situation. This type of "diagnostic house call" can provide information about caregiver burnout, elder mistreatment, use of medications that the primary physician is not aware of, and alcohol abuse. It can also be helpful when the treatment plan is unexpectedly not effective. For a house call program to be effective and financially viable it is imperative that the program be well planned. Current regulations allow for reimbursement to physicians, nurse practitioners, and physician assistants, but involvement of other health care services (e.g., laboratory and visiting nurses services) is essential. Choosing the right patients is also of paramount importance.

Strictly speaking, no one is homebound. There is always a way to bring a homebound person to the hospital or to a physician's office. However, except in the case of a medical emergency, transportation by ambulance is not covered by most health insurance plans, and ambulance trips cost several hundred dollars.

The definition of *homebound* that applies to the Centers for Medicare & Medicaid Services (CMS) eligibility criteria for formal home care (see Home Care in Appendix 1) does not concern house calls by physicians/practitioners. Many physicians who perform house calls use stricter criteria because their offices are better equipped to provide care than patients' homes. Therefore, a patient who is unable to leave his or her home unassisted because of dementia but has a relative who can provide transportation to the doctor's office may not be a suitable candidate for house calls, although the CMS criterion for homebound is met.

For practical purposes, a homebound person can be defined as someone who cannot leave the home, transiently (e.g., after surgery) or permanently, using personal or other resources readily available in the community (e.g., friends, relatives, taxi service, senior citizens' transportation, public transportation). Such a person should receive health services at home.

Some programs are designed to provide multidisciplinary geriatric assessments with patients' homes. There are no Medicare CPT reimbursement codes to pay providers for such service; therefore, the provision of care by a single provider is described.

THE HOUSE CALL

Most first visits at home are scheduled well in advance. Therefore, it is almost always possible for the informal caregiver (most frequently the patient's daughter) to be present during the visit. Even when a family provides care in shifts, arrangement can be made for a key member of the informal caregiving team to be present. When the patient's condition requires substantial nursing services (e.g., a patient with an active pressure ulcer), every effort should be made for the visiting nurse to be present during the visit; this will enable the whole team to discuss the plan of care.

Taking a history in the patient's home is no different in its content than a history taken in the office, but because it is done on the patient's turf, often over coffee and muffins, the interaction tends to be less formal. Permission should be requested to inspect the living quarters. What does the home look like? Is it clean? Is it orderly? Can the patient get around, go to the kitchen, go to the bathroom? Is the environment safe? Are there loose rugs, nightlights, rails in the bathroom? An office visit, no matter how comprehensive, cannot provide a complete understanding of the patient's daily routine. The cabinet or drawer that contains the medications should be inspected. Outdated and discontinued medications should be discarded immediately. The refrigerator and food cupboards should also be checked, especially when the homebound patient depends on others for his or her food supply. Aside from appearance, what does the home smell like? Incontinence may be immediately detected. Many elderly patients are reluctant to report incontinence in the office. It is more difficult to hide during a house call.

Observing the interaction between caregivers and patients is also a precious source of information. In the office, patients and families are generally on their best behavior and outbursts are unlikely to occur. In the home setting, people are less inhibited, even in the presence of the physician. Therefore, they are more likely to display their usual pattern of interaction. Moreover, the request for a house call is often placed at a time of crisis. Most often, the crisis is not a new medical problem but rather an exhausted caregiver who needs support or respite.

Although the goal of a house call will certainly vary, like any physician-patient interaction, the content of a home visit should include a number of staple items (Table A1-3). Because most candidates for home care are frail or disabled, a functional assessment should always be performed. This includes gathering information on physical function, such as activities of daily living (ADL), instrumental activities of daily living (IADL), mobility, and continence; social and role function, such as visits by friends and relatives, and interest in sexual activity; and mental function, such as cognition and affect. Unlike the office setting, where such assessment must be done formally by asking specific questions, much of this information can be collected by simple observation during a home visit. A more complete checklist describing the relation between the patient and the home environment is presented in Fig. A1-1.

Asking homebound elderly patients to discuss ethical issues such as care intensity should be a routine practice. In the hospital, a common and important question is whether to resuscitate. At home the equivalent issue is whether to hospitalize. Whatever decision is made, it is entered into the patient's record. Equally important is the question of surrogate decision makers. Competent patients are routinely requested to think about designating someone who will have durable power of attorney for medical decisions. This is also entered into the medical record.

Homebound patients and their informal caregivers should be given a list of community resources.

The physical exam is often less complete at home than in the office or at the hospital. Although technically feasible, a pelvic exam for cancer screening may not be indicated in an elderly patient with Alzheimer's dementia. Although a bimanual exam is possible, expecting to visualize a cervix with an elderly patient lying in a regular bed is unreasonable. Most patients who receive care at home do not expect the same comprehensive services routinely provided to ambulatory patients; nonetheless, it is best to be explicit and explain to patients the medical goals. Blood and urine tests and an occasional ECG can be obtained as readily in the home as in the office (or community-based laboratories). Portable x-rays can be obtained at great expense and poor quality. Typically, a situation that calls for x-rays or other diagnostic procedures requires evaluation in a hospital.

LOGISTICS AND TIME MANAGEMENT

The logistics of house calls may explain why many physicians, busy with their office and hospital work, find house calls an inefficient use of their time. There is obviously some validity to this argument. However, steps can be taken to reduce travel time. The physician with a substantial number of homebound patients can arrange to make routine visits to a cluster of patients who live in the same neighborhood. The fact that older members of our society tend to congregate in elderly housing makes clustering easy to accomplish. A photocopy of a map illustrating the location of the patient's home is placed in front of the patient's chart.

Except for first encounters, two to four house calls can be scheduled per hour when several visits are arranged in the same apartment building or neighborhood. In addition, routine house calls can be made to replace idle time caused by cancellations in the office. This can actually improve the efficiency of a geriatric practice (e.g., during bad weather).

House calls for urgent problems (e.g., a fever) may be impossible to plan in a physician's schedule. Urgent visits can be made at the end of the day on the way home from work. However, it should be made clear to homebound patients that emergencies cannot always be dealt with in the home. The willingness to make house calls should not eliminate use of traditional emergency services when necessary.

Physicians and practitioners who make house calls should specify the conditions under which they will provide this service. For example:

- Patients are eligible for the house calls program if they live within a 15-minute drive and are unable to leave their home.
- Scheduled visits are made every 3 to 4 months. A half-day of a physician's schedule per month may be reserved for these visits, and patients are also seen during last-minute unfilled cancellations in the ambulatory practice schedule. Unscheduled visits are made for more urgent problems at the request of the patient, a family member, or a home care nurse.
- On enrollment, patients and their caregivers should be given an information sheet stating that although efforts will be made to see patients with acute problems, the practice cannot guarantee the ability to make emergency visits and cannot provide home visits at night or during weekends.

Physicians and practitioners who provide house calls should have a tool kit ("doctor's bag") with the following equipment:

Basic Supplies
- Gloves
- Sphygmomanometer
- Oto-ophthalmoscope
- Stethoscope
- Thermometer
- Lubricating jelly
- Stool guaiac cards and developer
- Toenail clippers
- Ear syringe and/or cerumen curette
- Tongue depressors
- Hand disinfectant/wash
- Scale (in patient's home)
- Prescription pad
- Patient chart with directions
- Local street map
- Cell phone
- Dictaphone

Additional Advisable Supplies
- Voice amplifier
- Foley catheter
- Wound debridement kit
- Wound dressing materials
- Specimen cups
- Portable scale pulse oximeter
- Lancets and Glucometer with alcohol pads, 2x2 gauze, and bandages
- Urine dipsticks
- Peak flow meter

Supplies for Special Circumstances
- Punch biopsy kit
- Excisional biopsy kit
- Suture/staple removal kit

The chronic conditions that physicians can expect to manage during house calls are the same as those seen in the office for an age-matched population with a bias toward conditions that impair mobility such as dementia, post stroke, severe arthritis, and severe CHF and COPD.

Acute illnesses include the following:
- Infections, mostly respiratory and urinary
- Exacerbation of CHF or COPD
- Syncope
- Falls
- Delirium
- Wounds (pressure ulcers, venous ulcers, arterial ulcers, diabetic ulcers)
- Gastroenteritis and abdominal pain
- Acute musculoskeletal problems (injuries, arthralgia)
- Acute and chronic pain
- Failure to thrive
- End-of-life care

TABLE A1-3   Problems to Address during a Geriatric Home Visit

Safety
Household risks (e.g., loose rugs, nightlights, bathroom rails)
Security
Appliances, fire alarm
Dirt, dust, humidity
Access to telephone or other means of calling for help

Psychosocial Situation
Mental status
Affect (rule out depression)
Support (family, friends, rule out loneliness)
Financial resources

Ethical Issues
Intensity of care (especially terminal care)
Decision to (not to) hospitalize
Surrogate decision maker (durable power of attorney) or living will

Functional Status
Activities of daily living (ADL)
Instrumental activities of daily living (IADL)
Mobility
Vision and hearing assessment

Continence
Urine and stool

Nutrition
Availability of food
Ability to prepare and eat meals
Alcoholism

Medical Problems
Tertiary prevention (diagnose, treat, and monitor chronic diseases)
Primary prevention (vaccination, hygiene)
Diagnose and treat acute illness
Prognosis
Skin care, foot care

Primary Care
Access and availability of care
Coordination of team of health care professionals
Continuity of care

1. Type of dwelling   ( ) House   ( ) Apartment

2. Previous living situation   ( ) House   ( ) Apartment

3. Who lives at the residence: Name(s), Relation(s) _____
   ( ) Completely alone   ( ) Alone part of the day   ( ) Rarely/never alone

4. Stairs   ( ) None (or ramp)   ( ) Stairs to main floor   ( ) Stairs to upstairs

5. Mobility   ( ) Ambulatory without care   ( ) Ambulatory with care   ( ) Ambulatory with walker
   ( ) Chair bound   ( ) Bed bound

6. ADL

7. IADL

8. Function in the home (I, independent; A, assistance required; D, dependent; NA, not applicable)

A. General Obstacle Negotiation

	I	A	D	NA
Elevator				
Stairs				
Ramp				
Uneven terrain				
Thresholds				
Through doorways				
Can patient escape safely (e.g., fire)				

NOTE: Stair covering and railing, smoke alarms, emergency exits, extension cords

B. Entrance

	I	A	D	NA
Driveway				
Walkway				
Landing				
Unlock door				
Open door				
Access mail				

NOTE: Lighting, obstacles

C. Living/Family Room

	I	A	D	NA
Ability to maneuver through room				
Ability to transfer on/off chairs				
Ability to manage TV				
Ability to reach and use phone				

NOTE: Lighting, floors, emergency numbers by phone

D. Kitchen

	I	A	D	NA
Ability to maneuver through room				
Ability to use table and chair				
Ability to reach shelves/cabinet				
Ability to use appliances (refrigerator, stove, sink)				
Ability to prepare meals				

NOTE: Lighting, floors, reachability of utensils/dishes/food; the quantity and quality of the food

E. Bathroom

	I	A	D	NA
Ability to maneuver to and through room				
Ability to transfer on/off toilet				
Ability to transfer in/out of tub or shower				
Ability to reach sink, faucet, grooming supplies				

NOTE: Lighting (also between bedroom and bathroom); obstacles; nonskid surface (tub and shower); tub and shower bench; tub, shower or toilet rails; hot water temperature

F. Bedroom

	I	A	D	NA
Ability to maneuver to and through room				
Ability to transfer in/out of bed				
Ability to reach phone				
Ability to reach light switch				
Ability to use closets and drawers				

NOTE: Lighting, obstacles

G. Medications

	I	A	D	NA
Ability to identify medication				
Ability to follow instructions				
Ability to open containers				

NOTE: What medications are found; outdated, no longer prescribed?

FIGURE A1-1 Checklist for the traditional home evaluation. (From Ferri F, Fretwell MD, Wachtel TJ: *Practical Guide to Care of the Geriatric Patient*, ed 2, St. Louis, 1997, Mosby.)

PAYMENT FOR HOUSE CALLS

- Home visits (includes senior housing and independent living)
  - New patient CPT codes: 99341, 99342, 99343, 99344, 99345. The documentation requirements for these codes are similar to office-based new patient evaluation and management (E&M).
  - Established patient CPT codes: 99347, 99348, 99349, 99350; also similar to office visit codes (Table A1-4).
- Domicilliary visits (include assisted living and group homes)
  - New patient CPT codes: 99321, 99222, 99323. The documentation requirement for 99321 is a problem-focused history and examination and low-complexity decision making. For 99322, it is expanded problem-focused history and examination and moderate-complexity decision making. For 99323, it is detailed history and high-complexity decision making.
  - Established patient CPT codes 99331, 99332, and 99333 with the same documentation requirements as for follow-up nursing home patients.

- In addition, CMS pays physicians for overseeing the work done by home care agencies. The CPT codes for these services are:
  - G0180 certification for home care
  - G0179 recertification for home care
  - G0181 care plan overnight for home care (requires at least 30 minutes per month and ability to document the time spent)
  - G0182 care plan oversight for hospice (same time requirements)

SUGGESTED READINGS

American Academy of Home Care Physicians: Executive summary, public policy statement, 2005.

Boling P, Abbey L, Keenan J: Home care. In Ham R, Sloane P, Warshaw G (eds): *Primary Care Geriatrics,* ed 4, St. Louis, 2002, Mosby, pp 217-228.

Eleazer P: Community based care. In Cobbs E, Duthie E, Murphy JB (eds): *Geriatric Review Syllabus,* ed 5, Malden, MA, 2003, Blackwell.

Unwin B, Jerant A: The home visit, *Am Fam Physician* 60:1481-1488, 1999.

AUTHORS: **TOM J. WACHTEL, M.D.,** and **JOHN B. MURPHY, M.D.**

TABLE A1-4 CPT Codes and Approximate 2004 Medicare Allowable Charges

Code	Visit Type	2004 Medicare Allowable Charges (before geographic adjustments)
99341	New patient, low severity	$57.87
99342	New patient, moderate severity	$84.38
99343	New patient, moderate to high severity	$123.21
99344	New patient, high severity	$161.67
99345	New patient, unstable	$200.13
99347	Established patient, minor	$44.43
99348	Established patient, low to moderate severity	$75.42
99349	Established patient, moderate to high severity	$116.86
99350	Established patient, high severity	$169.89

INTRODUCTION

1. Definitions and Concepts
   a. Life expectancy is defined as the average length of life expected for a population of individuals of a given age. Life expectancy, not otherwise specified, is calculated from birth. Age-specific life expectancy is calculated for a group of individuals of a specific age.
   b. U.S. life expectancies based on the 2000 census are presented in Table A1-5.
   c. The calculation of life expectancy is based on the age configuration of the population at the time that a census is taken; therefore life expectancies are calculated as if an individual were able to live every year of his or her life in the present state of population mortality. This, of course, is not true; the younger a person is, the more likely to benefit from advances in community health and medical progress or be penalized by changes in morbidity prevalence (e.g., obesity) or other social calamities such as war.
   d. As people age, the differences between men and women or between African Americans and Caucasians attenuate.
   e. Maximum life span is defined as the length of the longest-lived members of a species. The longest recorded human life is 122 years (a French woman). Current research suggests that average human life span in the absence of premature death from disease or trauma approximates 85 years with a standard deviation of 4 to 5 years. Biotechnology may alter these statistics in the future.
   f. Life span is species-specific and is believed to be genetically determined; an almost perfect correlation exists between maximum cell doublings in tissue culture for a given species and the life span for that species. Therefore, it should not be surprising to find longevity running in certain families. However, the mechanism of aging (senescence) has not been identified; and although theories abound (e.g., accumulation of oxygen free radicals, growth hormone deficit), most interventions to correct them (e.g., antioxidants, growth hormone) have not been proven to be effective fountains of youth. The only promising means to increase longevity to date are food restriction (works in rats) and lowering body temperature (works in hamsters).
   g. Current thinking attributes the limit on life span to a progressive decline in organ reserve that begins for humans at age 20 to 30. Reserve function is needed to respond to lifetime stress. When reserve function has declined to about 20% above basal levels, routine daily perturbations cannot be overcome, homeostasis cannot be maintained, and death will occur with minor illnesses or trauma that would be trivial for vigorous individuals.

2. Compression of mortality (and morbidity) and the rectangularization of the population survival curve (Fig. A1-2)
   a. Although human life span has not varied during the past millenary, human life expectancy has increased dramatically. For example, life expectancy from birth in the United States in 1900 was 47 years; and in 2002 it was 77.3 years. This gain can be attributed to improvement in infant mortality and primary preventive measures such as sanitation and immunization. Progress in and increased access to medical care can also take some credit for the gains in life expectancy.
   b. The combination of a finite limit on life span and an increase in life expectancy results in more individuals achieving their maximum life potential of 85 ± 5 years in the population. This trend is demonstrated graphically by a narrowing bell-shaped curve of the number of deaths (Fig. A1-2, B).

TABLE A1-5 Life Expectancy by Race, Sex, and Age: U.S. 2002*

Age	ALL RACES			WHITE			BLACK		
	Total	Male	Female	Total	Male	Female	Total	Male	Female
0	77.3	74.5	79.9	77.7	75.1	80.3	72.3	68.8	75.6
1	76.8	74.1	79.4	77.2	74.6	79.7	72.4	68.8	75.6
5	72.9	70.2	75.4	73.3	70.7	75.8	68.5	65.0	71.7
10	67.9	65.3	70.5	68.3	65.7	70.8	63.6	60.1	66.8
15	63.0	60.3	65.5	63.4	60.8	65.9	58.7	55.2	61.8
20	58.2	55.6	60.7	58.6	56.1	61.0	53.9	50.5	57.0
25	53.5	51.0	55.8	53.8	51.4	56.1	49.3	46.0	52.1
30	48.7	46.3	51.0	49.0	46.7	51.2	44.7	41.6	47.4
35	44.0	41.6	46.1	44.3	42.0	46.4	40.1	37.1	42.7
40	39.3	37.0	41.4	39.6	37.4	41.6	35.6	32.8	38.1
45	34.8	32.6	36.7	35.0	32.9	36.9	31.3	28.5	33.7
50	30.3	28.3	32.2	30.5	28.5	32.4	27.3	24.6	29.5
55	26.1	24.1	27.7	26.2	24.3	27.9	23.4	21.0	25.4
60	22.0	20.2	23.5	22.1	20.3	23.6	19.9	17.6	21.6
65	18.2	16.6	19.5	18.2	16.6	19.5	16.6	14.6	18.0
70	14.7	13.2	15.8	14.7	13.3	15.8	13.5	11.8	14.7
75	11.5	10.3	12.4	11.5	10.3	12.3	10.9	9.5	11.7
80	8.8	7.8	9.4	8.7	7.7	9.3	8.6	7.5	9.2
85	6.5	5.7	6.9	6.4	5.7	6.8	6.6	5.8	7.0
90	4.8	4.2	5.0	4.7	4.1	4.9	5.1	4.5	5.3
95	3.6	3.2	3.7	3.4	3.0	3.5	3.9	3.6	4.0
100	2.7	2.5	2.8	2.4	2.3	2.5	3.0	2.9	3.0

Source: National Vital Statistics Reports, Vol. 53, No. 6, November 10, 2004.
*Race categories are consistent with the 1977 Office of Management and Budget guidelines.

3. Future Trends
   a. The rectangularization of population survival, the compression of morbidity, and the compression of senescence are predicated on the hypothesis of a finite limit of organ reserve (Fig. A1-3, *A*). As stated by Fries, "As the organ reserve decreases so does the ability to restore homeostasis, and eventually even the smallest perturbation prevents homeostasis to be restored. The inevitable result is natu-

   ral death, even without disease" or after a short acute illness (e.g., pneumonia).
   b. Alternately, progress in medical technology (e.g., artificial organs) could conceivably halt the trend toward rectangularization and simply move the entire survival curve to the right (Fig. A1-3, *B*).
   c. The secular trend toward rectangularization of population survival curves is not inconsistent with a (transient) con-

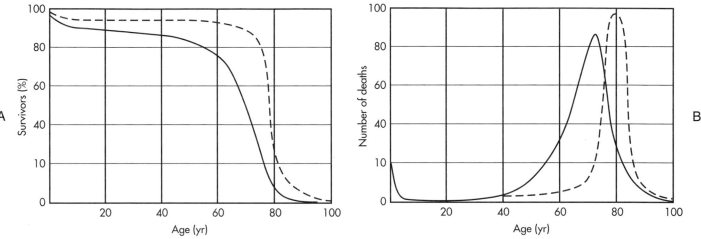

FIGURE A1-2   A, Proportion of survivors in the population (Y axis). **B,** Number of deaths per year in each 1-year age bracket. *Solid line*, present; *dotted line*, future. (From Ferri F, Fretwell MD, Wachtel TJ: *Practical Guide to Care of the Geriatric Patient*, ed 2, St. Louis, 1997, Mosby.)

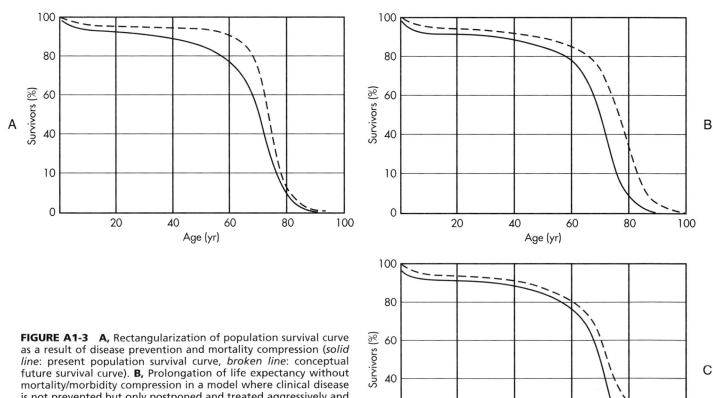

FIGURE A1-3   A, Rectangularization of population survival curve as a result of disease prevention and mortality compression (*solid line*: present population survival curve, *broken line*: conceptual future survival curve). **B,** Prolongation of life expectancy without mortality/morbidity compression in a model where clinical disease is not prevented but only postponed and treated aggressively and successfully in older people (*solid line*: present population survival curve, *broken line*: conceptual future survival curve). **C,** Change in a population survival curve where oldest segment of population is experiencing greatest decline in mortality (*solid line*: present population survival curve, *broken line*: conceptual future survival curve). (From Ferri F, Fretwell MD, Wachtel TJ: *Practical Guide to Care of the Geriatric Patient*, ed 2, St. Louis, 1997, Mosby.)

temporary widening of the period of morbidity and mortality associated with recent data that indicate that the elderly citizens of our population are enjoying the greatest decline in mortality (Fig. A1-3, *C*).

d. Possible reasons for the recent downturn in cardiovascular disease and related deaths can be attributed to reduced dietary saturated fat and cholesterol levels, positive developments in medical care for coronary heart disease and stroke, better treatment of hypertension, and improved access to health care for the elderly since 1965 because of the Medicare program.

4. Age-adjusted life expectancy is often underestimated for older individuals because clinicians are familiar with life expectancy figures from birth only. An 80-year-old woman has a life expectancy of 9.5 years: should she be in good general baseline health, an acute life-threatening, but reversible, illness should be treated as aggressively as in a younger person barring specific reasons not to (including patient preference).

Increasing life expectancy is the reason that the relentless issue of social security solvency keeps resurfacing on the political agenda. Indeed because it is funded by taxing working people, the declining ratio of working to retired people in the population can only lead to an increasing tax burden, a decrease in the benefit (payment), raising retirement age, or some combination of those (see Fig. A1-4). The same problem applies to the funding of the Medicare system.

SUGGESTED READINGS

Fries JF: Aging, natural death, and the compression of morbidity, *N Engl J Med* 303:130-135, 1980.

Olshansky SJ, Carnes BA, Cassel C: In search of Methuselah: estimating the upper limits to human longevity, *Science* 150:634-640, 1990.

Olshansky SR et al: A potential decline in life expectancy in the United States in the 21st century, *N Engl J Med* 352:1138-1145, 2005.

Wachtel TJ: The connection between health promotion and health care costs. Does it matter? *Am J Med* 94:451-454, 1993.

AUTHOR: **TOM J. WACHTEL, M.D.**

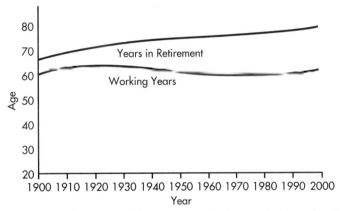

FIGURE A1-4 Impact of increasing life expectancy in the population ratio of time in retirement and time at work.

INTRODUCTION

In 1965, the Social Security Act established Medicare and Medicaid, Titles XVIII and XIX, respectively. When the Medicare program was enacted in 1966 it was a responsibility of the Social Security Administration (SSA), whereas the Medicaid program was administered by the Social and Rehabilitation Service (SRS). SSA and SRS were agencies in the Department of Health, Education, and Welfare (HEW). In 1977, the Health Care Financing Administration (HCFA) was created under HEW to effectively coordinate the Medicare and Medicaid programs. In 1980, HEW was divided into the Department of Education and the Department of Health and Human Services (HHS). In 2001, HCFA was renamed the Centers for Medicare & Medicaid Services (CMS).

MEDICARE

Medicare is a health insurance program for Americans age 65 or older. Currently, Medicare provides coverage to approximately 40 million persons. Certain people younger than age 65 can qualify for Medicare, including some individuals who have disabilities and all individuals who have end-stage kidney disease. The program helps with the cost of health care, but it does not cover all medical expenses or the cost of most long-term care.

Medicare is financed by payroll taxes paid by workers and employers, general tax dollars, and the monthly premiums of beneficiaries. Medicare has several parts, including hospital insurance (Medicare Part A) and medical insurance (Medicare Part B). These two parts of Medicare help pay for different kinds of health care costs. The sources of Medicare funding are different for each part. Part A is funded by the 1.45% payroll tax. Part B funding comes from two sources, 75% from general federal revenues and 25% from beneficiary premiums. In 2003 the source of funding for Medicare was 55% payroll taxes, 28% general tax revenues, 9% premiums, and 8% from interest and taxes on SS benefits.

MEDICARE PART A

Medicare Part A helps pay for inpatient care in a hospital or skilled nursing facility (SNF) following a hospital stay, some home health care, and hospice care. The specific components of Medicare Part A coverage are listed in Table A1-6. Although for most beneficiaries there is no premium for Part A, there are deductibles, co-pays, and limitations on the duration of coverage. The deductibles and co-pays for 2005 are listed in Table A1-7 along with the limitations in duration of coverage. The coverage is based on a benefit period, which is defined as 60 days out of the hospital.

MEDICARE PART B

Medical insurance (also called Medicare Part B) helps pay for doctors' services and many other medical services and supplies that are not covered by Part A. The specific components of Medicare Part B coverage are listed in Table A1-8. Unlike Medicare Part A, Part B requires the beneficiary to pay a monthly premium that will increase annually as the national cost of Medicare Part B increases. The monthly premiums, co-pays, and deductibles for Medicare Part B are listed in Table A1-9. Some of the items not covered by Medicare A or B are listed in Table A1-10.

MEDICARE PART C (MEDICARE MANAGED CARE PLANS)

Medicare Managed Care plans were previously known as Medicare Plus Choice and now as Medicare Advantage plans. They are health insurance programs offered by Medicare-qualified organizations to Medicare-eligible individuals, in lieu of Original Medicare plan coverage. The health plans receive 95% of the age-adjusted per capita cost (AAPCC) for Medicare beneficiaries in the region. The plans are at risk and can make a profit or loss. At a minimum they must provide the same benefits offered under Original Medicare plan coverage but may offer benefits beyond traditional Medicare. The programs generally "manage" the care offered to beneficiaries to minimize unnecessary services and diminish costs to the organization. They come in a variety of forms. Examples of Medicare Advantage plans include:

- HMO plans (health maintenance organization plans), which offer no coverage for providers or facilities outside the HMO network and almost always require a network primary care physician referral to access a network specialist.
- POS plans (point of service plans) offer a network of preferred providers, like HMO plans, but also provide reduced benefits for providers or facilities outside the HMO network.
- Regionally expanded preferred provider organization (PPO) plans are similar to POS plans but have broader geographic access to network providers in a larger service area, and reduced benefits outside the PPO network.
- PSO plans, otherwise known as provider-sponsored organizations, are similar to the POS plans but are usually organized with physicians that practice in a regional or community hospital.

TABLE A1-6   Medicare Part A Coverage Benefits

• **Hospital**	Semiprivate room, meals, general nursing, and other hospital services and supplies.
• **Inpatient Mental Health**	Limited to 190 days in a lifetime.
• **Skilled Nursing Facility**	Semiprivate room, meals, skilled nursing and rehabilitative services (after a related 3-day inpatient hospital stay).
• **Home Health Care**	Limited to reasonable and necessary part-time skilled nursing care and home health aide services as well as physical therapy, occupational therapy, and speech-language therapy.
• **Hospice Care**	For people with a terminal illness, includes drugs for symptom control and pain relief, medical and support services from a Medicare-approved hospice.
• **Blood**	Blood transfused in a hospital or skilled nursing facility during a covered stay.

TABLE A1-7   Medicare Part A Deductibles, Co-pays, and Limitations

• **Hospital Coverage (2005)**	$912 for a hospital stay of 1–60 days. $228 per day for days 61–90 of a hospital stay. $456 per day for days 91–150 of a hospital stay. (Lifetime Reserve Days do not recur per benefit period.) All costs for each day beyond 150 days (all costs beyond 90 days once Lifetime Reserve Days exhausted).
• **Skilled Nursing Facility**	Nothing for the first 20 days. $114 per day for days 21–100. All costs beyond the 100th day in the benefit period.
• **Hospice**	Nothing for Medicare-approved services. 20% of the Medicare-approved amount for durable medical equipment.

MEDICARE PART D

Beginning January 1, 2006, beneficiaries will choose one of at least two private plans or Medicare Advantage plans that offers drug coverage in their locale. The initial Medicare Part D drug benefit enrollment period begins November 15, 2005, and lasts until May 15, 2006. The Medicare Part D drug benefit is optional. However, Medicare beneficiaries who do not enroll in Part D during the initial enrollment period and who decide to enroll in Part D later will pay a higher premium. There are no provisions in the Medicare drug benefit law to contain drug costs. In fact, the legislation prohibits Medicare from using its purchasing power to negotiate lower drug prices for beneficiaries. The specifics of the Medicare Drug benefit are depicted in Fig. A1-5.

MEDIGAP POLICIES

A Medigap policy is a health insurance policy sold by a private insurance company to fill "gaps" in Original Medicare plan coverage. The Omnibus Budget Reconciliation Act (OBRA) of 1990 required that Medigap plans be standardized in as many as 10 different benefit packages offering varying levels of supplemental coverage. All policies sold since July 1992 (except in three exempted states) have conformed to 1 of these 10 standardized benefit packages, known as plans A through J. In 1999, about 10.7 million Medicare beneficiaries (more than one fourth of all beneficiaries) had a Medigap policy to help cover Medicare's cost-sharing requirements as well as some benefits not covered by Medicare parts A or B

MEDICAID

Title XIX of the Social Security Act is a federal/state entitlement program that pays for medical assistance for certain individuals and families with low incomes and resources. This program, known as Medicaid, became law in 1965 as a cooperative venture jointly funded by the federal and state governments to assist states in furnishing medical assistance to eligible needy persons. Medicaid is the largest source of funding for medical and health-related services for America's poorest people. Within broad national guidelines established by federal statutes, regulations, and policies, each state (1) establishes its own eligibility standards; (2) determines the type, amount, duration, and scope of services; (3) sets the rate of payment for services; and (4) administers its own program. Medicaid policies for eligibility, services, and payment are complex and vary considerably, even among states of similar size or geographic proximity. Thus, a person who is eligible for Medicaid in one state may not be eligible in another state, and the services provided by one state may differ considerably in amount, duration, or scope from services provided in a similar or neighboring state. In addition, state legislatures may change Medicaid eligibility, services, or reimbursement during the year.

The Balanced Budget Act (BBA) included a state option known as Programs of All-inclusive Care for the Elderly (PACE). PACE provides an alternative to institutional care for persons aged 55 or older who require a nursing facility level of care. The PACE team offers and manages all health, medical, and social services and mobilizes other services as needed to provide preventative, rehabilitative, curative, and supportive care.

TABLE A1-8 Components of Medicare Part B Coverage

- **Medical and Other Services**:
  - Doctors' services (not routine physical exams*)
  - Outpatient medical and surgical services and supplies
  - Diagnostic tests
  - Ambulatory surgery center facility fees for approved procedures
  - Durable medical equipment
  - Outpatient mental health care
  - Outpatient occupational and physical therapy, including speech-language therapy
- **Outpatient Hospital Services**
- **Blood Transfusions**
- **Preventive Services**
  - Bone mass measurements
  - Cardiovascular screening (starting January 1, 2005, fasting lipid profile)
  - Colorectal cancer screening
  - Diabetes services
  - Glaucoma testing
  - Pap test and pelvic examination (if indicated)
  - Prostate cancer screening
  - Screening mammograms
  - Vaccinations—influenza and Pneumovax
  - "Welcome to Medicare" physical examination includes
    - Measurement of height, weight, and blood pressure
    - An ECG
    - Education and counseling.

*Except a one-time comprehensive assessment at enrollment.

TABLE A1-9 Premiums, Deductibles, and Co-pays for Medicare Part B

- **Part B premium** $78.20 per month in 2005* (set at 25% of Medicare Part B cost).

- **Deductible** $110 (in 2005) deductible (once per calendar year).

- **Co-pays** 20% of the Medicare-approved amount after the deductible.
  20% for all outpatient physical, occupational, and speech-language therapy services.
  50% for most outpatient mental health care.

*Beginning in 2006 the Medicare Part B Premium will be means tested and the annual premium for beneficiaries will rise with income.
under $80,000 ($160,000 for couples), 25% of Part B costs.
between $80,000 and $100,000, 35% of Part B costs.
between $100,000 and $150,000, 50% of Part B costs.
between $150,000 and $200,000, 65% of Part B costs.
over $200,000, 80% of Part B costs ($3,000/year in 2005 dollars).

TABLE A1-10 Items Not Covered by Medicare Part A or B

- Acupuncture
- Dental care and dentures
- Cosmetic surgery
- Custodial care at home or in a nursing home
- Health care while traveling outside of the United States
- Hearing aids and hearing exams for the purpose of fitting a hearing aid
- Hearing exams (screening)
- Long-term care, such as custodial care in a nursing home
- Orthopedic shoes
- Outpatient prescription drugs (see Medicare D)
- Routine foot care
- Routine eye care and most eyeglasses
- Routine or yearly physical exams (except the "Welcome to Medicare" PE)
- Screening tests (except those listed above under preventive services)

Long-term care is an important provision of Medicaid that will be increasingly utilized as our nation's population ages. The Medicaid program paid for over 41% of the total cost of care for persons using nursing facility or home health services in 2001. National data for 2001 show that Medicaid payments for nursing facility services totaled $37.2 billion for more than 1.7 million beneficiaries of these services. With the percentage of our population who are elderly or disabled increasing faster than that of the younger groups, the need for long-term care is expected to increase.

Medicare beneficiaries who have low incomes and limited resources may also receive help from the Medicaid program. For such persons who are eligible for full Medicaid coverage, the Medicare health care coverage is supplemented by services that are available under their state's Medicaid program, according to eligibility category. These additional services may include, for example, nursing facility care beyond the 100-day limit covered by Medicare, prescription drugs, eyeglasses, and hearing aids.

For persons enrolled in both programs, any services that are covered by Medicare are paid for by the Medicare program before any payments are made by the Medicaid program, because Medicaid is always the "payer of last resort."

Starting January 2006, the new Medicare prescription drug benefit will provide drug coverage for Medicare beneficiaries, including those who also receive coverage from Medicaid. In addition, individuals eligible for both Medicare and Medicaid will also receive the low-income subsidy for both the Medicare drug plan premium and assistance with cost sharing for prescriptions. Medicaid will no longer provide drug benefits for Medicare beneficiaries.

SUGGESTED READING

Centers for Medicare & Medicaid Services: http://www.cms.hhs.gov/

AUTHOR: **JOHN B. MURPHY, M.D.**

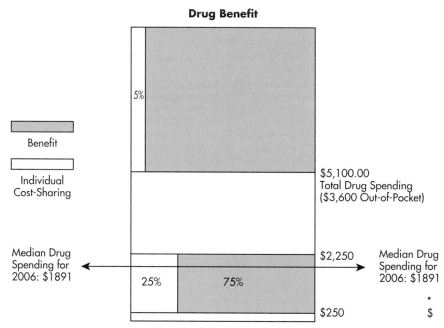

FIGURE A1-5   Medicare Part D drug benefit, as of January 1, 2006.

NURSING HOMES

Nursing homes have evolved from the Alms Houses of a century ago into highly regulated institutions providing care to primarily older individuals with profound medical, psychiatric, and social disabilities. In the last 10-20 years, the degree of regulation and the level of impairment of nursing home residents have increased dramatically. In the United States, there are roughly 17,000 nursing homes with 1.8 million beds that care for 1.6 million persons receiving custodial care (nursing facility, NF) or skilled care (skilled nursing facility, SNF). Most nursing homes provide both NF and SNF levels of care. Two thirds of the nation's nursing homes are for-profit facilities, and nearly 55% of all homes are part of large regional or national chains. Roughly 25% of nursing homes are voluntary not-for-profit facilities and about 10% are government affiliated. The average nursing home is about 100 beds and fewer than 10% have more than 200 beds.

NURSING HOME STAFFING

Nursing home staff include the following groups: nursing, social work, administration, therapists (may be full time or provided by an outside agency and include physical therapy, occupational therapy, and speech pathology), activities staff, dietary, housekeeping, and maintenance. Nursing universally accounts for the majority of the staff and minimally trained nurses aides make up the bulk of the nursing staff. Relatively few licensed nurses are present to conduct assessments, distribute medications, supervise nurses aides, communicate with physicians, and administer treatments. Only a small percentage of nursing homes, typically the largest nursing homes, have employed physicians. A 1996 Institute of Medicine report recommended increased staffing levels as an important step to increase quality of care in nursing homes, but the financial resources to achieve these increases are lacking. The recruitment and retention of nursing staff is a major challenge, with turnover rates for licensed nurses as high as 50% per year and still higher for nursing assistants.

NURSING HOME RESIDENTS

The lifetime risk of a nursing home stay is currently estimated to be 43%. The risk of being in a nursing home increases with age: 1.5% for Americans age 65-74 and 20% for those 85 and older. The average length of stay in a nursing home is about 2 years, with 25% having stays of 3 months or less, 50% with stays of 1 year or longer, and 20% staying as long as 5 years. As a group, nursing home residents are increasingly disabled. Only 2.8% of nursing home residents are independent in all activities of daily living (ADL) and 83% require assistance with three or more ADL. Dementia is one of the most frequent conditions of nursing home residents, estimated at a prevalence of 50%-70%. Behavioral problems are common (33%), as are communication problems that are seen in more than 50% of residents. Depression is also very common, estimated at a prevalence of 20%. Most nursing home residents suffer from many chronic illnesses. One half of nursing home residents are 85 years or older and less than 10% are younger than 65. Most nursing home residents are women (72%), and although 89% are white, black persons are actually at higher risk of a nursing home stay at earlier ages than white persons. Additional factors associated with admission to a nursing home are low income, poor family supports (particularly the lack of a daughter), and cognitive impairments.

FINANCING OF LONG-TERM CARE

Nursing home expenditures currently exceed $100 billion per year and are expected to top $150 billion by 2007. Public expenditures account for roughly two thirds of all nursing home spending; with Medicaid expenditures double that of Medicare. Medicare covers only short-term posthospital stays whereas Medicaid pays for custodial care for persons who have exhausted their personal finances. The remaining one third of nursing home costs are out-of-pocket expenditures, with a very small amount being covered by long-term care insurance. Nearly one third of persons who enter a nursing home paying privately will "spend down" and end up on Medicaid. Almost all facilities charge private-pay residents more than Medicaid, often twice as much. Thus, the nursing home with a high self-pay payer mix will be more financially able to provide higher quality services and is more likely to be profitable. The cost of physician payments for nursing home residents is covered by Medicare Part B and, when applicable, Medicaid. The typical nursing home base cost per year is in excess of $60,000, although there is considerable geographic variation.

QUALITY ASSURANCE

Beginning with the Federal Nursing Home Reform Act of 1987 (OBRA 87), there have been a number of initiatives to enhance quality. The federal government has established minimum staffing guidelines, training guidelines, basic resident rights, and comprehensive mandatory resident assessments. The standardized resident assessment is known as the minimum data set (MDS) and focuses on clinical issues of quality of care. The MDS will trigger resident assessment protocols (RAPs) for identified problems. Quality indicators (QIs) are a relatively new initiative to enhance quality of care in nursing homes. Each is described below.

MINIMUM DATA SET (MDS)

The minimum data set quantifies current or potential problems in medical, psychologic, or functional domains. The MDS is completed for residents admitted for a non Medicare stay within 14 days of admission, annually, and when a significant change in resident status occurs. In addition, an abbreviated MDS is conducted quarterly. For patients admitted for a stay covered by Medicare Part A, the MDS is completed more frequently. The MDS is completed by the nursing home staff and should be available for the physician to review, but unfortunately many physicians do not avail themselves of these data. When the MDS is completed, certain item responses identify or trigger one of a number of RAPs.

RESIDENT ASSESSMENT PROTOCOLS (RAPS)

The RAPs that are triggered by the MDS include issues common to nursing home populations and are listed below. The RAPs highlight areas that need attention and guide the care team through further assessment and intervention (care plan).

- Delirium
- Cognitive loss and dementia
- Visual functioning
- Activities of daily living (ADL)
- Functional rehabilitation potential
- Urinary incontinence and indwelling catheters
- Psychosocial well-being
- Mood
- Behavioral symptoms
- Activities
- Falls
- Nutritional status
- Feeding tubes
- Dehydration and fluid maintenance
- Dental care
- Pressure ulcers
- Psychotropic drug use
- Physical restraints

QUALITY INDICATORS (QIS)

QIs are designed to highlight existing or potential problems as a means to guide each facility's QA (quality assurance) program. QIs can cover a number of domains that include quality indicators. Examples are listed in Table A1-11. QIs may be compared among facilities that are similar, as a way to benchmark standards. Although each nursing home must conduct a QA program that represents all major disciplines, the design of such programs is not standardized.

ROLE OF THE PHYSICIAN

Medical care of nursing home residents offers unique challenges and demands exemplary clinical skills. The physician practicing in a nursing home must embrace interdisciplinary care and be sensitive to ethical issues. Nursing home care will include care that is preventative, curative, or palliative. The care requires a biopsychosocial approach. Table A1-12 lists the responsibilities of the physician practicing in the nursing home setting. These responsibilities reflect standards of care as well as specific regulations. The regulations encompass several domains, each of which corresponds to a regulatory code known as a tag number. The domains address physician services, resident assessment, resident rights, and quality of care. Tables A1-13 and A1-14 list suggested time management guidelines for efficient nursing home practice and the CPT codes for physician billing in the nursing home.

SUGGESTED READINGS

Donius M. Comprehensive assessment in an institutional setting. In Ostreweil D, Brummel-Smith, Beck J (eds): *Comprehensive Geriatric Assessment*, New York, 2000, McGraw-Hill, pp 225-251.

Katz P: Nursing home care. In Hazzard W et al: *Principles of Geriatric Medicine and Gerontology*, ed 5, New York, 2003, McGraw-Hill, pp 197-209.

Katz P, Karuza J: Nursing home care. In Cobbs E, Duthie E, Murphy JB (eds): *Geriatric Review Syllabus*, ed 5, Malden, MA, 2003, Blackwell.

Sloane P, Boustani M: Institutional care. In Ham R, Sloane P, Warshaw G (eds): *Primary Care Geriatrics*, ed 4, St. Louis, 2002, Mosby, pp 199-216.

AUTHOR: **JOHN B. MURPHY, M.D.**

TABLE A1-11 Examples of Nursing Home Quality Indicators

Domain	Quality Indicator
Accidents	Incidence of new fractures
	Incidence (prevalence) of falls
Nutrition	Prevalence of weight loss
	Prevalence of tube feeding
	Prevalence of dehydration
Psychotropic drug use	Prevalence of antipsychotic use without appropriate reason
	Prevalence of sedative/hypnotic use
Skin care	Prevalence of pressure ulcers, Stage 1-4

TABLE A1-12 Physician Responsibilities in the Nursing Home

1. Comprehensively assess each resident, assist in care plan development and coordination of all aspects of care. (Tag 272, 279)

2. Periodically review the care plan and assure that the goals and objectives for each care plan are rational and functionally relevant. (Tag 272, 279, F 250, F 309)

3. Implement treatments and services to enhance or maintain physical and psychologic function and to avoid accidents. (Tag F 502-512, F 310, F 311, F 323, F 324)

4. Physically attend to each resident in a manner consistent with state and federal guidelines (visit every 30 days for the first 90 days following admission, and at least every 60 days thereafter) while assuring that the appropriate diagnostic tests are performed and followed up in a timely manner. (Tag F 387, F 500-512)

5. Respond in a timely fashion to a resident's change in function or condition. (Tag F 157)

6. Inform residents of their health status and optimize ability for residents to exercise self-determination. (Tag F 151, 152, and 154.)

7. Determine each resident's decision-making capacity while establishing advance directives. (Tag F151 and F152)

8. Assure that residents are free from unnecessary drugs by periodic review of drug regimens and consultant pharmacist recommendations. (Tag F 329-331, F 428 and F 429)

TABLE A1-13 Time Management Guidelines

- Limit practice to only a few facilities.
- Employ a nurse practitioner or physician's assistant who can manage routine care and serve as a liaison between yourself and nursing staff and families.
- Establish regular days for rounding in a particular nursing home.
- Always cluster routine visits, avoid seeing a single patient on one visit.
- Develop protocols for common problems.
- Address advance directives with resident and family soon after admission.
- Establish strong relationships with nursing staff and nursing home administrative staff.
- Conduct rounds with the floor nurse to ensure acquisition of key information and to make sure plans are carried out appropriately.
- Train staff to limit after-hours calls to urgent medical problems and establish a system for conveying nonurgent information (e.g., regularly scheduled call).

TABLE A1-14 CPT Codes for Nursing Facility Services (New 2006 Codes)

COMPREHENSIVE NURSING FACILITY ASSESSMENTS, ADMISSIONS AND RE-ADMISSIONS

99304	Low complexity (e.g., simple annual assessment)
99305	Moderate complexity (e.g., complex annual assessment or simple admit/readmit)
99306	High complexity (e.g., complex admission or readmit)

SUBSEQUENT NURSING FACILITY CARE, ESTABLISHED PATIENT

99307	Low (e.g., stable, recertification)
99308	Moderate (e.g., change in treatment, new complaint, not responding)
99309	Serious medical event or several unstable medical conditions
99310	High (e.g., major medical event)
99315	Nursing facility discharge management, less than 30 minutes
99316	Nursing facility discharge management, more than 30 minutes
99318	Annual comprehensive assessment

INTRODUCTION

It is generally expected that patients will be cared for by their attending physician within the nursing home. The availability of consultants/specialists in nursing homes is variable and nursing home residents often need to be transported to specialist offices or hospitals for consultations. In the hospital setting, daily visits by the attending physician are appropriate, expected, and re-imbursed by third-party payers. Ambulatory patients are seen episodically by their primary care physician and have some degree of control over the frequency of their office visits. Nursing home patients do not usually need to be seen on a daily basis, but they should be visited by their attending physician according to some schedule.

The Centers for Medicare & Medicaid Services (CMS) has created such a schedule to assure "reasonable" physician visitation in the long-term care setting. The *Medicare Career Manual* describes payment of physician's visits to residents of nursing facilities and nursing facilities in section 15509.1:

- Nursing home visits must comply with federal regulations (42 CFR 483.40).

RESIDENT ASSESSMENTS

Medicare Part B pays for visits necessary to perform all Medicare-required assessments. Physicians should use the CPT codes for comprehensive nursing facility assessments (99304-99306 and 99318) to report these evaluation and management services. Comprehensive assessments must be coupled with the creation of a minimum data set (MDS) and resulting resident assessment protocols (RAPs). This occurs at the time of admission, readmission, once-a-year routinely, and whenever a change in condition requires a new MDS (e.g., a stroke).

SUBSEQUENT VISITS

Subsequent visits are classified as routine (or regulatory) and sick visits. These visits and all other medically necessary visits for the diagnosis or treatment of illness or injury or to improve the functioning of a body part are covered under Medicare Part B. Physicians should use CPT codes for subsequent nursing facility care (99307-99310) when reporting evaluation and management services that do not involve resident assessments. Medicare pays for visits required to monitor and evaluate residents once every 30 days for the first 90 days after admission and once every 60 days thereafter. Medical necessity of a service is a key criterion for payment. Medical necessity is assumed to exist when regulatory visits are performed. The schedule for those visits is determined by the date of admission rather than the previous visit. The timing can be difficult to comply with because auditors allow 10 days before or after the scheduled date is "consistent with the requirement," but a visit "off-schedule" or sick visit does not reset the clock. The physician or practitioner determines the necessity for sick visits. A patient with pneumonia who is managed in a nursing home can be seen appropriately every day while unstable. A patient with onychomycosis, treated with an antifungal agent, does not need daily visits to monitor progress. Providing unnecessary services is called Medicare abuse (fraud is billing for a service that was not provided).

DISCHARGE SERVICES

Assessment visits and subsequent regulatory or sick visits require face-to-face contact between the patient and the practitioner/physician. Discharge services (CPT codes 99315 and 99316) may not require face-to-face contact on the day of discharge (controversial): the billing date is the discharge date, but the service is typically provided over several days; it includes discharge forms, prescriptions, phone calls, a discharge summary, etc. It is a time-based service: 99315, 30 minutes or less; 99316, longer than 30 minutes. These codes can be used if the reason for discharge is death.

DOCUMENTATION

- The volume of documentation should not be the primary influence on which a specific level of service is billed. Documentation should simply support the level of service reported.
- Assessment documentation
  - See sample form, which can be used for admissions, readmissions, and annual comprehensive visits (Fig. A1-6).
- Follow-up regulatory visits
  - At the minimum, these notes must include:
  1. Date
  2. Reason for visit (e.g., follow-up for diabetes and CHF)
  3. Relevant interval history (may refer to nurses notes and telephone calls)
  4. Physical examination
  5. Interval diagnostic test result acknowledgment
  6. Assessment or impression or diagnosis
  7. Plan of care
  8. Legible identity (signature) of writer

The 30-day/60-day regulatory visit should address the medical problems that are under current active management. For example, blood sugar results should be mentioned in diabetic patients, blood pressure should be mentioned in hypertensive patients, mental function or behaviors should be mentioned in patients treated with psychoactive medication. Because most nursing home residents have multiple comorbid conditions, SOAP notes may not be the most efficient way to document care.

- Sick visits should be problem focused and would typically resemble daily progress notes in a hospital record.
  - Chief complaint/reason for visit
  - Symptoms
  - Examination
  - Diagnosis
  - Treatment

SOAP notes may be appropriate for such visits.

- What evaluation of management (E & M) CPT code to use? The national frequency of NH visit codes is presented in Table A1-15. Individual physician/practitioner coding profiles should generally reflect these statistics.

All E & M codes have performance and documentation requirements. Each code has standards that pertain to:

- History
- Examination
- Medical decision making

CPT codes 99304, 99305, 99306, and 99318 are typically straightforward because of the comprehensive nature of these visits. Documentation requirements for subsequent visit CPT codes 99307, 99308, 99309, and 99310 are complex. The same rules apply to regulatory visits and sick visits, which complicates the task of selecting the "correct" CPT code.

TABLE A1-15 **NH Visits—2000 CMS.gov***

Code	%
99301	2.0
99302	2.9
99303	4.8
99311	37.4
99312	41.4
99313	10.3
99315	1.0
99316	0.3

*These codes are now obsolete.

COMPREHENSIVE HISTORY & PHYSICAL EXAMINATION

ATTENDING PHYSICIAN _____ DATE _____
NAME: _____ AGE _____
REASON FOR ADMISSION:_____
_____
_____
_____

PAST MEDICAL HISTORY: _____
_____
_____
_____

Social History/Habits:
Marital Status: Living Situation:
Smoking:
Alcohol: Other:
Family History: _____

Functional Status:

Basic ADLs

	Independent	Dependent
Transfers	_____	_____
Feeding	_____	_____
Bathing	_____	_____
Dressing	_____	_____
Grooming	_____	_____

Ambulation:
__ unassisted __ with walker
__ with cane __ non-ambulatory
Urine:
continent __ incontinent __
Stool:
continent __ incontinent __

Informant: Patient __ Staff __ Family __

Review of Symptoms:

	NO	YES
Headache	☐	☐
Chest pain	☐	☐
Abdominal Pain	☐	☐
Pain in Limbs	☐	☐
Other Pain	☐	☐
SOB	☐	☐
Dizziness	☐	☐
Fall	☐	☐

	NL	ABN
Hearing	☐	☐
Vision	☐	☐
Urination	☐	☐
Bowel	☐	☐
Sleep	☐	☐
Appetite	☐	☐
Energy	☐	☐
Memory	☐	☐

EXAM:
Vital signs: BP _____ P _____
Ears: Hearing _____
          TM _____
Eyes: Vision (L) _____ (R) _____
          ROM _____ Fields _____
          Pupils _____
Nose: _____
Throat: _____
Neck: LN _____
        Thyroid _____
        Carotids _____
Breasts & Axillae: _____
Extremities:
        Pulses _____
        Edema _____
Skin: _____

Weight _____
Lungs _____
Heart _____
Abdomen _____
Rectal:
        Prostate _____
        Mucosa _____
        Stool _____
Ortho: _____
Neuro:
        Motor _____
        Reflexes _____
        Gait _____
Mental Status: _____
Affect: _____

Laboratory Data	Radiology
	ECG
	ECHO

Goals of Admission: Rehabilitation/postacute care ☐   Long-term care ☐
Advance Directives: _____
Assessment and Plan:

Attending Physician:_____ Date _____

FIGURE A1-6 Comprehensive History & Physical Examination

ASSESSMENT/COMPREHENSIVE VISITS

The work and documentation presented on the form included in this chapter will generally satisfy the requirement for these CPT codes:

- 99318 should be used for an overall annual review of the patient's medical problems. This service is not required, but it is desirable and allowed by Medicare. It should occur contemporaneously with a new MDS but Medicare does not specify how closely the two activities should coincide.
- 99306 is used for most new admissions and some readmissions to a long-term care facility (skilled or nonskilled).
- 99305 is used for occasional moderately complex admissions and many (skilled or nonskilled) readmissions following hospital stays that result in relatively little change in the patient's condition or plan of care (e.g., noncardiac chest pain or a urinary infection).
- 99304 is used for (unusual) simple admissions or re-admission (e.g., a physically healthy person with dementia only).

Admission and readmission visits should occur as soon as possible after the admission to the nursing home. The condition of the patient may or may not require a visit within 24-48 hours of admission, but waiting longer than 1 week is not advisable. Medicare allows up to 30 days to complete the admission. A sick visit may precede the admission visit. The CPT code for such sick visit is a subsequent visit code. Some states and the Joint Commission for the Accreditation of Hospitals (JCAHO) have more stringent time rules for admission visits.

SUBSEQUENT VISIT CODES

- History is divided into
  - History of present illness
  - Past medical history
  - Social history
  - Review of systems

and for each of the four categories into
  - Problem-focused
  - Expanded problem focused
  - Detailed
  - Comprehensive
- Examination is divided into
  - Problem focused
  - Expanded problem focused
  - Detailed
  - Comprehensive
- Medical decision making is divided into
  - Number of diagnoses and management options
  - Amount and complexity of data
  - Risk of complication, morbidity, and mortality

and for each of the following categories into
  - Straightforward
  - Low
  - Moderate
  - High

The various permutations of the above categories define the CPT level. 99307 requires (2 of 3) a problem-focused history, a problem-focused exam, and straightforward or low-complexity decision making. 99308 requires (2 of 3) an expanded problem-focused history, an expanded problem-focused exam, and moderate-complexity decision making. 99309 requires (2 of 3) a detailed history, a detailed exam, and moderate- or high-complexity medical decision making. 99310 requires (2 of 3) a detailed history, a detailed exam, and high-complexity medical decision making. The task of determining the correct CPT code is often more complicated than managing the patient. The fact that Medicare allows for a visit to document only a history and examination without decision making (assessment and plan) for these codes makes no clinical sense. Therefore, rather than present the scores of possible permutations, clinical vignettes should be more useful for clinicians.

REGULATORY SUBSEQUENT VISITS

- 99307: a stable patient with Alzheimer's dementia treated with donepezil
- 99308: a patient with dementia, hyperlipidemia, and hypertension who is doing well but whose medication must be adjusted to improve blood pressure control
- 99309: a patient with a past stroke, diabetes, hypertension, progressing renal failure, and osteoporosis who visited her nephrologist 2 weeks ago and requires a review of capillary glucose levels, the nephrology consultation, and changes in several chronic condition treatments.

SICK VISITS

- 99307: diagnosis and treatment of pink eye or eczema.
- 99308: evaluation and management of urinary tract infection, new pressure ulcer.
- 99309: evaluation and management of chest pain, new delirium, a new stroke, pneumonia.
- 99310 would generally be used for the evaluation and management of a life-threatening illness in the nursing home in lieu of the hospital.

The existence of comorbidities will often result in more work and a higher CPT code. For example, a UTI in a diabetic patient has additional clinical implications (e.g., impact of UTI on glycemic control) and would justify the use of CPT code 99309 instead of 99308 so long as the documentation accounts for the added complexity of the situation.

NOTES

- A change of physician does not allow for usage of a comprehensive CPT code even if the work is comprehensive.
- Advance practice nurses (nurse practitioner) are not allowed to perform the admission work for skilled patients. They can admit nonskilled patients. They can alternate the subsequent regulatory visits with the attending physician and there is no limitation on the number of sick visits they can perform. Nurse practitioners will be paid by Medicare for the services they are allowed to perform.
- All consultations must be ordered by the attending physician or practitioner who works with him or her.
- Even professionals with ample experience in coding will sometimes disagree about what CPT code to use. The choice among CPT codes is often difficult because of the interplay of multiple chronic conditions.

AUTHOR: **TOM J. WACHTEL, M.D.**

INTRODUCTION

Providing medical care to nursing home patients differs from both the hospital setting and the outpatient setting. Hospitalized patients are acutely ill and are seen every day. Subspecialists in many fields are available for consultation on short notice when help is needed. Ambulatory patients are seen episodically for chronic disease management, health maintenance, or acute conditions, but they are generally independent and mobile and can usually carry out their physicians' orders independently or with minimal formal or informal assistance.

Three concepts highlight the nature of nursing home medical care: interdisciplinary, geriatric, and regulated. Nursing home patients are typically sicker than ambulatory patients (postacute care) or more debilitated (long-term care), but their usual condition does not require daily visits. However, this patient population's usual condition requires the services of various professionals such as nurses, rehabilitation personnel, dietitians, social workers, personal care attendants, and others with whom the attending physician must interact by phone or face-to-face. This ongoing interaction is necessary both to receive information about the patient's status and to order care. Nursing home physicians must be comfortable with interdisci-plinary teamwork in order to perform effectively. In addition, nursing home physicians must be familiar with geriatric principles to practice competently in this environment. This requires familiarity with geriatric syndromes and with functional concepts (assessments and outcomes). Finally, nursing homes are highly regulated institutions. Many of the state and federal government regulations are the result of historical (and sometimes current) poor care. Attending physicians may not agree with every regulation (as we do not always agree with every speed limit), but failure to comply results in difficulties for the facility and its managing staff, including the medical director. By agreeing to accept responsibility for the medical care of a nursing home resident, the attending physician agrees implicitly or explicitly (Fig. A1-7) to comply with the various rules and regulations.

The nuts and bolts of the nursing home attending physician are described in the model practice agreement displayed in Fig. A1-7. The most notable difference from practice in other settings is the need to work as a member of a care team whose functional captain is the nurse, although the attending physician writes the orders and the nurses and other professionals carry them out. Because physician presence in the

MODEL PRACTICE AGREEMENT

The attending physician and the nursing facility share a common goal—the nursing facility expectation should be separated and signed off by the administrator or owner, the highest possible quality of life of the residents.

Achieving the highest attainable quality of life for the resident requires the joint efforts of multiple disciplines, which must operate collaboratively.

The attending physician provides medical care (primary function) and interacts with nursing, rehabilitation specialists, dietary, social services, and other professionals (collaborative function) in the context of a highly government-regulated environment (regulatory function). This complex structure requires physician knowledge, skills, attitudes, and activities that are not typically encountered in other practice settings. This must be understood and accepted.

Attending physicians agree to perform the following:
1. Approve orders on the day of admission (may be done by phone)
2. Visit new patients within 48 hours of admission, unless the patient was examined by a physician within the 5 days prior to admission (e.g., a hospital transfer). In the latter case, with documentation, the attending physician has 7 days to visit the patient.
3. The admission visit is comprehensive. It should include a history, a physical examination, a review/assessment of all the diagnoses, a plan of care for each of the diagnoses, a general goal/purpose for the nursing facility stay, and other matters that may need addressing (e.g., advance directives).
4. The attending physician agrees to visit the resident no less than every 30 days for the first 3 months, and then no less than every 60 days ("regulatory visits"). The attending physician also agrees to visit the resident when a change in condition or an accident requires such a visit ("sick visits"). Alternate regulatory visits and any sick visits may be performed by a nurse practitioner (NP) or a physician assistant (PA).
5. The progress notes must be legible, indicate the purpose of the visit, document the findings (H&P or S&O), and contain an assessment (diagnoses) and plan (treatments). The notes must be signed and dated.
6. Over the course of a year, all the resident's medical problems and treatments must be documented in progress notes. This can be done over the course of several visits, or the resident can have an annual "comprehensive visit."
7. The attending physician must be available 24/7 personally or through a coverage arrangement that will be disclosed to the nursing facility.
8. The attending physician agrees to sign all regulatory forms or contact the facility's medical director if he or she believes a form is incorrect or inappropriate.
9. The attending physician will participate in the discharge planning process of residents under care.
10. The attending physician will attend at least one annual meeting with the facility's medical director.
11. The nursing facility agrees to provide high quality services to its residents.
12. The nursing facility agrees to inform the attending physician and the resident's family of any change in condition in a timely manner.
13. The facility will inform the attending physician of patient-specific problems and systemic issues identified during usual care, quality improvement activities or state/federal inspections.
14. The nursing facility will make every effort to provide specialty consultants (e.g., psychiatry and podiatry) on site, and will arrange for transportation of residents for off-site consultations.
15. The attending physician will inform the medical director of any concerns regarding the care provided to residents by nursing home personnel.

FIGURE A1-7 Model Practice Agreement

facility is intermittent, nursing home nurses have been described as the "eyes and ears" of the physician, but the physician must be aware of the abilities of individual nurses in obtaining accurate clinical information. The most important factor in gauging the quality of this information is prior experience in working with a particular nurse. Interaction with residents' families (and friends) is equally important for transfer of information in both directions. Families need to know what to expect.

Transitions are a time of particular patient vulnerability because the patient is new to the care team, and because the transfer of information is often incomplete between institutions (e.g., hospital and nursing home). Ideally, direct communication between nurses and between the physicians from both institutions should take place, but in practice many obstacles prevent such interactions. The prevalence of dementia is near 50% among long-term care patients who cannot provide reliable medical histories. The quality of the recorded medical information is also variable for many reasons (multiple transitions, low priority, specialty care).

Regulations determine the frequency of routine physician visits, but there are no limitations on the number of "sick" visits that attending physicians can make so long as such visits are "necessary" in the judgment of the physician. There are also no regulatory limitations on consultations, but few specialists visit nursing home patients who therefore must be transported to consultants' offices. This requires nursing home attending physicians to be true generalists and often extend their scope of practice beyond what would be ordinary in their hospital or office practice.

SUGGESTED READING

Dimant J: Roles and responsibilities of attending physicians in skilled nursing facilities, *J Am Med Dir Assoc* 4:231-243, 2003.

AUTHOR: **TOM J. WACHTEL, M.D.**

INTRODUCTION

A medical director is a physician who is responsible for overseeing certain aspects of medical care and services for an organization or a health care system. Hospitals have department chairs, chiefs of staff, division directors, or vice presidents for medical affairs. As the needs and the care of nursing home residents became more complex, the expertise of physicians was needed to complement the knowledge and skills of the nursing staff. Medicare through the OBRA '87 regulations requires that all long-term care facilities designate a medical director. Interpretive guidelines describe some following duties:

- Ensure that the facility provides appropriate care.
- Ensure implementation of resident care policies.
- Provide oversight of physician services.
- Oversee overall clinical care and make sure it is adequate.
- Correct inadequate medical care when such is identified or reported.
- Consult with residents or their attending physicians when needed or requested.

GENERAL STATEMENT

The role of the medical director can be broken down into three categories:

- Domains of care that fall under physician expertise: physician/practitioner services including timeliness of visits, appropriateness of orders, credentialing of physician/practitioners, availability of needed consultants, infection control, formulating advance directives, employee health issues, medical record maintenance (e.g., admission notes, progress notes, discharge summaries), treatment protocols, etc. The medical director should be actively involved in collaboration with the facility's leadership (e.g., the administrator and the director of nursing) in the oversight of the above domains and shares responsibility with the leadership for satisfactory nursing home performance of those areas. If problems are discovered during inspections, quality assurance activities, or otherwise, the medical director should provide assistance and recommendations pertaining to corrective action plans. The medical director may need to intervene directly with staff physicians/practitioners who are not performing according to expectation.
- Domains of care that are the primary responsibility of other health professionals but require some degree of medical director input (e.g., nursing, physical therapy, dietary, social work): the medical director should be aware of those departments' policies and procedures and how they are fulfilling their function. If problems are identified internally (e.g., as a result of a mishap or during the quality assurance process) or by an external party (e.g., by state inspectors), the medical director should be informed and may be involved in helping the nursing home formulate plans to correct the problem(s), but should not be held responsible for the actual implementation of the corrective actions, given that the medical director has no authority over any nursing home employees and has no access to nursing home financial resources.
- Domains of services to nursing home residents that should not be under medical director oversight or responsibility include laundry services, food services, plumbing, fire, and safety: physicians have no training and should not be expected to have any expertise in these areas. Therefore, if problems are identified in those areas (e.g., as a "deficiency" during an inspection), the medical director can be informed of those problems (as may be required by the regulatory process), but there should be no expectation from anyone that the medical director has a role in the plan or correction or that she or he can be held responsible for such correction.

SPECIFIC MEDICAL DIRECTOR JOB DESCRIPTION

QUALIFICATIONS:

1. Licensed physician.
2. Two years of experience in long-term care or specialized training in geriatrics or chronic disease/impaired populations.
3. Desirable attributes:
   a. Medical director certification or equivalent training in management.
   b. Be the attending physician for a caseload of patients in the facility that one directs, e.g., 10%.

AREAS OF RESPONSIBILITY

1. General:
   a. Overall coordination, execution, and monitoring of physician/practitioner activities.
   b. Monitoring and evaluating the outcomes of the health care services (e.g., quality assurance [QA]).
2. Physician/practitioner oversight.
   a. Establish and implement a procedure to review physician/practitioner credentials and grant privileges to be or remain on the list of attending.
   b. Establish rules that govern the performance of physicians/practitioners.
   c. Make staff aware of those rules.
   d. Oversee physician/practitioner performance. Establish a formal procedure for such oversight (e.g., QA).
3. Define the scope of practice for physicians/practitioners (would usually use state/federal regulations).
4. Ensure physician performance in the following activities:
   a. Accept responsibility for the care of residents assigned to them.
   b. Perform timely admission procedures including review of medical records.
   c. Make periodic as well as other pertinent visits.
   d. Provide adequate ongoing medical coverage (i.e., 24/7).
   e. Provide appropriate medical care.
   f. Document care and do so legibly.
   g. Formulate and approve advance directives/end of life orders.
   h. Other (may be physician, resident, or facility specific).
5. Cover for the attending physician when the latter is unavailable or not performing appropriately. The medical director usually becomes the attending physician by default when no other physician on staff is available or willing to accept the patient. The medical director may become involved directly in the care of another physician's patient under the following circumstances:
   a. Request by resident/family.
   b. Request by nursing home staff (e.g., a nurse).
   c. Request by another physician.
   d. When aware of a quality of medical care concern.
   e. When aware of a risk management issue.
   f. The patient or proxy must consent to involvement by another physician or the medical director as rapidly as possible.
6. Policies and procedures: the medical director is responsible for the content of those policies and procedures that fall under the physician's domain. The medical director should "sign off" on those documents and monitor their implementation even though this is not required by law. The medical director should review policies and procedures that pertain to other types of health care professionals (e.g., nursing) but not be responsible for their implementation. Other policies and procedures should not be under medical director oversight.
7. Quality Improvement (QI): The medical director or her/his designee must attend the quality assurance meetings and be an active participant in the QI process. The medical director should review and sign the minutes produced during

those meetings. The medical director should participate in the facility's overall QI process including areas that are not in the medical domain because a physician is often the most knowledgeable member of the QA committee in the management and interpretation of statistical data among nursing home personnel.

8. Employee health oversight: nursing homes have varying policies concerning employee health. It is not expected that medical directors substitute for employees' primary care physicians. What is expected is that the medical director establish or approve policies that cover employee immunization programs, that address diagnosis and treatment of infectious illnesses that could be transmitted to residents or other employees, that deal with conditions that could affect the performance of the worker, and that ensure that occupational safety measures are consistent with regulatory requirements.

9. Infection control: the medical director is expected to advise and consult with designated nursing staff regarding communicable diseases, infection control, and isolation procedures, and interact when appropriate with public health officials.

10. Review the reports that describe the findings of formal inspections by the state department of health. When deficiencies are identified, the medical director must be involved in the plan of correction of problems that are in the medical domain (e.g., F tag 501). The medical director should acknowledge corrective actions concerning problems that exist in other health care domains but not be expected to be accountable for their actual corrections. Medical directors should not be party to corrective measures that have nothing to do with the practice of medicine.

11. Other:
   a. Staff education (physician and other personnel).
   b. Participate in hiring/interview of key management personnel (e.g., administrator and director of nursing).
   c. Participate in important project development (e.g., a respirator unit).
   d. Interact as needed with state's ombudsman.
   e. Interact as needed with resident families.

MEDICAL DIRECTOR OVERSIGHT PLAN AND AUTHORITY

The nursing home administrator and medical director will draft a plan that will describe how the medical director will carry out her/his responsibilities. This plan should be a written document that is part of the medical director's employment contract. This contract should define the authority of the medical director. The medical director reports to the administrator and usually serves in an advisory capacity. A formal procedure should be created and updated by facility management staff and by the medical director to document performance. Periodic medical director performance evaluations should be carried out.

MEDICAL DIRECTOR ACCOUNTABILITY

Medical directors are held accountable to perform the job described in this chapter. Nursing homes are subjected to considerable oversight by government agencies and other parties (ombudsman, families of residents, etc.). The frail nature of nursing home residents may lead to events such as death, injuries, pressure ulcers, malnutrition, medication errors, etc., which could generate complaints about nursing homes, their medical directors, and their physicians. The state's department of (public) health and the state's board of licensure and discipline may be asked to adjudicate those complaints. Therefore, medical directors should maintain a written record of their activities, for example, in the form of a quarterly report to the QA committee.

CAVEATS

The federal and state regulations define a broad outline of nursing home medical director responsibilities; however, those texts are so vague as to preclude a direct translation into a functional and realistic job description. Additionally, the breadth of the regulatory scope of responsibilities of the medical director job within the long-term care setting is unreasonable because it includes areas of involvement where physicians have no expertise. Finally, the authority bestowed on medical directors is limited by the part-time nature of the position and its advisory status without hire or firepower over any member of the nursing home employees.

Pursuant to the Federal Nursing Home Reform Act of 1987 and specifically, 42 C.F.R. 483.75(I), each nursing home covered by the act must designate an individual to serve as a medical director. The regulations further state that each medical director is responsible for (1) the implementation of resident care policies and (2) the coordination of medical care in the facility. Although these subtopics may appear simple and straightforward, it is the variety of responsibilities included within each subtopic that cause concern and call for interpretation. Indeed, taken literally, the job description implied by the regulatory language goes beyond the role of a hospital chief of staff or department chair. For example, a nursing home medical director's responsibility for the implementation of "resident care policies" has been interpreted to extend to "Admissions, transfers, and discharges; infection control; use of restraints; physician privileges and practice; responsibilities of non-physician health care workers in resident care; emergency care and resident assessment and care planning; accidents and incidents; ancillary services such as laboratory, radiology and pharmacy; use of medication; use and release of clinical information; and overall quality of care."

In addition, a director's responsibility as related to "the coordination of medical care" in the facility has been interpreted to encompass "Monitoring and ensuring implementation of resident care policies, and providing oversight and supervision of physician services and medical care of residents; overseeing the overall clinical care of residents to ensure that care is adequate and effective; evaluating reports of possible inadequate medical care and taking appropriate action to remedy problems; and assuring the support of essential medical consultants as needed."

Despite the vast amount of responsibility imposed on each director, the regulations do not provide each medical director with an equivalent amount of authority necessary to ensure compliance with the pertinent regulations. Furthermore, most medical director contracts only require that the director work at the facility for a minimal number of hours (e.g., 2-4) each week. In combination with the regulations, such arrangements make the director an easy target for liability purposes, investigation by state licensing boards, and even criminal prosecution, but do not provide an obvious mechanism whereby the director can enforce his or her ideas and strategies. A carefully worded medical director employment contract may offer some protection (Fig. A1-8).

SUGGESTED READING

Levenson S: The medical director: back to basics, *Caring for the ages* 46-51, 2004.

AUTHOR: **TOM J. WACHTEL, M.D.**

SAMPLE MEDICAL DIRECTOR CONTRACT FOR RHODE ISLAND NURSING HOMES

WHEREAS, Happy Care Health Center in order to participate in certain federal and/or state health care programs, is required to engage the services of a medical director and

WHEREAS, Octoplusdoc, MD, hereinafter also referred to as the medical director, is a doctor of medicine licensed to practice his/her profession under the laws of the State of Rhode Island, is willing to provide said services as medical director,

NOW, THEREFORE, said Happy Care Health Center and Dr. Octoplusdoc hereby and herewith mutually agree to the terms and conditions hereinafter set forth:

1. Happy Care Health Center designates Octoplusdoc, MD as medical director
2. The medical director shall devote XX hours per month (more or less) to the performance of his/her non-direct patient care duties under this agreement.
3. The medical director provides medical expertise and communicates regularly with the administrator, the director of nursing and other professional staff regarding clinical and administrative issues, specific patient care problems and professional staff needs.
4. The medical director will be involved and accountable in the development of medical treatment policies and procedures. The medical director should be aware of other health professionals' policies (e.g., nursing, rehabilitation, dietician, social work). Non-clinical policies and procedures (e.g., cleaning, kitchen, plumbing, fire codes) are not the medical director's responsibility.
5. The medical director participates in developing and is accountable for policies and procedures regarding the services of the medical and practitioner staff:
   5.1 Credentialing of physicians and advance practice nurses/physician assistants
   5.2 Define the scope of practice for physicians/practitioners
   5.3 Establish rules that govern physician/practitioner performance:
      • Accept responsibility for the care of residents assigned to them
      • Perform timely admission visits, including examinations and writing orders
      • Perform periodic and other pertinent visits
      • Provide appropriate state of the art medical care
      • Document care consistent with CMS documentation guidelines
      • Formulate/approve end of life orders
   5.4 In emergency situations, cover for the attending physician when unavailable or not performing appropriately
6. The medical director oversees the implementation of resident care policies and medical/practitioner staff performance
   6.1 Participate in on-going quality improvement/assurance activities by attending the QI/QA committee meetings and reviewing the minutes
   6.2 Advise on specific resident care problems identified during the normal process of delivering services to residents
   6.3 Advise about the identification and management of systemic medical problems that may occur from time to time (e.g., outbreaks and infection control issues).
7. The medical director assists the facility in identifying needs for new resident care or staff policies/procedures and reviews existing policies from time to time.
8. The medical director advises the administrator and other relevant organization leaders about employee health policies and issues
9. The medical director must review state and federal survey/inspection reports and help to prepare a response and/or plan of correction when needed.
10. The medical director helps the facility to coordinate the care provided to residents. This becomes particularly important when a long-term care facility identifies itself as specialized and needs a relevant specialist to provide consultation (e.g., respirator unit, dialysis patients, etc.). The medical director cannot be held responsible for certain services that are unavailable (e.g,. dental care)
11. The medical director will work with the facility to promote residents' rights and quality of life and interacts with ombudsman when needed.
12. The administrator and the director of nursing shall make themselves available to the medical director to discuss relevant matters as needed.
13. Facility personnel will inform the medical director about care issues in a timely manner as such issues arise.
14. The medical director provides a periodic report to the administrator and receives a periodic evaluation from the administrator.
15. This center shall pay to the medical director as a fee for his services, the amount of $XXXX per month. Said amount of money is compensation for his/her services as medical director only, and does not include any amounts due him/her for professional fees arising from his/her services to residents or others (e.g., employees) and payable to him/her by residents or third parties. In no case is the professional fee for individual care of a resident a part of the payment for services as medical director.
16. The medical director shall not be considered, and he/she is not, an employee of Happy Care Health Center, but is an independent contractor responsible for his/her own acts.
17. The medical director is expected to attend meetings, conferences, seminars or the like that may be concerned in whole or in part with medical direction in order to remain current with the job. The nursing home will cover up to $XXXX per year in expenses related to continuing education activities.
18. This agreement may be amended at any time by mutual agreement, in writing. This agreement shall be for a term of one year, but shall automatically renew on the anniversary date of its signing for an additional year each anniversary date thereafter. This agreement may be terminated by the medical director at any time with 60 days notice or by the nursing home at any time with 180 days notice (or continued payment for 180 days from the time of termination notice).
19. The medical director shall maintain malpractice insurance at all times in an amount not less than one million dollars ($1,000,000). This insurance will cover the medical director for his/her administrative duties (this is not typically included in standard medical malpractice policies). If the nursing home provides such coverage, the medical director will be identified by name in its policy.
20. Nothing in this contract shall be construed to prohibit either party from entering any other agreement with any other person or entity.

FIGURE A1-8 Sample Medical Director Contract for Rhode Island Nursing Homes

INTRODUCTION

Occupational therapy (OT) is a health profession designed to help people improve their ability to perform tasks in their activities of daily living (ADL) and working environments. Occupational therapists work with individuals who have conditions that are mentally, physically, developmentally, or emotionally disabling. Occupational therapists help persons improve their basic motor functions and reasoning abilities as well as compensate for permanent loss of function. Their goal is to help clients have independent, productive, and satisfying lives. Occupational therapists assist patients in performing activities of all types, ranging from using a computer to caring for daily needs such as dressing, cooking, and eating. Physical exercises may be used to increase strength and dexterity, whereas other activities may be chosen to improve visual acuity and the ability to discern patterns. Therapists instruct those with permanent disabilities, such as spinal cord injuries, cerebral palsy, or muscular dystrophy, in the use of adaptive equipment, including wheelchairs, splints, and aids for eating and dressing. Family and caregiver education are core components of the field.

EDUCATION AND LICENSING

- Currently a 4-year bachelor's degree is the minimum requirement to be an occupational therapist registered (OTR).
- Beginning in 2007, a master's degree will become the minimum requirement to qualify for an OTR.
- Occupational therapists must graduate from an accredited educational program and pass a national certification examination.
- Licensing is at a state level.
- Occupational therapy assistants have either a 2-year associate's degree or a 1-year certificate program.

SCOPE OF OCCUPATIONAL THERAPY ASSESSMENT AND TREATMENT TECHNIQUES

- Perceptual, sensory, and cognitive assessment.
- Assessment of activities of daily living (ADL).
- Assess work readiness.
- Assessment of need for assistive technology.
- Driving assessments.
- Design, fabrication, and training in the use of assistive technology and orthotic or prosthetic devices.
- Customized treatment programs to improve a person's ability to perform ADL.
- Comprehensive home and job site evaluations with adaptation recommendations.
- Cognitive retraining programs.
- Guidance to family members and caregivers.

PHYSICIAN REFERRAL TO OCCUPATIONAL THERAPISTS

- Referral can be for assessment, treatment, or both.
- Referral needs a specific diagnosis.
- Referral should include a statement requesting a specific treatment or that the therapist can evaluate and treat as he or she determines most appropriate.
  - Examples:
    1. Dx. Stroke, ICD-9CM 436: evaluate ability to self-feed and provide large-diameter grip eating utensils, a plate guard, and two-handed cup.
    2. Dx. Parkinson's disease, ICD-9CM 332.0: evaluate and treat as necessary.
- Occupational therapy is covered under Medicare and most health insurance plans with a physician's prescription.

SUGGESTED READINGS

American Medical Association: *Health Professions Career and Education Directory*, Chicago, 2002, Author, pp 248-249.

Hoenig H, Cutson T: Geriatric rehabilitation. In Hazzard W et al: *Principles of Geriatric Medicine and Gerontology*, ed 5, New York, 2003, McGraw-Hill, pp 285-302.

Mosqueda L, Brummel-Smith K: Rehabilitation. In Ham R, Sloane P, Warshaw G (eds): *Primary Care Geriatrics*, ed 4, St. Louis, 2002, Mosby, pp 149-163.

AUTHOR: **JOHN B. MURPHY, M.D.**

INTRODUCTION

In 1900 most Americans died of unexpected relatively acute medical illnesses, conditions, and accidents. Currently, most Americans die of complications of chronic illnesses. Palliative care as defined by the World Health Organization refers to "the active total care of patients whose disease is not responsive to curative treatments. Control of pain, of other symptoms, and psychological, social and spiritual problems is paramount. The goal of palliative care is achievement of the best possible quality of life for patients and their families." Although palliative care is imperative and most commonly provided at the end of life, it should be recognized that for those living with chronic illnesses and disability, palliative care should be an essential component of care even though they may not be imminently dying. Currently fewer than 20% of Americans are enrolled in hospice before death.

PROCESS OF CARE

- The physician needs to recognize that palliative care is appropriate. Such recognition should come from the physician's assessment of the patient's condition but may come to the physician's attention from other health professionals, patients, family, or friends.
- Following recognition that palliative care is appropriate, the physician needs to facilitate a discussion of palliative care and end of life decisions with the patient and family. This will frequently take more than one encounter and should include an assessment of what the patient and family understand, what their beliefs and wishes may be, and the provision of information regarding prognosis as well as a sense of confidence in the ability to provide relief from suffering.
- The physician needs to establish a plan of care and help the family continue to adhere to the goals of the plan as circumstances change. With adequate support, patients and families can stick to the initial plan and avoid the emotional roller coaster of constantly changing goals. Establishing a plan of care should include involvement of those resources necessary to accomplish the goals (e.g., referral to a hospice program, involvement of clergy).

COMPONENTS OF PALLIATIVE CARE

SYMPTOM CONTROL

- Pain
  - Pain assessment—use pain assessment scale

    I—I—I—I—I—I—I—I—I—I—I
    0   1   2   3   4   5   6   7   8   9 10
    No   Moderate   Worst
    pain   pain   possible
                              pain
  - Nonpharmacologic pain control—heat, cold, massage, cognitive behavioral interventions (relaxation, imagery, and psychotherapy)
  - Pharmacologic pain control
    1. Mild pain—acetaminophen, NSAIDs (including aspirin).
    2. Moderate pain—opioids: codeine, hydromorphone, morphine, hydrocodone, and oxycodone; administer extended release medications on schedule and short-acting medications for breakthrough pain.
- Anxiety
  - Nonpharmacologic—cognitive-behavioral interventions (relaxation, imagery, and psychotherapy).
  - Pharmacologic—intermediate acting benzodiazepam (lorazepam), morphine.

- Constipation—stool softener (e.g., docusate sodium), bowel stimulant (e.g., senna), and if needed osmotic laxative (e.g., lactulose).
- Nausea/Vomiting—treatment should be based on the site causing the nausea and vomiting:
  - Central chemoreceptor trigger center—use prochlorperazine or ondansetron.
  - Gut—use serotonin antagonists or antimotility agent.
  - Vestibular—use meclizine or scopolamine.
  - Cerebral cortex (raised intracranial pressure)—use dexamethasone.
- Diarrhea: frequently secondary to anticonstipation medications or fecal impaction; if true diarrhea try cholestyramine.
- Dyspnea—treat underlying cause, then oxygen and opioids.
- Anorexia
  - Nonpharmacologic—oral agents like artificial saliva, glycerin swabs, and Popsicles.
  - Pharmacologic—megestrol acetate and corticosteroids may be helpful early in the illness.
- Cough—treat underlying illness, then dextromethorphan and opioids.
- Delirium—identify reversible causes (e.g., infection, impaction, pain, hypoxia) and then use antipsychotics.
- Depression—SSRIs and possibly psychostimulants.

CAREGIVER SUPPORT

- Psychologic—assess for depression and anxiety and treat accordingly.
- Spiritual—assess spiritual needs, incorporate spiritual needs into care plan, and involve appropriate consultants.
- Social—assess for caregiver burnout, identify financial resources, consider respite care, and involve appropriate consultants (e.g., MSW).

SETTINGS

- Home—most formal hospice care is provided in individual's homes but this requires able family members or friends to provide the majority of custodial care.
- Inpatient hospice—typically for terminal care, acute control of symptoms, or as bridge in home hospice program.
- Nursing home—preferably provided with formal involvement of hospice program.
- Hospital—common, but not optimum, site for terminal care.

FINANCES

- Hospice—a benefit of Medicare that covers palliative care when elected by a patient and a physician certifies that the patient has a prognosis of 6 months or less (see Hospice in Appendix 1).
  - Covers physician services related to hospice diagnosis, nursing care, medications, durable medical equipment, social services, short-term respite care, chaplaincy services, physical and occupational therapy, bereavement services, and home health aid services.

SUGGESTED READINGS

AGS Panel on Chronic Pain in Older Persons: The management of chronic pain in older persons, *J Am Geriatr Soc* 46(5):635-652, 1998.

AGS Panel on Persistent Pain in Older Persons: The management of persistent pain in older persons, *J Am Geriatr Soc* 50:5205-5224, 2002.

Hlorenz K, Lynn J: Care of the dying patient. In Hazzard W et al: *Principles of Geriatric Medicine and Gerontology*, ed 5, New York, 2003, McGraw-Hill, pp 323-334.

AUTHOR: **JOHN B. MURPHY, M.D.**

INTRODUCTION

Physical therapy is a health profession concerned with the assessment, diagnosis, and treatment of disease and disability through physical means. Physical therapy is performed by a licensed practitioner who works with the physical aspects of a medical illness and specializes in the use of exercise to treat physical conditions. Physical therapy focuses primarily on assessment and treatment of persons with musculoskeletal, neurologic, and cardiopulmonary conditions. The physical therapist may use a variety of modalities and prescribe devices. The goals are to improve strength, mobility, and function; relieve pain; and prevent or minimize disability. Patient and family education are core components of the practice of physical therapy.

EDUCATION AND LICENSING

- Physical therapist has at minimum a 4-year college degree, often a master's degree, and occasionally a doctorate.
- Physical therapy assistant generally has a 2-year junior or community college associate's degree.
- Physical therapists are licensed at a state level but must pass a national exam administered at the state level.
- Evaluate and treat primarily under the prescription of a patient's physician.

SCOPE OF EVALUATION CAPABILITIES

- Joint range of motion
- Muscle strength and endurance
- Integrity of sensation and proprioception
- Muscle tone
- Functional ability
- Gait assessment
- Performance of activities of daily living (ADL)

PHYSICAL THERAPY TECHNIQUES

- Therapeutic exercise
- Joint mobilization and range of motion exercises
- Ambulation training
- Cardiovascular endurance training
- Relaxation exercises
- Therapeutic massage
- Biofeedback
- Training in ADL
- Pulmonary physical therapy

MODALITIES USED

- Traction
- Ultrasound
- Cryotherapy
- Diathermy
- Electrotherapy
- Hydrotherapy

PHYSICIAN REFERRAL TO PHYSICAL THERAPISTS

- Referral can be for assessment, treatment, or both.
- Referral needs a specific diagnosis.
- Referral should include a statement requesting a specific treatment or that the therapist can evaluate and treat as he or she determines most appropriate.
  - Examples:
    1. Dx. Parkinson's disease, ICD-9CM, 332.0: evaluate gait, prescribe and train patient in use of a wheeled walker.
    2. Dx. Adhesive capsulitis, ICD-9CM, 726.0: evaluate and treat as necessary.
- Physical therapy is covered under Medicare and most health insurance plans with a physician's prescription, but primarily for recovery, not for maintenance programs.

SUGGESTED READINGS

American Medical Association: *Health Professions Career and Education Directory,* Chicago, 2002, Author, pp 289-290.

Hoenig H, Cutson T: Geriatric rehabilitation. In Hazzard W et al: *Principles of Geriatric Medicine and Gerontology,* ed 5, New York, 2003, McGraw-Hill, pp 285-302.

Mosqueda L, Brummel-Smith K: Rehabilitation. In Ham R, Sloane P, Warshaw G (eds): *Primary Care Geriatrics,* ed 4, St. Louis, 2002, Mosby, pp 149-163.

AUTHOR: **JOHN B. MURPHY, M.D.**

DEFINITION

There is no universally accepted definition of quality of life. The World Health Organization defines quality of life as "an individual's perception of their position in life in the context of the culture and value systems in which they live and in relation to their goals, expectations, standards and concerns. It is a broad ranging concept affected in a complex way by the person's physical health, psychological state, personal beliefs, social relationships and their relationship to salient features of their environment." Quality of life is a subjective determination, thus two individuals with the same physical status may have different quality of life perceptions.

COMPONENTS OF QUALITY OF LIFE

Four domains have been found to affect the quality of life perceptions of older adults:

1. Physical: a composite of one's bodily status (well versus ill), bodily and mental capabilities, and satisfaction of needs necessary to sustain life (e.g., food, shelter).
2. Psychologic: determined by the ability or inability to cope emotionally with one's life situation.
3. Social: the presence of interpersonal relationships that form a network that is available to provide bodily and emotional support as needed.
4. Environmental: a composite of the location where an individual lives and the persons with whom the individual interacts in that location.

SYNONYMS

Well-being. Health-related quality of life (HRQOL) is a specific term used to define the impact of health status on quality of life.

EPIDEMIOLOGY

The factors found to be associated with quality of life vary from study to study. Some of the predictors associated with lower quality of life include hospitalization, poor health behaviors, impaired mobility, urinary incontinence, hemodialysis, and inability to complete basic or instrumental activities of daily living without assistance. Institutionalized older adults report lower quality of life compared with community-dwelling older adults. The association between gender or race and quality of life depends on the population examined. In two studies, women over the age of 75 reported lower quality of life than their male counterparts. African-American dialysis patients have been found to report higher quality of life compared with non—African-American dialysis patients. In contrast, a study conducted among terminally ill persons did not find any association between gender or race and quality of life perceptions.

PHYSICAL FINDINGS

There are no physical findings that are specific to perceived quality of life. Nonspecific physical findings that have been associated to lower quality of life include body mass index ≤ 20 and poor dentition (<20 teeth). A variety of symptoms including shortness of breath, chronic cough, anxiety, depression, fatigue, insomnia, and pain are also associated with lower quality of life.

EVALUATION OF QUALITY OF LIFE

1. Several generic and disease-specific instruments have been developed to assess quality of life. Generic instruments typically assess multiple domains and are applicable to individuals with a variety of illnesses. Disease-specific instruments assess domains that are presumed to relate directly to the target illness and are only applicable to individuals with the specific illness being targeted. Four quality of life instruments pertinent to older adults are described as follows. Please refer to Appendix 2 for more information.

   a. Medical Outcomes Study Short Form 36-Item Questionnaire (SF-36) is a generic health status instrument that is often used in research studies to assess quality of life. The instrument is easy to administer and has been found to be suitable as an interviewer-administered questionnaire for older outpatients. Poor performance in studies that enrolled hospitalized older adults suggests the instrument should not be administered to this population. Adults aged 75 years and over may have difficulty self-administering the SF-36.
   b. World Health Organization Quality of Life Instrument for Older Adults (WHOQOL-OLD) is a generic quality of life instrument that is currently under development by the World Health Organization. The WHOQOL-OLD is being designed as a research instrument for investigations that enroll older adults from a variety of cultures. The instrument will become available for general use in the near future.
   c. Missoula-VITAS Quality of Life Index (MVQOLI) is an instrument that was designed for use with hospice patients who are terminally ill because of any advanced disease process. As such, the questionnaire has an end of life focus. The instrument is suitable for older adults and individuals with a variety of educational backgrounds. The MVQOLI is applicable as either a clinical or a research tool and may be self-administered.
   d. Quality of Life in Alzheimer's Disease Scale (QOL-AD) is an instrument that was designed to assess the quality of life of persons with Mini Mental State Examination scores between 10 and 25. The QOL-AD incorporates information obtained directly from the patient and supplemental information provided by a caregiver. This instrument is short (13 items) and may easily be used in clinical practice or as part of a research investigation.
2. Global quality of life perceptions are commonly assessed through the use of a simple, direct question such as, "How would you rate your overall quality of life? Would you say Excellent, Very Good, Good, Fair, or Poor?" There is fair correlation between this single global item and the longer quality of life scales.

TREATMENT

Efforts to improve quality of life should be individualized and targeted toward the domains (physical, psychologic, social, environmental) that affect quality of life perceptions. Examples of domain-specific interventions that may improve quality of life are as follows:

- The physical domain may be improved by the alleviation of symptoms and improved disease management.
- The psychologic domain may be positively affected by pharmacologic interventions, such as antidepressant medications, and nonpharmacologic interventions, such as counseling.
- Efforts to improve upon a patient's social domain may require the recruitment of family or formal caregivers.
- A referral to a supervised housing complex may improve the environmental domain.

DIFFERENTIAL DIAGNOSIS

Poor quality of life can be associated with any acute or chronic illness; thus, a global quality of life assessment is warranted in any older adult.

The approach to management of an older adult with complaints of poor quality of life involves several steps. An exploration of the patient's perception of his or her physical, psychologic, social, and environmental domains may be assisted by the use of a generic or disease-specific instrument.

The remainder of the evaluation should focus on the problematic domains identified by the patient. Complaints of a physical nature suggest a comprehensive geriatric evaluation is warranted to determine whether treatment modifications are in order. Particular conditions for assessment include failure to thrive, malnutrition, and cancer.

Conditions to consider if deficits in the psychologic domain are revealed include depression, cognitive impairment, self-neglect, or physical abuse. Assistance from a geriatric case manager or social worker should be sought for individuals who present with deficits in their social or environmental domains.

REFERRAL

Older adults with poor quality of life may benefit from a referral to a geriatrics specialist. Referral to a geriatric psychiatrist should be considered for individuals that present with predominantly emotional problems.

PEARLS & CONSIDERATIONS

- Quality of life (QOL) is composed of four domains—physical, psychologic, social, and environmental. Health-related quality of life (HRQOL) is used to define the impact of an individual's health status on quality of life perceptions. The terms are occasionally used interchangeably.
- Quality of life is subjective. Thus quality of life determinations may not correspond to perceived or actual health status.
- Quality of life perceptions are dynamic and heavily influenced by expectations. The closer your actual existence is to your expectations for your life, the better your quality of life is likely to be.
- Quality of life is one component of quality end of life care. Quality end of life care is a major focus of palliative care. Refer to the chapter on palliative care for more detail on the interaction of quality of life with care at the end of life.

SUGGESTED READINGS

Borglin G et al: Self-reported health complaints and their prediction of overall and health-related quality of life among elderly people, *Int J Nursing Studies* 42:147-158, 2005.

Borowiak E, Kostka T: Predictors of quality of life in older people living at home and in institutions, *Aging Clin Exp Res* 16:212-220, 2004.

Byock IR: Measuring quality of life for patients with terminal illness: the Missoula-VITAS quality of life index, *Palliat Med* 12:231-244, 1998.

Detmar SB et al: Health-related quality of life assessment and patient-physician communication: a randomized controlled trial, *JAMA* 288:3027-3034, 2002.

Farquhar M: Elderly people's definitions of quality of life, *Soc Sci Med* 41:1439-1446, 1995.

Ferrucci L et al: Disease severity and health-related quality of life across different chronic conditions, *J Am Geriatr Soc* 48:1490-1495, 2000.

Hayes V et al: The SF-36 Health Survey Questionnaire: is it suitable for use with older adults? *Age Ageing* 24:120-125, 1995.

Katsura H et al: Both generic and disease specific health-related quality of life are deteriorated in patients with underweight COPD, *Resp Med* 99:624-630, 2005.

Lara-Munoz C, Feinstein AR: How should quality of life be measured? *J Investig Med* 47:17-24, 1999.

Nanda U, Andresen EM: Health-related quality of life: a guide for the health professional, *Eval Health Prof,* 21:179-215, 1998.

Parker SG et al: Measuring health status in older patients: the SF-36 in practice, *Age Ageing* 27:13-18, 1998.

Stenzelius K et al: Patterns of health complaints among people 75+ in relation to quality of life and need of help, *Arch Geron Geriat* 40:85-102, 2005.

Testa MA, Simonson DC: Assessment of quality-of-life outcomes, *N Engl J Med,* 334:835-840, 1996.

WHOQOL Group: http://www.who.int/evidence/assessment-instruments/qol/ql1.htm

AUTHOR: **LISA M. WALKE, M.D.**

INTRODUCTION

- Rehabilitation is critical to geriatric health care because disabling conditions are common among older persons and greatly affect quality of life, but are frequently amenable to treatment.
- Rehabilitation is based on a conceptual framework wherein a disease results in impairment, which is an alteration in physical function at the organ level. The impairment then causes a limitation in a person's activities of daily living (ADL), which is known as a disability. When a disability prevents a person from fully functioning in society, the person has a handicap. This framework is depicted with stroke as an example.
  Disease: Stroke
  Impairment: Left side weakness (organ level)
  Disability: Inability to transfer (person level)
  Handicap: Inability to live alone (societal level)
- Rehabilitation is an approach to care that can be applied anywhere and not just in special units.
- Rehabilitation is less involved in treating disease and more involved in enhancing function across all domains; physical, psychological, and social.
- Rehabilitation is based on comprehensive functional assessment and typically is interdisciplinary.

PROCESS FOR REHABILITATION

- Stabilize the primary problem (e.g., stroke).
  - Treat the hypertension or atrial fibrillation to prevent another stroke.
- Prevent secondary complications.
  - Prevent pressure ulcers, DVT, malnutrition, or a shoulder subluxation.
- Restore lost function.
  - Strength and endurance training: teach stand pivot transfers from bed to wheelchair and instruct in the use of a walker or wheelchair.
- Promote adaptation of the person to the environment.
  - Facilitate physical and psychological acceptance of the changes in function.
- Adapt the environment, physical and personal.
  - Build a ramp for entry into the house, widen doorways to allow a wheelchair to enter, install grab bars in the bathroom.
  - Assess family strengths, build on strengths, and provide supports to bolster weaknesses (e.g., respite care, elderly day care).

REHABILITATION PROFESSIONALS

- Physiatrist—physician trained in physical medicine and rehabilitation (PM&R).
- Rehabilitation nurse—provides nursing care, reinforces and adapts techniques taught by other rehabilitation team members, provides psychologic support, and trains family and other caregivers.
- Physical therapist—assesses strength, range of motion, endurance, and mobility. Focuses primarily on transfers and ambulation.
- Occupational therapist—focuses on assessing and addressing disabilities in activities of daily living (ADL) and some instrumental activities of daily living (IADL)
- Speech pathologist—evaluates and treats patients with aphasia, dysphagia, perceptual disorders, speech impairments, and cognitive problems.
- Recreational therapist—identifies and implements satisfying recreational activities to help patients adjust to their disability.
- Audiologist—assesses degree and characteristics of hearing loss, prescribes auditory aids (including hearing aids), and conducts aural rehabilitation.
- Psychologist—assesses psychologic function and treats psychologic conditions.
- Neuropsychologist—assesses complex neuropsychologic impairments and develops plans for treatment, frequently assisting other rehabilitation team members in adapting their interventions to meet the unique needs of cognitively impaired patients.
- Social worker—assesses social and psychologic strengths and weaknesses of patients and caregivers and identifies community resources needed for optimum family function.
- Orthotist—fashions complex rehabilitation aids such as a prosthesis or back brace.

REHABILITATION SETTINGS

- General principles
  - Provided in the least restrictive, most independent, and least costly setting
  - Provided only following a decrement of function, not for maintenance
  - Provided only as long as the patient continues to make progress
  - Provided only when a patient has sufficient cognitive capability to benefit from therapy
- Acute hospital
  - Immediate phase post illness or operation
  - Duration—brief, a few days to a week
  - Focuses on initial assessment and determination of where to provide subsequent care
  - Designed to prevent complications and bridge patient to next setting
  - Examples—immediate period post stroke or hip fracture
- Acute-level rehabilitation center
  - Patients with complex medical and/or rehabilitation needs that require an interdisciplinary team of rehabilitation specialists
  - Duration—intermediate, generally 1 to 3 weeks
  - Patient must require two or more therapies, be able to benefit from and participate in therapy for at least 3 hours per day
  - Unable to have needs met in a less intensive (expensive) setting
  - Example—stroke patient with good endurance, hemiparesis, mild cognitive deficits, and dysphagia
- Skilled nursing facility (SNF)
  - Patients with functional losses that would benefit from rehabilitation but cannot be cared for at home because of the extent of the functional impairments or the lack of support in the home who may benefit from an interdisciplinary team
  - Duration—intermediate, weeks to a few months
  - Must need a licensed professional (registered nurse, physical or occupational therapist, or speech pathologist) 5 days per week
  - Example—patient with hip fracture who lives alone
  - Medicare requires a hospitalization of at least 3 days in duration within the previous 30 days
- Home
  - Patients with functional losses that would benefit from rehabilitation who have adequate supports in the home or who have mild impairments
  - Duration—brief to long term, days to months
  - Rehabilitation does not require cumbersome equipment that cannot be provided in the home
  - Patient must be homebound (does not go out of the house except for medical care)
  - May require one or more therapies and may provide interdisciplinary team care

- ○ Example—patient who has a total hip replacement for osteoarthritis, is otherwise healthy and robust, who has excellent in-home support and a handicapped-accessible home
- Outpatient
  - ○ Straightforward rehabilitation needs, with one or more therapies, but commonly only one
  - ○ Duration—brief to long term
  - ○ May require access to sophisticated equipment
  - ○ Frequently follows acute hospital, rehabilitation center, SNF, or home rehabilitation program
  - ○ Example—gait assessment and prescription of adaptive mobility aid (e.g., cane or walker)

CONDITIONS NEEDING REHABILITATION AND LIKELY SETTING FOR PROVIDING SERVICES

- Acute-level rehabilitation unit
  - ○ Stroke, amputation, complex fracture (e.g., hip fracture in patient with previous stroke)
- Skilled nursing facility
  - ○ Routine hip fracture, total joint replacement, deconditioning

- Home
  - ○ Stroke or major joint repair with excellent in-home supports, deconditioning
- Outpatient
  - ○ Follow-up care after rehabilitation in another setting, small or medium joint surgery, assessment of unstable gait, prescription of adaptive mobility aid (e.g., walker, cane), adhesive capsulitis of shoulder.

SUGGESTED READINGS

Hoenig H: Geriatric rehabilitation: state of the art, *J Am Geriatr Soc* 45:1371, 1997.

Hoenig H, Cutson T: Geriatric rehabilitation. In Hazzard W et al: *Principles of Geriatric Medicine and Gerontology,* ed 5, New York, 2003, McGraw-Hill, pp. 285-302.

Mosqueda L, Brummel-Smith K: Rehabilitation. In Ham R, Sloane P, Warshaw G (eds): *Primary Care Geriatrics,* ed 4, St. Louis, 2002, Mosby, pp. 149-163.

AUTHOR: **JOHN B. MURPHY, M.D.**

INTRODUCTION

Speech pathology is the science concerned with the diagnosis and treatment of functional and organic speech defects and disorders. Speech and language pathologists evaluate and treat patients with aphasia, cognitive problems, perceptual disorders, and dysphagia.

EDUCATION AND LICENSING

- Minimum education is master's degree
- National certification exam administered by the Educational Testing Service (ETS)
- Licensing at the state level
- Frequently will work with an audiologist

COMMON CONDITIONS ASSESSED AND TREATED

- Dysphagia, including modified barium swallow examinations (MBS)
- Aphasias
- Stroke-associated cognitive and communication disorders
- Language perception disorders
- Hearing impairments and aural rehabilitation

PHYSICIAN REFERRAL TO SPEECH PATHOLOGISTS

- Referral can be for assessment, treatment, or both.
- A referral needs specific diagnosis.
- The services must be medically necessary.
- The plan of care needs to be established by either a speech-language pathologist or the physician.
- The patient must be under the care of a physician.
- Medicare requires physician review of the plan of care every 30 days but no longer stipulates frequency of physician visits.

SUGGESTED READINGS

Hoenig H, Cutson T: Geriatric rehabilitation. In Hazzard W et al: *Principles of Geriatric Medicine and Gerontology,* ed 5, New York, 2003, McGraw-Hill, pp 285-302.

Mosqueda L, Brummel-Smith K: Rehabilitation. In Ham R et al (eds): *Primary Care Geriatrics,* ed 4, St. Louis, 2002, Mosby, pp 149-163.

AUTHOR: **JOHN B. MURPHY, M.D.**

Tools of Geriatric Assessment

Michigan Alcoholism Screening Test (MAST)

Name: _____

Date: _____

Score: _____

			Yes	No
*1.	(2)	Do you feel you are a normal drinker? (By normal we mean you drink less than or as much as most other people)	❏	❏
2.	(2)	Have you ever awakened the morning after some drinking the night before and found that you could not remember part of the evening?	❏	❏
3.	(1)	Does your wife, husband, a parent, or other near relative ever worry or complain about your drinking?	❏	❏
*4.	(2)	Can you stop drinking without a struggle after one or two drinks?	❏	❏
5.	(1)	Do you ever feel guilty about your drinking?	❏	❏
*6.	(2)	Do friends or relatives think you are a normal drinker?	❏	❏
*7.	(2)	Are you able to stop drinking when you want to?	❏	❏
8.	(5)	Have you ever attended a meeting of Alcoholics Anonymous (AA)?	❏	❏
9.	(1)	Have you gotten into physical fights when drinking?	❏	❏
10.	(2)	Has your drinking ever created problems between you and your wife, husband, a parent, or other relative?	❏	❏
11.	(2)	Has your wife, husband, or other family member ever gone to anyone for help about your drinking?	❏	❏
12.	(2)	Have you ever lost friends because of your drinking?	❏	❏
13.	(2)	Have you ever gotten into trouble at work or school because of drinking?	❏	❏
14.	(2)	Have you ever lost a job because of drinking?	❏	❏
15.	(2)	Have you ever neglected your obligations, your family, or your work for two or more days in a row because you were drinking?	❏	❏
16.	(1)	Do you drink before noon fairly often?	❏	❏
17.	(2)	Have you ever been told you have liver trouble? Cirrhosis?	❏	❏
18.	(2)	After heavy drinking have you ever had Delirium Tremens (DTs) or severe shaking or heard voices or seen things that really weren't there?**	❏	❏

Continued on following page

Michigan Alcoholism Screening Test (MAST) *(Continued)*

19.	(5)	Have you ever gone to anyone for help about your drinking?	☐	☐
20.	(5)	Have you ever been in a hospital because of drinking?	☐	☐
21.	(2)	Have you ever been a patient in a psychiatric hospital or on a psychiatric ward of a general hospital where drinking was part of the problem that resulted in hospitalization?	☐	☐
22.	(2)	Have you ever been seen at a psychiatric or mental health clinic or gone to any doctor, social worker, or clergyman for help with any emotional problem where drinking was part of the problem?	☐	☐
23.	(2)	***Have you ever been arrested for drunk driving, driving while intoxicated, or driving under the influence of alcoholic beverages? If yes, how many times? _____	☐	☐
24.	(2)	Have you ever been arrested, or taken into custody, even for a few hours, because of other drunk behavior? If yes, how many times? _____	☐	☐

*Negative responses are alcoholic responses.
**5 points for each Delirium Tremens
***2 points for each arrest

From Selzer ML: The Michigan Alcoholism Screening Test: the quest for a new diagnostic instrument, *Am J Psychiatry* 127:1653-1658, 1971.

Blessed Dementia Scale and Information-Memory Concentration (IMC) Test

Name: _____

Date: _____

Address: _____

Phone: _____

D.O.B.: _____   Gender: Male   Female

Medical Record #: _____

Changes in performance of everyday activities

1. Inability to perform household tasks	1	½	0
2. Inability to cope with small sums of money	1	½	0
3. Inability to remember short list of items, e.g., in shopping	1	½	0
4. Inability to find way about indoors	1	½	0
5. Inability to find way about familiar streets	1	½	0
6. Inability to interpret surroundings (e.g., to recognize whether in hospital or at home, to discriminate between patients, doctors and nurses, relatives and hospital staff, etc.)	1	½	0
7. Inability to recall recent events (e.g., recent outings, visits of relatives or friends to hospital, etc.)	1	½	0
8. Tendency to dwell in the past	1	½	0

Changes in habits

9. Eating:

Cleanly with proper utensils	0
Messily with spoon only	2
Simple solids, e.g., biscuits	2
Has to be fed	3

10. Dressing:

Unaided	0
Occasionally misplaced buttons, etc.	1
Wrong sequence, commonly forgetting items	2
Unable to dress	3

11. Complete sphincter control

	0
Occasional wet beds	1
Frequent wet beds	2
Doubly incontinent	3

Changes in personality, interests, drive

No change	0
12. Increased rigidity	1
13. Increased egocentricity	1
14. Impairment of regard for feelings of others	1
15. Coarsening of affect	1
16. Impairment of emotional control, e.g., increased petulance and irritability	1
17. Hilarity in inappropriate situations	1
18. Diminished emotional responsiveness	1
19. Sexual misdemeanor (appearing de novo in old age)	1
Interests retained	0
20. Hobbies relinquished	1
21. Diminished initiative or growing apathy	1
22. Purposeless hyperactivity	1

Total _____

Ascertain from relative/friend. Applies to last 6 months. Score lies between 0 (fully preserved capacity) and +28 (extreme incapacity)

Information–Memory–Concentration Test

Information test—Score for correct response shown; incorrect responses score 0.

Name	1
Age	1
Time (hour)	1
Time of day	1
Day of week	1
Date	1
Month	1
Season	1
Year	1
Place—	
Name	1
Street	1
Town	1
Type of place (e.g,. home, hospital, etc.)	1
Recognition of persons (cleaner, doctor, nurse, patient, relative; any two available)	2

Total _____

Memory:

(1) personal

Date of birth	1
Place of birth	1
School attended	1
Occupation	1
Name of sibs or name of wife	1
Name of any town where patient had worked	1
Name of employers	1

(2) non-personal

Date of World War I[1]	1
Date of World War II[1]	1
Monarch[2]	1
Prime Minister[3]	1

(3) Name and address (5-minute recall)

Mr. John Brown	
42 West Street	
Gateshead[4]	5

Concentration

Months of year backwards	2	1	0
Counting 1-20	2	1	0
Counting 20-1	2	1	0

Total _____

Scores lie between 0 (complete failure) and +37 (full marks)
1. ½ for approximation within 3 years.
2. President in U.S. version.
3. Vice President in U.S. version.
4. Chicago in U.S. version.

From Blessed G, Tomlinson BF, Roth M: The association between quantitative measures of dementia and of senile change in the cerebral grey matter of elderly subjects, *Br J Psychiatry* 114:797-811, 1968.

Clock Drawing Test (CLOX)
An executive clock drawing task©

STEP 1: Turn this form over on a light-colored surface so that the circle below is visible. Have the subject draw a clock on the back. Instruct him or her to **"Draw me a clock that says 1:45. Set the hands and numbers on the face so that a child could read them."** Repeat the instructions until they are clearly understood. Once the subject begins to draw, no further assistance is allowed. Rate this clock (CLOX 1).

STEP 2: Return to this side and let the subject observe you draw a clock in the circle below. Place 12, 6, 3, and 9 first. Set the hands again to 1:45. Make the hands into arrows. Invite the subject to copy your clock in the lower right-hand corner. Score this clock (CLOX 2).

RATING			
Organization Elements	**Point Value**	**CLOX 1**	**CLOX 2**
Does figure resemble a clock?	1		
Outer circle present?	1		
Diameter > 1 inch?	1		
All numbers inside the circle?	1		
12, 6, 3, and 9 placed first?	1		
Spacing intact? (Symmetry on either side of the 12-6 axis?) If yes, skip next.	2		
If spacing errors are present, are there signs of correction or erasure?	1		
Only Arabic numerals?	1		
Only numbers 1–12 among the Arabic numerals present?	1		
Sequence 1–12 intact? No omissions or intrusions.	1		
Only two hands present?	1		
All hands represented as arrows?	1		
Hour hand between 1 and 2 o'clock?	1		
Minute hand longer than hour?	1		
None of the following:	1		
1) Hand pointing to 4 or 5 o'clock?			
2) "1:45" present?			
3) Intrusions from "hand" or "face" present?			
4) Any letters, words, or pictures?			
5) Any intrusion from circle below?			
	TOTAL		

CLOX scores range from 0–15. Lower scores reflect greater impairment.

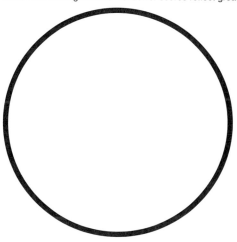

From Royall DR, Cordes JA, Polk M: CLOX: an executive clock drawing task, *J Neurol Neurosurg Psychiatry* 64:588–594, 1998. (http://jnnp.bmjjournals.com/cgi/reprint/64/5/588)

Hachinski Ischemic Score (HIS) for Multi-Infarct Dementia

Name: _____

Date: _____

Address: _____

Phone: _____

D.O.B.: _____ *Gender: Male   Female*

Medical Record #: _____

	Score
Abrupt onset	2
Stepwise deterioration	1
Fluctuating course	2
Nocturnal confusion	1
Relative preservation of personality	1
Depression	1
Somatic complaints	1
Emotional incontinence	1
History of hypertension	1
History of strokes	2
Generalized atherosclerosis	1
Focal neurological symptoms	2
Focal neurological signs	2

(A score of greater than 7 suggests a vascular component to the dementia.)

From Hachinski VC, Iliff LD, Silhka E, et al: Cerebral blood flow in dementia, *Arch Neurol* 32:632–637, 1975.

Mini-Cog Scoring Algorithm

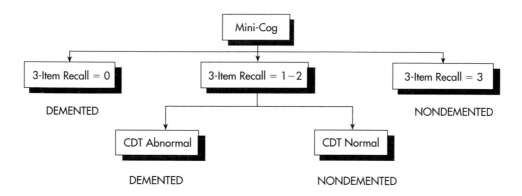

CDT, Clock drawing test.
From Borson S, Scanlon J, Brush M, Vitaliano P, Dokmak A: The mini-cog: a cognitive "vital signs" measure for dementia screening in multilingual elderly, *Int J Geriatr Psychiatry* 15:1021–1027, 2000.

Mini-Mental State Examination (MMSE)

The Mini-Mental State Examination (MMSE) is no longer available for text publication. The MMSE is now published and sold by Psychological Assessment Resources, Inc., 16204 N. Florida Ave, Lutz, FL 33549; phone: 1-800-331-8378 or 1-813-968-3003; website: http://www.parinc.com/.

The MMSE form published by Psychological Assessment Resources, Inc. is based on its original 1975 conceptualization, with minor subsequent modifications by the authors. MMSE kits are available and include an MMSE clinical guide, pocket norms card, user's guide, and test forms.

Targeted Population: Older adults.

Description: One of the most widely used tests of cognitive function, the MMSE is also well studied. The MMSE is a screening test only; diagnosis of dementia requires a full mental status examination with history and physical examination. The test contains 11 items in two parts. The first part requires verbal responses and assesses orientation, memory, and attention. The second part evaluates naming of objects, ability to follow oral and written commands, sentence writing, and ability to copy a complex polygon.

Scores: Points are assigned to correct responses. Total scores range from 0 to 30. The mean score for normal individuals is 27.6; for patients with dementia, the mean score is 9.7 (Folstein et al, 1975). The cutoff score ranges from 23 to 25 in multiple studies (McDowell & Newell, 1996). Cutoff scores may vary based on level of education. Scores at or less than the cutoff warrant further evaluation of cognitive function.

Accuracy: The MMSE has demonstrated good to excellent reliability (internal consistency, test–retest, and interrater) and validity (content and correlations with other cognitive function tests) in numerous studies (Tombaugh & McIntyre, 1992; McDowell & Newell, 1996). Predictive validity studies have shown that the MMSE has good ability to indicate when an individual becomes cognitively impaired. Some variation in scores was noted when educational levels were compared, with lower scores implying more cognitive impairment among those with higher education than among those with less education (Uhlmann & Larson, 1991). As education level increases, the specificity of the MMSE also rises, whereas the sensitivity decreases. Hence, cutoff scores may be lower in less educated persons. With the use of normative data, Crum et al (1993) provided cutoff scores of 19 for 0 to 4 years of education, 23 for 5 to 8 years of education, 27 for 9 to 12 years of education, and 29 for college level and beyond.

Administration Time: This test is not timed but takes approximately 10 minutes to administer.

Descriptive summary from Loretz L: *Primary Care Tools for Clinicians: A Compendium of Forms, Questionnaires, and Rating Scales for Everyday Practice*, St. Louis, 2005, Mosby.

Sample Material from the Mini-Mental State Examination (MMSE)

Orientation to Time
   "What is the date?"

Registration
   "Listen carefully. I am going to say three words. You say them back after I stop.
   Ready? Here they are...
   APPLE (pause), PENNY (pause), TABLE (pause). Now repeat those words back to me." (Repeat up to 5 times, but score only the first trial.)

Naming
   "What is this?" (Point to a pencil or pen.)

Reading
   "Please read this and do what it says." (Show examinee the words on the stimulus form.)
   CLOSE YOUR EYES

Severe Mini-Mental State Examination

Severe Mini-Mental State Examination Instrument

Name: (1 point if close; 3 if completely accurate)
First _____
Last _____

Birthday: (1 point if any elements correct; 2 points if completely accurate)
_____

Repeat three words: (1 point for each word)
Bird _____
House _____
Umbrella _____

Follow simple directions: (1 point for following command; 2 points for continuing to hold command [i.e., 5 seconds] until told to stop)
Raise your hand _____
Close your eyes _____

Name simple objects: (1 point for each object)
Pen _____
Watch _____
Shoe _____

Draw circle from command: (1 point)
Circle _____

Copy square: (1 point)
Square _____

Write name: (1 point if close; 2 points if completely accurate)
First _____
Last _____

Animal generation: (number of animals in 1 minute)
1 to 2 animals: 1 point
3 to 4 animals: 2 points
>4 animals: 3 points

Spell "CAT" forward: (1 point for each letter given in correct order)
C _____
A _____
T _____

Scoring Rules for the Severe Mini-Mental State Examination

Question 1: The patient is asked to state his or her first and last names. Three points are given for each correct answer. Women, if married, must give married name (if that is her legal name).

Question 2: The patient is asked to state the month, day, and year of birth. Any order is acceptable. Two points if completely correct. One point for any of the three items.

Question 3: The examiner tells the patient that he or she is going to say three words and then ask the patient to repeat them. The examiner then says, "bird, house, umbrella," and asks the patient to repeat them. One point is given for each correctly named item.

Question 4: The examiner shows the patient three items, one at a time, and asks the patient to name it. A pen, watch, and shoe are then shown to the patient. One point is given for each correctly named item.

Question 5: The patient is asked to follow a direction (for 5 seconds). The first direction is "shut your eyes;" the second is "raise your hand" (either one or both hands is acceptable). Two points are given for each direction if the patient follows and continues the command until told to stop by the examiner. One point is given for each command if the patient follows the command but does not maintain it until told to stop by the examiner.

Question 6: The patient is given a clean sheet of paper and a pen and is asked to write (printing or cursive acceptable) his or her first and last name. Two points are awarded for each item if totally correct and legible, one point if poorly legible or if letters are left out. Women must write their married last name.

Question 7: The patient is verbally asked to draw a circle. One point if the item drawn resembles a circle, i.e., it must be closed, may be somewhat elliptical, any size acceptable.

Question 8: A copy of a square is presented to the patient, and he or she is asked to copy it. The examiner should not identify the square orally. One point is given if the copy has four sides that touch; rectangular-appearing squares are acceptable.

Question 9: The patient is asked to generate as many animals as he or she can think of in 1 minute. One point is given for up to two animals, two points for up to four animals, three points for more than four animals.

Question 10: The patient is asked to spell the word "CAT." Letters must be in correct order. One point is given for each correct lettter.

From Harrell LE, Marson D, Chatterjee A, Parrish JA: The severe mini-mental state examination: a new neuropsychologic instrument for the bedside assessment of severely impaired patients with Alzheimer disease, *Alzheimer Dis Assoc Disord* 14(3):168–175, 2000.

Confusion Assessment Method (CAM)

The Confusion Assessment Method (CAM) Instrument

Acute onset
1. Is there evidence of an acute change in mental status from the patient's baseline?

Inattention
(The questions listed under this topic were repeated for each topic where applicable.)
2. A. Did the patient have difficulty focusing attention, for example, being easily distractible or having difficulty keeping track of what was being said?
   Not present at any time during interview
   Present at some time during interview, but in mild form
   Present at some time during interview, in marked form
   Uncertain
   B. (If present or abnormal) Did this behavior fluctuate during the interview, that is, tend to come and go or increase and decrease in severity?
   Yes
   No
   Uncertain
   Not applicable
   C. (If present or abnormal) Please describe his or her behavior:

Disorganized thinking
3. Was the patient's thinking disorganized or incoherent, such as rambling or irrelevant conversation, unclear or illogical flow of ideas, or unpredictable switching from subject to subject?

Altered level of consciousness
4. Overall, how would you rate this patient's level of consciousness?
   Alert (normal)
   Vigilant (hyperalert, overly sensitive to environmental stimuli, startled very easily). Lethargic (drowsy, easily aroused)
   Stupor (difficult to arouse)
   Coma (unarousable)
   Uncertain

Disorientation
5. Was the patient disoriented at any time during the interview, such as thinking that he or she was somewhere other than the hospital, using the wrong bed, or misjudging the time of day?

Memory impairment
6. Did the patient demonstrate any memory problems during the interview, such as inability to remember events in the hospital or difficulty remembering instructions?

Perceptual disturbances
7. Did the patient have any evidence of perceptual disturbances, for example, hallucinations, illusions, or misinterpretations (such as thinking something was moving when it was not)?

Psychomotor agitation
8. Part 1.
   At any time during the interview, did the patient have an unusually increased level of motor activity, such as restlessness, picking at bedclothes, tapping fingers, or making frequent sudden changes of position?

Psychomotor retardation
8. Part 2.
   At any time during the interview, did the patient have an unusually decreased level of motor activity, such as sluggishness, staring into space, staying in one position for a long time, or moving very slowly?

Altered sleep-wake cycle
9. Did the patient have evidence of disturbance of the sleep-wake cycle, such as excessive daytime sleepiness with insomnia at night?

Confusion Assessment Method (CAM) Diagnostic Algorithm
(Delirium is diagnosed when both features 1 and 2 are positive, along with either feature 3 or 4.)

Feature 1: Acute Onset and Fluctuating Course
This feature is usually obtained from a family member or nurse and is shown by positive responses to the following questions: Is there evidence of an acute change in mental status from the patient's baseline? Did the (abnormal) behavior fluctuate during the day, that is, tend to come and go or increase and decrease in severity?

Feature 2: Inattention
This feature is shown by a positive response to the following question: Did the patient have difficulty focusing attention, for example, being easily distractible or having difficulty keeping track of what was being said?

Feature 3: Disorganized Thinking
This feature is shown by a positive response to the following question: Was the patient's thinking disorganized or incoherent, such as rambling or irrelevant conversation, unclear or illogical flow of ideas, or unpredictable switching from subject to subject?

Feature 4: Altered Level of Consciousness
This feature is shown by any answer other than "alert" to the following question: Overall, how would you rate this patient's level of consciousness? (alert [normal], vigilant [hyperalert, overly sensitive to environmental stimuli, startled very easily], lethargic [drowsy, easily aroused], stupor [difficult to arouse], or coma [unarousable])

From Inouye AK, van Dyck Ch, Alessi CA: Clarifying confusion: the confusion assessment method, *Ann Intern Med* 113(12):941–948, 1990.

Confusion Assessment Method for the Intensive Care Unit (CAM-ICU)

Confusion Assessment Method for the Intensive Care Unit (CAM-ICU) Instrument
Delirium is diagnosed when both features 1 and 2 are positive, along with either feature 3 or 4.

Feature 1: Acute Onset of Mental Status Changes or Fluctuating Course
- Is there evidence of an acute change in mental status from the baseline?
- Did the (abnormal) behavior fluctuate during the past 24 hours, that is, tend to come and go or increase and decrease in severity?

Sources of information: Serial Glasgow Coma Scale or sedation score ratings over 24 hours as well as readily available input from the patient's bedside critical care nurse or family.

Feature 2: Inattention
- Did the patient have difficulty focusing attention?
- Is there a reduced ability to maintain and shift attention?

Sources of information: Attention screening examinations by using either picture recognition or Vigilance A random letter test (see Attention Screening Examinations [ASE] for the Intensive Care Unit). Neither of these tests requires verbal response, and thus they are ideally suited for mechanically ventilated patients.

Feature 3: Disorganized Thinking
- Was the patient's thinking disorganized or incoherent, such as rambling or irrelevant conversation, unclear or illogical flow of ideas, or unpredictable switching from subject to subject?
- Was the patient able to follow questions and commands throughout the assessment?
    1. "Are you having any unclear thinking?"
    2. "Hold up this many fingers." (Examiner holds two fingers in front of the patient.)
    3. "Now, do the same thing with the other hand" (not repeating the number of fingers).

Feature 4: Altered Level of Consciousness
- Any level of consciousness other than "alert."
- Alert—normal, spontaneously fully aware of environment and interacts appropriately
- Vigilant—hyperalert
- Lethargic—drowsy but easily aroused, unaware of some elements in the environment, or not spontaneously interacting appropriately with the interviewer; becomes fully aware and appropriately interactive when prodded minimally
- Stupor—difficult to arouse, unaware of some or all elements in the environment, or not spontaneously interacting with the interviewer; becomes incompletely aware and inappropriately interactive when prodded strongly
- Coma—unarousable, unaware of all elements in the environment, with no spontaneous interaction or awareness of the interviewer, so that the interview is difficult or impossible even with maximal prodding

Attention Screening Examinations (ASE) for the Intensive Care Unit
- (A) Picture Recognition ASE
- (B) Vigilance A Random Letter Test

(A) Picture Recognition ASE (Fig. A2-1)
Step 1: Five pictures
Say to the patient: "Mr. or Mrs. X, I am going to show you pictures of some common objects. Watch carefully and try to remember each picture because I will ask what pictures you have seen." Then show Step 1 of either Form A or Form B, alternating daily if repeat measures are taken.

Step 2: Ten pictures
Say to the patient: "Now I am going to show you some more pictures. Some of these you have already seen and some are new. Let me know whether or not you saw the picture before by nodding your head yes (demonstrate) or no (demonstrate)." Then show Step 2 of Form A or B, depending on which form was used in Step 1.

Form A (Step 1)	Form B (Step 1)
key	boot
cup	dog
car	knife
table	pants
hammer	paintbrush

Form A (Step 2)	Form B (Step 2)
key	boot
cup	dog
car	knife
table	pants
hammer	paintbrush
glass	fork
lock	cat
truck	dress
chair	toothbrush
saw	shoe

This test is scored by the number of correct "yes" or "no" answers (out of a possible 10) during the second step. To improve the visibility for elderly patients, the images are printed on 6 × 10-inch buff-colored paper and laminated with a flat finish. As did Hart et al, we showed each image for 3 seconds. When a patient had known visual impairment and no corrective lenses, we substituted the Vigilance A Random Letter Test (1, 2).

(B) Vigilance A Random Letter Test
Directions: Tell the patient: "I am going to read you a long series of letters. Whenever you hear the letter A, indicate by squeezing my hand." Read the following letter list in a normal tone at a rate of one letter per second.

    LTPEAOAICTDALAA
    ANIABFSAMRZEOAD
    PAKLAUCJTOEABAA
    ZYFMUSAHEVAARAT

Scoring: Currently, only preliminary standardized norms exist for this test. The average person should complete the task without error ($x = 0.2$); a sample of randomly selected brain-damaged patients made an average of ten errors. Examples of common organic errors are a) failure to indicate when the target letter has been presented (omission error); b) indication made when a nontarget letter has been presented (commission error); and c) failure to stop tapping with the presentation of subsequent nontarget letters (perseveration error) (3).

REFERENCES

1. Hart RP, Levenson JL, Sessler CN, Best AM, Schwartz SM, Rutherford LE: Validation of a cognitive test for delirium in medical ICU patients, *Psychosomatics* 37(6):533-546, 1996.
2. Hart RP, Best AM, Sessler CN, Levenson JL: Abbreviated cognitive test for delirium, *J Psychosom Res* 43(4):417-423, 1997.
3. Strub RL, Black FW: *The Mental Status Examination in Neurology,* ed 3, Philadelphia, 1993, FA Davis.

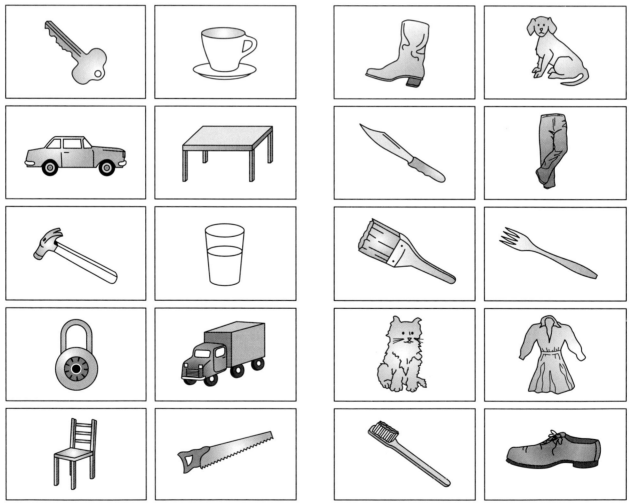

FIGURE A2-1 Form A and Form B, Picture Recognition Attention Screening Examination for the Intensive Care Unit.

Criteria Used by Delirium Experts

Criteria for delirium from *Diagnostic and Statistical Manual for Mental Disorders*—Reference standard evaluations were performed using all available information including patient examinations and interactions, nurse and family interviews, physicians' and nurses' notes, laboratory values, and any other chart data present.

A. Disturbance of consciousness (i.e., reduced clarity of awareness of the environment) with reduced ability to focus, sustain, or shift attention

B. A change in cognition (e.g., memory deficit, disorientation, language disturbance) or the development of a perceptual disturbance that is not better accounted for by a preexisting, established, or evolving dementia

C. Disturbance that develops over a short period of time (usually hours to days) and tends to fluctuate during the course of the day

D. Evidence from the history, physical examination, or laboratory findings that the disturbance is caused by one of the following:

    i. Direct physiologic consequences of a general medical condition

    ii. Direct result of medication use or substance intoxication (substance intoxication delirium)

    iii. Direct result of a withdrawal syndrome (substance withdrawal delirium)

    iv. Direct result of more than one of the preceding etiologies (delirium due to multiple etiologies)

The diagnosis of cognitive impairment involved careful observations of the abilities of the patient and knowledge of the patient's former level of functioning. To identify all cases of cognitive impairment, we adopted the following measures:

a) The preceding criteria from the *Diagnostic and Statistical Manual for Mental Disorders* and mental status definitions were employed consistently.

b) A delirium expert evaluation was conducted to determine which of these criteria were met by the patient. This involved a bedside evaluation and screening for cognitive and attention deficits.

c) Last, interviewing the family and nurse who provided the majority of patient care established baseline functioning and identified fluctuations.[1]

REFERENCE

1. American Psychiatric Association: *Diagnostic and Statistical Manual of Mental Disorders,* ed 4, Washington, DC, 1994, American Psychiatric Association.

From Ely EW, Margolin R, Francis J, et al: Evaluation of delirium in critically ill patients: validation of the Confusion Assessment Method for the Intensive Care Unit (CAM-ICU), *Crit Care Med* 29(7):1370–1379, 2001.

Center for Epidemiologic Studies Depression Scale (CES-D)

Name: _____

Date: _____

As I read the following statements, please tell me how often you felt or behaved this way.

IN THE LAST WEEK. Did you feel this way:

    0 = Rarely or none of the time (i.e., less than 1 day)?
    1 = Some or a little of the time (i.e., 1-2 days)?
    2 = Occasionally or a moderate amount of time (i.e., 3-4 days)?
    3 = Most or all of the time (i.e., 5-7 days)?
    — = No response

	Rarely	Some of of the time	Occasionally	Most of the time	No response
1. I was bothered by things that usually don't bother me	0	1	2	3	—
2. I did not feel like eating; my appetite was poor	0	1	2	3	—
3. I felt that I could not shake off the blues even with help from my family and friends	0	1	2	3	—
*4. I felt that I was just as good as other people	3	2	1	0	—
5. I had trouble keeping my mind on what I was doing	0	1	2	3	—
6. I felt depressed	0	1	2	3	—
7. I felt that everything I did was an effort	0	1	2	3	—
*8. I felt hopeful about the future	3	2	1	0	—
9. I thought my life had been a failure	0	1	2	3	—
10. I felt fearful	0	1	2	3	—
11. My sleep was restless	0	1	2	3	—
*12. I was happy	3	2	1	0	—
13. I talked less than usual	0	1	2	3	—
14. I felt lonely	0	1	2	3	—
15. People were unfriendly	0	1	2	3	—
*16. I enjoyed life	3	2	1	0	—
17. I had crying spells	0	1	2	3	—
18. I felt sad	0	1	2	3	—
19. I felt people disliked me	0	1	2	3	—
20. I could not get going	0	1	2	3	—

*Items are reverse-scored.
Range of scores 0–60, with higher scores indicating more depressive symptoms.

From Radloff LS: The CES-D Scale: a self-report depression scale for research in the general population, *Appl Psychol Measure* 2:385–401, 1977.

Cornell Scale for Depression in Dementia (CSDD)

Name: _____

Date: _____

Scoring (based on symptoms/signs occurring during the week prior to testing):

a = unable to evaluate; 0 = absent; 1 = mild or intermittent; 2 = severe.

Location: ☐ Nursing Home Resident   ☐ Outpatient   ☐ Inpatient

A. MOOD-RELATED SIGNS

1. ANXIETY ....a   0   1   2
    anxious expression, ruminations, worrying
2. SADNESS ....a   0   1   2
    sad expression, sad voice, tearfulness
3. LACK OF REACTIVITY TO PLEASANT EVENTS ....a   0   1   2
4. IRRITABILITY ....a   0   1   2
    easily annoyed, short tempered

B. BEHAVIORAL DISTURBANCES

5. AGITATION ....a   0   1   2
    restlessness, handwringing, hairpulling
6. RETARDATION ....a   0   1   2
    slow movements, slow speech, slow reactions
7. MULTIPLE PHYSICAL COMPLAINTS ....a   0   1   2
    (score 0 if gastrointestinal symptoms only)
8. LOSS OF INTEREST ....a   0   1   2
    less involved in usual activities (score only if change occurred
    acutely—in less than 1 month)

C. PHYSICAL SIGNS

9. APPETITE LOSS ....a   0   1   2
    eating less than usual
10. WEIGHT LOSS ....a   0   1   2
    (score 2 if greater than 5 lb in one month)
11. LACK OF ENERGY ....a   0   1   2
    fatigues easily, unable to sustain activities (score only if change occurred
    acutely—in less than 1 month)

D. CYCLIC FUNCTIONS

12. DIURNAL VARIATION ON MOOD ....a   0   1   2
    symptoms worse in the morning
13. DIFFICULTY FALLING ASLEEP ....a   0   1   2
    later than usual for this person
14. MULTIPLE AWAKENINGS DURING SLEEP ....a   0   1   2
15. EARLY MORNING AWAKENING ....a   0   1   2
    earlier than usual for this person

E. IDEATIONAL DISTURBANCES

16. SUICIDE ....a   0   1   2
    feels life is not worth living, has suicidal wishes, or makes suicidal attempt
17. POOR SELF-ESTEEM ....a   0   1   2
    self-blame, self-deprecation, feelings of failure
18. PESSIMISM ....a   0   1   2
    anticipation of the worst
19. MOOD-CONGRUENT DELUSIONS ....a   0   1   2
    delusions of poverty, illness, or loss

Score: _____

Total score ≥ 8 suggests significant depressive symptoms.

The Cornell Scale is administered in two steps. First, the clinician interviews the patient's caregiver on each of the 19 items of the Cornell Scale and then briefly interviews the patient. Symptoms and signs are described to the caregiver as they appear on the scale. For example, to rate the presence of anxiety, the clinician asks the caregiver whether or not he or she has observed the patient having an anxious expression, or whether or not the patient is ruminating or worrying. The clinician is free to use additional descriptions to help the caregiver understand the meaning of each item. The caregiver is instructed to base his or her report on observations of the patient's behavior during the week prior to interview. Two of the items, "loss of interest" and "lack of energy," require not only that the patient is less involved in usual activities or has less energy during the week prior to interview, but also that changes in these behaviors occurred relatively acutely, i.e., over a period of less than 1 month. In these two items, the caregiver is initially asked to describe the patient's behavior during the week prior to interview and then is asked to provide information about the onset of behavioral changes that may have occurred earlier. The item on "weight loss" is based entirely on information about the patient's weight during the month preceding the interview. During the interview with the caregiver, the clinician assigns preliminary scores to each item of the Corrnell Scale. Next, the clinician briefly interviews the patient using Cornell Scale items as a basis for inquiry and observation, but does not necessarily confine himself or herself to these questions. If there is a large discrepancy between the clinician's observations and the caregiver's report on any item, the clinician interviews the caregiver again and attempts to clarify the reason for disagreement. After this process, the Cornell Scale is scored on the basis of the clinician's final judgment.

The total time of administration and rating of the Cornell Scale is approximately 30 min (approximately 20 min interview with the subject's caregiver and about 10 min interview with the subject).

Geriatric Depression Scale (GDS)

Name: _____

Date: _____

Circle the best answer for how you felt over the past week.

1. *Are you basically satisfied with your life?...	Yes	No
2. Have you dropped many of your activities and interests?.............................	Yes	No
3. Do you feel that your life is empty?...	Yes	No
4. Do you often get bored?...	Yes	No
5. *Are you hopeful about the future?...	Yes	No
6. Are you bothered by thoughts you can't get out of your head?......................	Yes	No
7. *Are you in good spirits most of the time?...	Yes	No
8. Are you afraid something bad is going to happen to you?	Yes	No
9. *Do you feel happy most of the time?..	Yes	No
10. Do you often feel helpless?...	Yes	No
11. Do you often get restless and fidgety?..	Yes	No
12. Do you prefer to stay at home, rather than going out and doing new things?..........	Yes	No
13. Do you frequently worry about the future?..	Yes	No
14. Do you feel you have more problems with memory than most?......................	Yes	No
15. *Do you think it is wonderful to be alive now?.......................................	Yes	No
16. Do you often feel downhearted and blue?	Yes	No
17. Do you feel pretty worthless the way you are now?	Yes	No
18. Do you worry a lot about the past?..	Yes	No
19. *Do you find life very exciting?	Yes	No
20. Is it hard for you to get started on new projects?	Yes	No
21. *Do you feel full of energy?..	Yes	No
22. Do you feel that your situation is hopeless?	Yes	No
23. Do you think that most people are better off than you are?	Yes	No
24. Do you frequently get upset over little things?	Yes	No
25. Do you frequently feel like crying?	Yes	No
26. Do you have trouble concentrating?	Yes	No
27. *Do you enjoy getting up in the morning?..	Yes	No
28. Do you prefer to avoid social gatherings?..	Yes	No
29. *Is it easy for you to make decisions?..	Yes	No
30. *Is your mind as clear as it used to be?	Yes	No

Scoring: Assign one point for each 'yes' answer: 2, 3, 4, 6, 8, 10, 11, 12, 13, 14, 16, 17, 18, 20, 22, 23, 24, 25, 26, 28
     *Assign one point for each 'no' answer: 1, 5, 7, 9, 15, 19, 21, 27, 29, 30

Score: _____ Completed by: _____ Date: _____

Normal: 0 to 10; Mildly depressed: 11 to 20; Very depressed: 21 to 30

Adapted from Yesavage JA, Brink TL: Development and a validation of a geriatric depression screening scale: a preliminary report, *J Psychiatr Res* 17(1):37–49, 1983.

Hamilton Anxiety Rating Scale (HARS)

Name: _____

Rater: _____

Date: _____

The Hamilton Anxiety Scale (HARS, HAM-A) consists of 14 items, each defined by a series of symptoms. Each item is rated on a 5-point scale: 0-absent; 1-mild; 2-moderate; 3-severe; 4-incapacitating. Higher scores indicate increased anxiety.

SYMPTOMS

1. Anxious Mood   0 1 2 3 4
   - worries
   - anticipates worst

2. Tension   0 1 2 3 4
   - startles
   - cries easily
   - restless
   - trembling

3. Fears   0 1 2 3 4
   - fear of the dark
   - fear of strangers
   - fear of being alone
   - fear of animal

4. Insomnia   0 1 2 3 4
   - difficulty falling asleep or staying asleep
   - difficulty with nightmares

5. Intellectual   0 1 2 3 4
   - poor concentration
   - memory impairment

6. Depressed Mood   0 1 2 3 4
   - decreased interest in activities
   - anhedonia
   - insomnia

7. Somatic Complaints–Muscular   0 1 2 3 4
   - muscle aches or pains
   - bruxism

8. Somatic Complaints–Sensory   0 1 2 3 4
   - tinnitus
   - blurred vision

9. Cardiovascular Symptoms   0 1 2 3 4
   - tachycardia
   - palpitations
   - chest pain
   - sensation of feeling faint

10. Respiratory Symptoms   0 1 2 3 4
    - chest pressure
    - choking sensation
    - shortness of breath

11. Gastrointestinal Symptoms   0 1 2 3 4
    - dysphagia
    - nausea or vomiting
    - constipation
    - weight loss

12. Genitourinary Symptoms   0 1 2 3 4
    - urinary frequency or urgency
    - dysmenorrhea
    - impotence

13. Autonomic Symptoms   0 1 2 3 4
    - dry mouth
    - flushing
    - pallor
    - sweating

14. Behavior at Interview   0 1 2 3 4
    - fidgets
    - tremor
    - paces

TOTAL SCORE: _____

Adapted from Hamilton M: The assessment of anxiety states by rating, *Brit J Med Psychol* 32:50–55, 1959. Copyright 1959 The British Psychological Society. Reprinted with permission.

Abnormal Involuntary Movement Scale (AIMS)—
Screening for Tardive Dyskinesia

Patient Name: _____   *Examiner:* _____

Date of Visit: _____

Examination Procedure[a]   Either before or after completing the EXAMINATION PROCEDURE observe the patient unobtrusively, at rest (e.g., in the waiting room). The chair to be used in this examination should be a hard, firm one without arms.

1) Ask patient whether there is anything in his/her mouth (e.g., gum, candy, etc.) and if there is, to remove it.
2) Ask patient about the <u>current</u> condition of his/her teeth. Ask patient if he/she wears dentures. Do teeth or dentures bother patient now?
3) Ask patient whether he/she notices any movements in mouth, face, hands, or feet. If yes, ask to describe and to what extent they <u>currently</u> bother patient or interfere with his/her activities.
4) Have patient sit in chair with hands on knees, legs slightly apart, and feet flat on floor. (Look at entire body for movements while patient is in this position.)
5) Ask patient to sit with hands hanging unsupported: [for a male patient, hands hanging between his legs, and for a female patient wearing dress, hands hanging over her knees].[b] (Observe hands and other body areas.)
6) Ask patient to open mouth. (Observe tongue at rest within mouth.) Do this twice.
7) Ask patient to protrude tongue. (Observe abnormalities of tongue movement.) Do this twice.
8) Ask patient to tap thumb, with each finger, as rapidly as possible for 10-15 seconds, separately with right hand, then with left hand. (Observe facial and leg movements.)
9) Flex and extend patient's left and right arms (one at a time). (Note any rigidity.)
10) Ask patient to stand up. (Observe in profile. Observe all body areas again, hips included.)
11) Ask patient to extend both arms outstretched in front with palms down. (Observe trunk, legs, and mouth.)
12) Have patient walk a few paces, turn, and walk back to chair. (Observe hands and gait.) Do this twice.

Movement Ratings[a,b]   Complete EXAMINATION PROCEDURE (above) before making ratings for the MOVEMENT RATINGS, rate the highest severity observed.

0 = none
1 = minimal (may be extreme normal)
2 = mild
3 = moderate
4 = severe

FACIAL & ORAL MOVEMENTS:

❶ **Muscles of facial expression** (e.g., movements of forehead, eyebrows, periorbital area, cheeks; include frowning, blinking, smiling, grimacing [of upper face].)   0 1 2 3 4

❷ **Lips and perioral area** (e.g., puckering, pouting, smacking)   0 1 2 3 4

❸ **Jaw** (e.g., biting, clenching, chewing, mouth opening, lateral movement)   0 1 2 3 4

❹ **Tongue** (Rate only increase in movement both in and out of mouth, NOT inability to sustain a movement.)   0 1 2 3 4

EXTREMITY MOVEMENTS:

❺ **Upper** *(arms, wrists, hands, fingers)* Include choreic movements, (i.e., rapid, objectively purposeless, irregular, spontaneous), athetoid movements (i.e., slow, irregular, complex, serpentine). Do NOT include tremor (i.e., repetitive, regular rhythmic)   0 1 2 3 4

❻ **Lower** *(legs, knees, ankles, toes)* e.g., lateral knee movement, foot tapping, heel dropping, foot squirming, inversion & eversion of foot)   0 1 2 3 4

TRUNK MOVEMENTS:

❼ **Neck, shoulders, hips** (e.g., rocking, twisting, squirming, pelvic gyrations) Include diaphragmatic movements.   0 1 2 3 4

GLOBAL JUDGMENTS: [score based on highest single score on items 1-7 above]

❽ Severity of abnormal movement   0 1 2 3 4

❾ Incapacitation due to abnormal movement   0 1 2 3 4

❿ Patient's awareness of abnormal movement (Rate only patient's report.)   0 1 2 3 4

0 = no awareness;   1 = aware, no distress;   2 = aware, mild distress;
3 = aware, moderate distress;   4 = aware, severe distress.

Rate item 10 according to reported level of distress

DENTAL STATUS

⓫ Current problems with teeth and/or dentures   No: 0   Yes: 1

⓬ Does patient usually wear dentures?   No: 0   Yes: 1

[a]Munetz and Benjamin (1988) offer a detailed review of the Examination Procedure as well as a detailed proposal for how to score the Movement Ratings. The authors note the recommendation that the AIMS be administered twice per year beginning prior to the start of neuroleptic (antipsychotic) drug therapy (Baldressarini et al, 1980). They also note that although ratings above 0 may suggest tardive dyskinesia, it is important to determine if the abnormal movement is clinically significant. Also, nonmedication causes should be ruled out. The original AIMS scoring directed that movements (re: Examination Procedure items 8, 11, and 12) be scored 1 point less if they did not occur spontaneously. However, Munetz and Benjamin recommend not following this direction. Schooler and Kane (1982) propose the following criteria for a diagnosis of probable tardive dyskinesia: (a) exposure to neuroleptics for a total of at least 3 months, (b) score of 2 for at least 2 body areas, or score of 3 for at least 1 body area, and (c) rule out other causes for abnormal movement.

[b]AIMS text in brackets was added or rephrased by Munetz and Benjamin (1988).

From Guy W: *ECDEU Assessment Manual for Psychopharmacology,* revised edition, Washington, DC, 1976, US Department of Health, Education, and Welfare. Modified by Munetz MR, Benjamin S: How to examine patients using the Abnormal Involuntary Movement Scale, *Hospital Com Psychiatry* 39(11):1172–1177, 1988.

Berg Balance Scale

Name: _____

Date: _____

General Instructions

Please demonstrate each task and/or give instructions as written below. When scoring, please record the lowest response category that applies for each item.

In most items, the subject is asked to maintain a given position for a specific time. Progressively more points are deducted if the time or distance requirements are not met, if the subject's performance warrants supervision, or if the subject touches an external support or receives assistance from the examiner. Subjects should understand that they must maintain their balance while attempting the tasks. The choices of which leg to stand on or how far to reach are left to the subject. Poor judgment will adversely influence the performance and the scoring.

Equipment required for testing are a stopwatch or watch with a second hand and a ruler or other indicator of 2, 5, and 10 inches (5, 12.5, and 25 cm). Chairs used during testing should be of reasonable height. Either a step or a stool (of average step height) may be used for item #12.

Item	Description	Score (0-4)
1.	Sitting to standing	_____
2.	Standing unsupported	_____
3.	Sitting unsupported	_____
4.	Standing to sitting	_____
5.	Transfers	_____
6.	Standing with eyes closed	_____
7.	Standing with feet together	_____
8.	Reaching forward with outstretched arm	_____
9.	Retrieving object from floor	_____
10.	Turning to look behind	_____
11.	Turning 360 degrees	_____
12.	Placing alternate foot on stool	_____
13.	Standing with one foot in front	_____
14.	Standing on one foot	_____
	Total	_____

1. Sitting to Standing

INSTRUCTIONS: Please stand up. Try not to use your hands for support.

( ) 4   able to stand without using hands and stabilize independently
( ) 3   able to stand independently using hands
( ) 2   able to stand using hands after several tries
( ) 1   needs minimal aid to stand or to stabilize
( ) 0   needs moderate or maximal assist to stand

2. Standing Unsupported

INSTRUCTIONS: Please stand for two minutes without holding.

( ) 4   able to stand safely 2 minutes
( ) 3   able to stand 2 minutes with supervision
( ) 2   able to stand 30 seconds unsupported
( ) 1   needs several tries to stand 30 seconds unsupported
( ) 0   unable to stand 30 seconds unassisted

If a subject is able to stand 2 minutes unsupported, score full points for sitting unsupported. Proceed to item #4.

Berg Balance Scale *(Continued)*

3. Sitting with Back Unsupported But Feet Supported on Floor or on a Stool
INSTRUCTIONS: Please sit with arms folded for 2 minutes.

( ) 4   able to sit safely and securely 2 minutes
( ) 3   able to sit 2 minutes under supervision
( ) 2   able to sit 30 seconds
( ) 1   able to sit 10 seconds
( ) 0   unable to sit without support 10 seconds

4. Standing to Sitting
INSTRUCTIONS: Please sit down.

( ) 4   sits safely with minimal use of hands
( ) 3   controls descent by using hands
( ) 2   uses back of legs against chair to control descent
( ) 1   sits independently but has uncontrolled descent
( ) 0   needs assistance to sit

5. Transfers
INSTRUCTIONS: Arrange chair(s) for a pivot transfer. Ask subject to transfer one way toward a seat with armrests and one way toward a seat without armrests. You may use two chairs (one with and one without armrests) or a bed and a chair.

( ) 4   able to transfer safely with minor use of hands
( ) 3   able to transfer safely; definite need of hands
( ) 2   able to transfer with verbal cueing and/or supervision
( ) 1   needs one person to assist
( ) 0   needs two people to assist or supervise to be safe

6. Standing Unsupported with Eyes Closed
INSTRUCTIONS: Please close your eyes and stand still for 10 seconds.

( ) 4   able to stand 10 seconds safely
( ) 3   able to stand 10 seconds with supervision
( ) 2   able to stand 3 seconds
( ) 1   unable to keep eyes closed 3 seconds but stays steady
( ) 0   needs help to keep from falling

7. Standing Unsupported with Feet Together
INSTRUCTIONS: Place your feet together and stand without holding.

( ) 4   able to place feet together independently and stand for 1 minute safely
( ) 3   able to place feet together independently and stand for 1 minute with supervision
( ) 2   able to place feet together independently and to hold for 30 seconds
( ) 1   needs help to attain position but able to stand for 15 seconds with feet together
( ) 0   needs help to attain position and unable to hold for 15 seconds

8. Reaching Forward with Outstretched Arm While Standing
INSTRUCTIONS: Lift arm to 90 degrees. Stretch out your fingers and reach forward as far as you can. (Examiner places a ruler at end of fingertips when arm is at 90 degrees. Fingers should not touch the ruler while subject is reaching forward. The recorded measure is the distance forward that the fingers reach while the subject is in the most forward leaning position. When possible, ask subject to use both arms when reaching to avoid rotation of the trunk.)

( ) 4   can reach forward confidently >25 cm (10 inches)
( ) 3   can reach forward >12.5 cm safely (5 inches)
( ) 2   can reach forward >5 cm safely (2 inches)
( ) 1   reaches forward but needs supervision
( ) 0   loses balance while trying/requires external support

9. Pick Up Object from the Floor from a Standing Position
INSTRUCTIONS: Pick up the shoe/slipper that is placed in front of your feet.

( ) 4   able to pick up slipper safely and easily
( ) 3   able to pick up slipper but needs supervision
( ) 2   unable to pick up slipper but reaches 2-5 cm (1-2 inches) from slipper and keeps balance independently
( ) 1   unable to pick up slipper and needs supervision while trying
( ) 0   unable to try/needs assist to keep from losing balance or falling

10. Turning to Look Behind Over Left and Right Shoulders While Standing
INSTRUCTIONS: Turn to look **directly** behind you over toward left shoulder. Repeat to the right.
Examiner may pick an object to look at directly behind the subject to encourage a better twist turn.

( ) 4   looks behind from both sides and weight shifts well
( ) 3   looks behind one side only; other side shows less weight shift
( ) 2   turns sideways only but maintains balance
( ) 1   needs supervision when turning
( ) 0   needs assist to keep from losing balance or falling

11. Turn 360 Degrees
INSTRUCTIONS: Turn completely around in a full circle. Pause. Then turn a full circle in the other direction.

( ) 4   able to turn 360 degrees safely in 4 seconds or less
( ) 3   able to turn 360 degrees safely one side only in 4 seconds or less
( ) 2   able to turn 300 degrees safely but slowly
( ) 1   needs close supervision or verbal cueing
( ) 0   needs assistance while turning

12. Placing Alternate Foot on Step or Stool While Standing Unsupported
INSTRUCTIONS: Place each foot alternately on the step/stool. Continue until each foot has touched the step/stool four times.

( ) 4   able to stand independently and safely and complete 8 steps in 20 seconds
( ) 3   able to stand independently and complete 8 steps >20 seconds
( ) 2   able to complete 4 steps without aid with supervision
( ) 1   able to complete >2 steps; needs minimal assist
( ) 0   needs assistance to keep from falling/unable to try

13. Standing Unsupported One Foot in Front
INSTRUCTIONS: (Demonstrate to Subject) Place one foot directly in front of the other. If you feel that you cannot place your foot directly in front, try to step far enough ahead that the heel of your forward foot is ahead of the toes of the other foot. (To score 3 points, the length of the step should exceed the length of the other foot and the width of the stance should approximate the subject's normal stride width)

( ) 4   able to place foot tandem independently and hold 30 seconds
( ) 3   able to place foot ahead of other independently and hold 30 seconds
( ) 2   able to take small step independently and hold 30 seconds
( ) 1   needs help to step but can hold 15 seconds
( ) 0   loses balance while stepping or standing

14. Standing on One Leg
INSTRUCTIONS: Stand on one leg as long as you can without holding.

( ) 4   able to lift leg independently and hold >10 seconds
( ) 3   able to lift leg independently and hold 5-10 seconds
( ) 2   able to lift leg independently and hold = or >3 seconds
( ) 1   tries to lift leg; unable to hold 3 seconds but remains standing independently
( ) 0   unable to try or needs assist to prevent fall

( ) Total Score (Maximum = 56)

Timed Up and Go Test

Targeted Population: Older adults.

Description: The timed Up and Go test is a modified, timed version of the Get Up and Go test (Mathias et al, 1986), which evaluates gait and balance. The patient is observed and timed while rising from an armchair, walking 3 meters, turning, walking back, and sitting down again. No physical assistance is given. The patient wears regular footwear and uses any customary walking aid. A stopwatch or wrist-watch with a second hand is used to time this activity. The patient is allowed one practice trial and then three actual trials. The times from the three actual trials are averaged. This test is quick, requires no special equipment or training, and is easily included as part of the routine medical examination.

Scores: A score of < 10 seconds = freely mobile, < 20 seconds = mostly independent, 20 to 29 seconds = variable mobility, > 30 seconds = impaired mobility. A score of 30 seconds or greater indicates that the patient has impaired mobility, requires assistance, and is at a high risk for falls.

Accuracy: The authors reported that the time score was reliable (interrater and intrarater); correlated well with log-transformed scores on the Berg Balance Scale, gait speed, and Barthel Index of ADL; and appeared to predict the patient's ability to go outside alone safely. The authors suggest that the timed Up and Go test is a reliable and valid test for quantifying functional mobility, which may also be useful in monitoring clinical change over time.

Administration Time: < 2 minutes.

From Podsiadlo D, Richardson S: The timed "Up and Go:" a test of basic functional mobility for frail, elderly persons, *J Am Geriatric Soc* 39:142, 1991. Reprinted with permission Blackwell Publishing Ltd.

Descriptive summary from Loretz L: *Primary Care Tools for Clinicians: A Compendium of Forms, Questionnaires, and Rating Scales for Everyday Practice*, St. Louis, 2005, Mosby.

Tinetti Balance and Gait Evaluation
Performance-Oriented Assessment of Mobility

Name: _____

Date: _____

Address: _____

Phone: _____

D.O.B.: _____ *Gender: Male   Female*

Medical Record #: _____

Balance

Instructions: Subject is seated in a hard, armless chair. The following maneuvers are tested:

1. Sitting balance
   0 = Leans or slides in chair
   1 = Steady, safe

2. Arise
   0 = Unable without help
   1 = Able but uses arm to help
   2 = Able without use of arms

3. Attempts to arise
   0 = Unable without help
   1 = Able, but requires more than one attempt
   2 = Able to arise with one attempt

4. Immediate standing balance (first 5 seconds)
   0 = Unsteady (staggers, moves feet, marked trunk sway)
   1 = Steady but uses walker/cane or grabs other object for support
   2 = Steady without walker or cane or other support

5. Standing balance
   0 = Unsteady
   1 = Steady, but wide stance (medial heels > than 4″ apart) or uses cane/walker or other support
   2 = Narrow stance without support

6. Nudge (subject at maximum position with feet as close together as possible. Examiner pushes lightly on subject's sternum with palm of hand 3 times.)
   0 = Begins to fall
   1 = Staggers, grabs, but catches self
   2 = Steady

7. Eyes closed (at maximum position #6)
   0 = Unsteady
   1 = Steady

8. Turn 360°
   0 = Discontinuous steps
   1 = Continuous steps
   0 = Unsteady (grabs, staggers)
   1 = Steady

9. Sit down
   0 = Unsafe (misjudged distance; falls into chair)
   1 = Uses arms or not a smooth motion
   2 = Safe, smooth motion

_____ /16 _____   BALANCE SCORE

Continued on following page

Tinetti Balance and Gait Evaluation *(Continued)*

Gait
Instructions: Subject stands with examiner. Walks down hallway or across room, first at his/her usual pace, then back at a "rapid but safe" pace (using usual walking aid such as cane/walker).

10. Initiation of gait (immediately after told "go")
    0 = Any hesitancy or multiple attempts to start
    1 = No hesitancy

11. Step length and height (right foot swing)
    0 = Does not pass L. stance foot with step
    1 = Passes L. stance foot
    0 = R. foot does not clear floor completely with step
    1 = R. foot completely clears floor

12. Step length and height (left foot swing)
    0 = Does not pass R. stance foot with step
    1 = Passes R. stance foot
    0 = L. foot does not clear floor completely with step
    1 = L. foot completely clears floor

13. Step symmetry
    0 = R. and L. step length not equal (estimate)
    1 = R. and L. step length appear equal

14. Step continuity
    0 = Stopping or discontinuity between steps
    1 = Steps appear continuous

15. Path (estimated in relation to floor tiles, 12" wide. Observe excursion of one foot over about 10 feet of course.)
    0 = Marked deviation
    1 = Mild/moderate deviation or uses a walking aid
    2 = Straight without walking aid

16. Trunk
    0 = Marked sway or uses walking aid
    1 = No sway but flexion of knees or back or spreads arms out while walking
    2 = No sway, no flexion, no use of arms and no walking aid

17. Walk stance
    0 = Heels apart
    1 = Heels almost touching while walking

_____ **/12** _____ GAIT SCORE

_____ **/28** _____ TOTAL MOBILITY SCORE (BALANCE AND GAIT)

From Tinetti ME: Performance-oriented assessment of mobility problems in elderly patients, *J Am Geriatric Soc* 34:119–126, 1986. Reprinted with permission Blackwell Publishing, Ltd.

Hearing Handicap Inventory for the Elderly-Screening Version (HHIE-S)*

Name: _____

Date: _____

Address: _____

Phone: _____

D.O.B.: _____ Gender: Male   Female

Medical Record #: _____

	Yes (4)	Sometimes (2)	No (0)
E-1. Does a hearing problem cause you to feel embarrassed when meeting new people?	_____	_____	_____
E-2. Does a hearing problem cause you to feel frustrated when talking to members of your family?	_____	_____	_____
S-3. Do you have difficulty hearing when someone speaks in a whisper?	_____	_____	_____
E-4. Do you feel handicapped by a hearing problem?	_____	_____	_____
S-5. Does a hearing problem cause difficulty when visiting friends, relatives, or neighbors?	_____	_____	_____
S-6. Does a hearing problem cause you to attend religious services less often than you would like?	_____	_____	_____
E-7. Does a hearing problem cause you to have arguments with family members?	_____	_____	_____
S-8. Does a hearing problem cause you difficulty when listening to TV or radio?	_____	_____	_____
E-9. Do you feel that any difficulty with your hearing limits or hampers your personal or social life?	_____	_____	_____
S-10. Does a hearing problem cause you difficulty when in a restaurant with relatives or friends?	_____	_____	_____

E = emotional response S = social/situational response
*Range of total points, 0-40; 0-8, no self-perceived handicap; 10-22, mild to moderate handicap; 24-40, significant handicap

From Ventry IM, Weinstein BE: Identification of elderly people with hearing problems, *ASHA* July 25:37, 1983. Copyright by the American-Speech-Language-Hearing Association. Reprinted with permission.

Body Mass Index

	Normal						Overweight					Obese										Extreme Obesity															
BMI	19	20	21	22	23	24	25	26	27	28	29	30	31	32	33	34	35	36	37	38	39	40	41	42	43	44	45	46	47	48	49	50	51	52	53	54
Height (inches)												Body Weight (pounds)																								
58	91	96	100	105	110	115	119	124	129	134	138	143	148	153	158	162	167	172	177	181	186	191	196	201	205	210	215	220	224	229	234	239	244	248	253	258
59	94	99	104	109	114	119	124	128	133	138	143	148	153	158	163	168	173	178	183	188	193	198	203	208	212	217	222	227	232	237	242	247	252	257	262	267
60	97	102	107	112	118	123	128	133	138	143	148	153	158	163	168	174	179	184	189	194	199	204	209	215	220	225	230	235	240	245	250	255	261	266	271	276
61	100	106	111	116	122	127	132	137	143	148	153	158	164	169	175	180	185	190	195	201	206	211	217	222	227	232	238	243	248	254	259	264	269	275	280	285
62	104	109	115	120	126	131	136	142	147	153	158	164	169	175	180	186	191	196	202	207	213	218	224	229	235	240	246	251	256	262	267	273	278	284	289	295
63	107	113	118	124	130	135	141	146	152	158	163	169	175	180	186	191	197	203	208	214	220	225	231	237	242	248	254	259	265	270	278	282	287	293	299	304
64	110	116	122	128	134	140	145	151	157	163	169	174	180	186	192	197	204	209	215	221	227	232	238	244	250	256	262	267	273	279	285	291	296	302	308	314
65	114	120	126	132	138	144	150	156	162	168	174	180	186	192	198	204	210	216	222	228	234	240	246	252	258	264	270	276	282	288	294	300	306	312	318	324
66	118	124	130	136	142	148	155	161	167	173	179	186	192	198	204	210	216	223	229	235	241	247	253	260	266	272	278	284	291	297	303	309	315	322	328	334
67	121	127	134	140	146	153	159	166	172	178	185	191	198	204	211	217	223	230	236	242	249	255	261	268	274	280	287	293	299	306	312	319	325	331	338	344
68	125	131	138	144	151	158	164	171	177	184	190	197	203	210	216	223	230	236	243	249	256	262	269	276	282	289	295	302	308	315	322	328	335	341	348	354
69	128	135	142	149	155	162	169	176	182	189	196	203	209	216	223	230	236	243	250	257	263	270	277	284	291	297	304	311	318	324	331	338	345	351	358	365
70	132	139	146	153	160	167	174	181	188	195	202	209	216	222	229	236	243	250	257	264	271	278	285	292	299	306	313	320	327	334	341	348	355	362	369	376
71	136	143	150	157	165	172	179	186	193	200	208	215	222	229	236	243	250	257	265	272	279	286	293	301	308	315	322	329	338	343	351	358	365	372	379	386
72	140	147	154	162	169	177	184	191	199	206	213	221	228	235	242	250	258	265	272	279	287	294	302	309	316	324	331	338	346	353	361	368	375	383	390	397
73	144	151	159	166	174	182	189	197	204	212	219	227	235	242	250	257	265	272	280	288	295	302	310	318	325	333	340	348	355	363	371	378	386	393	401	408
74	148	155	163	171	179	186	194	202	210	218	225	233	241	249	257	264	272	280	287	295	303	311	319	326	334	342	350	358	365	373	381	389	396	404	412	420
75	152	160	168	176	184	192	200	208	216	224	232	240	248	256	264	272	279	287	295	303	311	319	327	335	343	351	359	367	375	383	391	399	407	415	423	431
76	156	164	172	180	189	197	205	213	221	230	238	246	254	263	271	279	287	295	304	312	320	328	336	344	353	361	369	377	385	394	402	410	418	426	435	443

Adapted from *Clinical Guidelines on the Identification, Evaluation, and Treatment of Overweight and Obesity in Adults: The Evidence Report.*

NESTLÉ NUTRITION SERVICES

Mini Nutritional Assessment (MNA)

Last name: _____   First name: _____   Sex: _____   Date: _____

Age: _____   Weight, kg: _____   Height, cm: _____   I.D. Number: _____

Complete the screen by filling in the boxes with the appropriate numbers.
Add the numbers for the screen. If score is 11 or less, continue with the assessment to gain a Malnutrition Indicator Score.

Screening

A Has food intake declined over the past 3 months due to loss of appetite, digestive problems, chewing or swallowing difficulties?
0 = severe loss of appetite
1 = moderate loss of appetite
2 = no loss of appetite   ☐

B Weight loss during last 3 months
0 = weight loss greater than 3 kg (6.6 lbs)
1 = does not know
2 = weight loss between 1 and 3 kg (2.2 and 6.6 lbs)
3 = no weight loss   ☐

C Mobility
0 = bed or chair bound
1 = able to get out of bed/chair but does not go out
2 = goes out   ☐

D Has suffered psychological stress or acute disease in the past 3 months
0 = yes   2 = no   ☐

E Neuropsychological problems
0 = severe dementia or depression
1 = mild dementia
2 = no psychological problems   ☐

F Body Mass Index (BMI) (weight in kg) / (height in m)^2
0 = BMI less than 19
1 = BMI 19 to less than 21
2 = BMI 21 to less than 23
3 = BMI 23 or greater   ☐

Screening score (subtotal max. 14 points)   ☐ ☐
12 points or greater   Normal – not at risk – no need to complete assessment
11 points or below   Possible malnutrition – continue assessment

Assessment

G Lives independently (not in a nursing home or hospital)
0 = no   1 = yes   ☐

H Takes more than 3 prescription drugs per day
0 = yes   1 = no   ☐

I Pressure sores or skin ulcers
0 = yes   1 = no   ☐

J How many full meals does the patient eat daily?
0 = 1 meal
1 = 2 meals
2 = 3 meals   ☐

K Selected consumption markers for protein intake
• At least one serving of dairy products (milk, cheese, yogurt) per day?   yes ☐   no ☐
• Two or more servings of legumes or eggs per week?   yes ☐   no ☐
• Meat, fish or poultry every day   yes ☐   no ☐
0.0 = if 0 or 1 yes
0.5 = if 2 yes
1.0 = if 3 yes   ☐ . ☐

L Consumes two or more servings of fruits or vegetables per day?
0 = no   1 = yes   ☐

M How much fluid (water, juice, coffee, tea, milk…) is consumed per day?
0.0 = less than 3 cups
0.5 = 3 to 5 cups
1.0 = more than 5 cups   ☐ . ☐

N Mode of feeding
0 = unable to eat without assistance
1 = self-fed with some difficulty
2 = self-fed without any problem   ☐

O Self view of nutritional status
0 = views self as being malnourished
1 = is uncertain of nutritional state
2 = views self as having no nutritional problem   ☐

P In comparison with other people of the same age, how does the patient consider his/her health status?
0.0 = not as good
0.5 = does not know
1.0 = as good
2.0 = better   ☐ . ☐

Q Mid-arm circumference (MAC) in cm
0.0 = MAC less than 21
0.5 = MAC 21 to 22
1.0 = MAC 22 or greater   ☐ . ☐

R Calf circumference (CC) in cm
0 = CC less than 31   1 = CC 31 or greater   ☐

Assessment (max. 16 points)   ☐ ☐ . ☐

Screening score   ☐ ☐

Total Assessment (max. 30 points)   ☐ ☐ . ☐

Malnutrition Indicator Score

17 to 23.5 points   at risk of malnutrition   ☐

Less than 17 points   malnourished   ☐

Ref.: Guigoz Y, Vellas B and Garry PJ. 1994. Mini Nutritional Assessment: A practical assessment tool for grading the nutritional state of elderly patients. *Facts and Research in Gerontology.* Supplement #2:15-59.
Rubenstein LZ, Harker J, Guigoz Y and Vellas B. Comprehensive Geriatric Assessment (CGA) and the MNA: An Overview of CGA, Nutritional Assessment, and Development of a Shortened Version of the MNA. In: "Mini Nutritional Assessment (MNA): Research and Practice in the Elderly". Vellas B, Garry PJ and Guigoz Y , editors. Nestlé Nutrition Workshop Series. Clinical & Performance Programme, vol. 1. Karger, Bâle, in press.

Pain Assessment

Visual Analog Scale

The Worst Imaginable Pain —————————————————————————————— No Pain

Verbal Descriptor Scale (VDS)

— The most intense pain imaginable

— Very severe pain

— Severe pain

— Moderate pain

— Mild pain

— Slight pain

— No pain

Numeric Rating Scale (NRS)

20	19	18	17	16	15	14	13	12	11	10	9	8	7	6	5	4	3	2	1	0

Instrumental Activities of Daily Living Scale (IADL)

Name: _____

Date: _____

D.O.B.: _____Gender: Male   Female

Medical Record #: _____

Circle one statement in each category A–H that applies to subject.

A. Ability to Use Telephone

1. Operates telephone on own initiative; looks up and dials numbers, etc.   1

2. Dials a few well-known numbers.   1

3. Answers telephone but does not dial.   1

4. Does not use telephone at all.   0

B. Shopping

1. Takes care of all shopping needs independently   1

2. Shops independently for small purchases   0

3. Needs to be accompanied on any shopping trip.   0

4. Completely unable to shop.   0

C. Food Preparation

1. Plans, prepares, and serves adequate meals independently.   1

2. Prepares adequate meals if supplied with ingredients.   0

3. Heats, serves, and prepares meals or prepares meals but does not maintain adequate diet.   0

4. Needs to have meals prepared and served.   0

D. Housekeeping

1. Maintains house alone or with occasional assistance (e.g., "heavy work domestic help").   1

2. Performs light daily tasks such as dishwashing, bed making.   1

3. Performs light daily tasks but cannot maintain acceptable level of cleanliness.   1

4. Needs help with all home maintenance tasks.   1

5. Does not participate in any housekeeping tasks.   0

E. Laundry

1. Does personal laundry completely.   1

2. Launders small items; rinses stockings, etc.   1

3. All laundry must be done by others.   0

F. Mode of Transportation

1. Travels independently on public transportation or drives own car.   1

2. Arranges own travel via taxi, but does not otherwise use public transportation.   1

3. Travels on public transportation when accompanied by another.   1

4. Travel limited to taxi or automobile with assistance of another.   0

5. Does not travel at all.   0

G. Responsibility for Own Medications

1. Is responsible for taking medication in correct dosages at correct time.   1

2. Takes responsibility if medication is prepared in advance in separate dosage.   0

3. Is not capable of dispensing own medication.   0

H. Ability to Handle Finances

1. Manages financial matters independently (budgets, writes checks, pays rent and bills, goes to bank), collects and keeps track of income.   1

2. Manages day-to-day purchases, but needs help with banking, major purchases, etc.   1

3. Incapable of handling money.   0

> OVERALL SCORE: 7-8 = high level independence
> 5-6 = moderate level independence
> 3-4 = moderate level dependence
> 1-2 = dependence

Adapted from Lawton MP, Brody EM: Assessment of older people: self-maintaining and instrumental activities of daily living, *Gerontologist* 9:179–186, 1969.

Katz Index of Activities of Daily Living

Date of Visit: _____

Patient Name: _____

Medical Record #: _____

Date of Birth: _____ *Age:* ____ *Gender:* Male   Female

For each area of functioning listed below, check description that applies. (The word "assistance" means supervision, direction, or personal assistance.)

BATHING—either sponge bath, tub bath, or shower.

☐	☐	☐
Receives no assistance (gets in and out of tub by self if tub is usual means of bathing)	Receives assistance in bathing only one part of the body (such as back or a leg)	Receives assistance in bathing more than one part of the body (or not bathed)

DRESSING—gets clothes from clothes closets and drawers—including underclothes and outer garments and uses fasteners (including braces if worn)

☐	☐	☐
Gets clothes and gets completely dressed without assistance	Gets clothes and gets dressed without assistance except for assistance in tying shoe	Receives assistance in getting clothes or in getting dressed or stays partly or completely undressed

TOILETING—going to the "toilet room" for bowel and urine elimination; cleaning self after elimination, and arranging clothes

☐	☐	☐
Goes to "toilet room," cleans self, and arranges clothes without assistance (may use object for support such as cane, walker, or wheelchair and may manage night bedpan or commode, emptying same in morning)	Receives assistance in going to "toilet room" or in cleansing self or in arranging clothes after elimination or in use of night bedpan or commode	Doesn't go to room termed "toilet" for the elimination process

TRANSFER

☐	☐	☐
Moves in and out of bed as well as in and out of chair without assistance (may be using object for support such as cane or walker)	Moves in and out of bed or chair with assistance	Doesn't get out of bed

CONTINENCE

☐	☐	☐
Controls urination and bowel movement completely by self	Has occasional "accidents"	Supervision helps keep control, catheter is used, or is incontinent

FEEDING

☐	☐	☐
Feeds self without assistance	Feeds self except for getting help in cutting meat or buttering bread	Receives assistance in feeding or is fed partly or completely by using tubes or intravenous fluids

From Katz S, Downs TD, Cash HR, et al: Progress in the development of the Index of ADL, *Gerontologist* 10:23, 1970.

The Index of Independence in Activities of Daily Living: Scoring and Definitions (Katz)

The Index of Independence in Activities of Daily Living is based on an evaluation of the functional independence or dependence of patients in bathing, dressing, going to toilet, transferring, continence, and feeding. Specific definitions of functional independence and dependence appear after the index.

A —Independent in feeding, continence, transferring, going to toilet, dressing, and bathing.

B —Independent in all but one of these functions.

C —Independent in all but bathing and one additional function.

D —Independent in all but bathing, dressing, and one additional function.

E —Independent in all but bathing, dressing, going to toilet, and one additional function.

F —Independent in all but bathing, dressing, going to toilet, transferring, and one additional function.

G —Dependent in all six functions.

Other —Dependent in at least two functions, but not classifiable as C, D, E, or F.

Independence means without supervision, direction, or active personal assistance, except as specifically noted as follows. This is based on actual status and not on ability. A patient who refuses to perform a function is considered as not performing the function, even though he is deemed able.

Bathing (sponge, shower, or tub)

Independent: assistance only in bathing a single part (as back or disabled extremity) or bathes self completely

Dependent: assistance in bathing more than one part of body; assistance in getting in or out of tub or does not bathe self

Dressing

Independent: gets clothes from closets and drawers; puts on clothes, outer garments, braces; manages fasteners; act of tying shoes is excluded

Dependent: does not dress self or remains partly undressed

Going to toilet

Independent: gets to toilet; gets on and off toilet; arranges clothes; cleans organs of excretion (may manage own bedpan used at night only and may or may not be using mechanical supports)

Dependent: uses bedpan or commode or receives assistance in getting to and using toilet

Transfer

Independent: moves in and out of bed independently and moves in and out of chair independently (may or may not be using mechanical supports)

Dependent: assistance in moving in or out of bed and/or chair; does not perform one or more transfers

Continence

Independent: urination and defecation entirely self-controlled

Dependent: partial or total incontinence in urination or defecation; partial or total control by enemas, catheters, or regulated use of urinals and/or bedpans

Feeding

Independent: gets food from plate or its equivalent into mouth (precutting of meat and preparation of food, as buttering bread, are excluded from evaluation)

Dependent: assistance in act of feeding (see above); does not eat at all or receives parenteral feeding

Stepwise Approach to Preoperative Cardiac Assessment

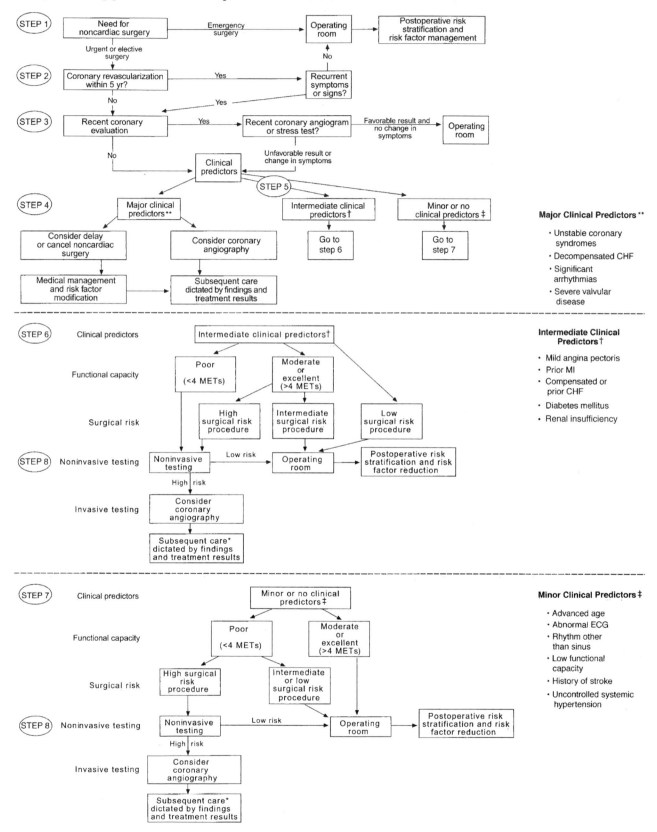

*Subsequent care may include cancellation or delay of surgery, coronary revascularization followed by noncardiac surgery, or intensified care. *CHF,* congestive heart failure; *ECG,* electrocardiogram; *MET,* metabolic equivalent; *MI,* myocardial infarction.

Eagle, K.A. et al. *Circulation.* 2002;105:1257-1267.

TABLE A2-1 Indications for Coronary Angiography* in Perioperative Evaluation Before (or After) Noncardiac Surgery

Class I†: Patients with suspected or known CAD:
- Evidence for high risk of adverse outcome based on noninvasive test results
- Angina pectoris unresponsive to adequate medical therapy
- Most patients with unstable angina pectoris
- Nondiagnostic or equivocal noninvasive test in a high-risk patient (Table A2-3) undergoing a high-risk noncardiac surgical procedure (Table A2-5)

Class II†:
- Intermediate-risk results during noninvasive testing
- Nondiagnostic or equivocal noninvasive test in a lower-risk patient (Table A2-3) undergoing a high-risk noncardiac surgical procedure (Table A2-5)
- Urgent noncardiac surgery in a patient convalescing from acute MI
- Perioperative MI

Class III†:
- Low-risk noncardiac surgery (Table A2-5) in a patient with known CAD and low-risk results on noninvasive testing
- Screening for CAD without appropriate noninvasive testing
- Asymptomatic after coronary revascularization, with excellent exercise capacity (≥7 METs)
- Mild stable angina in patients with good LV function, low-risk noninvasive test results
- Patient is not a candidate for coronary revascularization because of concomitant medical illness
- Prior technically adequate normal coronary angiogram within 5 years
- Severe LV dysfunction (eg, ejection fraction <20%) and patient not considered candidate for revascularization procedure
- Patient unwilling to consider coronary revascularization procedure

*If results will affect management.

†Class I: Conditions for which there is evidence for and/or general agreement that a procedure be performed or a treatment is of benefit. Class II: Conditions for which there is a divergence of evidence and/or opinion about the treatment. Class III: Conditions for which there is evidence and/or general agreement that the procedure is not necessary.

CAD, Coronary artery disease; LV, left ventricular; MET, metabolic equivalent; MI, myocardial infarction.

Adapted from ACC/AHA Guidelines for Coronary Angiography.

TABLE A2-2 Clinical Predictors of Increased Perioperative Cardiovascular Risk (Myocardial Infarction, Congestive Heart Failure, Death)

Major

Unstable coronary syndromes
- Acute or recent myocardial infarction* with evidence of important ischemic risk by clinical symptoms or noninvasive study
- Unstable or severe† angina (Canadian Class III or IV)‡

Decompensated congestive heart failure

Significant arrhythmias
- High-grade atrioventricular block
- Symptomatic ventricular arrhythmias in the presence of underlying heart disease
- Supraventricular arrhythmias with uncontrolled ventricular rate

Severe valvular disease

Intermediate

Mild angina pectoris (Canadian Class I or II)

Previous myocardial infarction by history or pathological Q waves

Compensated or prior congestive heart failure

Diabetes mellitus (particularly insulin-dependent)

Renal insufficiency

Minor

Advanced age

Abnormal ECG (left ventricular hypertrophy, left bundle branch block, ST-T abnormalities)

Rhythm other than sinus (eg, atrial fibrillation)

Low functional capacity (eg, inability to climb one flight of stairs with a bag of groceries)

History of stroke

Uncontrolled systemic hypertension

ECG, Electrocardiogram.

*The American College of Cardiology National Database Library defines *recent MI* as greater than 7 days but less than or equal to 1 month (30 days).

†May include "stable" angina in patients who are unusually sedentary.

‡Eagle, K.A. et al. *Circulation.* 2002;105:1257-1267.

TABLE A2-3 Estimated Energy Requirements for Various Activities

1 MET ↓ **4 METs**	Can you take care of yourself? Eat, dress, or use the toilet? Walk indoors around the house? Walk a block or two on level ground at 2-3 mph or 3.2-4.8 km/h? Do light work around the house like dusting or washing dishes?	**4 METs** ↓ **>10 METs**	Climb a flight of stairs or walk up a hill? Walk on level ground at 4 mph or 6.4 km/h? Run a short distance? Do heavy work around the house like scrubbing floors or lifting or moving heavy furniture? Participate in moderate recreational activities like golf, bowling, dancing, doubles tennis, or throwing a baseball or football? Participate in strenuous sports like swimming, singles tennis, football, basketball, or skiing?

TABLE A2-4 Cardiac Risk* Stratification for Noncardiac Surgical Procedures

High
(Reported cardiac risk often >5%)
- Emergent major operations, particularly in the elderly
- Aortic and other major vascular
- Peripheral vascular
- Anticipated prolonged surgical procedures associated with large fluid shifts and/or blood loss

Intermediate
(Reported cardiac risk generally <5%)
- Carotid endarterectomy
- Head and neck surgery
- Intraperitoneal and intrathoracic surgery
- Orthopedic surgery
- Prostate surgery

Low†
(Reported cardiac risk generally <1%)
- Endoscopic procedures
- Superficial procedure
- Cataract surgery
- Breast surgery

*Combined incidence of cardiac death and nonfatal myocardial infarction.
†Do not generally require further preoperative cardiac testing.

Eagle, K.A. et al. *Circulation*. 2002;105:1257-1267.

Braden Scale for Predicting Pressure Sore Risk

Patient's Name _____ Evaluator's Name _____ Date of Assessment _____

SENSORY PERCEPTION ability to respond meaningfully to pressure-related discomfort	**1. Completely Limited** Unresponsive (does not moan, flinch, or grasp) to painful stimuli, due to diminished level of consciousness or sedation. OR limited ability to feel pain over most of body.	**2. Very Limited** Responds only to painful stimuli. Cannot communicate discomfort except by moaning or restlessness. OR has a sensory impairment which limits the ability to feel pain or discomfort over ½ of body.	**3. Slightly Limited** Responds to verbal commands, but cannot always communicate discomfort or the need to be turned. OR has some sensory impairment which limits ability to feel pain or discomfort in 1 or 2 extremities.	**4. No Impairment** Responds to verbal commands. Has no sensory deficit which would limit ability to feel or voice pain or discomfort.			
MOISTURE exposed to moisture	**1. Constantly Moist** Skin is kept moist almost constantly by perspiration, urine, etc. Dampness is detected every time patient is moved or turned.	**2. Very Moist** Skin is often, but not always, moist. Linen must be changed at least once a shift.	**3. Occasionally Moist** Skin is occasionally moist, requiring an extra linen change approximately once a day.	**4. Rarely Moist** Skin is usually dry, linen only requires changing at routine intervals.			
ACTIVITY degree of physical activity	**1. Bedfast** Confined to bed.	**2. Chairfast** Ability to walk severely limited or non-existent. Cannot bear own weight and/or must be assisted into chair or wheelchair.	**3. Walks Occasionally** Walks occasionally during day, but for very short distances, with or without assistance. Spends majority of each shift in bed or chair.	**4. Walks Frequently** Walks outside room at least twice a day and inside room at least once every two hours during waking hours.			
MOBILITY ability to change and control body position	**1. Completely Immobile** Does not make even slight changes in body or extremity position without assistance.	**2. Very Limited** Makes occasional slight changes in body or extremity position but unable to make frequent or significant changes independently.	**3. Slightly Limited** Makes frequent though slight changes in body or extremity position independently.	**4. No Limitation** Makes major and frequent changes in position without assistance.			
NUTRITION usual food intake pattern	**1. Very Poor** Never eats a complete meal. Rarely eats more than ⅓ of any food offered. Eats 2 servings or less of protein (meat or dairy products) per day. Takes fluids poorly. Does not take a liquid dietary supplement OR is NPO and/or maintained on clear liquids or IV's for more than 5 days.	**2. Probably Inadequate** Rarely eats a complete meal and generally eats only about ½ of any food offered. Protein intake includes only 3 servings of meat or dairy products per day. Occasionally will take a dietary supplement. OR receives less than optimum amount of liquid diet or tube feeding.	**3. Adequate** Eats over half of most meals. Eats a total of 4 servings of protein (meat, dairy products) per day. Occasionally will refuse a meal, but will usually take a supplement when offered. OR is on a tube feeding or TPN regimen which probably meets most of nutritional needs.	**4. Excellent** Eats most of every meal. Never refuses a meal. Usually eats a total of 4 or more servings of meat and dairy products. Occasionally eats between meals. Does not require supplementation.			
FRICTION & SHEAR	**1. Problem** Requires moderate to maximum assistance in moving. Complete lifting without sliding against sheets is impossible. Frequently slides down in bed or chair, requiring frequent repositioning with maximum assistance. Spasticity, contractures, or agitation leads to almost constant friction.	**2. Potential Problem** Moves feebly or requires minimum assistance. During a move skin probably slides to some extent against sheets, chair, restraints, or other devices. Maintains relatively good position in chair or bed most of the time but occasionally slides down.	**3. No Apparent Problem** Moves in bed and in chair independently and has sufficient muscle strength to lift up completely during move. Maintains good position in bed or chair.				
				Total Score			

National Pressure Ulcer Advisory Panel (NPUAP) Staging System for Pressure Ulcerations

Stage I: Nonblanchable erythema of intact skin, the heralding lesion of skin ulceration. In individuals with darker skin, discoloration of the skin, warmth, edema, induration, or hardness may also be indicators.

Stage II: Partial-thickness skin loss involving epidermis, dermis, or both. The ulcer is superficial and presents clinically as an abrasion, blister, or shallow crater.

Stage III: Full-thickness skin loss involving damage to or necrosis of subcutaneous tissue that may extend down to, but not through, underlying fascia. The ulcer presents clinically as a deep crater with or without undermining of adjacent tissue.

Stage IV: Full-thickness skin loss with extensive destruction, tissue necrosis, or damage to muscle, bone, or supporting structures (e.g., tendon, joint capsule). Undermining and sinus tracts may also be associated with Stage IV pressure ulcers.

National Pressure Ulcer Advisory Panel, 1998. website: http://www.npuap.org

Norton Pressure Ulcer Prediction Scale

Name	Date	Physical condition		Mental condition		Activity		Mobility		Incontinent		Total score
		Good	4	Alert	4	Ambulant	4	Full	4	Not	4	
		Fair	3	Apathetic	3	Walk/help	3	Slightly limited	3	Occasional	3	
		Poor	2	Confused	2	Chairbound	2	Very limited	2	Usually/Urine	2	
		Very bad	1	Stupor	1	Stupor	1	Immobile	1	Doubly	1	

Interpretation: maximum score 20; minimum score 5; at risk for pressure ulcer if score ≤ 14.

Doreen Norton, Rhoda McLaren and A N Exton-Smith, An Investigation of Geriatric Nursing Problems in Hospital 8 National Corporation for the Care of Old People (now Centre for Policy on Ageing), London, 1962.

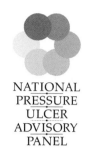

NATIONAL
PRESSURE
ULCER
ADVISORY
PANEL

Pressure Ulcer Scale for Healing (PUSH)
PUSH Tool 3.0

Patient Name_____ Patient ID#_____

Ulcer Location _____ Date _____

Directions:

Observe and measure the pressure ulcer. Categorize the ulcer with respect to surface area, exudate, and type of wound tissue. Record a sub-score for each of these ulcer characteristics. Add the sub-scores to obtain the total score. A comparison of total scores measured over time provides an indication of the improvement or deterioration in pressure ulcer healing.

LENGTH X WIDTH (in cm²)	0	1	2	3	4	5	Sub-score
	0	< 0.3	0.3 – 0.6	0.7 – 1.0	1.1 – 2.0	2.1 – 3.0	
	6	7	8	9	10		
	3.1 – 4.0	4.1 – 8.0	8.1 – 12.0	12.1 – 24.0	> 24.0		
EXUDATE AMOUNT	0 None	1 Light	2 Moderate	3 Heavy			Sub-score
TISSUE TYPE	0 Closed	1 Epithelial Tissue	2 Granulation Tissue	3 Slough	4 Necrotic Tissue		Sub-score
							TOTAL SCORE

Length x Width: Measure the greatest length (head to toe) and the greatest width (side to side) using a centimeter ruler. Multiply these two measurements (length x width) to obtain an estimate of surface area in square centimeters (cm²). Caveat: Do not guess! Always use a centimeter ruler and always use the same method each time the ulcer is measured.

Exudate Amount: Estimate the amount of exudate (drainage) present after removal of the dressing and before applying any topical agent to the ulcer. Estimate the exudate (drainage) as none, light, moderate, or heavy.

Tissue Type: This refers to the types of tissue that are present in the wound (ulcer) bed. Score as a "4" if there is any necrotic tissue present. Score as a "3" if there is any amount of slough present and necrotic tissue is absent. Score as a "2" if the wound is clean and contains granulation tissue. A superficial wound that is reepithelializing is scored as a "1". When the wound is closed, score as a "0".

   4 – Necrotic Tissue (Eschar): black, brown, or tan tissue that adheres firmly to the wound bed or ulcer edges and may be either firmer or softer than surrounding skin.

   3 – Slough: yellow or white tissue that adheres to the ulcer bed in strings or thick clumps, or is mucinous.

   2 – Granulation Tissue: pink or beefy red tissue with a shiny, moist, granular appearance.

   1 – Epithelial Tissue: for superficial ulcers, new pink or shiny tissue (skin) that grows in from the edges or as islands on the ulcer surface.

   0 – Closed/Resurfaced: the wound is completely covered with epithelium (new skin).

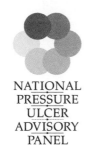

NATIONAL
PRESSURE
ULCER
ADVISORY
PANEL

Pressure Ulcer Scale for Healing (PUSH)
PUSH Tool 3.0

Patient Name_____ Patient ID# _____

Ulcer Location _____ Date _____

Directions:

Observe and measure pressure ulcers at regular intervals using the PUSH Tool.
Date and record PUSH sub-scores and Total Scores on the Pressure Ulcer Healing Record below.

Pressure Ulcer Healing Record												
Date												
Length x Width												
Exudate Amount												
Tissue Type												
PUSH Total Score												

Graph the PUSH Total Scores on the Pressure Ulcer Healing Graph below.

PUSH Total Score	Pressure Ulcer Healing Graph											
17												
16												
15												
14												
13												
12												
11												
10												
9												
8												
7												
6												
5												
4												
3												
2												
1												
Healed = 0												
Date												

Medical Outcomes Study Short Form 36 (MOS SF-36)

Targeted Population: Adolescents (age 14 and older) and adults.

Description: Developed from the work at the Rand Corporation in Santa Monica, California, the MOS SF-36 measures health status and outcomes from the patient's point of view. The MOS SF-36 contains 36 items that measure eight dimensions: physical activities (10 items), role limitations caused by physical health problems (4 items), role limitations caused by emotional problems (3 items), social limitations (2 items), pain (2 items), general health perceptions (5 items), vitality and fatigue (4 items), and mental health (5 items). There is one question in which subjects are asked to compare current health to that of one year previous to provide an estimate of change in health status. The MOS SF-36 is one of the most well-known health status instruments and is used around the world.

Scores: Each item has a different scoring format, ranging from a simple "yes/no" response to Likert-type scales. An equation with weighted scores is used to obtain item scores; mean scores may be calculated for subscales. The scoring method is complex, is described fully in the user's manual, and can be done with automated software. An overall score is not reported.

Accuracy: The MOS SF-36 and MOS SF-12 are well-developed, concise instruments with excellent core descriptions of reliability and validity (McHorney et al, 1993, 1994). Many studies detailing the good to excellent reliability and validity of these tools are reviewed by McDowell and Newell (1996) and Bowling (1997). The MOS SF-36 has become a standard against which other instruments are measured.

Administration Time: 5 to 15 minutes by self-administration or by trained interviewer.

Co-copyright and trademark holders for the Medical Outcomes Study Short Form 36 (MOS SF-36) and Medical Outcomes Study Short Form 12 (MOS SF-12) are the Medical Outcomes Trust (MOT), the Health Assessment Lab, and QualityMetric Incorporated. Information regarding licensing, use, and ordering may be found online at http://www.qualitymetric.com/products/descriptions/sflicenses.shtml. The forms may be viewed at http://www.qualitymetric.com/products/sfsurveys.aspx. The MOS SF-36, MOS SF-12, and other quality-of-life forms may also be viewed at http://www.rand.org/health/surveys.html.

Missoula-VITAS
Quality of Life Index (MVQOLI)

Improving quality of life for patients is the primary goal for hospice care and for end-of-life care in any setting. The Missoula-VITAS Quality of Life Index (MVQOLI) is specifically designed to evaluate the patient's experience of quality of life during advanced illness.

Based on Dr. Ira Byock's model of growth and development at the end of life, the MVQOLI is used both as an assessment tool to inform care planning and as an outcome measure. The instrument produces a quality of life profile for each individual patient that graphically reveals the influence of 5 domains of experience on quality of life.

The instrument contains 25 items that assess 5 dimensions of a person's subjective experience—symptoms, functional status, interpersonal relations, emotional well-being, and transcendence.

MISSOULA-VITAS QUALITY OF LIFE INDEX (TM)

V - 25

INSTRUCTIONS:

Indicate the extent to which you agree or disagree with the following statements by marking in one of the circles below the question. For items with two statements, indicate agreement with one or the other or if they are equally true, choose "Neutral." If you make a mistake or change your mind, place an X through the wrong answer and mark the circle indicating your correct answer.

Patient's Name: _____ Today's Date: _____

GLOBAL

How would you rate your overall quality of life?

○	○	○	○	○
Worst Possible	Poor	Fair	Good	Best Possible

SYMPTOM

1. My symptoms are adequately controlled.

○	○	○	○	○
Agree Strongly	Agree	Neutral	Disagree	Disagree Strongly

2. I feel sick all the time.

○	○	○	○	○
Agree Strongly	Agree	Neutral	Disagree	Disagree Strongly

3. I accept my symptoms as a fact of life.

○	○	○	○	○
Agree Strongly	Agree	Neutral	Disagree	Disagree Strongly

4. I am satisfied with current control of my symptoms.

○	○	○	○	○
Agree Strongly	Agree	Neutral	Disagree	Disagree Strongly

5. Despite physical discomfort, in general I can enjoy my days. **OR** Physical discomfort overshadows an opportunity for enjoyment.

○	○	○	○	○
Agree Strongly	Agree	Neutral	Disagree	Disagree Strongly

FUNCTION

6. I am still able to attend to most of my personal needs by myself. **OR** I am dependent on others for my personal care.

○	○	○	○	○
Agree Strongly	Agree	Neutral	Disagree	Disagree Strongly

7. I am still able to do many of the things I like to do. **OR** I am no longer able to do many of the things I like to do.

○	○	○	○	○
Agree Strongly	Agree	Neutral	Disagree	Disagree Strongly

8. I am satisfied with my ability to take care of my basic needs.

○	○	○	○	○
Agree Strongly	Agree	Neutral	Disagree	Disagree Strongly

9. I accept the fact that I can not do many of the things I used to do. **OR** I am disappointed that I cannot do many of the things I used to do.

○	○	○	○	○
Agree Strongly	Agree	Neutral	Disagree	Disagree Strongly

10. My contentment with life depends upon being active and being independent in my personal care.

○	○	○	○	○
Agree Strongly	Agree	Neutral	Disagree	Disagree Strongly

INTERPERSONAL

11. I have recently been able to say important things to the people close to me.

○	○	○	○	○
Agree Strongly	Agree	Neutral	Disagree	Disagree Strongly

12. I feel closer to others in my life now than I did before my illness. **OR** I feel increasingly distant from others in my life.

○	○	○	○	○
Agree Strongly	Agree	Neutral	Disagree	Disagree Strongly

13. In general, these days I am satisfied with relationships with family and friends.

○	○	○	○	○
Agree Strongly	Agree	Neutral	Disagree	Disagree Strongly

14. At present, I spend as much time as I want to with family and friends.

○	○	○	○	○
Agree Strongly	Agree	Neutral	Disagree	Disagree Strongly

Continued on following page

INTERPERSONAL *(Continued)*

15. It is important to me to have close personal relationships.

○	○	○	○	○
Agree Strongly	Agree	Neutral	Disagree	Disagree Strongly

WELL-BEING

16. My affairs are in order;   OR   My affairs are not in order; I could die today with a clear mind.   I am worried that many things are unresolved.

○	○	○	○	○
Agree Strongly	Agree	Neutral	Disagree	Disagree Strongly

17. I feel generally at   OR   I am unsettled and peace and prepared   unprepared to leave this to leave this life.   life.

○	○	○	○	○
Agree Strongly	Agree	Neutral	Disagree	Disagree Strongly

18. I am more satisfied with myself as a person now than I was before my illness.

○	○	○	○	○
Agree Strongly	Agree	Neutral	Disagree	Disagree Strongly

19. The longer I am ill,   OR   The longer I am ill, the the more I worry   more comfortable I am about things "getting   with the idea of "letting go." out of control."

○	○	○	○	○
Agree Strongly	Agree	Neutral	Disagree	Disagree Strongly

20. It is important to me to be at peace with myself.

○	○	○	○	○
Agree Strongly	Agree	Neutral	Disagree	Disagree Strongly

TRANSCENDENT

21. I have a greater sense   OR   I feel more disconnected of connection to all   from all things now than things now than I did   I did before my illness. before my illness.

○	○	○	○	○
Agree Strongly	Agree	Neutral	Disagree	Disagree Strongly

22. I have a better sense   OR   I have less of a sense of of meaning in my life   meaning in my life now now than I have had   than I have had in the past. in the past.

○	○	○	○	○
Agree Strongly	Agree	Neutral	Disagree	Disagree Strongly

23. As the end of my life   OR   As the end of my life approaches, I am   approaches, I am uneasy comfortable with the   with the thought of my thought of my own death.   own death.

○	○	○	○	○
Agree Strongly	Agree	Neutral	Disagree	Disagree Strongly

24. Life has become more   OR   Life has lost all value for precious to me; every   me; every day is a burden. day is a gift.

○	○	○	○	○
Agree Strongly	Agree	Neutral	Disagree	Disagree Strongly

25. It is important to me to feel that my life has meaning.

○	○	○	○	○
Agree Strongly	Agree	Neutral	Disagree	Disagree Strongly

Did you complete this questionnaire by yourself?

○	○
Yes	No

Nottingham Health Profile (NHP)

Targeted Population: Adults.

Description: The Nottingham Health Profile (NHP) provides a brief indication of a patient's perceived emotional, social, and physical health problems (Hunt et al, 1981, 1985). It serves to identify how people feel when they experience ill health. There are 45 items, 38 in Part I and 7 in Part II. Six domains consist of items for physical mobility (8 items), pain (8 items), social isolation (5 items), emotional reactions (9 items), energy (3 items), and sleep (5 items). This tool, which is more frequently used in Europe, is suitable for use in primary care clinical settings.

Scores: Each item is weighted on the basis of findings from previous studies. The maximum sum of the items in each domain is 100. The higher the score, the greater is the health problem. Scores are presented as profiles rather than overall scores. A mean score may be calculated across all items within each domain. The overall score is the mean across all items.

Accuracy: Extensive testing has indicated good reliability, test-retest/reproducibility, internal consistency, and validity for the NHP (MacDowell & Newell, 1996; Jenkinson et al, 1988). Disadvantages revolve around its limitations in measurement of function (some disabilities are not measured), inadequate index of mental distress, and inability to detect small improvements in health (Bowling, 1997).

Administration Time: 5 to 10 minutes by self-administration.

Contact S. McKenna for permission for use: Dr. Stephen McKenna, Galen Research, Enterprise House, Manchester Science Park, Lloyd Street North, Manchester M15 6SE, UK. This tool may be viewed online at http://www.medal.org/ch1.html.

Descriptive summary from Loretz L: *Primary Care Tools for Clinicians: A Compendium of Forms, Questionnaires, and Rating Scales for Everyday Practice*, St. Louis, 2005, Mosby.

Functional Independence Measure (FIM™) Instrument

LEVELS		NO HELPER
	7 Complete Independence (timely, safely) 6 Modified Independence (device)	**NO HELPER**
	Modified Dependence 5 Supervision (subject = 100%) 4 Minimal Assistance (subject = 75%+) 3 Moderate Assistance (subject = 50%+) **Complete Dependence** 2 Maximal Assistance (subject = 25%+) 1 Total Assistance (subject = less than 25%)	**HELPER**

Self-Care   ADMISSION   DISCHARGE   FOLLOW-UP
A. Eating
B. Grooming
C. Bathing
D. Dressing—Upper Body
E. Dressing—Lower Body
F. Toileting

Sphincter Control
G. Bladder Management
H. Bowel Management

Transfers
I. Bed, Chair, Wheelchair
J. Toilet
K. Tub, Shower

Locomotion
L. Walk/Wheelchair   W Walk   W Walk   W Walk
M. Stairs   C Wheelchair   C Wheelchair   C Wheelchair
   B Both   B Both   B Both

Motor Subtotal Score

Communication   A Auditory   A Auditory   A Auditory
N. Comprehension   V Visual   V Visual   V Visual
O. Expression   B Both   B Both   B Both
   A Auditory   A Auditory   A Auditory
   V Visual   V Visual   V Visual
   B Both   B Both   B Both

Social Cognition
P. Social Interaction
Q. Problem Solving
R. Memory

Cognitive Subtotal Score

TOTAL FIM™ SCORE

NOTE: Leave no blanks. Enter 1 if patient is not testable due to risk.

Functional Independence Measure (FIM): Items and Levels of Function

SELF-CARE

Eating. Includes use of suitable utensils to bring food to mouth, chewing, and swallowing, once meal is appropriately prepared.

Grooming. Includes oral care, hair grooming, washing hands and face, and either shaving or applying makeup.

Bathing. Includes bathing the body from the neck down (excluding the back), tub, shower, or sponge/bed bath. Performs safely.

Dressing—Upper Body. Includes dressing above the waist as well as donning and removing prosthesis or orthosis when applicable.

Dressing—Lower Body. Includes dressing from the waist down as well as donning or removing prosthesis or orthosis when applicable.

Toileting. Includes maintaining perineal hygiene and adjusting clothing before and after toilet or bed pan use. Performs safely.

SPHINCTER CONTROL

Bladder Management. Includes complete intentional control of urinary bladder and use of equipment or agents necessary for bladder control.

Bowel Management. Includes complete intentional control of bowel movement and use of equipment or agents necessary for bowel control.

MOBILITY

Transfers: Bed, Chair, Wheelchair. Includes all aspects of transferring to and from bed, chair, and wheelchair, and coming to a standing position, if walking is the typical mode of locomotion.

Transfer: Toilet. Includes getting on and off a toilet.

Transfers: Tub or Shower. Includes getting into and out of a tub or shower stall.

LOCOMOTION

Walking or Using Wheelchair. Includes walking, once in a standing position, or using a wheelchair, once in a seated position, on a level surface.

Check most frequent mode of locomotion. If both are about equal, check W *and* C. If initiating a rehabilitation program, check the mode for which training is intended.
( ) W = Walking ( ) C = Wheelchair

Stairs. Goes up and down 12 to 14 stairs (one flight) indoors.

COMMUNICATION

Comprehension. Includes understanding of either auditory or visual communication (e.g., writing, sign language, gestures).

Check and evaluate the most usual mode of comprehension. If both are about equally used, check A *and* V.
( ) A = Auditory ( ) V = Visual

Expression. Includes clear vocal or nonvocal expression of language. This item includes both intelligible speech or clear expression of language using writing or a communication device.

Check and evaluate the most usual mode of expression. If both are about equally used, check V *and* N.
( ) V = Vocal ( ) N = Nonvocal

SOCIAL COGNITION

Social Interaction. Includes skills related to getting along and participating with others in therapeutic and social situations. It represents how one deals with one's own needs together with the needs of others.

Problem Solving. Includes skills related to solving problems of daily living. This means making reasonable, safe, and timely decisions regarding financial, social, and personal affairs and initiating, sequencing, and self-correcting tasks and activities to solve the problems.

Memory. Includes skills related to recognizing and remembering while performing daily activities in an institutional or community setting. It includes ability to store and retrieve information, particularly verbal and visual. A deficit in memory impairs learning as well as performance of tasks.

DESCRIPTION OF THE LEVELS OF FUNCTION AND THEIR SCORES

INDEPENDENT—Another person is not required for the activity (NO HELPER).

7 COMPLETE INDEPENDENCE—All of the tasks described as making up the activity are typically performed safely, without modification, assistive devices, or aids, and within a reasonable time.

6 MODIFIED INDEPENDENCE—Activity requires any one or more than one of the following: an assistive device, more than reasonable time, or there are safety (risk) considerations.

DEPENDENT—Another person is required for either supervision or physical assistance in order for the activity to be performed, or it is not performed (REQUIRES HELPER).

MODIFIED DEPENDENCE—The subject expends half (50%) or more of the effort. The levels of assistance required are:

5 Supervision or setup—Subject requires no more help than standby, cuing or coaxing, without physical contact. Or, helper sets up needed items or applies orthoses.

4 Minimal contact assistance—With physical contact the subject requires no more help than touching, and subject expends 75% or more of the effort.

3 Moderate assistance—Subject requires more help than touching, or expends half (50%) or more (up to 75%) of the effort.

COMPLETE DEPENDENCE—The subject expends *less* than half (*less* than 50%) of the effort. Maximal or total assistance is required, or the activity is not performed. The levels of assistance required are:

2 Maximal assistance—Subject expends less than 50% of the effort, but at least 25%.

1 Total assistance—Subject expends less than 25% of the effort.

**Androgen Deficiency in Aging Males
(ADAM) Questionnaire**

Name: _____

Date: _____

Choose the answers below that best describe how you have been feeling. Answers will help your health care provider and you to better manage your medical needs.

1. Do you have a decrease in libido (sex drive)?	Yes	No
2. Do you have a lack of energy?	Yes	No
3. Do you have a decrease in strength and/or endurance?	Yes	No
4. Have you lost height?	Yes	No
5. Have you noticed a decreased "enjoyment of life?"	Yes	No
6. Are you sad and/or grumpy?	Yes	No
7. Are your erections less strong?	Yes	No
8. Have you noticed a recent deterioration in your ability to play sports?	Yes	No
9. Are you falling asleep after dinner?	Yes	No
10. Has there been a recent deterioration in your work performance?	Yes	No

Any man answering yes to #1, #7, or any three others has a high likelihood of having a low testosterone level.

From Morley JE, Perry HM: Androgen deficiency in aging men, *Med Clin North Am,* 83(5):127–289, 1999.

Burke Dysphagia Screening Test

1. Has the patient had a bilateral stroke?	Yes	No
2. Has the patient had a stroke involving the brainstem?	Yes	No
3. Does the patient have a history of pneumonia during the acute stroke phase?	Yes	No
4. Does the patient have coughing associated with feeding or during a 3-ounce water swallow test?	Yes	No
5. Does the patient persistently fail to consume at least one half of meals?	Yes	No
6. Is prolonged time required for feeding the patient?	Yes	No
7. Is a non-oral feeding program in progress for the patient?	Yes	No

Score: A "yes" response to one or more items is a positive screen.

From DePippo KL, Holas MA, Reding MJ: The Burke dysphagia screening test: validation of its use in patients with stroke, *Arch Phys Med Rehabil* 75(2):1284-1286, 1994. Reprinted with permission from American Congress of Rehabilitation Medicine and the American Academy of Physical Medicine and Rehabilitation. Also described online at http://www.medal.org/ch8.html.

American Urological Association (AUA) Symptom Index

Last Name	First Name	Date

Mark the response correct for you and type in your score in the far right box for all SEVEN questions.

1. **Incomplete emptying:** Over the past month, how often have you had a sensation of not emptying your bladder completely after you finished urinating?

Not at all	Less than 1 time in 5	Less than half the time	About half the time	More than half the time	Almost always	Your Score
0	1	2	3	4	5	

2. **Frequency:** Over the past month, how often have you had to urinate again less than 2 hours after you finished urinating?

Not at all	Less than 1 time in 5	Less than half the time	About half the time	More than half the time	Almost always	Your Score
0	1	2	3	4	5	

3. **Intermittency:** Over the past month, how often have you found that you stopped and started again several times when you urinated?

Not at all	Less than 1 time in 5	Less than half the time	About half the time	More than half the time	Almost always	Your Score
0	1	2	3	4	5	

4. **Urgency:** Over the past month, how often have you found it difficult to postpone urination?

Not at all	Less than 1 time in 5	Less than half the time	About half the time	More than half the time	Almost always	Your Score
0	1	2	3	4	5	

5. **Weak stream:** Over the past month, how often have you had a weak stream?

Not at all	Less than 1 time in 5	Less than half the time	About half the time	More than half the time	Almost always	Your Score
0	1	2	3	4	5	

6. **Straining:** Over the past month, how often have you had to push or strain to begin urination?

Not at all	Less than 1 time in 5	Less than half the time	About half the time	More than half the time	Almost always	Your Score
0	1	2	3	4	5	

7. **Nocturia:** Over the past month or so, how many times did you get up to urinate from the time you went to bed until the time you got up in the morning?

None	1 time	2 times	3 times	4 times	5 or more times	Your Score
0	1	2	3	4	5	

Add up your scores for total AUA score = _____

Quality of Life Due to Urinary Symptoms: If you were to spend the rest of your life with your urinary condition just the way it is now, how would you feel about that? (Bold, Highlight, or Underline)

Delighted   Pleased   Mostly satisfied   Mixed   Mostly dissatisfied   Unhappy   Terrible

Scores: Items are scored as follows: 0 points = not at all, 1 point = less than 1 in 5 times (<20%), 2 points = less than half the time (<50%), 3 points = about half the time (50%), 4 points = more than half the time (>50%), 5 points = almost always (>80%). Scores for the seven items are summed for a total score. Suggested interpretation for total scores is as follows: < 7 = mild benign prostatic hyperplasia (BPH) symptoms; 8 to 19 = moderate BPH symptoms; >20 = severe BPH symptoms.

The American Urological Association (AUA) Symptom Index is widely available online for downloading and can be found at http://www.prostate-cancer.org/tools/forms/aua_symptom_form.html.

Incontinence Impact Questionnaire (IIQ-7)

Name: _____

Date: _____

Has urine leakage affected your:

("X" one for each question)

	Not at all	Slightly	Moderately	Greatly
1. Ability to do household chores (cooking, housecleaning, laundry)?	☐	☐	☐	☐
2. Physical recreation such as walking, swimming, or other exercise?	☐	☐	☐	☐
3. Entertainment activities (movies, concerts, etc.)?	☐	☐	☐	☐
4. Ability to travel by car or bus more than 30 minutes from home?	☐	☐	☐	☐
5. Participation in social activities outside your house?	☐	☐	☐	☐
6. Emotional health (nervousness, depression, etc.)?	☐	☐	☐	☐
7. Feeling frustrated?	☐	☐	☐	☐

Urogenital Distress Inventory (UDI-6)

Do you experience, and if so, how much are you bothered by:

("X" one for each question)

	Not at all	Slightly	Moderately	Greatly
1. Frequent urination?	☐	☐	☐	☐
2. Urine leakage related to the feeling of urgency?	☐	☐	☐	☐
3. Urine leakage related to physical activity, coughing, or sneezing?	☐	☐	☐	☐
4. Small amounts of urine leakage drops?	☐	☐	☐	☐
5. Difficulty emptying your bladder?	☐	☐	☐	☐
6. Pain or discomfort in the lower abdominal or genital area?	☐	☐	☐	☐

From Shumaker SA, Wyman JF, Uebersax JS, et al: Health-related quality-of-life measures for women with urinary incontinence, *Qual Life Res* 3(5);291–306, 1994.

ROSENBAUM POCKET VISION SCREENER

	Point	Jaeger	distance equivalent
95			$\frac{20}{800}$
874			$\frac{20}{400}$
2 8 4 3	26	16	$\frac{20}{200}$
6 3 8 E Ш Ǝ X O O	14	10	$\frac{20}{100}$
8 7 4 5 Ǝ Ш Ш O X O	10	7	$\frac{20}{70}$
6 3 9 2 5 ш E Ǝ X O X	8	5	$\frac{20}{50}$
4 2 8 3 6 5 Ш E ш O X O	6	3	$\frac{20}{40}$
3 7 4 2 5 8 Ǝ Ш Ǝ X X O	5	2	$\frac{20}{30}$
9 3 7 8 2 6 ш ш E X O O	4	1	$\frac{20}{25}$
4 2 8 7 3 9 E ш ш o o x	3	1+	$\frac{20}{20}$

Card is held in good light 14 inches from eye. Record vision for each eye separately with and without glasses. Presbyopic patients should read through bifocal segment. Check myopes with glasses only.

DESIGN COURTESY J. G. ROSENBAUM, M.D.

PUPIL GAUGE (mm.)

2 3 4 5 6 7 8 9

Page numbers followed by b indicate boxes;
f, figures; t, tables.